A Practical Approach to Cardiac Arrhythmias

Second Edition

A Practical Approach to Cardiac Arrhythmias

Stephen C. Vlay, M.D.

Professor of Medicine, Division of
Cardiology, State University of New York at
Stony Brook, Health Sciences Center
School of Medicine; Director of the Stony
Brook Arrhythmia Study and Sudden
Death Prevention Center; Director of the
Coronary Care Unit, University Hospital,
Stony Brook, New York

Little, Brown and Company
Boston New York Toronto London

Library of Congress Cataloging-in-Publication Data
Vlay, Stephen C.
    A practical approach to cardiac arrhythmias / Stephen C. Vlay.—2nd ed.
        p.   cm.
    Rev. ed. of: Manual of cardiac arrhythmias / edited by Stephen C. Vlay. 1987.
    Includes bibliographical references and index.
    ISBN 0-316-91483-5
    1. Arrhythmia. I. Manual of cardiac arrhythmias. II. Title.
    [DNLM: 1. Arrhythmia—diagnosis. 2. Arrhythmia—therapy. WG 330
V867p 1995]
RC685.A65V56   1995
616.1'28—dc20
DNLM/DLC
for Library of Congress   95-23368
                                                                                                          CIP

Printed in the United States of America

SEM

Editorial: Nancy Megley, Richard L. Wilcox
Production Editor: Katharine S. Mascaro
Production Services: Julie Sullivan
Production Supervisor: Cate Rickard

To my family:

To my wife Linda, who has filled my life with happiness

to Colleen

and

to the memory of my parents, Rose and Stephen Vlay

Contents

Preface

In the mere eight years since publication of the first edition of this book, the advances in clinical electrophysiology have been astronomical. Ablation of accessory pathways, once only possible through surgery, can now be performed percutaneously through catheter techniques. Internal cardioverter defibrillators have taken a quantum leap, now providing antitachycardia pacing, cardioversion, defibrillation, pacing, and extensive telemetry, in addition to serving as a noninvasive electrophysiology laboratory.

The original purpose of this book is unchanged—to serve as an intermediate-level text focused on the clinical aspects of patients with cardiac arrhythmias. In addition, it goes beyond the basic facts to provide the reader with a solid foundation in arrhythmia management. The latest recommendations from national organizations regarding indications for treatment are included. This book is written for the clinician, who sees the patient in the office, emergency room, coronary care or telemetry unit, electrophysiology or cardiac catheterization laboratory, in the operating room, and on the medical or surgical service.

After a review of sudden cardiac death, the latest guidelines for cardiopulmonary resuscitation are reviewed. The chapter on basic electrophysiology contains new information on anatomic features of the conduction system and focuses on the role of ion channels, currents, receptors, and pumps. New clinical clues to the diagnosis of cardiac arrhythmias are provided in another chapter. A new section on the important clinical problem of syncope provides details about tilt table testing.

Three chapters describe supraventricular, preexcitation, and ventricular arrhythmias. The treatments of choice have changed significantly for all of these arrhythmias with less emphasis on pharmacologic therapy. Recommendations for the treatment of arrhythmias and conduction disturbances in the acute phase of acute myocardial infarction have been revised.

The noninvasive and invasive techniques for arrhythmia evaluation are covered in detail. There are new chapters on signal averaging techniques and radiofrequency catheter ablation—techniques that have revolutionized arrhythmia therapy.

While the number of available antiarrhythmic drugs has not increased significantly (and actually has decreased), the approach to pharmacologic therapy has changed through a greater appreciation of the effect of drugs on basic electrophysiologic mechanisms. The new classification scheme, The Sicilian Gambit, is discussed and compared with the prior Vaughan Williams scheme.

There are still unresolved issues in arrhythmia management. These controversies are discussed in detail in two chapters. Technological advances have made pacemakers and internal cardioverter defibrillators (ICDs) more versatile. The ICD chapter was updated multiple times with information about the latest devices in order to contain the most current information at press time. Surgical approaches to arrhythmia management are described and illustrated in detail.

The understanding of arrhythmias would be incomplete without a comprehensive evaluation of the psychiatric and neurologic aspects of the illness. Last, but certainly not least, is a section on counseling the arrhythmia patient and the family. This aspect of medical care cannot be neglected, and, in fact, is often part of the reason we became health care providers.

The evaluation and treatment of cardiac arrhythmias is a challenging field that continues to grow in complexity. The newer modalities of treatment have resulted in an improved lifestyle, outcome, and survival for many patients with disabling arrhythmias. In this field we are consistently learning more every day. We must use the new technology wisely and appropriately.

This text is written by clinicians for clinicians. I thank my contributing authors for again taking the time from their busy schedules to write and update their chapters.

Today the demands of clinical practice in a time of health care crisis make it more and more difficult to find the time for an academic endeavor. We hope that the readers will develop a better understanding of the concepts of clinical electrophysiology and arrhythmia management.

S. C. V.

Contributing Authors

Gust H. Bardy, M.D.

Associate Professor of Medicine, University of Washington School of Medicine; Electrophysiology Attending, Arrhythmia Services, University Medical Center, Seattle

Lou-Anne M. Beauregard, M.D.

Assistant Professor of Medicine, Division of Cardiology, University of Medicine and Dentistry of New Jersey, Robert Wood Johnson Medical School; Director of Heart Station and Pacemaker Follow-up Center, Cooper Hospital/University Medical Center, Camden, New Jersey

G. Lee Dolack, M.D.

Assistant Professor of Medicine, University of Washington School of Medicine; Electrophysiology Attending, Arrhythmia Services, University Medical Center, Seattle

Anne H. Dougherty, M.D.

Associate Professor of Medicine, University of Texas Medical School at Houston; Associate Director of Electrophysiology, Hermann Hospital, Houston

Gregory L. Fricchione, M.D.

Associate Professor of Psychiatry, Harvard Medical School; Director of Consultation Psychiatry, Brigham and Women's Hospital, Boston

Gerald V. Naccarelli, M.D.

Professor of Medicine and Chief, Division of Cardiology, Pennsylvania State University College of Medicine; Director of Pennsylvania State Cardiovascular Center, The Milton S. Hershey Medical Center, Hershey, Pennsylvania

Philip J. Podrid, M.D.

Professor of Medicine, Department of Cardiology, Boston University School of Medicine; Director of Arrhythmia Service, Department of Cardiology, University Hospital, Boston

James A. Reiffel, M.D.

Professor of Clinical Medicine, Division of Cardiology, Columbia University College of Physicians and Surgeons; Attending Physician and Director of Clinical Electrophysiology Programs, Columbia-Presbyterian Medical Center, New York

Andrea M. Russo, M.D. Assistant Professor of Medicine, University of Medicine and Dentistry of New Jersey, Robert Wood Johnson Medical School; Director of Clinical Electrophysiology Laboratory, Cooper Hospital/University Medical Center, Camden, New Jersey

Henry M. Spotnitz, M.D. Professor of Cardiothoracic Surgery, Columbia University College of Physicians and Surgeons; Attending-Vice Chairman of Cardiothoracic Surgery, Columbia-Presbyterian Medical Center, New York

Eric Taylor, Jr., M.D. Cardiology Fellow, Department of Medicine, Johns Hopkins University School of Medicine; Attending Physician, Division of Cardiology, Johns Hopkins Hospital, Baltimore

Levi Watkins, Jr., M.D. Associate Dean of Postdoctoral Programs, Johns Hopkins University School of Medicine; Professor of Cardiac Surgery, Johns Hopkins Hospital, Baltimore

Harvey L. Waxman, M.D. Professor of Medicine, University of Medicine and Dentistry of New Jersey, Robert Wood Johnson Medical School; Director of Cardiology, Cooper Hospital/University Medical Center, Camden, New Jersey

Linda C. Vlay, R.N., M.S., C.S., N.P.P. Clinical Instructor of Medicine, Division of Cardiology, State University of New York at Stony Brook, Health Sciences Center School of Medicine; Coordinator of Clinical Trials and Arrhythmia Center, Division of Cardiology, University Hospital at Stony Brook, New York

Stephen C. Vlay, M.D. Professor of Medicine, Division of Cardiology, State University of New York at Stony Brook, Health Sciences Center School of Medicine; Director of the Stony Brook Arrhythmia Study and Sudden Death Prevention Center; Director of the Coronary Care Unit, University Hospital, Stony Brook, New York

A Practical Approach to Cardiac Arrhythmias

Notice

The indications and dosages of all drugs in this book have been recommended in the medical literature and conform to the practices of the general medical community. The medications described do not necessarily have specific approval by the Food and Drug Administration for use in the diseases and dosages for which they are recommended. The package insert for each drug should be consulted for use and dosage as approved by the FDA. Because standards for usage change, it is advisable to keep abreast of revised recommendations, particularly those concerning new drugs.

1

Sudden Cardiac Death: An Overview

Stephen C. Vlay

Cardiovascular mortality continues to be the leading cause of death in the United States. Many of these deaths occur suddenly, with the number of these events estimated at 300,000 to 500,000 annually. There are few other events as devastating to the family and to society as the unexpected death of an individual thought to be in good health. The loss has a profound impact personally, socially, occupationally, and economically. In order to obtain a conservative approximation of financial loss, let us assume that only 250,000 victims of sudden cardiac death had income. If the income averaged $8,000, the annual loss is $2 billion. Certainly this is an underestimation and does not account for funds that must be expended to provide for the needs of the decedent's family. Thus, sudden cardiac death has a major impact. If we use the figure of 500,000 per annum, it translates into one sudden cardiac death every minute. Often the family member is told, "The cause of death was a massive heart attack." In fact, that is frequently not true. Although the majority of sudden cardiac death victims have underlying coronary artery disease, only a small minority suffer an acute transmural myocardial infarction.

As public education about cardiopulmonary resuscitation grows and paramedic teams become widespread, some victims of sudden cardiac arrest are fortunate enough to be resuscitated and brought to the hospital for medical evaluation. We have learned much about the mechanism of sudden cardiac death from these survivors, and this knowledge has changed the practice of cardiology. Aggressive evaluation and treatment, including noninvasive techniques, invasive electrophysiologic testing, arrhythmia surgery, and electronic devices, permit not only continued survival but resumption of routine and occupational activities.

I. **Definition: sudden cardiac death (SCD).** A number of definitions of sudden cardiac death have been offered over the past 25 years. To be considered primarily cardiac, the event must be nonviolent and nontraumatic. It is unexpected and usually instantaneous, but uniformly fatal within 1 hour of the onset of terminal symptoms. If the death is not witnessed, the individual would have to have been seen alive in the past 24 hours for the death to be considered an SCD.

The underlying rhythm disturbance in the vast majority of SCD victims is ventricular tachycardia (VT) or ventricular fibrillation (VF). VT usually precedes VF, whereas VF without even a few beats of VT is rare. Sudden death can result from complete heart block or asystole, but such deaths are less common. In fact, insertion of permanent pacemakers in some individuals with complete heart block does not prevent subsequent death since it may be due to a second problem, VT. The subsequent discussion emphasizes sudden cardiac death caused by malignant VT. The following formula provides a basis for further understanding: SCD = Anatomic Substrate + Trigger Factor.

II. **Epidemiology.** Who is at risk of SCD, and how can we prevent it? The former can be answered; the latter remains problematic. Figure 1-1 classifies sudden death as cardiac, probable cardiac, or noncardiac. Kannel examined the experience of the Framingham population [1]. Although the older individual with overt heart disease has an increased risk of SCD, 50% of the fatalities in men and 64% in women occur in the absence of known coronary artery disease (CAD). The victim of SCD is likely to be male and over 45 years of age. The incidence of SCD in women is delayed by 20 years compared to men. SCD in younger individuals, below age 45 years, is less frequent.

In patients with CAD, half the mortality is due to SCD. Interestingly there is a higher percentage of SCD in individuals without overt coronary disease than in patients with known disease (75% versus 20–34%). In men, 18% of acute myocardial infarction is associated with SCD; in women, the percentage is 24%. For patients with known CAD, left ventricular dysfunction is one of the most important risk factors. For those without

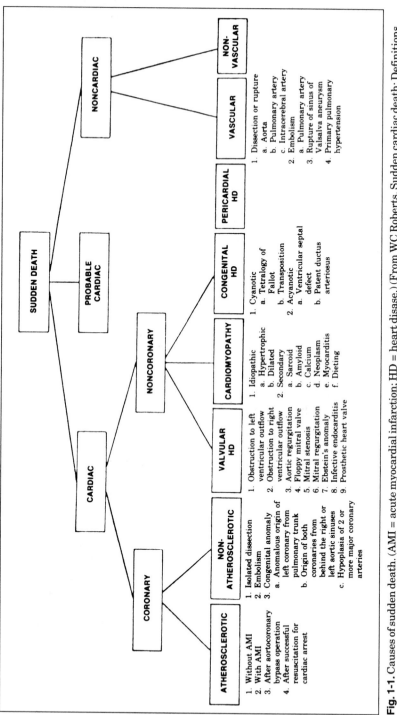

Fig. 1-1. Causes of sudden death. (AMI = acute myocardial infarction; HD = heart disease.) (From WC Roberts. Sudden cardiac death: Definitions and causes. Editorial. *Am J Cardiol* 57:1411, 1986.)

overt CAD, the coronary risk factors (smoking, hypertension, low high-density lipoprotein (HDL) and high low-density lipoprotein (LDL) cholesterol, diabetes mellitus, obesity), in addition to vital capacity and ECG abnormalities, can be used to estimate the risk of SCD by means of a multivariate equation.

Although long-term studies of individuals who have modified all of their significant risk factors are not available, it would seem reasonable to make certain recommendations in the hope of preventing SCD. The population that stands to gain the most benefit is the younger age group, in whom CAD has not yet developed or progressed. Recommendations include avoidance of cigarette smoking, control of blood pressure, a reasonable diet (low fat, low cholesterol), and exercise to prevent obesity. The population older than age 45 will also benefit from these measures.

Diabetes mellitus is an independent risk factor that increases cardiovascular mortality. Strict control of the serum glucose with diet, oral hypoglycemic drugs, or insulin decreases the incidence of vascular complications of diabetes. Patients with elevated cholesterol levels despite diet therapy benefit from specific lipid-lowering drugs and may have regression of atherosclerosis. Sudden cardiac death also occurs in the pediatric population [2, 3]. In the reported series, the incidence ranges from 1.3 to 8.5 per 100,000, but not all of the deaths can definitely be ascribed to a specific cardiac cause.

The Mayo Clinic identified risk factors including exercise-associated syncope, nonvasodepressor syncope, and familial history of sudden cardiac death or hypertrophic cardiomyopathy. Other centers have called attention to the occurrence of sinus node and atrioventricular node dysfunction, prolonged Q–T intervals, and accessory pathway conduction with Wolff-Parkinson-White syndrome in children and adolescents with sudden cardiac death. In addition, patients with ventricular arrhythmias after surgical treatment of Fallot's tetralogy may be at risk for sudden cardiac death.

III. **Anatomic substrates of sudden cardiac death.** Epidemiologic studies have taken into account the major risk factors in the population that contribute to the most common underlying cause of SCD, coronary artery disease. Yet there remain a wide variety of underlying cardiac abnormalities that are not identified by this type of analysis. It would be ideal to attribute SCD to one causative factor that would be easy to identify and predictive of outcome. This is unlikely, yet there may be a number of common end points of the various disease processes, such as left ventricular (LV) dysfunction, that act as markers for increased risk. In addition, a variety of different trigger factors may be capable of inducing a sustained arrhythmia. These factors are discussed later in this chapter.

The occurrence of an arrhythmia, such as asymptomatic nonsustained ventricular tachycardia (NSVT), may have different prognostic and therapeutic implications in individuals with different underlying problems. For example, consider congestive cardiomyopathy, CAD, and mitral valve prolapse. The patient with cardiomyopathy and NSVT may be difficult to treat, and SCD may occur even if a drug regimen capable of suppressing the arrhythmia is found. The patient may do well for a number of years without antiarrhythmic drug therapy. The patient with CAD and NSVT may be easier to evaluate and treat, particularly if LV function is preserved. Asymptomatic patients with mitral valve prolapse and NSVT may need no therapy (except perhaps a beta blocker) and still have an excellent prognosis. Thus, different underlying conditions may manifest a common arrhythmia (in this example, ventricular tachycardia) but require completely different approaches. At this time, an anatomic substrate that is predictive of SCD and is common to all contributing cardiac abnormalities has not been identified. However, there may be common factors within individual categories, such as CAD, that suggest an anatomic substrate predictive of outcome.

A. **Coronary artery disease.** The clinical outcome of patients with CAD has been studied by Holter monitoring, by cardiac catheterization, and at autopsy. A relationship was described between the presence of complex ventricular ectopy on ambulatory ECG recording and abnormalities of LV contraction or the severity of CAD. The prevalence and grade of ventricular ectopy increase with multivessel disease, elevated LV and diastolic pressure, and asynergy.

Longitudinal studies of survivors of myocardial infarction demonstrated that patients with VT have an increased risk of sudden cardiac death. VT was found to be an independent risk factor. The role of Holter monitoring and its predictive value are discussed and a detailed analysis of the various investigations is presented in Chap. 9. Multivariate analyses of patients with CAD undergoing cardiac catheterization identified additional variables predictive of survival: low ejection fraction, the number of diseased vessels, prior myocardial infarction, and proximal left anterior descending (LAD) coronary artery stenosis [4–7]. Studies suggest that clinical outcome in survivors of sudden cardiac arrest is related to the degree of narrowing in the anterior descending artery prior to the first septal perforator artery. As the degree of narrowing in this segment increases, the proportion surviving decreases [8, 9]. This finding has been corroborated in the general population, as well as in survivors of sudden cardiac arrest [10]. Other investigators have also noted the importance of proximal LAD disease [11–15].

Continued attempts at defining an anatomic substrate predictive of outcome in patients with CAD have included the addition of variables from electrophysiologic studies. An adverse outcome was associated with a high New York Heart Association functional type, failure of therapy identified as potentially effective during electrophysiologic studies, easy inducibility with a single ventricular extrastimulus, a prolonged H-V interval, LV aneurysm, an increased number of narrowed coronary arteries, male gender, more arrhythmia episodes, and extensive regional wall motion abnormalities.

Goldstein has evaluated the relationship of sudden cardiac death with a number of contributory factors. In 1972, he observed that patients with a history of CAD and a higher risk of death appeared to procrastinate most before seeking medical attention [16]. This delay is extremely detrimental since 15% to 45% of patients whose death is related to acute myocardial infarction die within the first hour. A later secondary prevention trial, the Aspirin Myocardial Infarction Study, noted that cardiac arrhythmia was the mechanism of death in 83% of all deaths within 24 hours [17]. Patients with the most severe underlying heart disease were at the highest risk.

Hinkle and Thaler studied the relationship between death caused by arrhythmia and death caused by circulatory failure [18]. In 58% of 743 cases, abrupt collapse and cessation of pulse and blood pressure were observed (arrhythmic death). In the remaining 42%, cessation of the pulse followed circulatory failure. One-third of the arrhythmic deaths and 10% of deaths related to circulatory failure were thought to be related to an acute ischemic event. Chronic congestive heart failure, indicating severe myocardial impairment, preceded arrhythmic deaths in 45%. The mechanism of death seemed to determine the location of death: Out-of-hospital deaths were arrhythmic (88%); in-hospital deaths were due to circulatory failure (71%).

Goldstein observed that patients with a primary arrhythmic event, rather than cardiac arrest in the presence of acute myocardial ischemia or infarction, had poorer survival and more underlying myocardial impairment [19]. Complex and frequent ventricular ectopy were additive risk factors [20]. Digitalis was implicated, but the need for this drug may reflect the severity of myocardial dysfunction. This controversy over the contribution of digitalis to subsequent sudden death has not been completely resolved.

Pathologists have observed the relationship between diseased coronary arteries and sudden cardiac death. Patients dying suddenly had more severe and more widespread coronary artery narrowings than patients dying of other causes [21]. A subsequent comparison of 31 previously symptomatic with 39 previously asymptomatic victims of sudden cardiac death revealed more severely narrowed coronary arteries in the symptomatic group. More ventricular scarring was observed in those with severe coronary disease [22]. In addition, more severe coronary narrowing was associated with increased heart weight. Of the 70 patients, only 13 had a coronary thrombus, but there were no other differences in regard to severity of coronary artery or myocardial disease [23].

Another study found a high incidence of coronary thrombus: 74 of 100 subjects [24]. There was no difference among those who died in the first 15 minutes, those who died in the first 45 minutes, and those who died after 1 hour. Plaque fissuring without thrombus was observed in 21 of 26 cases. Sixty-five percent of the thrombi were observed at sites of severe coronary narrowing. Arterial intimal injury was involved in 95% of the study population. The discrepancy in thrombus formation between the last two studies is unresolved [23, 24].

Despite this multitude of data from investigations at numerous centers, a precise anatomic definition of the underlying substrate in CAD predictive of sudden cardiac death or survival has not met with universal agreement [25]. Certainly the patient with poor LV function and additional variables mentioned above would seem to be at higher risk of VT or VF. But why do not all such individuals have this terminal outcome? Why does it occur, recur, or not occur? It is possible that another set of conditions related to ischemia, hypoxia, electrolyte imbalance, drug toxicity, or other trigger factors must also be met.

Nevertheless, to identify individuals who seem to be at higher risk, it may be reasonable to use the variables known to be associated with a poor prognosis. These individuals are candidates for further evaluation and treatment. These considerations are particularly important today, since the importance of silent myocardial ischemia has been established.

B. Cardiomyopathy. Disease of the heart muscle may be manifest in a variety of forms. Most commonly, some patients with CAD and myocardial infarction or ischemia will progress to an ischemic cardiomyopathy [26]. The association with ventricular arrhythmias and sudden death has been discussed. Dilated congestive cardiomyopathy is the most common nonischemic myopathy that physicians encounter in practice. Often it has a poor prognosis despite therapy directed at heart failure or the arrhythmia. Hypertrophic cardiomyopathy is the third major disorder in this category that sometimes goes unrecognized. A variety of disorders, including hypertension, valvular heart disease, and certain congenital cardiac abnormalities, may result in pressure-volume overload of the ventricles, producing a cardiomyopathic state. Rheumatic heart disease may include a myocarditis that affects the heart muscle primarily, in addition to scarring the valves. Finally, a variety of systemic illnesses, including diseases of metabolism, heredofamilial disorders, and infiltrative processes (such as amyloidosis or sarcoidosis), may result in a cardiomyopathy. Rare and unusual problems such as arrhythmogenic right ventricular dysplasia may be particularly difficult to manage.

No specific anatomic abnormalities are common to all of these conditions, but all have altered LV function. Paradoxically, LV dysfunction is manifest by both ends of the spectrum. In congestive cardiomyopathy, contractility is severely impaired. In hypertrophic cardiomyopathy, systolic function is hyperkinetic, although diastolic relaxation is impaired. Is the amount of heart muscle important? In 1914, Garrey's work suggested that fibrillation was more likely to occur in large sections of heart muscle. Clinically, left ventricular hypertrophy (LVH) is one of the most frequent findings at autopsy in victims of sudden cardiac death. It is unclear whether an increased mass of myocardium merely provides more abnormal tissue (increased number of pathways for circulating wave front) to sustain a tachyarrhythmia, or whether local changes occur, creating more arrhythmogenic foci. Both or more factors may be operative. Interestingly the VF threshold is lower in a large heart. But why do not all patients with large hearts and altered LV function die suddenly? Note the excellent cardiovascular performance of the athlete's heart with increased muscle mass but little risk of sudden cardiac death. Another important variable in the equation may be the presence of one or more trigger factors that precipitate VT or VF. The major cardiomyopathies are now briefly discussed.

1. **Congestive cardiomyopathy.** Dilated congestive cardiomyopathy is characterized by an insidious process that results in progressive deterioration of LV contractility and dilatation of the cardiac chambers [27, 28]. Sometimes there is a preceding myocarditis, but usually the cause remains obscure and is labeled idiopathic. The most common manifestation is congestive heart failure, but the rate of its progression varies with the individual.

   Ventricular ectopy is frequent and complex in patients with dilated congestive cardiomyopathy. Nonsustained VT is common, but its importance is incompletely resolved. The majority of studies indicate a poor correlation between the presence of nonsustained VT on Holter monitoring and clinical outcome. Although some studies have demonstrated a relationship between nonsustained VT and the severity of LV dysfunction as measured by cardiac index, diastolic pressure, and ejection fraction, others have failed to substantiate such a relationship. No study has demonstrated that antiarrhythmic drug therapy prevents sudden cardiac death. Amiodarone or an internal cardioverter-defibrillator may benefit some patients awaiting cardiac transplant. Current recommendations for treatment are discussed in Chap. 7.

2. **Hypertrophic cardiomyopathy.** Hypertrophic cardiomyopathy, a disorder of diastolic relaxation and hypercontractile systolic function, is characterized by LV hypertrophy and myocardial fiber disarray. There is a high incidence of ventricular ectopy in patients with this disorder, frequently manifest as nonsustained VT. In fact, the presence of nonsustained VT seems to identify a subgroup at high risk for sudden cardiac death [29, 30]. The mechanism of sudden death may vary, however; cardiac asystole, myocardial infarction, increased outflow

gradient or reduction in cardiac output owing to hemodynamic alteration, and rapid ventricular response in those with an accessory bypass tract (Wolff-Parkinson-White syndrome)—in addition to VT or VF—may cause death.

Studies from the Hammersmith Hospital suggest that risk factors for sudden cardiac death in those with hypertrophic cardiomyopathy include young age (14 years or younger), syncope at diagnosis, severe dyspnea, and a malignant family history (high incidence of SCD in other family members with hypertrophic cardiomyopathy). Other studies suggest that hemodynamic alterations, including low peak filling rate, large end systolic volume, and high ejection fraction, place the patient at a higher risk of SCD.

3. **Other cardiomyopathies.** The other cardiomyopathies that manifest a major problem with VTs are mentioned briefly. It is beyond the scope of this text to discuss each myopathy in detail.

In South America, Chagas' disease, caused by *Trypanosoma cruzi*, produces extensive scarring of the myocardium. The problem is not infrequent, and the disease is associated with atrial fibrillation, VT, and VF. SCD is not uncommon.

In patients with sarcoidosis, infiltration of the myocardium with granuloma can cause irritable foci, resulting in symptomatic VT. Arrhythmias in this disorder are notoriously difficult to manage with suppressive antiarrhythmic therapy. Even if surgical extirpation were possible, the risk of recurrence remains. Electronic devices such as implantable cardioverter-defibrillators may provide the answer. Myopathies may be localized to the right ventricle as well. Arrhythmogenic right ventricular dysplasia is a disorder manifested by a thin, dilated, poorly contractile right ventricle that may have multiple arrhythmia zones. Medical treatment is often unsuccessful, and surgical ventriculotomy may be necessary.

These three cardiomyopathies are examples of other processes in which ventricular tachyarrhythmias may result from localized abnormalities of the myocardium. Thus, it becomes clear that in the category of cardiomyopathy, SCD may be associated with an abnormality of ventricular myocardium, but there may be no common anatomic feature. It is also important to note that although LV hypertrophy may be a frequent autopsy finding in victims of SCD, the incidence of sudden death among all patients with LVH is not that impressive.

C. **Valvular disease.** Valvular abnormalities are commonly associated with abnormalities of ventricular function and contractility. Thus, they are similar to the cardiomyopathies in regard to an anatomic substrate for SCD. However, in certain situations, death may result primarily from a mechanical event or bradyarrhythmia rather than an irritable focus causing a ventricular tachyarrhythmia.

Aortic stenosis may be associated with extensive calcification. If this calcium penetrates the conduction system, heart block may occur. If the individual has advanced critical aortic stenosis and a severe gradient across the valve, death may be due primarily to the pressure overload and obstruction to outflow, even though VF may be the terminal arrhythmia.

The longer the duration and severity of the pressure-volume overload with any valvular abnormality (regurgitation or stenosis), the more likely there will be abnormalities of the affected myocardium. Associated with these abnormalities, arrhythmias may occur. In mitral stenosis, atrial arrhythmias are most common, and the incidence of ventricular tachyarrhythmias is minimal. In mitral regurgitation, both atrial and ventricular arrhythmias may be observed.

Mitral valve prolapse is a disorder that has been associated with ventricular ectopy as well as SCD. One possible mechanism was thought to be increased tension on the papillary muscle from the floppy mitral valve, resulting in ventricular premature beats. Another possibility is an associated cardiomyopathy. Some believe that the association between mitral valve prolapse and VF is fortuitous since the incidence of mitral valve prolapse is high and the incidence of SCD is low. Mitral valve prolapse in some of these patients may be a coincidental finding. These patients may have VT or VF caused by another primary process (e.g., primary electrical disease). However, in certain individuals, there may be a relationship. This issue is incompletely resolved.

Patients who have undergone valve replacement represent still another population at risk for a cardiac death—sudden or nonsudden. Many of these patients have abnormalities of ventricular function because of the primary disorder, and some suffered an insult during the time of surgery. Postoperative complications such as endocarditis, thrombosis, or prosthetic valve dysfunction may cause sudden death that is not primarily the result of ventricular tachy- or bradyarrhythmia.

Again, the common marker for ventricular arrhythmias and sudden cardiac death is an abnormality of LV function; however, no specific anatomic feature is common to all disorders.

D. **Abnormalities of the cardiac nervous system.** A number of disorders of cardiac innervation are associated with sudden cardiac death. Perhaps the most familiar is the **prolonged QT syndrome.** In fact, this disorder is more unrecognized than uncommon. The syndrome may be congenital or acquired. There are two congenital varieties: (1) the Jervell and Lange-Nielsen syndrome (associated with deafness) with autosomal recessive inheritance and (2) the autosomal dominant Romano-Ward syndrome. Most frequently, the acquired form is related to type 1 antiarrhythmic drugs (e.g., quinidine, disopyramide), tricyclic antidepressants, or phenothiazines. It may occur during acute myocardial infarction. Metabolic abnormalities such as hypokalemia may be associated with Q–T prolongation. Rarely, diseases of the central or peripheral nervous system (autonomic dysfunction) or cardiac ganglionitis will cause Q–T lengthening. Prolonged Q–T has been implicated in the sudden deaths of individuals on liquid-protein diets. A syndrome of sudden unexpected death was observed in patients eating a liquid-protein modified-fast diet [31]. Semistarvation seemed to be associated with Q–T interval prolongation. Similar findings were observed in patients with anorexia nervosa [32]. Possibly biochemical changes in the myocellular membrane resulted in prolongation of the Q–T interval.

On the ECG, the diagnosis is made by measuring a Q–T interval (corrected for heart rate) longer than 440 msec. The terminal arrhythmia is torsades de pointes leading to VF. In patients in whom the disorder is associated with autonomic dysfunction, the problems are thought to be related to an excess of sympathetic tone by the left stellate ganglion. Ganglionectomy has been performed, with varying degrees of success.

The role of other abnormalities of the cardiac nervous system is starting to be recognized. Infiltrative or degenerative lesions may occur anywhere in the cardiac conduction system or in the plexus of cardiac nerves. The effect of acute myocardial infarction on the discharge of local intracardiac nerves and subsequent arrhythmias is poorly understood. Thus, more work is necessary in this field. It is obvious that these abnormalities represent a completely different type of underlying anatomic substrate than previously described for coronary disease or cardiomyopathy. In fact, LV function in most patients with a prolonged Q–T syndrome is normal (unless other disease processes are also present). Owing to the absence of other signs or symptoms, cardiac neuropathies may go unrecognized until a life-threatening arrhythmia occurs.

E. **Other disorders of conduction associated with sudden cardiac death.** Sudden cardiac death may be related to both tachy- and bradyarrhythmias. Advanced degrees of heart block without appropriate escape rhythms may lead to poor perfusion, asystole, or, in some cases, an escape VT degenerating into VF. The most common reasons for advanced heart block are degeneration of the cardiac conduction system and block caused by CAD. With degeneration (Lenègre's disease) or infiltration by calcium (Lev's disease), the remaining heart muscle function may be relatively normal. With coronary disease, there may be associated scarring.

Another conduction abnormality associated with SCD is accessory bypass tract conduction (in particular, the Wolff-Parkinson-White syndrome). If conduction during atrial fibrillation occurs antegrade down the accessory pathway (bypassing the rate-limiting atrioventricular node), the ventricle may be stimulated at rates faster than 300/minute. This rapid stimulation (in fact, a VT) may degenerate into VF. In the individual with CAD, ischemia may occur, resulting in myocardial infarction or ischemia-related arrhythmias. The shorter the effective refractory period of the accessory pathway is, the greater is the risk for SCD. Thus, we document other underlying substrates of SCD without associated LV dysfunction.

F. **Sudden death not primarily caused by electrical instability.** In other underlying cardiac abnormalities associated with sudden death, the primary problem is mechanical, not electrical. These include disorders such as acute pericardial tamponade, atrial myxoma, anomalous coronary artery, and other congenital anomalies causing hypoxia or hemodynamic abnormalities. Although VF may be the terminal arrhythmia, it is clearly the result of a mechanical catastrophe requiring primary correction (even if sinus rhythm could be restored).

G. **Rare causes of sudden cardiac death.** Rarely, sudden death is totally unexpected and not associated with any known risk factors. A number of reports have focused on the syndrome in the Southeast Asian population [33]. Often the victims are young, have a cardiac arrest caused by VF in the early morning hours, and demonstrate no cardiac disease at autopsy. The syndrome is called *bangungut* in the Philippines, *pok-kuri* in Japan, and *nonlaitai* in Laos.

IV. **Summary.** The underlying cardiac abnormalities of sudden cardiac death and malignant ventricular tachyarrhythmias have been examined. There are no common features among all categories, although there are features within selected groups that place an individual at higher risk. This may be particularly true for coronary disease and hypertrophic cardiomyopathy. Victims of SCD may be divided into those with and those without LV dysfunction. Patients with disorders of the cardiac nervous system and certain conduction abnormalities may have apparently normal LV function. In patients with CAD, cardiomyopathy, or valvular dysfunction, LV dysfunction is common. Poor ejection fraction and elevated LV end diastolic pressure, resulting from abnormalities of the left ventricle, are predictors of an unfavorable outcome in these groups of patients. Nevertheless, LV dysfunction is probably not the single reason for the ultimate demise but rather a marker for the ravages of the underlying process.

What about the victims of SCD without any detectable heart disease? They appear in almost every reported series of ventricular tachyarrhythmias. Two possible explanations may provide a clue. First, the disease process may be in a very early stage of development, and the finding may be missed during evaluation or at autopsy. Second, diagnostic tools may not be sophisticated enough to detect very subtle abnormalities. Myocardial biopsy studies of apparently normal individuals with ventricular tachyarrhythmias have shown lymphocytic infiltrates in some, suggesting myocarditis [34].

Why do certain individuals with serious underlying heart disease continue to do well and respond to treatment, while others with apparently similar problems die suddenly? Certainly within a group, such as those with CAD, specific variables may place an individual at higher risk. In addition, VT or VF may be precipitated by one or more trigger factors (possibly harmless in the absence of the anatomic substrate).

V. **Trigger factors in sudden cardiac death.** Victims of SCD often have an underlying anatomic abnormality. Yet why did the individual die at that particular moment? What else happened to precipitate the malignant ventricular tachyarrhythmia? A number of variables are known to promote arrhythmias, and some remain undefined. Local changes in myocardium may alter the electrical properties of the tissue, which may, in turn, further alter the dispersion of refractoriness and make the tissue more vulnerable to arrhythmias. The next premature beat may then encounter tissue capable of maintaining a sustained arrhythmia. It is important to remember that participation of some of the trigger factors is better documented than that of others, whose role remains more theoretical and speculative.

Myocardial ischemia is certainly a factor operative in many patients with CAD and arrhythmias. It has become apparent that not all episodes of myocardial ischemia are associated with chest pain, and some may remain "silent." Myocardial ischemia may alter the anatomic substrate, make the heart more irritable (i.e., cause more ventricular ectopy), and result in further biochemical alterations at the cellular level. Ischemia may be caused by a variety of mechanisms, including atherosclerosis, spasm, or a combination of both. It may result from hemodynamic alterations such as tachycardia or hypotension, all affecting the myocardial blood supply-demand relationship.

Metabolic abnormalities, particularly **hypokalemia** and **hypomagnesemia,** have been well documented as associated with VT. In fact, correction of these two particular abnormalities may result in control of the arrhythmia. The **calcium** ion is another important ion in the genesis of rhythm disturbances. **Acidosis** or **alkalosis** may alter the local metabolic status and the concentration of the various ions. **Hypoxia** affects metabolic processes and creates more ischemia. **Anemia** or blood loss decreases the ability to circulate oxygen and also results in a tachycardia. Fever, infection, sepsis, hypertension, hypotension, and dehydration are systemic disorders producing hemodynamic abnormalities that may result in myocardial ischemia or metabolic alterations.

Drug toxicity is an extremely common trigger factor producing VT. The clinician must carefully determine who does and who does not require antiarrhythmic drugs, since these agents may cause sudden cardiac death in certain cases. **Digitalis toxicity** is commonly associated with arrhythmias, particularly in the presence of hypokalemia. Most type 1 antiarrhythmic drugs have a 5% to 10% incidence of exacerbating arrhythmias. Quinidine and disopyramide may result in torsades de pointes if administered to patients with a prolonged Q-T interval. "Quinidine syncope" has been well publicized, but perhaps not all of the cases are due to quinidine alone. In some cases, multiple drug toxicity is at fault. Consider the situation in which the patient is taking digitalis and quinidine. Quinidine raises the digoxin level and prolongs the Q–T interval. If the patient takes too much digitalis and his or her serum potassium is low, increased ventricular ectopy may result as the first manifestation of toxicity. More ventricular ectopic beats falling in a prolonged vulnerable period may increase the risk of VT.

All antiarrhythmic agents have the potential to cause proarrhythmia and result in SCD. **Phenothiazines** and **tricyclic antidepressant drugs** have also been observed to exacerbate arrhythmias. Alcohol, although not always considered by the general public to be a drug, may precipitate both atrial and ventricular arrhythmias. (Taken in large concentration over a long period of time, ethanol may result in a cardiomyopathy in susceptible individuals.) Terfenadine and certain antibiotics can cause torsades.

In patients with CAD, local metabolic changes may occur because of interactions of **platelets** and **platelet aggregation** on an atherosclerotic plaque. What are the effects of the **prostaglandins** (e.g., prostacyclin, thromboxane), **serotonin, endothelin,** and **bradykinin** regarding the genesis of arrhythmias? At this time, understanding of their role remains incomplete. Continued research may provide new insights.

Neural influences may provide a stabilizing or destabilizing factor under certain circumstances. Vagal tone seems to have a protective role, while excess sympathetic tone may lead to an increased risk of ventricular tachyarrhythmias. **Cardiac reflexes,** particularly those in response to myocardial ischemia or myocardial infarction, may play a role—sometimes protective, sometimes not—in the ultimate survival of patients with these conditions.

Finally, **psychosocial factors** and **emotional stress** must receive attention. Emotional stimulation may trigger a variety of physiologic responses: tachycardia, hypertension, and vasovagal syncope, to name just a few. In addition, arrhythmias may result as a response to these physiologic changes (many owing to sympathetic stimulation), neuroendocrine arousal, or other mechanisms less well understood. The association of life crisis in certain individuals with subsequent arrhythmias is well recognized. In particular, the recent loss of a loved one has been reported to be a finding in some victims of SCD. Psychologic factors are also operative in the patient who has been successfully resuscitated from sudden cardiac arrest and faces an extensive evaluation. This issue is addressed in Chaps. 20–21.

VI. **Overview.** The mechanisms of SCD are complex and multifactorial. There are a variety of underlying anatomic substrates as well as a number of trigger factors, some undefined. Within certain categories, such as CAD, certain abnormalities may increase the risk of sudden cardiac death. LV dysfunction is a marker for an increased likelihood of a malignant arrhythmia; however, it is a reflection of the severity of the underlying disease rather than a direct cause of the rhythm disturbance. The scope of this book has allowed only a brief mention of many of the anatomic substrates and trigger factors and their relationship to SCD. Readers are encouraged to consult the references and subsequent chapters that deal with specific problems in more depth.

Attention should be focused on identifying the individual who is at risk of VT or VF but may not have any clinical symptoms. If risk stratification is possible, high-risk individuals can receive specific treatment—either pharmacologic or electronic (pacemakers or defibrillators). Unfortunately, there are many financial and logistic problems. One cannot screen an entire population easily or cost-effectively with sophisticated and expensive tests. It may be possible to evaluate further certain subgroups, such as survivors of myocardial infarction with LV dysfunction and certain other anatomic abnormalities that place them at high risk of VF. Even this approach may be fraught with difficulties, particularly as economic resources for health care become more limited.

For the patient who has overt arrhythmias or has been resuscitated from sudden cardiac arrest, approaches to the problem have been established. Certainly approaches differ, and some remain controversial. Nevertheless, with the increased availability of antiarrhythmic drugs, electrophysiologic testing, arrhythmia surgery, pacemakers, and cardioverter-defibrillators, the mortality of those at risk of recurrent VT or VF has been reduced. It is the responsibility of the physician to determine which patients will benefit from these measures and to refer those patients to appropriate centers.

Therapy must be directed not only at the arrhythmia but at the underlying substrate and trigger factors. Just as the mechanisms of SCD are multifactorial, the evaluation and treatment must be multifaceted. The underlying cardiac problem must be identified and treated. The approach, noninvasive or invasive, appropriate to the specific arrhythmia and individual patient, must be selected. Conventional drug therapy must be evaluated before investigational agents can be used. In chapters dealing with individual arrhythmias, both the conventional drugs and investigational agents for refractory patients are discussed. The advantages and disadvantages of using electrophysiologic evaluation as opposed to drug testing by ambulatory monitoring are debated in Chaps. 15–16. The indications for and results of arrhythmia surgery, pacemakers, and automatic defibrillators are discussed in subsequent chapters. With continued investigation of and attention to the major public health problem of SCD, it may be possible to reduce significantly its mortality in the future.

References

1. Kannel WB, Schatzkin A. Sudden death: Lessons from subsets in population studies. *J Am Coll Cardiol* 5:141B–149B, 1985.
2. Driscoll DJ, Edwards WD. Sudden unexpected death in children and adolescents. *J Am Coll Cardiol* 5:118B–121B, 1985.
3. Garson A, et al. Ventricular arrhythmias and sudden death in children. *J Am Coll Cardiol* 130B–133B, 1985.
4. Weaver WD, et al. Angiographic findings and prognostic indicators in patients resuscitated from sudden cardiac death. *Circulation* 54:895–900, 1976.
5. Swerdlow CD, Winkle RA, Mason JW. Determinants of survival in patients with ventricular tachyarrhythmias. *N Engl J Med* 308:1436–1442, 1983.
6. Spielman SR, et al. Predictors of the success or failure of medical therapy in patients with chronic recurrent sustained ventricular tachycardia: A discriminant analysis. *J Am Coll Cardiol* 1:401–408, 1983.
7. Swerdlow CD, et al. Clinical factors predicting successful electrophysiologic-pharmacologic study in patients with ventricular tachycardia. *J Am Coll Cardiol* 1:409–416, 1983.
8. Vlay SC, et al. Relationship of specific coronary lesions and regional left ventricular dysfunction to prognosis in survivors of sudden cardiac death. *Am Heart J* 108:1212–1220, 1984.
9. Vlay SC, et al. Anatomic substrate and clinical outcome in survivors of sudden cardiac death: A multivariate analysis. *Cardiovasc Rev Rep* 7:861–875, 1986.
10. Vlay SC, et al. Prediction of sudden cardiac arrest: Risk stratification by anatomic substrate. *Am Heart J* 126:807–815, 1993.
11. Samaha JK, et al. Natural history of left anterior descending coronary artery obstruction: Significance of location of stenoses in medically treated patients. *Clin Cardiol* 8: 415–422, 1985.
12. Califf RM, et al. "Left main equivalent" coronary artery disease: Its clinical presentation and prognostic significance with nonsurgical therapy. *Am J Cardiol* 53:1489–1495, 1984.
13. Schuster EH, Griffith LSC, Bulkley BH. Preponderance of acute proximal left anterior descending coronary arterial lesions in fatal myocardial infarction: A clinicopathologic study. *Am J Cardiol* 47:1189–1196, 1981.
14. Abedin Z, Dack S. Isolated left anterior descending coronary artery disease: Choice of therapy. *Am J Cardiol* 40:654–657, 1977.
15. Rahimtoola SH. Left main equivalence is still an unproved hypothesis but proximal left anterior descending artery disease is a "high risk" lesion. *Am J Cardiol* 53:1719–1721, 1984.
16. Goldstein S, Moss AJ, Green W. Sudden death in acute myocardial infarction. Relationship to factors affecting delay in hospitalization. *Arch Intern Med* 129:720–724, 1972.
17. Goldstein S, Friedman L, Hutchinson R. Timing, mechanism and clinical setting of witnessed deaths in postmyocardial infarction patients. *J Am Coll Cardiol* 3:1111–1117, 1984.
18. Hinkle LE, Thaler HT. Clinical classification of cardiac deaths. *Circulation* 65:457–464, 1982.
19. Goldstein S, et al. Characteristics of the resuscitated out-of-hospital cardiac arrest victim with coronary heart disease. *Circulation* 64:977–984, 1981.
20. Goldstein S, Landis JR, Leighton R. Predictive survival models for resuscitated victims of out-of-hospital cardiac arrest with coronary heart disease. *Circulation* 71:873–880, 1985.
21. Roberts WC, Jones AA. Quantitation of coronary arterial narrowing at necropsy in sudden coronary death. Analysis of 31 patients and comparison with 25 control subjects. *Am J Cardiol* 44:39–45, 1979.
22. Warnes CA, Roberts WC. Sudden coronary death: Relation of amount and distribution

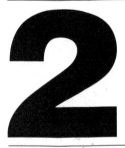

Cardiopulmonary Resuscitation, Techniques of Temporary Pacing, Cardioversion, and Defibrillation

Stephen C. Vlay

Cardiopulmonary resuscitation (CPR) is a technique that should be learned by the general public, in addition to physicians, nurses, and paramedical professionals. Training is divided into basic life support (BLS) and advanced life support (ALS). Standards for training and certification in these techniques have been defined by the American Heart Association. The 1992 National Conference on Cardiopulmonary Resuscitation and Emergency Cardiac Care recommendations have been published [1]. Every physician should obtain a copy and keep it for reference. This chapter is based in part on those recommendations. The last part of this chapter deals with techniques of temporary pacing, cardioversion, and defibrillation.

I. **Basic life support: adult.** After identification of a victim of sudden cardiovascular collapse, additional aid should be summoned immediately by dialing 911 or another emergency number and CPR instituted. The patient should be properly positioned and attention paid to airway, breathing, and circulation. It should be observed whether a pulse is present (even if weak) and whether the patient has spontaneous respirations.
    A. **Airway.** The airway may be obstructed by the tongue. Consequently, it is imperative to relieve the blockage by tilting the head backward and lifting the chin or the neck. **Place the hand on the victim's forehead and apply firm backward pressure with the palm,** so the victim's head is tipped back maximally. Then proceed with the chin-lift maneuver (Fig. 2-1). **Place the fingers of the other hand under the bony part of the lower jaw near the chin and lift, bringing the chin forward, supporting the jaw, and helping to tilt the head back.** Do not compress the soft tissues under the chin. Continue to press on the forehead to tilt the head back. Avoid closing the mouth completely. The thumb is not usually used but may help depress the victim's lower lip to keep the mouth open. If the patient has dentures, they may be left in place (making a mouth-to-mouth seal easier for rescue breathing) unless they are loose and unmanageable.
        Should the head tilt with chin lift be unsuccessful in opening the airway, the jaw thrust may be necessary. **Grasp the angles of the victim's lower jaw on both sides of the head and lift with both hands, displacing the mandible forward while tilting the head backward.** If the victim is suspected of having a neck injury, the head should be supported without extending the neck.
    B. **Breathing.** Once it is ascertained that the airway is not obstructed and the victim is without spontaneous respiration, rescue breathing should commence. **Gently pinch the nostrils closed** (to prevent escape of air) with the hand on the forehead. **Take a deep breath, open your mouth wide, and place it outside the victim's mouth, creating a tight seal. Blow air into the victim's mouth** for 1.5 seconds and **observe whether the victim's chest rises.** Then turn your head toward the victim's chest, take a breath of fresh air, and continue with one more breath (total of two) without allowing for full lung deflation between breaths. After the initial two breaths, breathing is cycled with chest compression.
        If CPR is being performed by **one rescuer, administer two rapid full breaths, without allowing for full deflation, after every 15 compressions.** If CPR is being performed by **two rescuers, deliver one breath every 5 seconds, interposed during the upstroke of the fifth chest compression.** If the victim has a pulse and chest compression is unnecessary, administer one breath every 5 seconds.
        If mouth-to-mouth resuscitation cannot be performed adequately, mouth-to-nose resuscitation may be necessary. For patients with a tracheostomy tube, one must breathe into the tube. Be aware that artificial resuscitation will also blow air into the stomach, causing gastric distention and predisposing to regurgitation. If this

of coronary narrowing at necropsy to previous symptoms of myocardial ischen ventricular scarring and heart weight. *Am J Cardiol* 54:65–73, 1984.

23. Warnes CA, Roberts WC. Sudden coronary death: Comparison of patients witl without coronary thrombus at necropsy. *Am J Cardiol* 54:1206–1211, 1984.
24. Davies MJ, Thomas A. Thrombosis and acute coronary artery lesions in sudden (ischemic death. *N Engl J Med* 310:1137–1140, 1984.
25. Rosenthal ME, et al. Sudden cardiac death following acute myocardial infarctic *Heart J* 109:865–876, 1985.
26. Vlay SC. Innovations in the management of ischemic cardiomyopathy. *Am H* 127:235–242, 1994.
27. Huang SK, Messer JV, Denes P. Significance of ventricular tachycardia in idio dilated cardiomyopathy: Observations in 35 patients. *Am J Cardiol* 51:507–512,
28. Follansbee WP, Michelson EL, Morganroth J. Nonsustained ventricular tachycai ambulatory patients: Characteristics and association with sudden cardiac deatl *Intern Med* 92:741–747, 1980.
29. Savage DD, et al. Prevalence of arrhythmias during 24 hour electrocardiographic toring and exercise testing in patients with obstructive and nonobstructive l trophic cardiomyopathy. *Circulation* 59:866–875, 1979.
30. McKenna WJ, et al. Prognosis in hypertrophic cardiomyopathy: Role of age and cl electrocardiographic and hemodynamic features. *Am J Cardiol* 47:532–538, 1981.
31. Isner JM, et al. Sudden, unexpected death in avid dieters using the liquid-protein ified-fast diet. *Circulation* 60:1401–1412, 1979.
32. Isner J, et al. Anorexia nervosa and sudden death. *Ann Intern Med* 102:49–52, 198
33. Otto CM, et al. Ventricular fibrillation causes sudden death in Southeast Asian i grants. *Ann Intern Med* 100:45–47, 1984.
34. Sugrue DD, et al. Cardiac histologic findings in patients with life-threatening vent lar arrhythmias of unknown origin. *J Am Coll Cardiol* 4:952–957, 1984.

Bibliography

Further references will be found in Chap. 7 and in the following sources.

James TN, Chairman. 15th Bethesda conference report: Sudden cardiac death. *J Coll Cardiol* 5 Supplement 1B–198B, June 1985.

Myerburg RJ (comp). Risk factors and epidemiology, pathology and pathophysiol *Circulation* 64:1070–1074, 1984.

Myerburg RJ (comp). Clinical, intervention, survival, neurophysiologic and p chophysiologic factors, and miscellaneous. *Circulation* 64:1291–1296, 1984.

Myerburg RJ, Kessler KM, Castellanos A. Sudden cardiac death: Epidemiology, tra sient risk, and intervention assessment. *Ann Intern Med* 119:1187–1197, 1993.

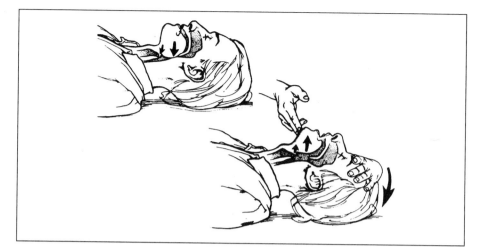

Fig. 2-1. Opening the airway. *Top:* Airway obstruction produced by tongue and epiglottis. *Bottom:* Relief by head tilt-chin lift. (Reprinted with permission from Guidelines for cardiopulmonary resuscitation and emergency cardiac care. *JAMA* 268:2186, 1992. Copyright 1992, American Medical Association.)

Table 2-1. Airway obstruction caused by foreign body

Conscious choking victim or victim who becomes unconscious
1. Identify complete airway obstruction (ask victim to speak).
2. Apply the Heimlich maneuver until object is expelled or patient loses consciousness.
3. When patient is unconscious, perform the finger sweep.
4. Open the airway and attempt to ventilate.
5. If unsuccessful, attempt Heimlich maneuver another 6–10 times.
6. Repeat steps 3–5.

Unconscious victim when the cause is unknown
Establish unresponsiveness, call for assistance, initiate CPR. If unable to ventilate:
1. Reposition the head; try to ventilate.
2. Apply the Heimlich maneuver.
3. Apply the finger sweep. Remove dentures if necessary.
4. Reposition the head; try to ventilate. If unsuccessful, repeat steps 2–4.

Source: Modified from Standards and guidelines for cardiopulmonary resuscitation and emergency cardiac care. *JAMA* 255:2924, 1986. Copyright 1986, American Medical Association.

occurs, turn the victim on the side to prevent aspiration, wipe out the mouth, and then reposition to resume CPR.

C. **Inability to establish patent airway.** An inability to establish a patent airway by positioning or the sudden onset of choking after eating suggests foreign body obstruction. Depending on the degree of consciousness, several maneuvers can be performed. The sequence of events recommended by the National Conference is listed in Table 2-1.

The subdiaphragmatic abdominal thrust (Heimlich maneuver) is a thrust to the upper abdomen or lower chest, forcing air out of the lungs. It is considered the preferred method in adults. **Never** place the hands on the xiphoid process or lower margins of the rib cage; rather, place them below this landmark but above the navel. Care must be taken to avoid injury to internal organs (Fig. 2-2).

The **finger sweep,** performed by grasping the tongue and lower jaw (between the thumb and fingers) and lifting, is performed only in unconscious victims with suspected airway obstruction, and **not** in patients who are breathing spontaneously. The index finger is inserted into the base of the throat to attempt to dislodge a foreign body. Do not push the object deeper into the airway. Only professionals trained

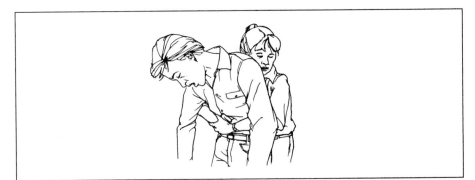

Fig. 2-2A. Heimlich maneuver administered to conscious victim of foreign body airway obstruction who is sitting or standing. (Reprinted with permission from Guidelines for cardiopulmonary resuscitation and emergency cardiac care. *JAMA* 268:2193, 1992. Copyright 1992, American Medical Association.)

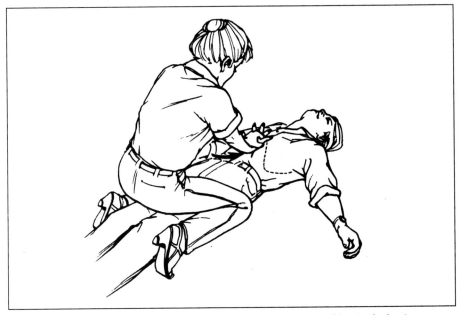

Fig. 2-2B. Heimlich maneuver administered to unconscious victim of foreign body airway obstruction who is lying down. (Reprinted with permission from Guidelines for cardiopulmonary resuscitation and emergency cardiac care. *JAMA* 268:2193, 1992. Copyright 1992, American Medical Association.)

in the use of devices to remove foreign bodies, including the Kelly clamp or Magill forceps, may use them if the foreign body can be seen. The **back blow** is a sharp blow to the spine, between the shoulder blades, delivered with the heel of the hand. It may be performed with the victim sitting, standing, or lying. The back blow is recommended for infants but **not** for adults.

D. **Circulation.** When the patient is pulseless, external chest compression must be started immediately. **Make certain that the victim is horizontal. Compress the sternum 1.5–2.0 inches (4–5 cm). Place a board beneath the victim's back if there is no firm surface.**

   Place the heel of one hand on the lower half of the sternum and the second hand over the first. The fingers are directed away from the rescuer and off the chest wall. **Straighten the elbows by locking them.** Position the shoulders over the hands so that the thrust is directly downward. After compression, release the pressure completely, but do not remove the hands from the chest. Arterial pressure during chest compression is maximal when the duration of compression is 50% of the compression-release cycle, with prolonged chest compression to be encouraged.

If there is only one rescuer, perform 15 chest compressions at a rate of 80–100/minute; then open the airway and provide two slow rescue breaths (1.5–2 seconds each). Reassess the patient after four complete cycles. With a second rescuer, the compression rate is 80–100/minute with a compression-ventilation ratio of 5:1 and a pause for inspiration of 1.5–2 seconds. Palpate the carotid pulse after the first minute of CPR and then every few minutes to determine the efficacy of CPR or the return of spontaneous pulses. CPR should be continued until the victim's circulation and ventilation have been restored (Table 2-2).

For special situations, such as stroke, near-drowning, traumatic injury, electrical shock, lightning strike, and hypothermia, refer to the National Conference recommendations [1].

II. **Advanced cardiac life support: adult.** Advanced cardiac life support consists of basic plus special techniques, devices, and aids (Table 2-3) for maintaining the circulation and respiration. It includes the use of specific cardiac drugs and cardioversion and defibrillation techniques.

Ventilation may be facilitated with a well-fitting **mask** or a **bag-valve-mask** device. Supplemental oxygen will improve myocardial and cerebral oxygenation. In cardiac arrest, the initial concentration of oxygen should be 100%. **Only if** the patient is unconscious, an oropharyngeal airway will assist in keeping the airway open. An esophageal obturator airway and esophageal gastric tube airway are available to prevent gastric distention and regurgitation during resuscitative efforts.

Should the patient not respond immediately to initial resuscitative efforts but remain apneic and pulseless, **endotracheal intubation** should be performed by a rescuer skilled in this technique. When this procedure is performed, ventilation should not be interrupted for longer than 30 seconds. After the tube is inserted, ventilation should contin-

Table 2-2. Reasons to discontinue cardiopulmonary resuscitation and basic life support

Effective spontaneous circulation and ventilation have been restored.

Care is transferred to emergency medical responders or another trained person, who continues BLS.

Care is transferred to ALS emergency medical personnel.

Care is transferred to a physician who determines that resuscitation should be discontinued.

Reliable criteria for the determination of death are recognized.

The rescuer is too exhausted to continue resuscitation, environmental hazards endanger the rescuer, or continued resuscitation would jeopardize the lives of others.

A valid no-CPR order is presented to the rescuers. Ethically and legally, there is no distinction between discontinuing CPR and not starting it in the first place.

BLS = basic life support; ALS = advanced life support; CPR = cardiopulmonary resuscitation.
Source: Emergency Cardiac Care Committee and Subcommittees, American Heart Association. Guidelines for cardiopulmonary resuscitation and emergency cardiac care. *JAMA* 268:2285, 1992. Copyright 1992, American Medical Association.

Table 2-3. Adjunctive equipment for advanced cardiac life support

Conventional pressure-cycled automatic resuscitators
Suction devices
Bed board
Mechanical devices for chest compression
Medical antishock garments
Intraaortic balloon counterpulsation
Electrocardiographic monitoring

ue manually with a bag-valve device until a respirator is available. Transtracheal catheter ventilation and cricothyrotomy are techniques of ventilation that require special skill to perform.

Venous access to the circulation is imperative, with a **central venous line** particularly desirable. Rather than interrupt CPR to cannulate the jugular or subclavian vein, the antecubital vein is the access of choice. If circulation is not restored quickly, a central line is necessary, to allow administration of fluids and medication. The techniques of central venous catheter placement are discussed later in this chapter.

Electrocardiographic monitoring of the rhythm should be instituted as soon as possible. If the rhythm is sinus and the patient remains pulseless and apneic, CPR is continued. If a life-threatening arrhythmia such as ventricular tachycardia (VT) or ventricular fibrillation (VF) is observed, electrical cardioversion or defibrillation should be performed as soon as a defibrillator is available. CPR is continued until that is possible.

Ventricular tachycardia may respond to a precordial thump, performed by delivering a blow to the sternum with the closed fist. Today it is considered an optional technique performed by those trained in ACLS in the situation of a witnessed cardiac arrest when the patient is **pulseless** and a defibrillator is not immediately available. It should not delay electrical defibrillation. The precordial thump may be ineffective or cause deterioration of the rhythm; consequently, it should not be used if the patient has a pulse unless a defibrillator and pacemaker are available.

No maneuvers should delay electrical cardioversion or defibrillation when it is immediately available. Techniques of cardioversion and defibrillation are discussed later in this chapter (**VII**).

A. Specific drug therapy. Drug therapy is discussed in subsequent chapters, but the essentials for cardiopulmonary resuscitation, including some of the newer drugs, are mentioned here. The drugs must be used as applicable in each individual situation.

1. **Oxygen.** Administer oxygen as soon as possible in 100% concentration.

2. **IV fluids.** Administer at a rate to keep a line open—usually dextrose 5% in water (D5W)—unless the patient is hypovolemic. If volume depletion is diagnosed, volume expansion with 0.9% saline or Ringer's lactate is the first step. Depending on the presenting problem, blood and normal serum albumin are additional considerations.

3. **Morphine sulfate.** Administer morphine sulfate in small intravenous (IV) doses for appropriate indications, but no more than 1–3 mg IV every 5 minutes. (If it proves to be too much of a respiratory depressant, reversal with naloxone may be necessary.) Additional morphine is given as required to control pain (of myocardial infarction). Morphine is useful in the treatment of pulmonary edema because of its venodilator capability. Venous return to the heart decreases, reducing end-diastolic volume and pressure. There is also a small effect on systemic vascular resistance, reducing afterload.

4. **Lidocaine.** If ventricular ectopy needs treatment or if the patient has life-threatening ventricular tachyarrhythmias (VT or VF), lidocaine is the drug of first choice.

   Administer a 1.0–1.5 mg/kg bolus (usual dose 50–100 mg), followed by a 2–4 mg/minute constant infusion. The rate of the constant infusion is increased from 2 mg/minute as necessary, to a maximal dose of 4 mg/minute. Additional boluses (0.5–1.5 mg/kg) can be given every 5–10 minutes if necessary (to a total of 3 mg/kg) to establish an adequate initial blood level. (A dose of 225–300 mg should not be exceeded. In fact, some patients exhibit CNS toxicity at that dose.) Elderly patients and those with heart failure or hepatic dysfunction start to manifest toxicity at lower doses. These individuals should not receive the second bolus, and the maintenance dose should be halved.

5. **Procainamide.** If lidocaine fails to control life-threatening ventricular arrhythmias, add procainamide. Administer 50–100 mg IV q5min (20 mg/minute) up to a total of 17 mg/kg. The loading should be stopped if the arrhythmia is controlled, if the patient becomes hypotensive, or if the QRS widens to 50% greater than baseline. If the arrhythmia is controlled by loading, maintenance infusion at a rate of 1–4 mg/minute (or lower in renal failure) is started.

6. **Bretylium.** When lidocaine or procainamide fails to control life-threatening ventricular arrhythmias, bretylium becomes the next drug to use. Some clinicians have administered bretylium initially to patients in VF in the hope that it will facilitate electrical defibrillation. However, it is not better than lidocaine, and it is limited by its attendant hypotensive effects, which may necessitate the addi-

tion of a drug such as phenylephrine. It is recommended after defibrillation, epinephrine, and lidocaine have failed to convert VF or its recurrence; after lidocaine and procainamide have failed to control VT; or after lidocaine and adenosine have failed to control wide-complex rhythms. Administer bretylium tosylate 5 mg/kg IV as a bolus, and then perform electrical defibrillation. If VF persists, increase the dose to 10 mg/kg, and repeat electrical defibrillation. If there is no response, continue to administer bretylium tosylate at 15- to 30-minute intervals, with recurrent attempts at electrical defibrillation. The maximum dosage is 30–35 mg/kg. For refractory VT that does respond to bretylium tosylate, a continuous infusion of 1–2 mg/minute is started.

7. **Beta blockers.** Beta blockers are useful as an adjunctive treatment of myocardial ischemia/infarction and reduce the incidence of VF. Three agents have shown benefit in trials: atenolol, metoprolol, and propranolol. Recommended doses are:

   Atenolol: 5–10 mg IV/5 minutes.
   Metoprolol: 5–10 mg IV/5 minutes, to a total of 15 mg.
   Propranolol: Total dosage of 0.1 mg/kg by slow IV push divided into 3 equal doses at 2–3-minute intervals (not more than 1 mg/minute).

   In patients with asthma or congestive heart failure, these drugs can be hazardous. See Chap. 11 for further details on their pharmacology.

8. **Atropine.** Atropine is useful in sinus bradycardia and high-degree atrioventricular (AV) block that occurs at the level of the AV node. Administer 0.5–1.0 mg IV, and repeat at 3–5-minute intervals until the desired rate is achieved. (A maximal dosage is 0.04 mg/kg.) A total dosage of 3.0 mg results in full vagal blockade. Dosages less than 0.5 mg may result in bradyarrhythmias due to a parasympathomimetic effect. A resultant tachycardia may be extremely detrimental in patients with acute myocardial ischemia or infarction. In certain situations, temporary pacing may be preferable.

9. **Isoproterenol.** Isoproterenol has potent inotropic and chronotropic properties. It can exacerbate arrhythmias and ischemia. The current indications are for refractory torsades de pointes and immediate control of bradyarrhythmias in denervated hearts of heart transplant patients. Add 1 mg of isoproterenol to 500 ml D5W (2 µg/ml) or 1 mg to 250 ml D5W (4 µg/ml). Infuse at a rate of 2–10 µg/minute, and titrate to the desired heart rate. The positive inotropic effect will increase the imbalance between myocardial oxygen supply and demand, possibly exacerbating myocardial ischemia or infarction. A pacemaker is preferable to prolonged administration of isoproterenol for bradycardia.

10. **Verapamil and diltiazem.** Verapamil and diltiazem are calcium channel blockers with negative dromotropic effects that slow conduction at the AV node. Verapamil may be used to terminate paroxysmal supraventricular tachycardia but is no longer the drug of choice. The dosage is 2.5–5 mg initially over 2 minutes and 5–10 mg given 15–30 minutes later (maximum dosage, 20 mg) if the arrhythmia persists. Be prepared for the rare occurrence of asystole or high-degree AV block. Hypotension may be reversed by 0.5–1.0 g of IV calcium chloride. For control of a fast ventricular response to atrial fibrillation, IV diltiazem at a dose of 0.25 mg/kg followed by a dose of 0.35 mg/kg is equivalent to verapamil. Maintenance therapy consists of a continuous infusion of diltiazem at a rate of 5–15 mg/hour.

11. **Adenosine.** Adenosine is the drug of choice for paroxysmal supraventricular tachycardia involving the AV node or sinoatrial node. It is a purinergic receptor blocker with a very short half-life (<10 seconds). It must be administered quickly, with an initial dose of 6 mg IV/1–3 seconds followed by a 20-ml saline flush. If unsuccessful, it can be repeated 1–2 minutes later with a 12-mg bolus. Side effects include flushing, dyspnea, and chest pain but are self-limited due to the short half-life. Theophylline and caffeine block the purinergic receptor (preventing its efficacy), and dipyridamole blocks its uptake (potentiating its effect).

12. **Magnesium.** Magnesium deficiency may result in ventricular arrhythmias and sudden cardiac death. Many physicians recommend starting replacement even before the laboratory value becomes known. Magnesium sulfate 1–2 g is diluted in 100 ml D5W and administered over 1–2 minutes if the arrhythmia is VT or VF. It is a treatment of choice in torsades de pointes. The routine use of magnesium for patients with acute myocardial infarction has not been conclusively demonstrated. For patients with documented magnesium deficiency, 1–2 g has been

administered over 5–60 minutes in 50–100 ml D5W, followed by 0.5–1.0 g/hour for up to 24 hours.

13. **Epinephrine.** Epinephrine stimulates both alpha- and beta-adrenergic receptors. During CPR, it elevates perfusion pressure, may increase cardiac contractility, may stimulate spontaneous cardiac contractions, and usually will coarsen fine VF. Coarse VF may be more amenable to electrical defibrillation and restoration of sinus rhythm.

Epinephrine is administered IV during CPR at a dose of 1.0 mg (10 ml of 1:10,000 solution). If no suitable IV access is available, the epinephrine may be administered into the tracheobronchial tree through the endotracheal tube. For tracheobronchial injection, the dose is at least 2 to 2.5 times the peripheral IV dose. Since epinephrine has a short half-life, it **must be administered every 3–5 minutes as long as CPR continues.**

Intracardiac injection is not routinely recommended because of potential morbidity. Nevertheless, some physicians claim that it is effective when other routes fail. The reason for success may be the stimulatory trauma to the ventricle rather than a specific effect of the epinephrine. This route should be used only as a last resort.

If the patient remains hypotensive after sinus rhythm is restored, vasopressor support may be necessary. Epinephrine is not the drug of choice. If indicated, the infusion is started at 1 µg/minute (1 mg epinephrine in 500 ml D5W or normal saline) and titrated to the desired hemodynamic effect (usually 2–10 µg/minute).

14. **Norepinephrine.** Norepinephrine has both alpha- and beta- receptor effects. It is a potent vasoconstrictor that raises the blood pressure but may severely compromise the renal and mesenteric circulation. The drug is particularly useful if the peripheral vascular resistance is low.

Norepinephrine bitartrate is administered IV with a 16-mg/liter or 16-µg/ml solution (8 mg norepinephrine bitartrate in 500 ml D5W or normal saline or 16 mg in 1000 ml) and the rate of administration titrated to achieve the desired blood pressure. The usual dose is 0.5–1.0 µg/minute titrated to the desired hemodynamic response. Norepinephrine is preferentially administered into a central venous line, as extravasation into the tissues results in ischemic necrosis and sloughing. Although phentolamine, 5–10 mg in 10–15 ml normal saline, infiltrated into the extravasated area may reduce the local injury, serious scarring may still result.

15. **Dopamine.** Dopamine, a chemical precursor of norepinephrine, has both alpha- and beta-adrenergic effects, as well as dopaminergic activity. In low dose (1–2 µg/kg/minute) it dilates renal and mesenteric beds with little increase in heart rate or blood pressure. Cardiac output increases with doses of 2–10 µg/kg/minute (beta effect). The alpha effect is prominent at high dose (10 µg/kg/minute) and results in vasoconstriction with BP elevation. At doses higher than 20 µg/kg/minute, renal and mesenteric blood flow diminishes greatly. Administration starts at a dose of 2.5–5 µg/kg/minute (400 mg dopamine hydrochloride [HCl] in 250 ml D5W = 1600 µg/ml, or 800 mg dopamine HCl in 250 ml D5W = 3200 µg/ml). Dopamine is inactivated in alkaline solution. Consequently it must not be added to solutions of sodium bicarbonate.

16. **Dobutamine.** Dobutamine, a beta stimulant, increases myocardial contractility but has less of an effect on BP or heart rate than does dopamine HCl. Administer dobutamine at 2–20 µg/kg/minute (dobutamine 250 mg in 500 ml D5W or normal saline = 500 µg/ml). Dobutamine is incompatible with alkaline solutions.

17. **Amrinone.** Amrinone is a positive inotropic agent with vasodilator activity. It is indicated for the short-term management of heart failure. Therapy is initiated with a 0.75–mg/kg bolus IV over a period of 2–3 minutes. Maintenance infusion is 5–15 µg/kg/minute. Thrombocytopenia has been reported in 2.4% of patients.

18. **Milrinone.** Milrinone is a newer positive inotrope with vasodilator activity and has the same indication as amrinone. Therapy is initiated with a loading dose of 50 µg/kg administered slowly over 10 minutes. Maintenance infusion is 0.375–0.75 µg/kg/minute. Milrinone does not have the same risk of thrombocytopenia as does amrinone; however, ventricular arrhythmias were reported in 12.1% of phase II and III clinical trials.

19. **Metaraminol.** Metaraminol is a potent alpha and beta stimulant whose actions are partially mediated via release of catecholamine stores. It is indicated for the prevention and treatment of hypotension occurring with general anesthesia, as

well as an adjunctive treatment for hypotension in other situations. For shock, administer metaraminol 0.5–5.0 mg followed by an infusion (15–100 mg metaraminol in 500 ml D5W or normal saline) as necessary.

20. **Methoxamine.** Methoxamine is a pure alpha stimulant. It may be particularly useful for the hypotensive patient with hypertrophic obstructive cardiomyopathy, in whom beta stimulation would be hazardous. The drug is also used in anesthesia. The usual IV dose is 3–5 mg injected slowly.

21. **Calcium chloride.** Calcium increases cardiac contractility and automaticity. It is indicated in cardiac arrest related to hyperkalemia, hypocalcemia, or toxic reaction to calcium-channel-blocking drugs. Administer 2 ml of 10% solution of calcium chloride (2–4 mg/kg) for the specific indications, and repeat as necessary.

22. **Digitalis.** Digitalis is infrequently called for during CPR unless there is a problem with atrial fibrillation and a rapid ventricular response. The need for digitalis has been replaced by IV diltiazem and IV verapamil.

23. **Nitroprusside.** Nitroprusside is a direct peripheral vasodilator, particularly useful in hypertensive crises and pulmonary edema. Administration of nitroprusside is usually started at 0.1–5 µg/kg/minute (50–100 mg nitroprusside in 250 ml D5W or normal saline = 200–400 µg/ml). The average dose is 3 µg/kg/minute. Since nitroprusside is light sensitive, the tubing must be wrapped with opaque material (usually aluminum foil).

24. **Nitroglycerin.** Nitroglycerin is a vasodilator. It may be given for relief of angina or for the treatment of congestive heart failure during acute myocardial infarction. Administer initially at a rate of 10–20 µg/minute (50–100 mg nitroglycerin in 250 ml D5W or normal saline). At doses of 30–40 µg/minute, the greatest effect is on the venous circulation. At higher doses (150–500 µg/minute, arteriolar dilatation occurs. Some preparations of nitroglycerin may be affected by the tubing (adsorption); the rate of administration must be adjusted accordingly.

25. **Sodium bicarbonate.** Bicarbonate is used to correct acidosis. In the past, it was common to administer bicarbonate routinely during CPR. Bicarbonate shifts the oxyhemoglobin saturation curve and inhibits the release of oxygen. Hypernatremia and hyperosmolarity result. Paradoxical acidosis from the production of carbon dioxide can diffuse into myocardium and cerebral cells, depressing function. Adverse effects may occur from extracellular alkalosis and central venous acidosis. The action of catecholamines may be diminished. Therefore, the current recommendations are to proceed with defibrillation, chest compression, ventilation, and pharmacologic therapy **before** using bicarbonate. After the combined interventions including more than one trial of epinephrine, bicarbonate may be given at the discretion of the physician in charge. Preexisting acidosis or hyperkalemia is an indication for bicarbonate. Administer 1 mEq/kg IV initially and then 0.5 mEq/kg q10min if necessary during continued cardiac arrest. Most ampules contain 44.6 or 50.0 mEq.

26. **Furosemide.** Furosemide is a diuretic that is useful for the treatment of pulmonary edema; it may have some benefit for cerebral edema that occurs after cardiac arrest. Administer 0.5–1.0 mg/kg IV slowly. If the patient has chronically taken large doses of furosemide, higher doses may be necessary.

27. **Ethacrynic acid.** Ethacrynic acid is another loop diuretic and is used infrequently today. Administer 0.5–1.0 mg/kg IV (usual dose is 50 mg).

28. **Bumetanide.** Bumetanide is a third loop diuretic. Administer 0.5–1.0 mg IV.

B. **Treatment of specific arrhythmias.** The treatment of arrhythmias is addressed individually in Chaps. 6 and 8. Figures 2-3 through 2-6 present algorithms recommended by the national conference for VT, VF, asystole, and electromechanical dissociation.

C. **Postresuscitative care.** Once the patient's vital signs have been restored, attention must be directed at maintaining them, determining the cause of the arrest, and assessing any damage. Specifically, the ventilatory capability and cardiac status of the victim must be reassessed:

Is a respirator required, or can the victim breathe spontaneously and maintain adequate oxygenation?
Did the victim suffer a myocardial infarction?
Has pulmonary edema been satisfactorily treated?
Is a Swan-Ganz pulmonary artery catheter necessary?
Are there any laboratory abnormalities that need correction?
Are the arrhythmias likely to recur?

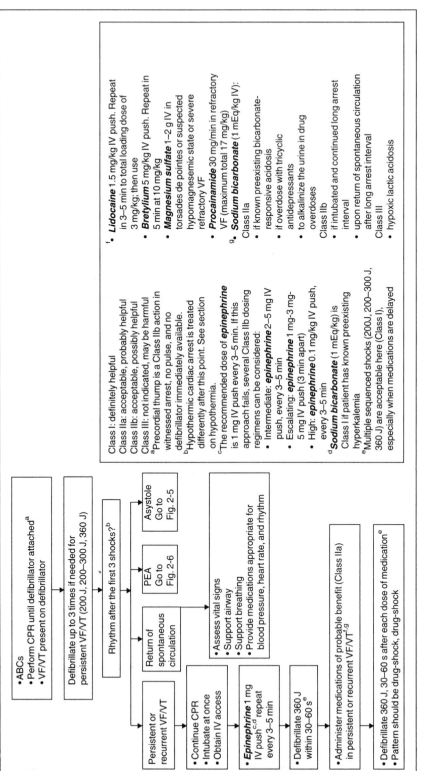

Fig. 2-3. Algorithm for ventricular fibrillation (VF) and pulseless ventricular tachycardia (VT). (Reprinted with permission from Guidelines for cardiopulmonary resuscitation and emergency cardiac care. *JAMA* 268:2217, 1992. Copyright 1992, American Medical Association.)

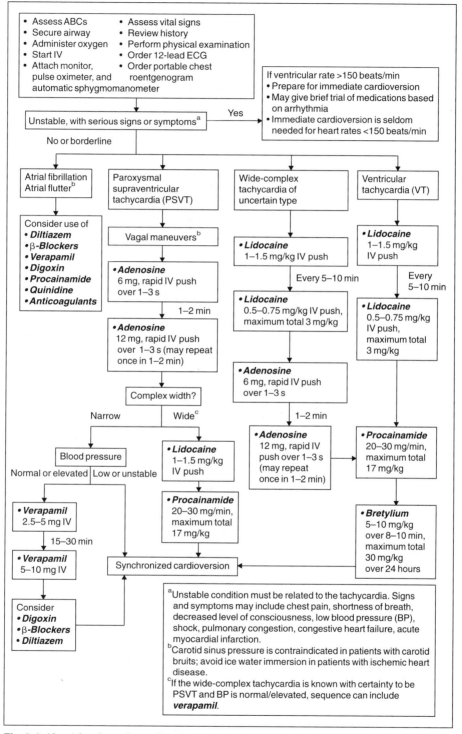

Fig. 2-4. Algorithm for tachycardia. (Reprinted with permission from Guidelines for cardiopulmonary resuscitation and emergency cardiac care. *JAMA* 268:2223, 1992. Copyright 1992, American Medical Association.)

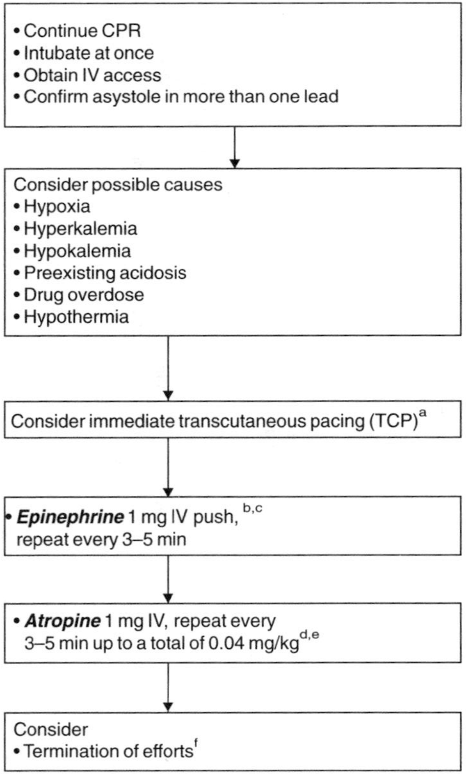

- Continue CPR
- Intubate at once
- Obtain IV access
- Confirm asystole in more than one lead

Consider possible causes
- Hypoxia
- Hyperkalemia
- Hypokalemia
- Preexisting acidosis
- Drug overdose
- Hypothermia

Consider immediate transcutaneous pacing (TCP)[a]

- *Epinephrine* 1 mg IV push, [b,c] repeat every 3–5 min

- *Atropine* 1 mg IV, repeat every 3–5 min up to a total of 0.04 mg/kg[d,e]

Consider
- Termination of efforts[f]

Class I: definitely helpful
Class IIa: acceptable, probably helpful
Class IIb: acceptable, possibly helpful
Class III: not indicated, may be harmful

[a]TCP is a Class IIb intervention. Lack of success may be due to delays in pacing. To be effective TCP must be performed early, simultaneously with drugs. Evidence does not support routine use of TCP for asystole.

[b]The recommended dose of *epinephrine* is 1 mg IV push every 3–5 min. If this approach fails, several Class IIb dosing regimens can be considered:
- Intermediate: *epinephrine* 2–5 mg IV push, every 3–5 min
- Escalating: *epinephrine* 1 mg-3 mg-5 mg IV push (3 min apart)
- High: *epinephrine* 0.1 mg/kg IV push, every 3–5 min

[c]*Sodium bicarbonate* 1 mEq/kg is Class I if patient has known preexisting hyperkalemia.

[d]Shorter *atropine* dosing intervals are Class IIb in asystolic arrest.
[e]*Sodium bicarbonate* 1 mEq/kg:
Class IIa
- if known preexisting bicarbonate-responsive acidosis
- if overdose with tricyclic antidepressants
- to alkalinize the urine in drug overdoses
Class IIb
- if intubated and continued long arrest interval
- upon return of spontaneous circulation after long arrest interval
Class III
- hypoxic lactic acidosis
[f]If patient remains in asystole or other agonal rhythms after successful intubation and initial medications and no reversible causes are identified, consider termination of resuscitative efforts by a physician. Consider interval since arrest.

Fig. 2-5. Algorithm for asystole. (Reprinted with permission from Guidelines for cardiopulmonary resuscitation and emergency cardiac care. *JAMA* 268:2220, 1992. Copyright 1992, American Medical Association.)

PEA includes
- Electromechanical dissociation (EMD)
- Pseudo-EMD
- Idioventricular rhythms
- Ventricular escape rhythms
- Bradyasystolic rhythms
- Postdefibrillation idioventricular rhythms

- Continue CPR
- Intubate at once
- Obtain IV access
- Assess blood flow using Doppler ultrasound

Consider possible causes
(Parentheses = possible therapies and treatments)
- Hypovolemia (volume infusion)
- Hypoxia (ventilation)
- Cardiac tamponade (pericardiocentesis)
- Tension pneumothorax (needle decompression)
- Hypothermia
- Massive pulmonary embolism (surgery, *thrombolytics*)
- Drug overdoses such as tricyclics, digitalis, β-blockers, calcium channel blockers
- Hyperkalemia[a]
- Acidosis[b]
- Massive acute myocardial infarction

- *Epinephrine* 1 mg IV push,[a,c] repeat every 3–5 min

- If absolute bradycardia (<60 beats/min) or relative bradycardia, give *atropine* 1 mg IV
- Repeat every 3–5 min up to total of 0.04 mg/kg[d]

Class I: definitely helpful
Class IIa: acceptable, probably helpful
Class IIb: acceptable, possibly helpful
Class III: not indicated, may be harmful
[a]*Sodium bicarbonate* 1 mEq/kg is Class I if patient has known preexisting hyperkalemia.
[b]*Sodium bicarbonate* 1 mEq/kg:
  Class IIa
  - if known preexisting bicarbonate-responsive acidosis
  - if overdose with tricyclic antidepressants
  - to alkalinize the urine in drug overdoses
  Class IIb
  - if intubated and long arrest interval
  - upon return of spontaneous circulation after long arrest interval
  Class III
  - hypoxic lactic acidosis
[c]The recommended dose of *epinephrine* is 1 mg IV push every 3–5 min
If this approach fails, several Class IIb dosing regimens can be considered
  - Intermediate: *epinephrine* 2–5 mg IV push, every 3–5 min
  - Escalating: *epinephrine* 1 mg-3 mg-5 mg IV push (3 min apart)
  - High: *epinephrine* 0.1 mg/kg IV push, every 3–5 min
[d]Shorter *atropine* dosing intervals are possibly helpful in cardiac arrest (Class IIb).

Fig. 2-6. Algorithm for electromechanical dissociation (pulseless electrical activity). (Reprinted with permission from Guidelines for cardiopulmonary resuscitation and emergency cardiac care. *JAMA* 268:2219, 1992. Copyright 1992, American Medical Association.)

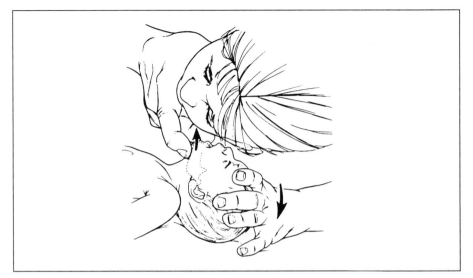

Fig. 2-7A. Opening the airway with the head tilt–chin lift maneuver. One hand is used to tilt the head, extending the neck. The index finger of the rescuer's other hand lifts the mandible outward by lifting on the chin. Head tilt should not be performed if cervical spine injury is suspected. (Reprinted with permission from Guidelines for cardiopulmonary resuscitation and emergency cardiac care. *JAMA* 268:2253, 1992. Copyright 1992, American Medical Association.)

Next, the physician must determine the extent of injury to other systems:

Is there adequate urine output?
Will the patient develop acute tubular necrosis owing to prolonged hypotension?
Is there hypovolemia to account for poor urine output?
What is the extent of the insult to the CNS during the time of hypotension?
Will there be any deficit? Is there any damage to the GI tract?
Is a nasogastric tube necessary?

Many of these issues are addressed when the patient arrives in the coronary care or intensive care unit.

    D. Termination of CPR. If cardiopulmonary resuscitation is unsuccessful, a physician must make the decision to terminate resuscitative efforts (see Table 2-2). The definition of **unresuscitatable** is "refractory to available BLS and ACLS measures adequate to test the responsiveness of the victim's cardiovascular system." Details are available from the National Conference recommendations [1].

III. Basic life support: infants and children. Cardiopulmonary resuscitation principles in infants (aged less than 1 year) and children (aged 1–8 years) are the same as in adults, although techniques may vary. The rescuer must establish that the victim is unresponsive or having respiratory difficulty. Aid is summoned and the victim correctly positioned. If found face down, the infant or child must be rolled over as a unit, with one hand supporting the head and neck so they do not roll or twist. If the rescuer is alone, the emergency medical service should be called after 1 minute of respiratory support (20 breaths including compressions). The airway is established and rescue breathing initiated. Chest compression is started if the pulse is absent.

    A. Airway. The airway must be opened if the victim is not breathing or is cyanotic and struggling to breathe. Perform the **head tilt–chin lift** technique. **Place one hand** on the **child's forehead** and **tilt the head gently back** into a **neutral or slightly extended position.** Then **place the fingers** under the **bony part of the lower jaw, lifting the mandible upward and outward (the jaw-thrust maneuver). Place two or three fingers of each hand under the lower jaw at its angle, lifting it upward and outward.** The mouth should remain partially open (Fig. 2-7).

    B. Breathing. If the victim remains apneic after the airway is cleared, rescue breathing must commence. **In the case of an infant, cover both the mouth and**

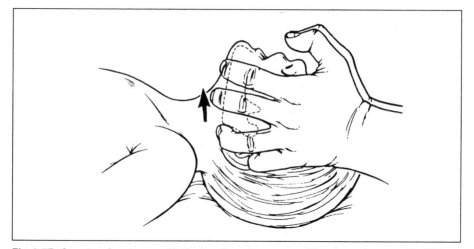

Fig. 2-7B. Opening the airway with the jaw-thrust maneuver. The airway is opened by lifting the angle of the mandible. The rescuer uses two or three fingers of each hand to lift the jaw, while the other fingers guide the jaw upward and outward. (Reprinted with permission from Guidelines for cardiopulmonary resuscitation and emergency cardiac care. *JAMA* 268:2254, 1992. Copyright 1992, American Medical Association.)

nose to make a seal. If a tight seal is not possible in a larger child, pinch the nostrils together. Then **deliver two slow breaths (1–1.5 seconds each), pausing after the first breath to take a breath and maximize oxygen content and minimize carbon dioxide.** The volume should be sufficient to make the chest rise. Since the infant or child has smaller lungs than an adult, smaller volumes are required. The initial two breaths open small sacs in the lung and determine airway patency. **If the lungs do not inflate, recheck the airway and adjust your position if necessary.** In some situations, gastric distention may be so pronounced as to prevent effective ventilation. Minimize gastric distention by providing slow breaths.

If the airway cannot be cleared, there is a possibility of foreign body obstruction (e.g., by a peanut, toy). This must be differentiated by history from an infectious cause of airway obstruction such as epiglottis or croup. Patients with these latter problems require immediate transfer to the nearest ACLS facility, while the former may respond to measures designed to remove the foreign body. Back blows and chest thrust may be used, but abdominal thrusts in this age group have the potential for injury to internal organs and should be avoided.

To clear a foreign body, the rescuer straddles the infant (abdomen down) over his or her arm, with the victim's head lower than the trunk. **Support the head with a hand around the jaw and chest. Rest the forearm on the thigh for additional support. Rapidly deliver up to five back blows with the heel of the hand between the infant's shoulder blades,** using less force than needed in an adult. Immediately thereafter, **place the free hand on the back, supporting the head and neck with the other hand and turn the victim. Place the infant on your thigh with the head lower than the trunk,** and **deliver five quick downward chest thrusts** (as in external chest compression).

If the unconscious victim is a larger child, **the Heimlich maneuver should be attempted. Position the child face up. Kneel at the child's feet or straddle the hips; place the heel of one hand on the child's abdomen in the midline (above the navel but below the rib cage). Place the second hand on top of the first, and exert a quick upward thrust into the abdomen. Repeat if necessary up to five times, and then attempt rescue breathing. If the obstruction remains, repeat the maneuver.**

Avoid blind finger sweeps in infants and children, which may push foreign bodies downward. After performing back blows and chest thrusts, lift the victim's lower jaw and tongue forward, open the mouth by placing the thumb into the mouth over the tongue (with the other fingers wrapped around the jaw), and remove the foreign

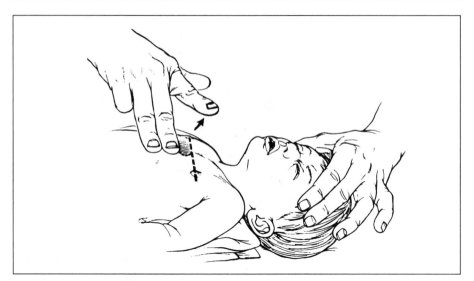

Fig. 2-8. Locating proper finger position for chest compression in infant. Note that the rescuer's other hand is used to maintain the victim's head position to facilitate ventilation. (Reprinted with permission from Guidelines for cardiopulmonary resuscitation and emergency cardiac care. *JAMA* 268:2256, 1992. Copyright 1992, American Medical Association.)

body if visualized. If the attempt is unsuccessful, try again. If the attempt is successful and the victim remains apneic, start rescue breathing. Ventilatory rates are 20/minute (once every 3 seconds).

   C. **Circulation.** Once the airway is clear and two breaths delivered, it must be determined whether the infant or child has had a respiratory arrest, a cardiac arrest, or both. In this age group, respiratory arrests owing to foreign body obstruction with or without cardiac arrest are more common than primary cardiac arrest. **Check the pulse. In a child, palpate the carotid artery. In an infant, palpate the brachial pulse** since the carotid artery may be difficult to appreciate because of the short neck.

   If there is no pulse, external chest compression should commence. Since infants and children are smaller than adults, the point and force of compression are different. For the infant, the correct area for compression is the lower third of the sternum. For the child, the correct area is determined by locating the notch where the ribs meet the sternum with the middle finger and placing the index finger next to it on the sternum. The area above the index finger is the point of compression in the child.

   Compress the sternum ¼–1 inch with two or three fingers in the infant (Fig. 2-8). **In the child, the heel of one hand may be necessary to affect compression. Use only the heel, keeping the fingers off the chest,** and increase the depth of compression to 1–1½ inches. **The rate of compression should be 100/minute for an infant or a child.**

   Coordinate external chest compression with rescue breathing. The ratio of compressions to respirations is 5:1, whether there are one or two rescuers. Further details are in the recommendations of the National Conference [1].

IV. **Advanced life support: infants and children.** Advanced cardiac life support in infants and children is similar to that for adults; however, the doses of drugs are different (Table 2-4). Similarly the size of the endotracheal tube, IV lines, and rates of infusion are less than in the adult. There are special considerations for the care of the neonate, but they are not addressed here. The reader is referred to the recommendations of the National Conference [1].

V. **Potential means for improvement of CPR.** The goals of CPR are to restore a regular rhythm and spontaneous breathing, while maintaining adequate perfusion to the vital organs. Despite current techniques, CPR is often unsuccessful; even if it is successful, other organs may have been compromised. New techniques for CPR continue under investigation. Initial observations that coughing during VF is capable of maintaining BP and consciousness suggest the importance of changes in intrathoracic pressure for maintaining the circulation.

Increases in intrathoracic pressure result in forward flow to the carotid arteries, but a pressure gradient is maintained in the venous system by valves in the jugular vein. Thus, this extrathoracic arteriovenous pressure gradient results in forward flow of blood. Efforts have been made to enhance pressure to increase flow. Simultaneous com-

Table 2-4. Drugs used in pediatric advanced life support

Drug	Dose	Remarks
Adenosine	0.1–0.2 mg/kg Maximum single dose: 12 mg	Rapid IV bolus
Atropine sulfate	0.02 mg/kg per dose	Minimum dose: 0.1 mg Maximum single dose: 0.5 mg in child, 1.0 mg in adolescent
Bretylium	5 mg/kg; may be increased to 10 mg/kg	Rapid IV
Calcium chloride 10%	20 mg/kg per dose	Give slowly
Dopamine hydrochloride	2–20 µg/kg per min	Alpha-adrenergic action dominates at ≥15–20 µg/kg per minute
Dobutamine hydrochloride	2–20 µg/kg per minute	Titrate to desired effect
Epinephrine for bradycardia	IV/IO: 0.01 mg/kg (1:10,000) ET: 0.1 mg/kg (1:1000)	Be aware of effective dose of preservatives administered (if preservatives are present in epinephrine preparation) when high doses are used
For asystolic or pulseless arrest	First dose: IV/IO: 0.01 mg/kg (1:10,000) ET: 0.1 mg/kg (1:1000) Doses as high as 0.2 mg/kg may be effective Subsequent doses: IV/IO/ET: 0.1 mg/kg (1:1000) Doses as high as 0.2 mg/kg may be effective	Be aware of effective dose of preservative adminis- tered (if preservatives present in epinephrine preparation) when high doses are used
Epinephrine infusion	Initial at 0.1 µg/kg per minute Higher infusion dose used if asystole present	Titrate to desired effect (0.1–1.0 µg/kg per minute)
Lidocaine	1 mg/kg per dose	
Lidocaine infusion	20–50 µg/kg per min	
Sodium bicarbonate	1 mEq/kg per dose or 0.3 × kg × base deficit	Infuse slowly and only if ventilation is adequate

IV = intravenous route; IO = intraosseous route; ET = endotracheal route.
Source: Emergency Cardiac Care Committee and Subcommittees, American Heart Association. Guidelines for cardiopulmonary resuscitation and emergency cardiac care. *JAMA* 268:2268, 1992. Copyright 1992, American Medical Association.

pression-ventilation, abdominal binding, and epinephrine have been used in an attempt to enhance cerebral and carotid perfusion. Techniques that increase blood flow to these beds may not, however, improve myocardial blood flow. Some studies suggest improved survival using intermittent abdominal compression during the relaxation phase of chest compression. Improvement in survival has not been seen with simultaneous ventilation and compression.

Only the established techniques of CPR can be accepted as standard medical practice, while research continues. In the electrophysiology laboratory, we utilize the cough technique routinely if a patient is induced into VT. This technique often maintains the circulation while we proceed with overdrive pacing. If this is unsuccessful and cardioversion or defibrillation is necessary, we instruct the patient to stop coughing before the electrical discharge. If the patient loses consciousness for 5–10 seconds, he or she usually does not remember the countershock.

VI. **Techniques of temporary pacing.** A temporary pacemaker is frequently required during cardiac arrest or in the diagnosis and treatment of cardiac arrhythmias. **Transcutaneous pacing** may be most suitable for the emergency situation. The ability to pace transcutaneously is dependent on electrode size and placement, chest size and shape, and occasionally the presence of a pericardial effusion. If pacing is successful and the patient requires it for a longer period of time, it may be necessary to place a transvenous lead. Transcutaneous pacing is uncomfortable at best and quite often painful. For transvenous pacing, a controlled setting using fluoroscopy is ideal and should be used when available. Fluoroscopy is particularly desirable when inserting an electrode (or even Swan-Ganz pulmonary artery catheter) in a patient with left bundle branch block (LBBB). The movement of the electrode in the right ventricle may cause a transient right bundle branch block (RBBB), which, in the presence of LBBB, will create complete heart block. It may be difficult to find blindly an area in the ventricle that the pacemaker will capture, particularly if the ventricle is scarred. Visualization of the catheter under fluoroscopy will minimize the risk of VT caused by blind probing of the ventricle with the electrode. In some cases, it is difficult to manipulate the electrode into the heart without fluoroscopy.

Some pulmonary artery monitoring catheters have a right ventricular port that allows the insertion of a temporary pacemaker into the right ventricle. If the catheter is already in position, insertion of the pacemaker is relatively straightforward and does not require fluoroscopy. If the patient does not have a stable rhythm and is hemodynamically unstable, insertion of the pulmonary artery catheter itself may be difficult.

Venous access is accomplished via a peripheral or central vein. Both routes have advantages and disadvantages. Peripheral insertion via the basilic or femoral vein has no risk of pneumothorax but requires fluoroscopic guidance for positioning. Maintenance of a pacemaker electrode in the femoral vein is associated with a risk of thromboembolism if the patient's blood is not anticoagulated. The femoral vein approach is usually reserved for emergencies when other access routes are not possible. While insertion into the femoral vein is percutaneous, the basilic vein approach usually is performed by a cutdown. The patient's arm must be immobilized, and the procedure carries the risk of thrombophlebitis. Central venous access may be achieved via the internal and external jugular veins or the subclavian vein. If properly performed, the jugular approach should avoid the risk of pneumothorax but involves a blind probe of the neck with a needle, with the risk of entering the carotid artery (particularly in an elderly patient with tortuous atherosclerotic arteries). Often it is quite difficult to manipulate an electrode down the external jugular vein, and the vein may tear. Thus, the internal jugular and subclavian veins are preferable, particularly in an emergency situation when rapid access is vital. The subclavian approach has the risk of pneumothorax and of entering the subclavian artery with a needle. If the situation is not an emergency and the clinician wishes to avoid probing the neck or chest with a needle (or if a pneumothorax would be catastrophic in the patient's condition), it is reasonable to consider the basilic vein approach. All pacemaker electrodes (and central catheters) must be inserted under strict sterile technique to minimize the risk of infection.

A. **Basilic vein approach.** In the forearm, the cephalic vein runs laterally along the brachialis muscle. The median cubital (or median basilic) vein courses in the middle portion of the arm until it crosses medially to join the basilic vein. A distal branch of the basilic vein runs medially until it joins the main branch (Fig. 2-9). Both the cephalic and the median cubital veins can usually be entered percutaneously. Since the cephalic vein runs laterally and may decrease in size before entering the axillary vein, attempting to advance a pacemaker electrode or catheter is difficult. Therefore

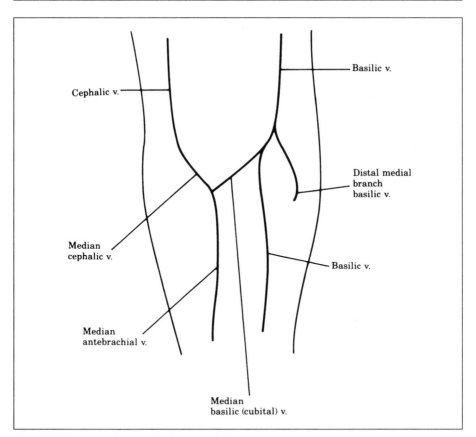

Fig. 2-9. Schematic of antecubital venous system.

it is preferable to enter the basilic vein, through either the median cubital vein or the distal medial branch of the basilic vein.

Often the median cubital vein is utilized for an IV line or is thrombosed because of multiple venipunctures, making it unsuitable for use. In this case, the distal medial branch should be considered. This involves cutdown, since this branch is not always obvious from the surface. Nevertheless, it is very superficial and does not require deep probing. A satisfactory vein is discovered in more than 95% of attempts.

Palpate the median epicondyle of the humerus. Find a point 2 cm lateral to it. After local anesthesia, make a horizontal incision ½ cm in each direction (total 1 cm). The vein will usually be found just below the surface, by using a small retractor.

Once the vein is entered (either the median cubital or distal medial branch of the basilic vein), the pacing electrode is threaded up into the basilic vein and advanced into the axillary vein, down into the subclavian vein, superior vena cava, and right side of the heart.

B. **Internal jugular vein approach.** Cannulation of the internal jugular vein usually allows rapid access with minimal complications. If the entry site is too low (thus becoming a clavicular approach), the risk of pneumothorax increases. The patient should be supine, with the legs slightly elevated to distend the veins. This position is not possible in some situations (such as pulmonary edema). Palpate the sternocleidomastoid muscle and locate its midportion. After local anesthesia, insert a probe needle behind the muscle, and direct it downward at a shallow angle to the neck, aiming between the jugular notch and the nipple. The syringe is under constant aspiration, so that it is ascertained immediately when a vessel is entered. Once the general direction is known, a larger needle (through which a guide wire is capable of passing) is used to enter the vein. A small scalpel incision at the site where the wire penetrates the skin will facilitate entry of the catheter sheath. The use of a catheter sheath with a side arm for the administration of fluids is preferred. Pass the catheter sheath and dilator over the wire (always holding one end of wire) and into the vein. Remove the dilator and guide wire. The pacing electrode may then be inserted and advanced to the right side of the heart.

C. **Subclavian vein approach.** Cannulation of the subclavian vein has the highest risk of complication and should be performed only by a clinician skilled in this technique.

The patient is placed in a supine position and the clavicle palpated. After local anesthesia is administered, a probe needle is inserted at the midpoint of the clavicle and gently advanced to the bone. It is carefully inserted under the clavicle and advanced in the direction of the jugular notch, while constant aspiration is maintained. Once the vein is located, a larger needle (with a lumen large enough for a guide wire) is advanced into the vein and the guide wire threaded. Then a catheter sheath and dilator are inserted over the wire, after which the wire and dilator are removed. The pacing electrode may then be inserted and advanced to the right side of the heart.

D. **Femoral vein approach.** The femoral vein approach should be used only by a clinician skilled in cardiac catheterization. The femoral vein is medial to the femoral artery and is entered via the Seldinger technique after local anesthesia. A catheter sheath and dilator are advanced over a guide wire with removal of the dilator and wire. The pacing electrode can then be inserted; it is advanced into the inferior vena cava and then into the right side of the heart.

E. **Pacemaker insertion.** Most temporary pacemakers are packaged by the manufacturer with all the appropriate sheaths, dilators, and other accessories. The physician must select the size, which usually ranges between 4–6 French. The smaller ones (4F, 5F) are more flexible and sometimes difficult to manipulate. The larger ones (6F) are more rigid and easier to position but have a slightly higher risk of irritation and perforation. Some pacing electrodes now have balloon tips to facilitate entry into the heart.

The pacing electrode should be advanced into the right ventricular apex by fluoroscopy when available. If fluoroscopy is unavailable, the electrode is connected to the V lead of the ECG by an alligator clamp. As the electrode enters the right atrium, the V lead on the ECG will demonstrate a large atrial deflection. Occasionally it will be difficult to determine which deflection is atrial and which is ventricular, particularly if the patient is having an arrhythmia.

By obtaining a bipolar recording (connect each of the atrial electrodes to the right arm and left arm leads of the ECG; monitor limb lead I), electrical activity in the chamber will be magnified on the rhythm strip. When the electrode enters the ventricle, ventricular activity will become very large. The physician then must determine the optimal site for pacing in terms of low threshold, stable location, and lack of ventricular irritability. If the pacemaker has been floated in via a balloon-tip catheter or a blind ECG sensing approach, the position should be confirmed by fluoroscopy or x ray once the situation is no longer emergent.

Finally, one other technique must be mentioned. It is used primarily in an emergency situation when fluoroscopy is unavailable and there is a problem hooking the pacing electrode to the ECG. The electrode is connected to the external pacemaker generator, set at the desired pacing rate with a relatively high output, and advanced until the ventricle captures. This is the least desirable method because of the lack of control and risk of inducing arrhythmias.

Once a suitable site is located (complete capture, no ventricular ectopy), the output of the pacemaker is turned down to check the threshold. If the threshold is above 1.0 mA, another site should be sought, unless the clinical situation contraindicates further manipulation at the time. An ideal threshold is between 0.5 and 1.0 mA. The output should be set at two and a half to three times the threshold, as it will increase daily. The threshold and output setting must be checked at least once daily. Finally, the sensitivity of the pacemaker should be adjusted to allow for appropriate sensing. Only in rare situations is it necessary to maintain the asynchronous mode (e.g., continuous overdrive suppression of an arrhythmia). After the procedure is completed, the electrode sutured into position, and the site sterilely protected, a chest x ray should be obtained to document the position of the electrode and exclude pneumothorax. Most often the pacemaker electrode is placed into the ventricle. On occasion, it may be necessary to perform atrial pacing. Atrial positions are usually less stable and may have higher thresholds.

If there is loss of capture by the pacemaker, it may be due to a requirement for a higher threshold, but most often results from migration of the electrode from its initial position. Usually the smaller the electrode (4F, 5F) is, the more likely this may occur. Repositioning must be performed immediately if pacing remains necessary. The clinician must be certain that perforation did not occur (possibly resulting in pericardial effusion or tamponade).

In addition to loss of optimal position by the pacing electrode, the problems commonly associated with temporary pacing include venous thrombophlebitis or thrombosis (particularly when a peripheral vein is used), infection at the entry site, and pneumothorax during entry into a central vein. It is important to insert the correct end of the electrode into the vein, since both ends are similar in appearance. The position of the electrodes is different, and pacing is possible only with the proper connection. Some of the pacemaker electrodes are color coded, with the end to be attached to the connecting cable appropriately matched. Other sources of problems during insertion are poor connections, faulty cables, generator battery depletion, and incorrect setting of parameters. All of these possibilities should be checked before replacing the pacing electrode.

   F. **Transthoracic pacemaker.** The transthoracic approach is the last resort when the patient remains asystolic during a cardiac arrest and does not respond to drugs such as atropine, epinephrine, or isoproterenol. Quite often the transvenous approach is not possible because of the position of the rescuers and the additional time it requires. Also, the transthoracic pacing electrode may not be readily available.

The substernal area is sterilely prepared, and a cardiac needle is inserted (usually at the junction of the ribs, sternum, and xiphoid process). The needle is directed toward the left shoulder. Aspiration of blood into the syringe indicates that the right ventricle has been entered. The syringe is removed, and the transthoracic pacemaker electrode is inserted into the needle and advanced into the right ventricle. These electrodes usually have a J-shaped tip, allowing contact with the endocardium when the electrode is withdrawn. The needle is removed and the electrode connected to the pacemaker generator. High voltage may be required.

If the patient survives and continues to require a pacemaker, a transvenous pacemaker should be inserted when his or her condition is stable. Transthoracic insertion of a pacemaker carries the risk of lacerating a coronary artery or causing a pneumothorax. Some physicians advocate discontinuation of this approach.

VII. Cardioversion and defibrillation. Electrical countershock to terminate an arrhythmia may be necessary in an emergency situation, or it may be performed electively for a less life-threatening condition. This section discusses the techniques of cardioversion and defibrillation. Subsequent chapters discuss the indications.

If cardioversion is being performed electively, the patient should fully understand the risks and benefits of the procedure. Ideally an anesthesiologist should be present during the procedure in case intubation becomes necessary. A short-acting barbiturate or similar drug is recommended for sedation. Although diazepam has been used, it has the disadvantage of prolonged sedation. Shorter-acting benzodiazepines, such as midazolam hydrochloride, may be useful.

The patient is supine, with surface electrodes connected to the cardioverter-defibrillator and an electrocardiograph. It is important for the patient to fast for 8 hours before the procedure to minimize any risk of aspiration. Blood chemistry should be checked to exclude electrolyte imbalance. If the patient is receiving digoxin chronically, the dose is usually withheld until the cardioversion is completed. It is not necessary to discontinue the drug long before cardioversion, as long as there are no signs or symptoms of digitalis toxicity. Oxygen may be administered via nasal cannula before and during the procedure. Before the patient starts to receive the sedative, a bed board may be placed under the back to prepare for any emergency.

The cardioverter-defibrillator is carefully checked to determine whether a clear signal is received on the monitor. For elective cardioversion, the synchronization switch is turned on to ensure that the shock will be delivered during the QRS complex. Either a dot or a line will appear above the QRS complex. For emergency defibrillation, synchronization is not used. Electrode gel is applied to the paddles, and they are positioned firmly on the chest to minimize transthoracic impedance. Two sets of paddles are available. The set of two traditional paddles is positioned on the chest, with paddle 1 to the right of the sternum (level of second rib) and paddle 2 to the left of the nipple, with the center of the electrode in the midaxillary line (at the fourth or fifth interspace). Alternatively, one paddle may be placed anteriorly over the left precordium and the other posteriorly behind the heart in the right infrascapular position.

Once the patient has been adequately sedated, the paddles positioned, and the synchronization feature checked and on, the cardioverter-defibrillator is charged to the desired energy. The physician warns everyone to remain clear of the patient and then delivers the countershock. The rhythm is recorded, and the patient's vital signs are checked. If the countershock is unsuccessful, the physician may elect to increase the energy and try another countershock. If the procedure is successful, the patient must be carefully monitored until fully conscious and breathing spontaneously. Mechanical ventilation via a face mask and bag may be necessary for a few minutes.

The energy required varies with the arrhythmia being treated. Atrial flutter requires the least energy and frequently is terminated by 50 joules with restoration of sinus rhythm. Supraventricular arrhythmias other than atrial fibrillation will usually respond to 50–100 joules. Low energy may also be used to terminate VT, but it is unwise to start below 100 joules if the patient is hemodynamically compromised or the tachycardia rate is rapid. For the patient with hypotensive VT, 100 or 200 joules should be used initially. If 100 joules fails to terminate VT, repeat the countershock with 200 joules. If that fails, use 300 joules, in a stepwise progression. Atrial fibrillation usually will not respond to less than 100 joules.

If the cardioversion is emergent and not elective, as in the patient with recurrent VT, further points require attention. Acidosis and hypoxia must be corrected. Since VT may recur, appropriate antiarrhythmic drugs (such as lidocaine) should be administered. Rare patients with extreme electrical instability (so-called electrical storm), often in the presence of acute myocardial injury, may require multiple cardioversions and defibrillations.

Cardioversions should not be attempted in the presence of digitalis toxicity. Even if the arrhythmia is corrected, it may recur. More important, cardioversion attempts when the patient has digitalis toxicity may precipitate VT or VF.

If the patient has VF, higher energies must be used, starting with 200 joules. For the second shock, 300 joules is appropriate, and for the third shock 360 joules. If the procedure is unsuccessful, continue CPR. For infants and children, the recommended energy for defibrillation is 2 joules/kg. If the shock is unsuccessful, the energy is doubled to 4 joules/kg. Synchronization is usually not possible in VF. In all cases of VT or VF, it is imperative that the patient's condition be fully evaluated when stable to determine risk of recurrence and the appropriate therapy.

After an arrhythmia is terminated by cardioversion or defibrillation, the initial recovery rhythm may be a sinus tachycardia or occasionally a sinus bradycardia. The physician must be prepared to treat the bradycardia if sustained and hemodynamically embarrassing. Sinus tachycardia usually slows relatively quickly. After termination of VF, a variety of supraventricular arrhythmias, including paroxysmal supraventricular tachycardia and accelerated junctional rhythms, may be present. The important objective of restoring BP has usually been achieved, and these arrhythmias usually spontaneously revert back to sinus rhythm once metabolic abnormalities are corrected.

The major risk in electrical cardioversion is embolization. Consequently patients at risk of thromboembolism should receive anticoagulants for an appropriate period before the procedure. Anticoagulation after successful cardioversion is usually continued for another 10–14 days in patients with atrial fibrillation since some may not have immediate restoration of effective mechanical contraction. The physician should be aware that even carefully performed cardioversions with correct synchronization may rarely result in VT or VF, requiring another countershock at higher energy. My policy is to monitor patients 12–24 hours after elective cardioversion to observe for any electrical instability. Monitoring for the full 24 hours is the conservative approach. Automatic external defibrillators using diagnostic algorithms have been introduced into the community and are available in many office buildings and ambulances. These involve application of adhesive electrodes by a family member, other bystander, or an emergency medical technician. The decision to deliver countershock is determined by computerized analysis of the rhythm. If VF or VT is detected, the rescuer delivers up to three sequential shocks for persistent or immediately recurrent VF/VT using energy levels of 200 joules, 200–300 joules, and 360 joules. Early defibrillation is extremely essential for survival.

VIII. **New issues in CPR: infection.** The risk of disease transmission in the performance of CPR or even in training has become a concern with the problems of human immunodeficiency virus (HIV), hepatitis B (HBV), and most recently drug-resistant tuberculosis. The National Conference has stated that "the probability that a rescuer (lay or professional) will become infected with HBV or HIV as a result of performing CPR is minimal." However, "the emergence of multidrug-resistant tuberculosis is a cause for concern."

Guidelines established by the Centers for Disease Control and the Occupational Safety and Health Administration include the use of barriers (latex gloves, mechanical ventilation devices including bag-valve masks that divert expired air from the rescuer) that decrease the risk of transmission. They further advise that "rescuers who have an infection that may be transmitted by blood or saliva should not perform mouth-to-mouth resuscitation if circumstances allow other immediate or effective methods of ventilation." "If a rescuer refuses to initiate mouth-to-mouth ventilation, he or she should at least access the EMS system, open the airway, and perform chest compressions until a rescuer arrives who is willing to perform ventilation or until ventilation can be initiated by skilled rescuers with the necessary barrier devices" [1].

IX. **Ethical issues.** This important topic covered by the National Conference deals with issues of when not to perform CPR, when to stop CPR, and the importance of advance directives (living will, health care proxy, durable power of attorney), which simplify matters for the health care provider and the family, particularly at the times of extreme emotional stress, when a patient is dying [1].

Reference

1. Emergency Cardiac Care Committee and Subcommittees, American Heart Association. Guidelines for cardiopulmonary resuscitation and emergency cardiac care. *JAMA* 268:2171–2302, 1992.

Bibliography

Criley JM, Blaufuss AH, Kissel E. Cough-induced cardiac compression. *JAMA* 236: 1246–1250, 1976.

Cummins RO, Eisenberg MS, Stults KR. Automatic external defibrillators: Clinical issues for cardiology. *Circulation* 73:381–384, 1986.

Kerber RE, et al. Evaluation of a new defibrillation pathway: Tongue-epigastric/tongue-apex route. II. Impedance characteristics in human subjects. *J Am Coll Cardiol* 4: 253–258, 1984.

Stults KR, Brown DD, Kerber RE. Efficacy of an automated external defibrillator in the management of out-of-hospital cardiac arrest: Validation of the diagnostic algorithm and initial clinical experience in a rural environment. *Circulation* 73:701–709, 1986.

Weaver WD, et al. Ventricular defibrillation: A comparative trial using 175-J and 320-J shocks. *N Engl J Med* 307:1101–1106, 1982.

Weisfeldt ML, Chandra N. Key references: Cardiopulmonary resuscitation. *Circulation* 66:898–900, 1133–1135, 1982.

Weisfeldt ML, Halperin HR. Cardiopulmonary resuscitation: Beyond cardiac massage. *Circulation* 74:443–448, 1986.

Principles of Basic Electrophysiology

Stephen C. Vlay

The interpretation and treatment of cardiac arrhythmias begin with an understanding of the anatomy and electrophysiology of the cardiac electrical system. Cleverly designed, it consists of a series of pacemaker cells with rapid discharge proximally and slower pacemaker cells distally to create a cascade type of system. If the higher pacemaker slows or fails, lower pacemakers provide a backup mechanism to maintain electrical activation of the heart. Since the higher or proximal pacemaker cells have faster rates, they depolarize the lower or distal cells before they would normally fire. Under certain conditions, a lower pacemaker may have a faster rate and thus usurp the position of the dominant pacemaker.

Under normal conditions, the dominant pacemaker is the sinoatrial (SA) node, which occupies the most superior position and discharges at a rate of 70–80/minute. Through a series of internodal pathways, the electrical impulse travels down to the atrioventricular (AV) node, which has an intrinsic rate of 40–60/minute. After passing through the AV node, the impulse continues down into the bundle of His, the bundle branches, the Purkinje fibers, and finally the ventricular myocardium. Purkinje fibers have an intrinsic rate of 15–40/minute (Fig. 3-1).

Cardiac muscle is a syncytium with intercalated disks separating individual cardiac cells and acting as low-resistance cell membranes. Activation of the cell results in an action potential, which moves from cell to cell and spreads over the entire mass of atrium or ventricle, in turn, stimulating contraction of the atria and ventricles.

I. **Anatomy of the conduction system**
   A. **Sinoatrial node.** The SA node, a crescent-shaped strip of specialized muscle, is located high in the right atrium adjacent to the superior vena cava. The length is 10–15 mm, the width 3–5 mm, and the thickness 2–3 mm. The SA node receives its blood supply from the SA artery, which can arise from the right (55%) or left circumflex (45%) coronary artery. In the SA node, there are a variety of cells, some of them with the property of rhythmic discharge, a pacemaker function. After leaving the SA node, the impulses penetrate the atria and continue to the AV node via the internodal pathways.
   B. **Internodal pathways.** Specialized conduction tracts that carry the sinus impulse to the AV node have been debated but have never been demonstrated as a discrete anatomic entity. Possibly, preferential conduction may occur through a functional pathway of atrial cells. The three previously described functional pathways are the anterior internodal tract (Bachmann's bundle and a descending branch), middle internodal tract (Wenckebach's bundle), and the posterior internodal tract (Thorel's pathway).
   C. **Atrioventricular node.** The AV node is situated between the ostium of the coronary sinus and tricuspid valve anulus. The length is 22 mm, the width 10 mm, and the thickness 2–3 mm. The AV node receives its blood supply from the AV nodal artery, a branch of the posterior descending artery (PDA). The PDA may arise from the right (90%) or circumflex (10%) coronary artery. The AV node continues distally as the bundle of His. When examined histologically, Purkinje fibers connecting the AV node to the bundle of His are larger than AV nodal fibers and have faster transmission velocities.
   D. **Bundle of His.** Purkinje fibers in the bundle of His are organized in parallel bands, unlike the interwoven mesh of cells in the AV node. The bundle of His penetrates the interventricular septum, dividing into right and left bundle branches. The electrophysiologist records the His spike from a pacing electrode in this position (see Fig. 12-4).

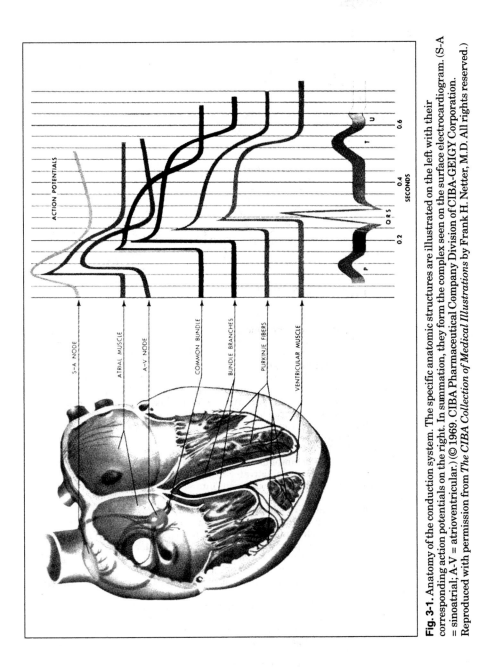

Fig. 3-1. Anatomy of the conduction system. The specific anatomic structures are illustrated on the left with their corresponding action potentials on the right. In summation, they form the complex seen on the surface electrocardiogram. (S-A = sinoatrial; A-V = atrioventricular.) (© 1969. CIBA Pharmaceutical Company Division of CIBA-GEIGY Corporation. Reproduced with permission from *The CIBA Collection of Medical Illustrations* by Frank H. Netter, M.D. All rights reserved.)

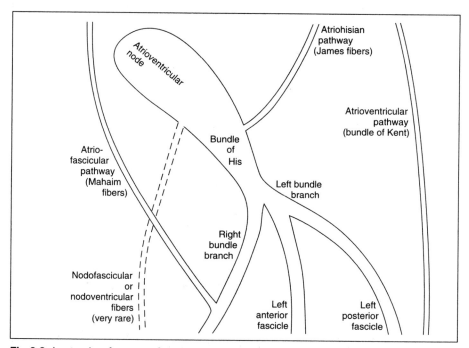

Fig. 3-2. Anatomic substrates of preexcitation. The various accessory pathways are outlined.

    E. Right bundle branch. The right bundle branch continues to course down the interventricular septum to the base of the anterior papillary muscle. The proximal third of the right bundle branch is supplied by the AV nodal artery; the distal two-thirds, by the left anterior descending artery.

    F. Left bundle branch. The left bundle branch divides after entering the interventricular septum. There are two well-recognized fascicles, the anterior and posterior, and some recent evidence to suggest a third, or central, fascicle. The anterior fascicle derives its blood supply from the left anterior descending coronary artery and activates the anterior and superior left ventricle. The posterior fascicle has a dual blood supply, from both the anterior descending and posterior descending coronary arteries. Consequently, the development of left posterior hemiblock after acute myocardial infarction indicates compromise of two major circulations and is a poor prognostic sign. The posterior fascicle activates the posterior and inferior left ventricle. Distally, all branches divide continuously into smaller branches that run intramyocardially.

    G. Accessory bypass tracts. In addition to the normal conducting system, some individuals have additional conduction system pathways that bypass the normal route. Often they have major clinical importance when active and involved in reciprocating tachycardia. An AV bypass tract is the **bundle of Kent,** a muscular bridge connecting the atria and ventricles. An individual patient may have more than one bundle of Kent. These bundles may be capable of antegrade or retrograde activation or both. The clinical syndrome associated with this tract (the **Wolff-Parkinson-White syndrome**) is considered in great detail in Chap. 7. Another accessory pathway, the **James** fibers, are an atrio-Hisian connection and insert into the bundle of His or distal AV node (bypassing the entire or proximal AV node). Clinical supraventricular tachyarrhythmias associated with this tract are described as the **Lown-Ganong-Levine** syndrome. It is important to note that ventricular activation remains normal. Finally, Mahaim fibers have recently been shown to represent atriofascicular connections (Fig. 3-2) and have the property of decremental conduction. Nodofascicular or nodoventricular fibers exist but are extremely rare.

  II. Electrophysiology. Definition of certain elementary electrophysiologic terms is important.

Excitability: The ability of a cell to respond to a stimulus. Both pacemaker and nonpacemaker cells have this property.

Automaticity: The ability to initiate and maintain a rhythmic discharge, thus functioning as a pacemaker. Automaticity is related to phase 4 diastolic depolarization of the action potential, with a spontaneous increase from the resting potential until a threshold level is achieved. Pacemaker cells in the heart include the SA node, AV node, and ventricles (and occasionally ectopic foci in the atria). Each may control the rhythm of the heart under specific circumstances.

Conductivity: The ability of a cell to carry an impulse to adjacent cells. Conduction velocity is dependent on the type of cell. Factors include the rate of depolarization, amplitude of the action potential, cellular interconnections, dimension and geometry of the cells, cable properties, and excitability of the membrane. Conduction is most rapid in the Purkinje fibers, at 4000 mm/second. Other cells have slower conduction velocities: atria, 1000 mm/second; ventricles, 400 mm/second; AV node, 200 mm/second. Conduction is much slower in the AV node, which serves a protective function in limiting the rate of ventricular response. Clinically this is especially important when the patient is in atrial fibrillation. In addition, the AV node has the property of **decremental conduction:** as the cycle length shortens (faster rate), the conduction time increases. Patients with accessory pathways that bypass the AV node have no rate-limiting steps. If the patient has an arrhythmia such as atrial fibrillation, a very rapid ventricular response is possible.

Refractoriness: The time period when the cell will not respond to a stimulus (Fig. 3-3). The refractory period is a function of the action potential duration and configuration, membrane potential, threshold potential, cell geometry, cable properties, and conduction block.

Absolute refractory period: Period when no stimulus, regardless of strength, can stimulate the cell.

Relative refractory period: Period subsequent to absolute refractory period when a stimulus stronger than usual may be able to stimulate the cell.

Effective refractory period: Interval between onset of action potential and stimulus, producing a propagated response.

Functional refractory period: Shortest interval between two successive propagated responses at a site distal to stimulus site when second response is premature.

Total refractory period: Interval between onset of action potential and end of relative refractory period.

Full recovery time: Period between onset of action potential and complete recovery of conductivity, excitability, and major action potential characteristics.

Table 3-1 describes these terms as they are applied in the electrophysiology laboratory. Refractory periods vary with the tissues, with the shortest refractory period in the atria and the longest in the AV node. Refractory periods are also directly related to cycle length or heart rate. The longer the cycle length (the slower the heart rate) is, the longer is the refractory period. Neural influences may alter refractory periods as well. Sympathetic stimulation shortens it, and parasympathetic (vagal) stimulation has varying effects. For example, vagal stimulation prolongs AV nodal refractory periods but shortens atrial refractory periods.

III. Cellular electrophysiology. Although this book is primarily directed at the clinical management of cardiac arrhythmias, it is useful to examine briefly electrophysiologic activity at the cellular level. Major advances in the treatment of arrhythmias derive from advances in this area. The major channels, pumps and carriers, and receptors are summarized in Tables 3-2, 3-3, and 3-4.

Microelectrode work in cardiac cells has demonstrated an 80- to 90-mV difference between intracellular and extracellular electrical fields, with an excess of negatively charged ions intracellularly. Since there is a membrane that is not easily permeable to the movement of charged ions, it is possible for this difference, or **transmembrane potential,** to exist; it is defined as the **resting potential.** Specific channels available for ion transport allow selective movement of sodium, potassium, or calcium to penetrate into or out of the cell. At rest, the potential is determined by the concentration gradient for potassium. With depolarization, the initial upstroke is dependent on the concentration gradient for sodium. Normally, intracellular potassium concentration is 140 mM, and extracellular potassium is 4 mM. For sodium, the intracellular and extracellular concentrations are reversed, with 150 mM extracellularly and 10 mM intracellularly. When potassium channels open, there is an outward ionic flow of potassium. When sodium (or calcium) channels open, there is an inward ionic flow of those ions. The net

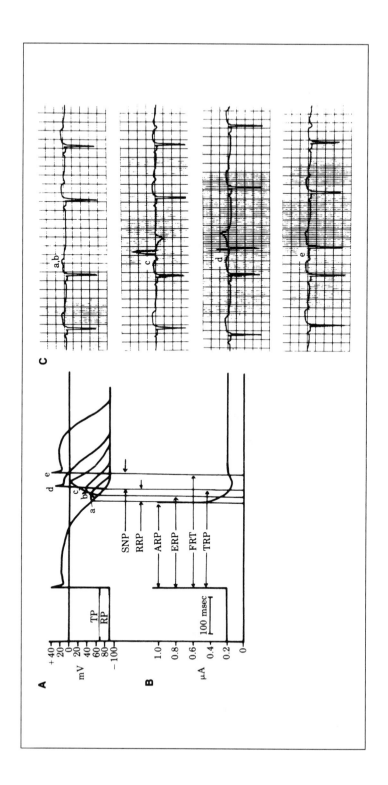

Fig. 3-3. The refractory periods of the action potential. **A.** The earliest responses (*a* and *b*) arise at such low levels of membrane potential and are so small and slowly rising that they do not propagate. The earliest propagated response (*c*) defines the end of the effective refractory period (*ERP*). Although response *d* arises during the supernormal period (*SNP*) of excitability, it is still smaller and more slowly rising than response *e*, which occurs after repolarization is complete and the normal level of resting potential (*RP*) restored. The first normal response (*e*) defines the end of the full recovery time (*FRT*). The level of the threshold potential (*TP*) is shown. **B.** Threshold current requirements are indicated in microamperes (µA). The fiber becomes inexcitable coincident with the inscription of phase 0 of the action potential. Recovery of excitability, as indicated by changes in threshold, progresses slowly during phase 3. The terminal portion of phase 3 is associated with a period of supernormal excitability. The diagram also illustrates the approximate duration of the absolute refractory period (*ARP*), the effective refractory period (*ERP*), relative refractory period (*RRP*), total refractory period (*TRP*), full recovery time (*FRT*), and the period of supernormal excitability (*SNP*). Vertical lines connecting *A* and *B* indicate the relationships between the time course of repolarization and refractoriness, and excitability. **C.** The electrocardiographic strips of atrial premature beats correspond to the different periods during repolarization. Beats *a* and *b* occur too early—either not conducting at all or resulting in a nonconducted atrial premature beat. Beats *c* and *d* occur later in the recovery phase, but with aberration since recovery is incomplete. Beat *c*, being earlier, is conducted more aberrantly. Beat *e* occurs after full recovery and is conducted normally. (From WJ Mandel, ed, *Cardiac Arrhythmias*. Philadelphia: Lippincott, 1980. P. 214.)

Table 3-1. Electrophysiologic definitions of refractoriness

S_1, A_1, H_1, V_1: stimulus artifact; atrial, His bundle, and ventricular electrograms of basic drive

S_2, A_2, H_2, V_2: stimulus artifact; atrial, His bundle, and ventricular electrograms of premature beat

Antegrade refractory periods

Effective refractory period (ERP) of the atrium: the longest S_1–S_2 interval that fails to result in atrial depolarization

ERP of the AV node: the longest A_1–A_2 interval measured in the His bundle electrogram that fails to propagate to the His bundle

ERP of the His-Purkinje system (HPS): the longest H_1–H_2 interval that fails to result in ventricular depolarization

ERP of the atrioventricular conduction system (AVCS): the longest S_1–S_2 interval that fails to result in ventricular depolarization

Functional refractory period (FRP) of the atrium: the shortest A_1–A_2 interval in response to any S_1–S_2 interval

FRP of the AV node: the shortest H_1–H_2 interval in response to any A_1–A_2 interval

FRP of the HPS: the shortest V_1–V_2 interval in response to any H_1–H_2 interval

FRP of the AVCS: the shortest V_1–V_2 interval in response to any S_1–S_2 interval

Relative refractory period (RRP) of the atrium: the longest S_1–S_2 interval at which the S_2–A_2 interval exceeds the S_1–A_1 interval (latency)

RRP of the AV node: the longest A_1–A_2 interval at which the A_2–H_2 interval exceeds the A_1–H_1 interval

RRP of the HPS: the longest H_1–H_2 interval at which the H_2–V_2 interval exceeds the H_1–V_1 interval or results in an aberrant QRS complex

Retrograde refractory periods

ERP of the ventricle: the longest S_1–S_2 interval that fails to evoke a ventricular response

ERP of the HPS: the longest S_1–S_2 or V_1–V_2 interval at which S_2 or V_2 blocks below the bundle of His. This measurement can be made only if H_2 is recorded prior to the occurrence of retrograde block

ERP of the AV node: the longest S_1–H_2 or H_1–H_2 interval at which H_2 fails to propagate to the atrium

ERP of the ventriculoatrial conduction system (VACS): the longest S_1–S_2 interval that fails to propagate to the atrium

FRP of the ventricle: the shortest V_1–V_2 interval as measured on the surface ECG or local ventricular electrogram in response to any S_1–S_2 interval

FRP of the HPS: the shortest S_1–H_2 or H_1–H_2 interval in response to any V_1–V_2 interval

FRP of the AVN: the shortest A_1–A_2 interval in response to any H_1–H_2 interval

FRP of VACS: the shortest A_1–A_2 interval in response to any S_1–S_2 interval

RRP of the ventricle: the longest S_1–S_2 interval at which the S_2–V_2 interval exceeds the S_1–V_1 interval. The V is measured from the surface ECG or a local electrogram at the site of ventricular stimulation

RRP of VACS: the longest S_1–S_2 interval at which the S_2–A_2 interval exceeds the S_1–A_1 interval

AV = atrioventricular.
Source: From ME Josephson, SF Seides (eds). *Clinical Cardiac Electrophysiology: Techniques and Interpretations* (2nd ed). Philadelphia: Lea & Febiger, 1993. P. 42.

Table 3-2. Channels

Inward currents

I Na

Inward excitatory current carried by Na$^+$ through a voltage-activated sodium channel

Produces rapid depolarization and current to drive action potential of impulse propagation in atrial, His-Purkinje, and ventricular cells

Not usually found in SA or AV cells

I Na B

Proposed background Na$^+$ current though voltage-independent channel in SA nodal cells

Although offset by outward potassium current in phase 4, may still contribute to pacemaker behavior

I Ca L

Activated regeneratively from a relatively depolarized threshold potential to produce depolarization and propagation in SA and AV nodal cells

Present in atrial, His-Purkinje, and ventricular cells, contributing to plateau and triggering calcium release from sarcoplasmic reticulum

Target of calcium blocking drugs

Modulated by neurotransmitters

I Ca T

Occurs though a different voltage-gated channel activated at potentials intermediate between thresholds for I Na and I Ca L.

Contributes to inward current to stage 4 depolarization in SA node and His-Purkinje cells

Absent in ventricular cells

May contribute to abnormal automaticity in atria

I f

Inward current carried by Na$^+$ through a nonspecific cationic channel activated by polarization to high membrane potentials in SA and AV nodal cells and His-Purkinje cells

Contributes to phase 4 depolarization and pacemaker function

Modulated by neurotransmitters

I NS

Channel gated by Ca^{++}

Cationic nonselective channel

If activated at resting potential, produces inward Na$^+$ current

May be activated by Ca^{++} release from sarcoplasmic reticulum during Ca^{++} overload

Contributes to delayed afterdepolarizations

Outward currents

I K1

Potassium current responsible for monitoring resting potential near K$^+$ equilibrium potential in atrial, His-Purkinje, and ventricular cells ("inward rectifier")

Shuts off during depolarization

I K

Potassium current carried through voltag- gated channels with slow activation kinetics ("delayed rectifier")

Turns on slowly during action potential plateau

Major current causing repolarization

After repolarization, turns off slowly to contribute to phase 4 depolarization

I to

Potassium current that turns on rapidly after depolarization and then inactivates

One type is voltage mediated and modulated by neurotransmitters

Other type is activated by Ca^{++}

Modifies action potential duration

Contributes to heterogeneity of repolarization

Table 3-2 (continued)

I K (ACh) or I K (Ado)
  Potassium current whose channel is activated by muscarinic (M2) receptor via GTP
    regulatory protein signal transduction
  Shuts down during depolarization (inward rectification)
  Contributes outward current at rest and during action potential
  Important in SA, AV nodes, and atria
  Can cause hyperpolarization
  Opened by activation of purinergic receptor
I K (ATP)
  Potassium current carried through metabolically regulated channel
  Blocked by ATP
  Activated by hypoxia
  May shorten action potential in ischemia
I Cl
  Chloride current that can be greatly increased by adrenergic receptor activation
    (favors repolarization)
  May generate inward current and contribute to pacemaker depolarization
I K (Ca)
  Potassium current carried through a channel activated by Ca^{++}
  Requires high levels of Ca^{++}

Gap junctions (Connexons)
  Large channels that electrically and chemically couple cardiac cells
  Form a large pore to permit passage of ions and small molecules

Ryanodine receptor
  Calcium channel in the sarcoplasmic reticulum that can be triggered to release Ca^{++}
    by calcium entry through I Ca L

SA = sinoatrial; AV = atrioventricular; GTP = guanosine triphosphate; ATP = adenosine
triphosphate.
Source: Data from The Sicilian gambit. *Circulation* 84:1831–1851, 1991.

Table 3-3. Pumps and Carriers

Active transport
ATP-dependent pumps in sarcolemma
  Na-K pump
    Blocked by digitalis
    Each cycle transports three Na^+ out and two K^+ into the cell, generating a small
      outward current
  Calcium pump

Carriers
Facilitate exchange of ions or substrate or pump them using energy
  Na/Ca countertransport system (sarcolemma)
    Generates I Na/Ca : exchanges one Ca^{++} for three Na^+
    Chief means of Ca^{++} efflux through sarcolemma
  Mitochondria
    Na/H exchanger
    Na/K/Cl cotransporter
    Cl/HCO_3 exchanger

Source: Data from The Sicilian gambit. *Circulation* 84:1831–1851, 1991.

flow (or charge) determines the changes in the resting potential as it becomes an action potential. An active transport system using magnesium-stimulated adenosinetriphosphatase (ATPase) maintains the concentration gradient across the cell membrane. Thus, with ATP as an energy source, sodium is pumped out, and potassium is pumped into the cell. There is a net outward charge movement since the amount of sodium pumped out exceeds the amount of potassium pumped in.

An action potential is created as a result of ionic currents across the cell membrane that occur through specific channels. Flow in these channels is controlled by a set of gates. The first gate, or activation (m) gate, opens in response to a depolarization, and sodium rapidly flows into the cell. The second gate, or inactivation (h) gate, closes in response to the depolarization, limiting the time that the sodium current can flow. Sodium conductance does not recur until the h gates are reopened. A second channel, with slower current flow, is also present. The activation (d) gate of this channel opens during the upstroke of the action potential, allowing sodium and calcium to flow into the cell (resulting in the plateau phase). Inactivation (f) gates close this channel (Fig. 3-4).

Table 3-4. Receptors

Beta-adrenergic receptor-effector coupling system
Modulates:
  L-type channels (can induce afterdepolarizations and triggered activity)
  I f channel (increase rate of sinus node pacemaker, latent atrial and ventricular pacemakers)
  Various potassium channels (I K, I to)
  I Cl
  Under certain conditions: Na channels
Increases intracellular cAMP
Activates cAMP-dependent protein kinase
Phosphorylates a peptide associated with the L-type Ca^{++} channel
Increases Ca^{++} current and contractility
Increased cAMP shifts activation curve of pacemaker current I f toward more positive potentials
Increases Na-K pump function (hyperpolarizes cardiac fibers, particularly those depolarized in ischemia)
Enhances voltage-dependent K^+ and voltage-independent Cl^- currents
Comments
  Both Ca^{++} and K^+ channel effects combine to accelerate AV nodal conduction and shorten AV nodal refractoriness
  Ion channel effects result in tachycardia and Q–T shortening associated with sympathetic stimulation

Alpha-adrenergic receptor-effector coupling system
Two to three alpha-1 adrenergic receptor subtypes in the heart are linked via G proteins to:
  Na-K pump (decrease rate of impulse initiation by automatic fibers)
  K channels (decreases in I K1, I K to, prolonging repolarization)
Induce triggered rhythms via delayed or early afterdepolarizations and abnormal automatic rhythms

Muscarinic receptor-effector coupling system
M2 receptor: dominant cardiac muscarinic receptor
Density is 2–5× higher in atria than in ventricle
M2 receptor coupled directly to ligand-operated I K (ACh) by G protein G K
M2 receptors inhibit adenylate cyclase via G 1
  Affects currents modulated by cAMP-dependent protein kinase (I Ca L, I f, I K)

Purinergic receptor-effector coupling system
Cardiac purinergic receptor = A1
Coupled by G K to ligand-operated potassium channel (I K[Ado])

---

cAMP = cyclic adenosine monophosphate; AV = atrioventricular.
Source: Data from The Sicilian gambit. *Circulation* 84:1831–1851, 1991.

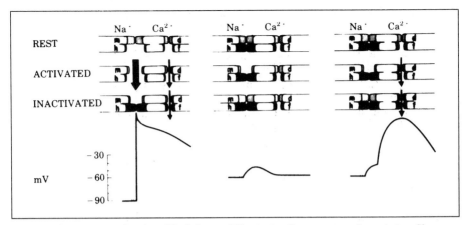

Fig. 3-4. The gating mechanism. The left panel illustrates the sequence of events in a fiber with a normal resting potential of -90 mV. The inactivation gates of the Na^+ channel (h) and the slow Ca^{2+}-Na^+ channel (f) are both open at rest. During activation (when the cell is stimulated) the m gates of the Na^+ channel open, and the resting inward current of sodium ions depolarizes the cell, giving rise to the upstroke of the action potential depicted below. The h gates then close the channel, thereby inactivating the Na^+ conductance. During the upstroke of the action potential, the membrane potential exceeds the more positive threshold potential of the slow channel; the activation (d) gates of the channel then open, and Ca^{2+} and Na^+ flow into the cell, giving rise to the plateau phase of the action potential. The f gates, which inactivate the Ca^{2+}-Na^+ channel, close much more slowly than the h gates, which inactivate the Na^+ channel. The middle panel shows the behavior of the channels when the resting potential is reduced to below -60 mV. The majority of the inactivation gates of the Na^+ channel remain closed as long as the membrane remains depolarized. When the cell is stimulated, the resulting inward Na^+ current is too small to cause an action potential. The inactivation (f) gates of the slow channel, however, are not closed, and, as shown in the right panel, excitation of the cell that is sufficient to open the slow channel, permitting the flow of slow inward current, may cause a slow response action potential to occur. (From AL Wit, JT Bigger, Possible electrophysiological mechanisms for lethal arrhythmias accompanying myocardial ischemia and infarction. *Circulation* 51 [Suppl.] and 52:III–96, 1975.)

The resting potential inside the cell is -90 mV. Depolarization owing to the rapid inward sodium current results in a rapid upstroke and is termed *phase 0*. When sufficient sodium channels have opened to allow the cell to reach the threshold potential, the current completes depolarization. Phase 1 represents early and rapid repolarization. The gating mechanism and duration of the action potential determine the prolonged refractory period, or phase 2. This plateau phase (phase 2) represents the absolute refractory period. Phase 3 corresponds to the relative refractory period and is a period of rapid repolarization when some sodium channels can be activated (h gates return to open position). Phase 4 is the interval from the end of repolarization until another action potential is generated. The membrane potential is back at -90 mV. The time spent between action potentials corresponds to diastole.

The cell remains at the resting potential until another stimulus occurs that is capable of reducing the resting potential to a critical level. If the cell has pacemaker capability, the resting potential spontaneously becomes less negative, until depolarization occurs (phase 4 diastolic depolarization) (Fig. 3-5). **Hyperpolarization** refers to the state in which the resting potential is more negative than usual (Fig. 3-6).

A. Sodium channels. The influx of Na^+ ions through voltage-sensitive pores (selective for Na^+) or channels results in the upstroke of the cardiac action potential. The gating mechanism in these channels allows rapid activation (opening) and slow closure. Sodium conductance is voltage dependent, creating an all-or-none type of phenomenon in regard to the propagated action potential.

Repolarization then causes restoration of the activation and inactivation mechanisms back to the resting condition. Membrane conductance is now thought to represent the product of random activity of single channels, some of which may be in the resting, open, inactivated states as a function of time and voltage dependence.

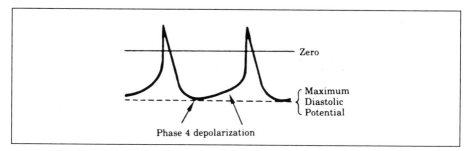

Fig. 3-5. Phase 4 depolarization. Membrane potentials recorded from a spontaneously active fiber. During the interval between the repolarization of one action potential and the upstroke of the next, there is a continuous progressive depolarization, which is referred to as phase 4 depolarization or diastolic depolarization. The broken line indicates the level of maximum negativity attained during the cycle; this is the maximum diastolic potential. (From PF Cranefield, *The Conduction of the Cardiac Impulse*. Mt. Kisco, NY: Futura, 1975. P. 9.)

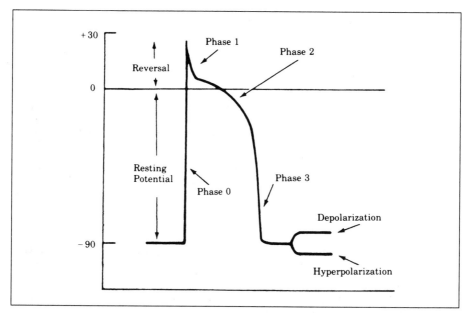

Fig. 3-6. Hyperpolarization and depolarization as depicted by a diagram of the action potential of a Purkinje fiber. When the fiber is quiescent the inside of the cell is −90 mV negative with respect to the outside (resting potential). At the peak of the action potential the interior of the cell becomes about 30 mV positive with respect to the outside so that there is a "reversal" or "overshoot." The upstroke is referred to as phase 0, the initial repolarization as phase 1, the plateau or period of persisting depolarization as phase 2, and the period of more rapid repolarization as phase 3. A change in membrane potential away from the resting potential toward zero is a depolarization; a change in the membrane potential that makes the inside of the cell more negative is a hyperpolarization. (From PF Cranefield, *The Conduction of the Cardiac Impulse*. Mt. Kisco, NY: Futura, 1975. P. 6.)

Sodium channels may also be modified through interaction with beta-adrenergic receptors. Catecholamines such as isoproterenol or phosphodiesterase inhibitors result in decreased sodium conductance, possibly through the action of a G protein, acting directly on the channel and/or through cAMP-dependent phosphorylation of the channel. Activation of beta-adrenergic receptors can inhibit Na^+ current and depress conduction, the latter dependent on both membrane depolarization and catecholamine concentration. This situation may occur clinically in myocardial ischemia or infarction and result in ventricular fibrillation.

Control of arrhythmias has been attempted with local anesthetic-type agents, which block impulse activity originating from damaged or depolarized tissue. Block may be tonic (independent of stimulation) or use dependent (increases with stimulus frequency, strength, and duration).

B. Potassium channels. Potassium current may be carried through a variety of channels, some of which have unique properties. I K1 is described as the *inward rectifier* because current flows preferentially in the inward direction. It activates on hyperpolarization and inactivates at very negative potentials. I K1 is responsible for the resting potential in atrial, ventricular, and Purkinje cells.

The *delayed rectifier* I K activates slowly after the upstroke of the action potential and is a major contributor to the action potential duration. It provides increasing outward current at the plateau of the action potential. As the heart rate accelerates, action potential duration shortens in a progressive manner, related in part to sustained activation of delayed rectifier conductance (i.e., I K does not deactivate completely due to the fast heart rate).

Another potassium current mediates stimulation of parasympathetic nerves to the heart, which release acetylcholine. This current, designated I K ACh, has similarities to I K1, including inward rectification modulated by potassium (external) and magnesium (internal). Activation of I K ACh by adenosine and muscarinic receptors may be mediated through G proteins.

Other potassium currents are described in Table 3-2.

C. Calcium channels. In the sarcolemma of cardiac cells, the inward current carried through open calcium channels determines a number of critical aspects of cardiac rhythm, including action potential duration, refractory period, and diastolic depolarization in pacemaker cells. In nodal cells, it determines the action potential upstroke and conduction velocity. These channels are also vital for cardiac contractility through their action on excitation-contraction coupling.

Two types of channels exist: one with large conductance and long-lasting current (**L type**) and the other with tiny conductance and transient current (**T type**). The L-type current is increased by Ca^{++} agonists, inhibited by verapamil, diltiazem, and the dihydropyridine-type antagonists, and stimulated by beta-adrenergic stimulation. The L type is the major channel providing inward current to the action potential plateau. The rate of rise of slow action potentials in the depolarized region of the AV node is determined by the L-type channel. Excitation-contraction is also mediated by these channels.

T-type channels are insensitive to dihydropyridine agonists or antagonists or to beta-adrenergic agonists. They may be important in determining the threshold for firing in Purkinje fibers and myocardial cells.

D. Gap junction channels. These channels provide the electrical and metabolic connections necessary for coordination of cellular function within a tissue. They function via a gating mechanism and have both high permeability and low selectivity.

E. Hyperpolarization-activated current I f. This current, sometimes referred to as the pacemaker current, is a time-dependent inward current, which may initiate slow diastolic depolarization. It is activated during hyperpolarization to the diastolic range. I f is modulated by cholinergic and adrenergic neurotransmitters.

F. Sodium/potassium pump. This pump sends sodium out the cells in exchange for potassium through the action of adenosinetriphosphatase.

IV. Mechanisms of arrhythmias. Treatment of arrhythmias may be facilitated if the mechanism is understood. Two basic concepts account for the majority of arrhythmias: abnormal impulse conduction and abnormal impulse generation. Abnormal conduction may be manifest by slowing and block; unidirectional block and reentry, with reentry either random or ordered; and reflection. Abnormal generation includes abnormal automaticity and triggered activity.

A. Reentry. Reentry may account for the majority of arrhythmias seen by the clinician. For reentry to occur, there must be a common pathway, unidirectional block, and the

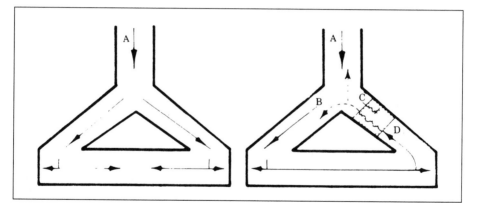

Fig. 3-7. The Schmitt-Erlanger model of reentry. The left diagram depicts a terminal segment of the conducting system that bifurcates before penetrating into the myocardium. There is a common initial pathway and communicating distal pathway. The right diagram demonstrates the situation when unidirectional block is present. Antegrade conduction cannot proceed through the shaded area and the impulse is blocked (*C*). Conduction proceeds normally down the other limb (*B*) and eventually is able to propagate in a retrograde direction to the area initially blocked (*D*). If it is not blocked (bidirectional block), but is able to penetrate through the area (unidirectional block), it may again be able to stimulate the normal tissue (*A, B*) if it has repolarized. If certain conditions are satisfied, a reentrant circuit may lead to sustained tachyarrhythmia. (From OS Narula, ed, *Cardiac Arrhythmias: Electrophysiology, Diagnosis and Management*. Baltimore: Williams & Wilkins, 1979. P. 9. © 1979, the Williams & Wilkins Co., Baltimore.)

ability of an area activated late to reexcite an area activated earlier. To understand this phenomenon in greater detail, one must consider a common initial pathway that divides into two pathways and then is reunited distally. In the normal condition, impulse conduction travels down both parallel pathways. With unidirectional block, however, conduction down one pathway is blocked in the antegrade direction. When the impulse that has traveled down the other pathway enters the common pathway and encounters excitable tissue in the blocked pathway, it can activate it in a retrograde fashion. The impulse travels up this pathway, and if the proximal tissue has had time to repolarize, it can again be depolarized. Therefore, if certain conditions are satisfied—appropriate timing, length of circuit, conduction velocity, refractoriness, and unidirectional block—an endless loop or circus movement rhythm may be sustained (Fig. 3-7).

Anisotropic conduction refers to the difference in conduction velocity in the long axis as compared to the short axis in tissue. When tissue is abnormal, differences will be magnified, interfering with or interrupting the normal flow of activation by the electrical wave front, resulting in the potential for reentry.

Reentry may occur over a small or large circuit, giving rise to the terms **microreentry** and **macroreentry.** Macroreentry may involve large circuits in the AV node, bundle branches, or accessory bypass tracts. Occasionally bundle branch reentry is seen during electrophysiologic testing. If a ventricular stimulus encounters the right bundle branch at a time when it is refractory, the stimulus may be able to cross the septum, excite the left bundle branch in retrograde fashion, penetrate the bundle of His, and excite the right bundle branch if now repolarized. This results in another ventricular depolarization. On the His bundle electrogram, the retrograde His deflection may be observed. Bundle branch reentry is considered a physiologic phenomenon, although it is seen infrequently in patients with ventricular tachycardia. Microreentry is usually considered to be a pathologic phenomenon. A microcircuit capable of sustaining a reentrant arrhythmia may exist in a diseased portion of the myocardium or conduction system. If it exists in the ventricle, it may be described as intraventricular reentry, which may be the mechanism of the majority of the ventricular tachycardias. Identification of the site of this microreentrant circuit by electrophysiologic mapping may allow surgical or nonsurgical extirpation.

Reflection is a form of reentry that does not require separate parallel pathways and thus produces no circus movement. One model of reflection considers unbranched Purkinje fiber bundles with depressed resting and action potentials with slow conduction. Excitation occurs slowly in one direction along a bundle of fibers, followed by excitation occurring in the opposite direction. Thus, the reflected impulse may result from reentry caused by longitudinal dissociation.

B. **Automaticity.** Automaticity, the ability to depolarize spontaneously and maintain a rhythmic discharge, is seen in cells in the sinus node, occasionally parts of the atria, the AV junctional region, and the His-Purkinje system. The SA node assumes the position of dominant pacemaker because it has the fastest rate. Subsidiary pacemakers are suppressed since the propagated impulse excites them before they can spontaneously depolarize. The rate of an automatic focus may be slowed by parasympathetic stimulation since acetylcholine decreases the slope of phase 4 depolarization by causing hyperpolarization. Drugs or SA disease may also slow the rate of sinus discharge, occasionally allowing another pacemaker to become dominant.

Automaticity may be considered abnormal when it occurs in fibers that are depolarized. The resting potential is reduced to less than -60 mV. The slow inward current may play a key role in abnormal automaticity since verapamil inhibits and epinephrine enhances this phenomenon.

In the clinical electrophysiology laboratory, automatic arrhythmias respond differently from reentry arrhythmias. Reentrant tachycardias may be initiated and terminated by programmed stimulation. Automatic tachycardias cannot, although an impulse that penetrates the automatic focus may reset the timing. Pacing at a rate faster than the automatic tachycardia will capture; however, the automatic rhythm resumes control when the pacing rate is slowed or terminated.

C. **Triggered activity.** Triggered activity is a third mechanism capable of initiating arrhythmias. It is not a spontaneous depolarization as seen in automaticity and is not due to a stimulus's exciting a repolarized cell. Rather, it is dependent on the previous action potential, when oscillations in the membrane potential depolarize the cell to threshold. These oscillations are defined as afterdepolarizations, that is, second subthreshold depolarizations that occur during repolarization or after it is complete. If the event occurs during phase 3 of the action potential, it is considered an early depolarization. Delayed afterdepolarizations occur after repolarization and at a higher membrane potential (Fig. 3-8).

Delayed afterdepolarizations may occur in the presence or absence of digitalis or catecholamines and are associated with a large increase in intracellular calcium ions due to the repetitive release of calcium from the sarcoplasmic reticulum. They result in an inward depolarizing current. Digitalis may induce delayed afterdepolarizations and triggered activity via inhibition of the sodium-potassium pump, increasing intracellular sodium, reducing the activity of the Na^+/Ca^{++} exchanger, and increasing intracellular calcium. Catecholamines may induce delayed afterdepolarizations and triggered activity by stimulating adrenergic receptors or augmenting digitalis- or ischemia-related delayed afterdepolarizations.

Like reentrant mechanisms, delayed afterdepolarization arrhythmias may be initiated and terminated by programmed stimulation. Triggered rhythms are more easily induced with rapid pacing than with extra stimuli. The coupling interval of the first ectopic beat of the triggered rhythm has a direct relation to the pacing cycle length. Tachycardia can be accelerated by overdrive stimulation. More ectopic beats are noted at faster heart rates. Although these arrhythmias may be somewhat more difficult to initiate, they are relatively easy to terminate. They may be blocked by both sodium or calcium blockers.

Thus, delayed afterdepolarizations result in extrasystoles and digitalis toxic arrhythmias, as well as catecholamine-dependent atrial and ventricular tachycardias. They may be responsible for some arrhythmias caused by ischemia and reperfusion. Mechanistic treatment would be directed at the calcium overload, using calcium channel blockers (verapamil, nifedipine, manganese) or by blocking the inward sodium (I NS) current (lidocaine, procainamide, quinidine, mexiletine, amiodarone) or increasing the outward current (increasing potassium conductance).

Early afterdepolarizations result from a change in net membrane inward current's delaying or interrupting repolarization. Mechanisms may include a reduction in the normal repolarizing current (I K), abnormal prolongation of inward current (Na^+ or Ca^{++} channels), or the simultaneous operation of enhanced inward and reduced outward currents. Afterdepolarizations may arise at slow heart or stimulation rates. In addition, afterdepolarizations occur after long pauses when the action potential duration is prolonged due to decreased extracellular K^+ or due to drugs that block I K or I K1. Clinically, afterdepolarizations may be associated with hypox-

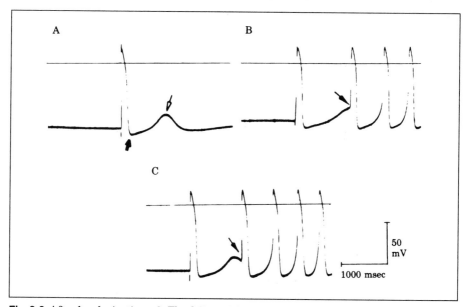

Fig. 3-8. Afterdepolarizations. **A.** The driven action potential is followed by an after hyperpolarization (*solid arrow*) and a delayed afterdepolarization (*open arrow*). **B.** The driven action potential is followed by a delayed afterdepolarization that reaches threshold, and a nondriven action potential (*arrow*) arises from the peak of the afterdepolarization. The triggered impulse is then followed by a "train" of nondriven triggered activity. **C.** The afterdepolarization that follows the driven action potential reaches a peak and then begins to decline before the occurrence of the nondriven impulse indicated by the arrow. Triggering presumably occurred in a fiber other than the one from which the transmembrane potential was being recorded, and that triggered impulse propagated to the impaled fiber, followed by triggered activity. (From OS Narula, ed, *Cardiac Arrhythmias: Electrophysiology, Diagnosis and Management.* Baltimore: Williams & Wilkins, 1979. P. 15. © 1979, the Williams & Wilkins Co., Baltimore.)

ia, electrolyte abnormalities, certain drugs, or injury. Afterdepolarizations can induce torsades de pointes and may be associated with reperfusion arrhythmias. Mechanistic treatment includes drugs that increase extracellular K^+, increasing heart rate, beta-adrenergic receptor activation, and suppression of triggering inward currents (e.g., drugs blocking calcium or sodium currents, alpha or beta receptors or Mg^{++}).

V. Effect of antiarrhythmic drugs on the action potential. Cardiac drugs are discussed in detail in Chap. 14, but the manner in which they alter the action potential is briefly described here. From the diagram of the action potential (see Fig. 3-6), it is obvious that the ability to achieve the threshold can be modified in several ways. First, if the cell has pacemaker capability and exhibits phase 4 depolarization, drugs that decrease the rate of spontaneous depolarization will delay achievement of threshold. Hyperpolarization at the cellular level or an increase in the threshold will also delay this event. Similarly, enhanced automaticity may result from an increase in the rate of spontaneous depolarization or a lowering of the threshold (Fig. 3-9).

Drugs that decrease conduction velocity will depress phase 0 and prolong the action potential. The effective refractory period may also be increased. The combination of effects on the action potential duration and effective refractory period may also affect the rate of depolarization. Finally, drugs that act on the slow inward current, the calcium antagonists, will slow conduction, prolong refractoriness, and decrease automaticity in the AV and SA nodes.

VI. General principles of drug action. Drugs used to treat specific arrhythmias may have multiple electrophysiologic effects on channels, pumps, and receptors, resulting in an alteration of the electrophysiologic substrate and affecting conduction, refractoriness, and automaticity.

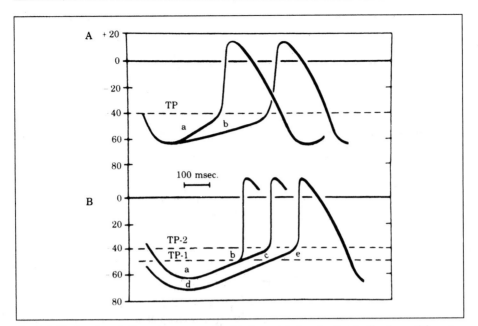

Fig. 3-9. Mechanisms influencing pacemaker discharge. **A.** A reduction in the slope of the pacemaker potential from *a* to *b* will diminish the frequency. **B.** An increase in the threshold (from TP-1 to TP-2) or an increase in the magnitude of the resting potential (from *a* to *d*) will also diminish the frequency. (From BF Hoffman, PF Cranefield, *Electrophysiology of the Heart*. New York: McGraw-Hill, 1960. Reproduced with permission.)

Tonic block develops in the absence of excitation. **Phasic block** refers to the additional reduction of sodium current when the heart rate or rate of stimulation increases. **Use dependence** refers to preferential association of the drug with the channel during activation to the open state or the prolonged plateau phase when inactivated. **Voltage dependence** is a function of the fraction of sodium channels activated in response to a depolarizing pulse and becoming accessible to the blocking action of the drug. It also reflects the direct effect of voltage on the ionized form of the drug. **Reverse use dependence** indicates that the prolongation of repolarization is greatest at the slowest heart or stimulation rates and decreases progressively as stimulation increases. **Heart rate dependence** refers to the fact that effects may vary at different heart rates, being antiarrhythmic at one rate and even proarrhythmic at another.

VII. **Glossary of other terms used to describe arrhythmias and electrophysiologic phenomena.** The following brief definitions represent a partial list of terms that have been used to describe arrhythmias and electrophysiologic phenomena (some are included for historical perspective).

Aberration, aberrant ventricular conduction: Abnormal intraventricular conduction of an impulse originating in the atria or AV junction. Quite often due to unequal refractoriness in the bundle branch system with a longer refractory period of the right bundle branch. May be acceleration or deceleration dependent. May also refer to conduction down accessory bypass tract.

Abnormal automaticity: Spontaneous impulse generated in fibers partially depolarized as a result of a pathologic process. Effects are a function of the magnitude of membrane depolarization. Arrhythmias include ectopic atrial tachycardia, accelerated idioventricular tachycardia, and ventricular tachycardia. Mechanistic treatment of these arrhythmias may be directed at the reduced maximum diastolic (resting) potential and may respond to K^+ channel activation or to Na^+-K^+ pump stimulation.

Accrochage: A relationship between two pacemaker foci during AV dissociation. The two pacemakers discharge at similar rates and remain in phase with each other, possibly because of electrophysiologic influences. Short periods of this mutual relationship are referred to as *accrochage*. Long in-phase periods are referred to as *synchronization*. Isorhythmic dissociation is an example of this phenomenon.

Anisotropic conduction: Conduction velocity in cardiac muscle depends on the direction relative to the fiber axis. Refers to the difference in conduction in the longitudinal and transverse directions across tissue.

Ashman's phenomenon, Ashman beat: Aberration during ventricular conduction, with a short cycle following a long cycle. Occurs frequently in atrial fibrillation (see Fig. 4-11).

Automaticity: Spontaneous impulse initiation by cardiac fibers due to phase 4 depolarization (inward Na^+ current I f).

Circus movement: Impulse propagation that traverses a reentrant loop. Central and lateral boundaries must be adequate. The length of the path must exceed the wavelength determined by effective refractoriness. Unidirectional block is present.

Concealed conduction: Conduction of an impulse that cannot be detected on the surface ECG as a discrete deflection but results in disturbed conduction of the subsequent beat. This disturbance may be manifest as a prolonged conduction time or failure to conduct the next beat. Often seen with penetration of impulse into the AV node.

Concertina effect: Varying degrees of preexcitation in a patient with an accessory bypass tract. Depending on factors such as heart rate and the presence of antiarrhythmic drugs, there may be more or less early activation via the bypass tract. This phenomenon is noted on the ECG by more or less delta wave activity.

Coronary sinus rhythm: Ectopic atrial pacemaker that activates the atria in a retrograde fashion, resulting in inverted P waves in ECG leads II, III, and aVF.

Delayed afterdepolarization: A result of calcium overload resulting in an inward depolarizing current. May result in digitalis-toxic arrhythmias, catecholamine-dependent atrial and ventricular tachycardias, and reperfusion arrhythmias.

Early afterdepolarization: A result of a change in net membrane inward current, delaying or interrupting repolarization. May induce torsades de pointes and be associated with reperfusion arrhythmias.

Electrotonus: Passive spread of current in the heart, as opposed to an active effect, such as an action potential.

Enhanced normal automaticity: Enhancement of slow phase 4 depolarization, for example, by adrenergic stimulation. Hyperpolarization due to an increase in K^+ currents results in hyperpolarization that will increase the rate. (Hyperpolarization alone slows the rate, but the additional effect on shortening the action potential duration and activating I f earlier results in a net increase in the rate.) Examples of arrhythmias include inappropriate sinus tachycardia, atrial tachycardias, and accelerated idioventricular tachycardia.

Entrainment: Increase in the rate of tachycardia to equal a faster pacing rate. The original tachycardia rate resumes when pacing is terminated (transient entrainment).

Escape capture bigeminy: Supraventricular conduction disturbance in which prolonged conduction to the ventricles results in an escape ventricular (or junctional) beat followed by a sinus beat that is then able to penetrate. Seen on the ECG as an escape beat followed by a conducted beat.

Excitable gap: In a reentry circuit, the tissue between the head and tail of circulating wave front is not refractory and can be depolarized. The extent of the excitable gap is dependent on conduction velocity, length of the circuit, and the refractory period. The excitable gap becomes important in the termination of an arrhythmia when an appropriately timed impulse can invade the circuit and cause bidirectional block.

Fusion: Impulse formation resulting from activation by two different pathways. Seen on the ECG to have characteristics of both originating foci. For example, a sinus beat partially exciting the ventricle in conjunction with a ventricular premature beat (VPB) will usually have an intermediate appearance between the normal narrow-complex supraventricular beat and the wide-complex VPB.

Gap phenomenon: Refers to failure of AV conduction during atrial extrastimulus assessment of refractory periods and resumption of AV conduction with further prematurity of the impulse.

Heart rate dependence: Refers to drug action. Interventions that can be antiarrhythmic at one heart rate may be ineffective or even provoke arrhythmias at a different heart rate.

Interference: Collision of two impulses, usually resulting in abolition of the circulating wave front.

Irritability: Condition or state facilitating the development of an arrhythmia.

Parasystole: Abnormal impulse initiation, thought to be automatic, whose expression is determined by the presence and extent of entrance and exit block. Recognized on the ECG by nonfixed coupling intervals, a mathematical relationship between ectopic beats, and fusion beats. May occur in the atrium or ventricle (see Fig. 8-16).

Phasic block: Refers to drug action. Additional reduction of sodium current by local anesthetic antiarrhythmic drugs when heart rate or rate of stimulation increases. Attributed to intermittent accessor variable affinity for channel binding sites, dependent on the gating state of the channel.

Reciprocation: Circus movement or reentry of an impulse resulting in recurrent activation of a cardiac chamber. Requires an additional pathway that allows the impulse to return to the originating chamber and reexcite it. For example, a supraventricular beat excites the ventricles via the AV node and His-Purkinje system, encounters an accessory bypass tract capable of retrograde conduction, and reexcites the atrium.

Reflection: Electrotonic transmission occurs across an inexcitable segment in a linear bundle. Delay in impulse transmission allows fibers proximal to the inexcitable segment to recover excitability and be available for excitation by current flowing retrogradely across the inexcitable zone.

Reverse use dependence: Refers to drug action. Prolongation of repolarization is greatest at the slowest heart or stimulation rates and progressively decreases as the rate of stimulation increases. Attributed to reduction in potassium channel blockade during plateau or at positive potentials so that block decreases as use increases.

Rule of bigeminy: Tendency of VPBs to follow a long preceding RR interval. Since the compensatory pause of the VPB causes another long RR interval, the cycle may repeat itself.

Sinoventricular rhythm: Activation of the ventricles via the specialized atrial internodal tracts without activation of the atria. Seen in hyperkalemia.

Supernormal conduction: Short period in the early phase of the cardiac recovery cycle when conduction is better than expected. A very early impulse may conduct, whereas later ones will not. Occurs just at the end of phase 3 of the action potential. Most often seen on the ECG as paradoxical AV conduction during periods of high-degree AV block. Seen only in depressed myocardium.

Tonic block: Refers to drug action. Block that develops in the absence of excitation. Characteristic of local anesthetic antiarrhythmic drugs with continuous access to drug binding sites. Correlates with lipid solubility.

Torsades de pointes ("twisting of the points"): An atypical ventricular tachycardia (VT) characterized by spindle-shaped groupings of VT beats. Usually occurs in the presence of prolonged Q–T (see Fig. 8-14).

Treppe phenomenon: "Warm-up" phenomenon of a pacemaker cell until a constant discharge rate is established.

Triggered activity: Dependent on afterdepolarizations in which the depolarization is dependent on the prior impulse.

Use dependence: Refers to drug action. Association of the drug with the channel occurs preferentially during activation to the open state of or during the prolonged plateau period when inactivated.

Voltage dependence: Refers to drug action. Function of the fraction of sodium channels that activate in response to a depolarizing pulse, becoming accessible to the blocking action of the drug and the direct effects of voltage on the ionized form of the drug.

Vulnerable period: Period during relative refractory period when the heart is at risk of fibrillation if stimulated. Corresponds to the apex of the T wave on the ECG. Represents the basis of the R-on-T phenomenon.

Wedensky effect: A subthreshold stimulus that is usually unable to evoke a response but can initiate a response if preceded by maximum stimulus.

Wedensky facilitation: An impulse arriving at a blocked zone enhances the excitability of nerve beyond the block. Most often noted as a conducted sinus beat following an escape beat in high-degree AV block.

Bibliography

Antzelevich C, Sicouri S. Clinical relevance of cardiac arrhythmias generated by afterdepolarizations. *J Am Coll Cardiol* 23:259–277, 1994.

Cranefield PF. *The Conduction of the Cardiac Impulse*. Mt. Kisco NY: Futura, 1975.

Josephson ME (ed). *Clinical Cardiac Electrophysiology* (2nd ed). Philadelphia: Lea & Febiger, 1993.

Narula OS (ed). *Cardiac Arrhythmias: Electrophysiology, Diagnosis and Management*. Baltimore: Williams & Wilkins, 1979.

Pick A, Langendorf R. *Interpretation of Complex Arrhythmias*. Philadelphia: Lea & Febiger, 1979.

Surawicz B, Reddy CP, Prystowsky EN (eds). *Tachycardias*. Boston: Martinus Nijhoff, 1984.

Task Force: The Sicilian gambit: A new approach to the classification of antiarrhythmic drugs based on their actions on arrhythmogenic mechanisms. *Circulation* 84:1831–1851, 1991.

Zipes DP, Jalife J (eds). *Cardiac Electrophysiology and Arrhythmias*. Orlando FL: Grune & Stratton, 1985.

Zipes DP, Jalife J (eds). *Cardiac Electrophysiology: From Cell to Bedside*. Philadelphia: Saunders, 1990.

Specific chapters of special interest:

Anderson RH, Becker AE. Anatomy of the conduction tissues and accessory atrioventricular connections (pp 240–248).

DiFrancesco D. Current I f and the neuronal modulation of heart rate (pp 28–35).

Gadsby DC. The Na/K pump of cardiac myocytes (pp 35–49).

Hess P. Cardiac calcium channels (pp 10–17).

Kirsch GE, Brown AM. Cardiac sodium channels (pp 1–10).

Pennefather P, Cohen IS. Molecular mechanisms of cardiac K^+ channel regulation (pp 17–28).

Veenstra RD. Physiology of cardiac gap junction channels (pp 62–69).

4

Clinical Recognition of Cardiac Arrhythmias

Stephen C. Vlay

Daily, the clinician is asked to diagnose cardiac arrhythmias in patients in the hospital and in the office. The diagnosis often is readily apparent, but occasionally he or she must use clues from the physical examination, and response to maneuvers or drugs, or special electrodes in addition to the ECG. This chapter presents the measures the physician utilizes at the bedside. Specific techniques in electrophysiology laboratory are discussed in Chap. 12.

I. **Hemodynamic compromise.** Is the patient hemodynamically compromised? Is the compromise due to the arrhythmia? These two questions must be answered immediately. Misdiagnosis of a sinus tachycardia as either atrioventricular (AV) nodal reentrant tachycardia or ventricular tachycardia (VT) leads to inappropriate treatment with drugs or cardioversion while the precipitating factor is ignored. In addition, the treatment of sinus tachycardia must be directed at its cause: volume depletion, hemorrhage, fever, hypoxia, sepsis, hyperthyroidism, or sympathetic stimulation owing to a variety of causes.

When ventricular tachyarrhythmias cause hemodynamic embarrassment, specific measures must be immediately undertaken. If the patient is in sustained VT or ventricular fibrillation (VF), the course of action is quite clear: cardiopulmonary resuscitation and electrical cardioversion or defibrillation. Certainly, rare patients have nonhypotensive sustained VT and may respond to other maneuvers, but the integrity of the systemic circulation must not be jeopardized.

With atrial tachyarrhythmias, the decision-making process is more difficult. For example, if a patient with **chronic** atrial fibrillation and a ventricular response usually controlled by digitalis develops an intercurrent illness, sympathetic discharge may speed the ventricular response. The patient may become hypotensive, particularly if the underlying cause is sepsis, blood loss, or volume depletion. Attempts at electrical cardioversion are unlikely to restore sinus rhythm and may be associated with embolization if the patient is not receiving anticoagulants chronically. Additional digitalis or diltiazem may assist in slowing the rate; nevertheless, treatment must be directed at the underlying cause. If, however, an **acute** atrial tachyarrhythmia, such as atrial flutter or atrial fibrillation with a rapid ventricular response, results in a greatly decreased cardiac output, electrical cardioversion is the treatment of choice. In certain situations, particularly in the case of a postoperative cardiac patient with transthoracic pacing electrodes in the atria, overdrive pacing for atrial flutter may be preferable to countershock.

Bradyarrhythmias may also cause hemodynamic embarrassment. The clinician must quickly determine whether the arrhythmia is a vasovagal episode, severe sinus bradycardia, AV block, junctional rhythm (perhaps with digitalis toxicity), or idioventricular rhythm. In this situation, a decision must be made as to the choice of therapy. Is it appropriate to administer atropine or isoproterenol, or is it necessary to use temporary pacing by the transvenous, transthoracic, or external thoracic method? Specific therapies are discussed for each arrhythmia (see Chaps. 6 and 8).

II. **Rate.** Heart rate will aid in the differentiation of one arrhythmia from another; however, there may be considerable overlap. When one considers rate, one evaluates the ventricular response first, but the atrial rate must not be ignored. Table 4-1 describes arrhythmias by the rate of the ventricular response. As can be appreciated, the clinician must use additional clues to arrive at the diagnosis. The next point to consider is regularity.

III. **Regularity.** Is the rhythm absolutely regular, fairly regular but with some minor variation, irregular, or irregularly irregular? The majority of the rhythms encountered are regular. The most common reason for minor variation is respiratory variation, in some cases overt enough to be called a sinus arrhythmia (Fig. 4-1). Thus, in a patient with sinus tachycardia, the rhythm will be essentially regular, but minor variation in rate may be seen during minutes or hours of observation. VT is fairly regular but also displays some variation, this time not related to alterations in sinus discharge (Fig. 4-2).

Atrial flutter and atrial tachycardia with block are generally regular but will be irregular with varying degrees of block (Fig. 4-3). Similarly, AV nodal reentry and reciprocating tachycardias utilizing an accessory pathway will be regular, except at the times of initiation or termination, when both may be irregular. AV junctional rhythms and tachycardias as well as accelerated idioventricular rhythms are fairly regular but also may be irregular (Fig. 4-4).

The most common reason for an irregular pulse is the presence of premature beats— atrial, junctional, or ventricular. When they are very frequent and occur in no set pattern, the pulse may incorrectly be thought to be atrial fibrillation until an ECG is obtained. If the premature beats occur in a fixed pattern, say, every other or every third beat, the pulse will display a bigeminal or trigeminal pattern (Fig. 4-5, p. 58). This type of rhythm is irregular but may be regularly irregular.

The rhythm that consistently is irregularly irregular is atrial fibrillation (Fig. 4-6, p. 58). The atrial rate ranges from 400–600 beats/minute, but the ventricular response is controlled via decremental conduction down the AV node (see Chap. 3). The ventricular response is grossly irregular and may be modified by the action of certain cardiovascular drugs that exert a negative chronotropic or negative dromotropic effect. These include digitalis, beta blockers, and certain calcium antagonists. One very important situation in which to recognize atrial fibrillation is in a patient with Wolff-Parkinson-White syndrome. If conduction is antegrade down the accessory pathway (see Chap. 7), the patient will display a wide-complex tachycardia at a rate of 300 beats/minute that is irregularly irregular with atrial fibrillation (Fig. 4-7, p. 59). One must differentiate this rhythm from VT tachycardia or flutter. The irregularity may provide the answer. VF is a chaotic rhythm, but assessment of regularity is not necessary to make this diagnosis.

Table 4-1. Arrhythmia differentiation by ventricular response

Ventricular rate	Diagnosis
Bradyarrhythmias	
<60	Sinus bradycardia
40–60	AV junctional rhythm
30–50	Idioventricular rhythm
50–110	Accelerated idioventricular rhythm
30–100	AV block
Rhythms with rates 60–100	
60–100	Sinus rhythm
60–100	Atrial fibrillation with slow to moderate ventricular response
75–175	Atrial flutter with varying block
75–200	Atrial tachycardia with varying block
70–130	AV junctional tachycardia (nonparoxysmal)
50–119	Accelerated idioventricular rhythm
Tachyarrhythmias	
100–180	Sinus tachycardia
100–180	Atrial fibrillation with a fast ventricular response
150–250	AV nodal reentrant tachycardia
75–150	Atrial flutter with varying block
75–200	Atrial tachycardia with varying block
150–300	Reciprocating tachycardias (including atrial fibrillation) utilizing accessory pathway
70–130	Accelerated AV junctional tachycardia (nonparoxysmal)
50–119	Accelerated idioventricular rhythm
120–250	Ventricular tachycardia
150–300	Ventricular flutter
400–600	Ventricular fibrillation

AV = atrioventricular.

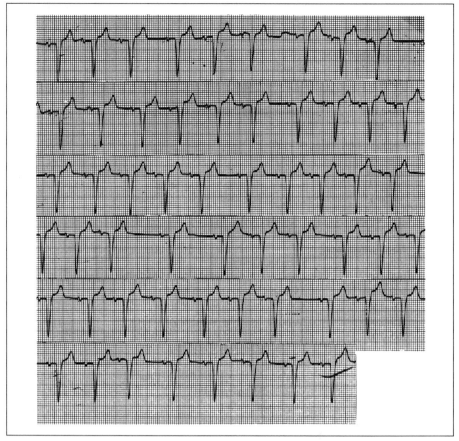

Fig. 4-1. Sinus arrhythmia. Slight variations in regularity are often related to respiratory variation.

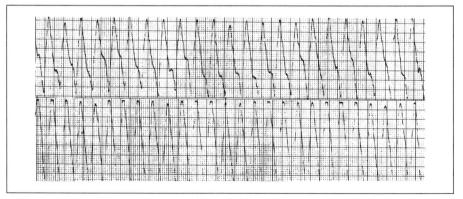

Fig. 4-2. Ventricular tachycardia, rate 188 beats/minute. Note the slight irregularity and later acceleration.

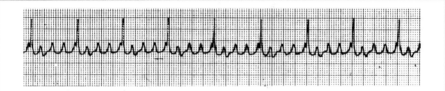

Fig. 4-3. Atrial flutter with 4:1 block. The flutter rate is 300 beats/minute. The ventricular response is 75 beats/minute.

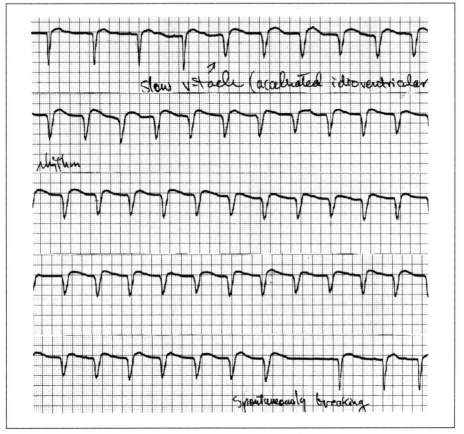

Fig. 4-4. Accelerated idioventricular rhythm (AIVR), rate 80 beats/minute, usurps dominance from the sinus node and later spontaneously terminates. Note the P waves that march through the AIVR. This rhythm occurred in an 83-year-old man admitted for acute myocardial infarction.

Finally, in cases of second-degree heart block, the rhythm may be irregular unless the block is unchanging (e.g., 2:1 block). The typical Wenckebach periodicity with type I second-degree AV block or high-degree variable block with Mobitz-type II second-degree AV block both will produce an irregular rhythm. Complete heart block will be fairly regular.

IV. Clues on the electrocardiogram

    A. QRS duration. One of the most obvious features on the ECG is the width of the QRS complex. Is it a wide-complex or narrow-complex arrhythmia? Quite often this information will exclude certain possibilities, but the diagnosis will remain difficult in certain cases.

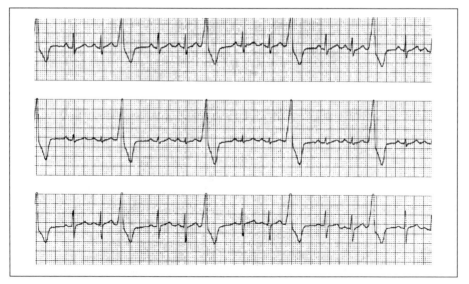

Fig. 4-5. Ventricular trigeminy. Two sinus beats are followed by a ventricular premature beat in a recurrent trigeminal pattern.

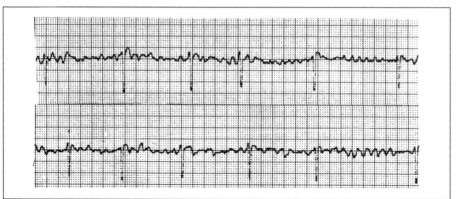

Fig. 4-6. Atrial fibrillation. Note coarse fibrillatory waves and an irregularly irregular slow ventricular response.

There are three prime causes of a wide QRS complex: aberrant or accessory pathway conduction, bundle branch block, and ventricular origin of the impulse. In the absence of clear P waves and other morphologic clues, the physician occasionally may have to resort to an intracardiac electrogram to establish the diagnosis. While some clinicians consider a QRS duration exceeding 140 msec to favor a ventricular origin of the tachycardia, this certainly is not definitive.

B. **QRS morphology.** The morphology of the QRS complex on the ECG depends on the epicardial breakthrough site. At one time it was thought that different morphologies of the QRS always represented different foci of origin. However, it was subsequently demonstrated that a single endocardial focus may have multiple pathways to the epicardium, depending on such factors as heart rate, refractoriness of the myocardium, timing of the premature beat, and modification by drugs. Thus, it is better to describe morphologically different ventricular premature beats as multiform rather than multifocal. Patients with scarred myocardium certainly may have multiple foci as well, but endocardial mapping is necessary to demonstrate this.

With this caveat in mind, one must approach with caution the tendency to label what appears to be a ventricular premature beat as left ventricular or right ventric-

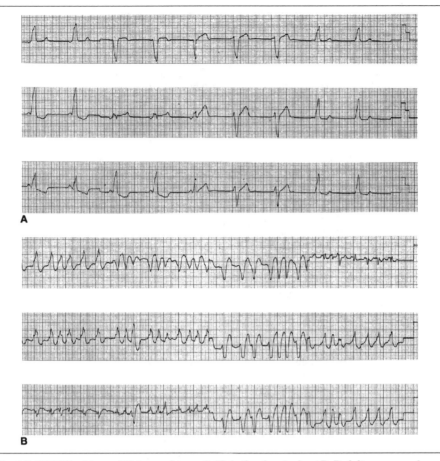

Fig. 4-7. Wolff-Parkinson-White syndrome. **A.** Note the classic short P–R, delta wave, and prolonged QRS when the patient is in sinus rhythm. **B.** Electrocardiogram of the same patient during atrial fibrillation and antegrade conduction to the ventricles via the accessory pathway. This rhythm must be distinguished from ventricular tachycardia. The marked irregularity suggests atrial fibrillation.

ular ectopy. The first question is whether it is, in fact, ventricular ectopy rather than aberration. Normally, if a supraventricular impulse occurs too early, and the AV node, bundle of His, and bundle branches have not yet repolarized (are in the refractory period), there will be no conduction to the ventricles. If the conducting system is partially repolarized, the impulse may be conducted to the ventricle, but not necessarily by the usual route. This abnormal conduction is designated as aberration. Marriott provides 10 criteria (Table 4-2) that favor ventricular ectopy [1]. As can be seen from his graphic illustration (Table 4-3), these morphologic descriptions may favor either aberration or ectopy, and Marriott states the odds from his experience. It must again be emphasized that the **morphologic criteria are not definitive.**

QRS axis and fusion beats are discussed shortly, but a few more comments on Table 4-2 are appropriate. **Rosenbaum's normal pattern** is the typical pattern of left bundle branch block (LBBB) in V_6; however, atypical for LBBB are the associated right axis deviation in the limb leads and "fat little R waves in V_1 and sometimes V_2" (Fig. 4-8). **Marriott's swinging pattern** is the change from an upright pattern to negative complexes that may imperceptibly occur during a run of VT (Fig. 4-9).

If the patient has atrial fibrillation as the underlying rhythm rather than sinus, one cannot utilize the presence of P waves to help distinguish aberration from ectopy. Table 4-4 lists Marriott's clues for this problem. **Undue prematurity** describes the situation in which the occurrence of a premature beat conducted aberrantly is unlikely because of the presence of AV block. **Fixed coupling** favors ventricular ectopy since it would be unexpected with aberrant beats. The **longer-shorter sequence** in atrial fibrillation refers to the possibility of **Ashman's phenomenon** (Fig. 4-10). Most commonly, the right bundle branch system has the longer refractory period. Thus, an early supraventricular impulse may be conducted down the left bundle branch with right bundle branch block (RBBB) morphology. In addition, the refractory periods of the bundle branches are directly proportional to the length of the preceding R–R interval. Long refractory periods occur after long preceding cycle lengths (slow heart rates). Short refractory periods occur after short preceding cycle lengths (fast heart rates). Thus, if a long cycle is followed by a short cycle, there is a

Table 4-2. Features favoring ventricular ectopy

Left "rabbit ear" taller in V_1
QS or RS in V_6
Bizarre frontal plane axis
Concordant V leads, positive or negative
Deepest QS in V_4 through V_5
Rosenbaum's "normal" pattern
R interrupting T
"Swinging" pattern
Fusion beats
Early nonaberrant capture beats

Source: From HJL Marriott, *Workshop in Electrocardiography*. Oldsmar, FL: Tampa Tracings, 1972. P. 218.

Table 4-3. Ventricular aberration versus ectopy: Morphologic clues

Manifestation		Favors	Odds
RSR′ variant in V_1 or MCL$_1$		Aberration	10:1
qRs in V_6 or MCL$_6$		Aberration	20:1
R or qR in V_1 or MCL$_1$ with taller left "rabbit ear"		LV ectopy	10:1
R or qR in V_1 or MCL$_1$ with taller right "rabbit ear"		Neither	
QS in V_6 or MCL$_6$		LV ectopy	20:1
rS in V_6 or MCL$_6$ (**nO** q)		LV ectopy	7:3
LBBB pattern with wide r in V_1 or MCL$_1$		RV ectopy	10:1

MCL = modified chest lead; LV = left ventricular; LBBB = left bundle branch block; RV = right ventricular.
Source: From HJL Marriott, *Workshop in Electrocardiography*. Oldsmar, FL: Tampa Tracings, 1972. P. 241.

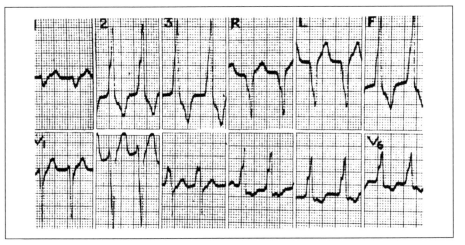

Fig. 4-8. Rosenbaum's normal pattern, which includes typical pattern of left bundle branch block in V_6, right axis deviation in the limb leads, and fat r waves in V_1 and V_2. (From HJL Marriott, *Workshop in Electrocardiography*. Oldsmar, FL: Tampa Tracings, 1972. P. 226.)

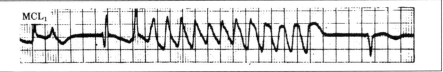

Fig. 4-9. Marriott's swinging pattern. Note the change from upright to negative complexes. (MCL_1 = modified chest lead.) (From HJL Marriott, *Workshop in Electrocardiography*. Oldsmar, FL: Tampa Tracings, 1972. P. 228.)

greater chance that part of the conducting system is refractory and the impulse is conducted aberrantly. What may favor a diagnosis of ventricular ectopy rather than aberration is the presence in the same ECG strip of **longer-shorter sequence** in which the beat following the shorter cycle is conducted normally. This would suggest that wide-complex beats with longer intervals are ectopic. Finally, wide-complex beats ending long cycle lengths would not be expected to be aberrant. Therefore, if the preceding cycle length is shorter, the beat following the longer cycle is likely to be ectopic. Table 4-5 summarizes Marriott's clues to aberration. A preceding P′ wave suggests an early beat finding incomplete repolarization. The RBBB morphology and triphasic contour have been discussed. Quite commonly, the initial vector of aberrantly conducted beats will be similar to that of the normally conducted beats. If only the second beat of a group of rapidly conducted beats displays an anomalous pattern, it is likely to be aberrant since it follows the longer-shorter rule, and the subsequent beats follow short cycles.

Electrophysiologic testing provides definitive diagnosis of the origin of arrhythmias that defy diagnosis by ECG. Wellens, Bar, and Lie correlated morphologic ECG evidence with data obtained with a His bundle electrogram (Table 4-6) [2]. As noted

Table 4-4. Features favoring ventricular ectopy in atrial fibrillation

Undue prematurity
Fixed coupling
Longer-shorter sequence without aberration
Shorter preceding cycle

Source: From HJL Marriott, *Workshop in Electrocardiography*. Oldsmar, FL: Tampa Tracings, 1972. P. 230.

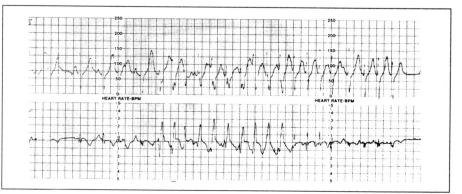

Fig. 4-10. Atrial fibrillation with areas of very rapid ventricular response and consecutively occurring aberrant ventricular conduction that closely simulates ventricular tachycardia. In V_1, the complexes demonstrate a right bundle branch block pattern.

above, definitive diagnosis cannot be made using morphology alone. In fact, Table 4-7 clearly demonstrates that the chances of aberration versus VT with certain configurations are 50-50. Thus, the clinician must look for additional clues such as left axis deviation, wide QRS, and AV dissociation. Interestingly, capture or fusion beats during VT were seen in only 4 of 33 episodes of sustained tachycardia in the Wellens, Bar, and Lie series [2]. Thus, although morphology is helpful, definitive diagnosis in certain cases can be made only with a His bundle electrogram. Figure 4-11 (p. 65) illustrates the utility of the morphologic clues, particularly in association with a change in the resting ECG. In 1991, Brugada and colleagues described another approach to the differential diagnosis of a regular wide-complex tachycardia (Fig. 4-12, p. 66) [3]. A diagnosis of VT is made when an RS complex cannot be identified in any precordial lead. If one is present and the R–S interval is longer than 100 msec, the diagnosis of VT is made. If the R–S interval is shorter than 100 msec, one looks for AV dissociation. If it is present, the diagnosis is VT. If it is absent, morphology criteria are analyzed in V_1 and V_6. In patients with a RBBB-like QRS, the diagnosis of VT is favored by a monophasic R, QR, or R–S in V_1 and R–S less than 1, QS or QR in V_6. In both cases a triphasic complex favors SVT. In patients with an LBBB-like QRS, the diagnosis of VT is favored by R greater than 30 msec or more than 60 msec to nadir S, or a notched S in V_1 or V_2. In V_6 a QR or QS favors VT. If both leads fulfill the criteria for VT, the diagnosis is established; otherwise the diagnosis is likely supraventricular tachycardia with aberration.

Table 4-5. Hallmarks of aberration

Preceding P' wave
RBBB pattern
Triphasic contour in lead V_1 (rsR') and V_6 (qRs)
Initial vector identical with that of flanking conducted beats
Second beat in a group

RBBB = right bundle branch block.
Source: From HJL Marriott, *Practical Electrocardiography* (5th ed). Baltimore: Williams & Wilkins, 1972. P. 178. © 1972, the Williams & Wilkins Co., Baltimore.

Table 4-6. Criteria for ventricular origin of tachycardia

QRS >140 msec
Left axis deviation
Certain configurational characteristics of QRS
Atrioventricular dissociation

Source: From HJJ Wellens, FWHM Bar, KI Lie, The value of the electrocardiogram in the differential diagnosis of a tachycardia with a widened QRS complex. *Am J Med* 64:27–33, 1978.

For patients with Wolff-Parkinson-White syndrome, the location of the accessory pathway may be ascertained by review of the QRS morphology and the delta wave.

The old classification into type A and type B is outdated. Originally it was based on a positive R in V_1 for left-sided pathways and a negative R in V_1 for right-sided pathways. As can be seen from Fig. 4-13 (p. 67), the multiple locations of pathways make this scheme an oversimplification. Fananapazir and colleagues based this map on morphologic criteria of the delta wave and QRS complex obtained at the time of surgery for patients with preexcitation [4]. Furthermore, they identified a combination of findings during atrial fibrillation, rapid atrial pacing, and endocardial mapping that identified patients with multiple accessory pathways. In patients with posteroseptal plus right-free-wall accessory pathways, 75% had markedly negative delta waves in leads II, III and aVF and a QS or rS pattern in leads V_1 through V_6. Half of patients with left lateral and left anterior accessory pathways had positive delta waves in leads II, III, and aVF, a negative delta wave in aVL, an rR pattern in V_1, and an R pattern in V_2 through V_6.

Arruda et al. described another scheme based on the results of mapping and ablation (Fig. 4-14, p. 68) [5].

If the delta wave in lead I is isoelectric or negative, or if R/S ratio is greater than 1 in V_1, the pathway is on the left free wall. Then if the delta wave in aVF is positive,

Table 4-7. Electrocardiographic clues in wide-complex tachycardia

Mean QRS axis in the frontal plane during tachycardia

	$<-30°$	$-30°\geqslant -<+90°$	$\geqslant +90°$	Undetermined
Ectopy				
LBBB configuration	15	6	4	
RBBB configuration	33	2	8	2
Aberrant				
LBBB configuration	3	19		
RBBB configuration	2	14	30	2

Configuration of right bundle branch block–shaped QRS complexes in lead V_1 during tachycardia

Type complex		QRS configuration in lead V_1	
		Aberrant	Ventricular tachycardia
1	⋀	·	12
2	⋀	7	9
3	⋀	12	2
4	⋀	28	2
5	⋀		4
6	⋀	1	12
7	⋁		4
		48	45

Table 4-7 (continued)

Configuration of right bundle branch block–shaped QRS complexes in lead V$_6$ during tachycardia

Type complex		Aberrant	Ventricular tachycardia
1		31	2
2		15	10
3		2	18
4			11
5			3
6			1
		48	45

Configuration in lead V$_6$ in patients with left bundle branch block–shaped QRS complexes during tachycardia

Type complex		Aberrant	Ventricular tachycardia
1		10	11
2		12	10
3		—	3
4		—	1
		22	25

LBBB = left bundle branch block; RBBB = right bundle branch block.
Source: From HJJ Wellens, FWHM Bar, KI Lie, The value of the electrocardiogram in the differential diagnosis of a tachycardia with a widened QRS complex. *Am J Med* 64:27–33, 1978.

the location is left lateral or anterolateral. But if the delta wave in aVF is equivocal or negative, the location is left posterior or left posterolateral.

If the delta wave in lead II is negative, the location of the accessory pathway is at the coronary sinus or middle cardiac vein.

If the delta wave in lead V$_1$ is equivocal or negative, the location of the accessory pathway is septal. Then if the delta wave in aVF is positive and the QRS axis is over 0, the location is anteroseptal. But if the delta wave in lead aVF is positive and the QRS axis is below 0, the location is midseptal. If the delta wave in aVF is equivocal, the location is left posteroseptal. If the delta wave in aVF is negative, the location is right posteroseptal.

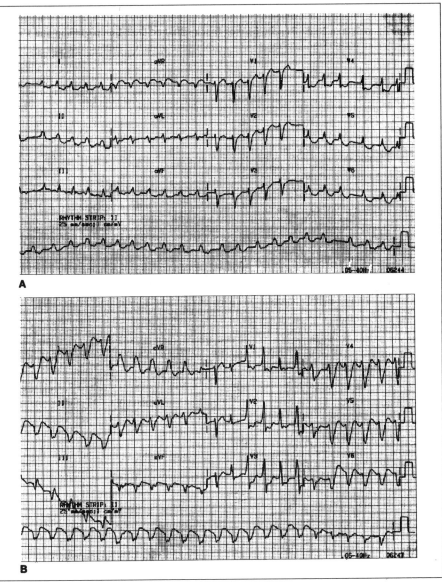

Fig. 4-11. A. Atrial fibrillation with a rapid ventricular response. Note the intraventricular conduction delay. **B.** When the patient later developed a symptomatic wide-complex tachycardia, the QRS interval and QRS axis changed dramatically. The rhythm is now ventricular tachycardia.

    In the remaining cases, the location is right free wall. If the delta waves in aVF and II are positive, the location is right anterolateral, right anterior paraseptal, or right anterolateral. If the delta wave in aVF is equivocal and the delta wave in II is positive, the location is right lateral. If the delta waves in both aVF and II are equivocal, the location is right posterior or right posterolateral.

   C. QRS axis. Normally, the QRS axis ranges between −30 and +120 degrees. Pathologic deviation of the axis leftward ranges between −30 and −90 degrees and rightward +120 and +180 degrees. The segment from +180 to −90 degrees (or northwest axis) may result from severe left or right axis deviation. With normal conduction, the cardiac impulse is transmitted down the septum and fans out to both ventricles

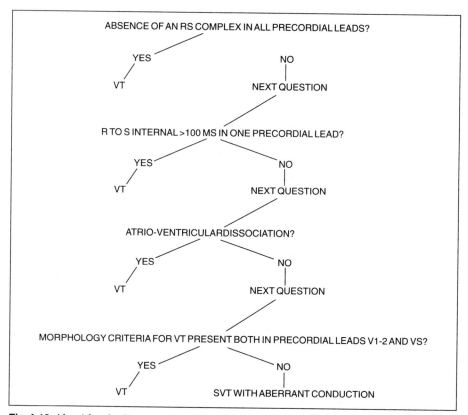

ABSENCE OF AN RS COMPLEX IN ALL PRECORDIAL LEADS?

YES — VT

NO — NEXT QUESTION

R TO S INTERNAL >100 MS IN ONE PRECORDIAL LEAD?

YES — VT

NO — NEXT QUESTION

ATRIO-VENTRICULAR DISSOCIATION?

YES — VT

NO — NEXT QUESTION

MORPHOLOGY CRITERIA FOR VT PRESENT BOTH IN PRECORDIAL LEADS V1-2 AND VS?

YES — VT

NO — SVT WITH ABERRANT CONDUCTION

Fig. 4-12. Algorithm for diagnosis of a tachycardia with a widened QRS complex. (From P Brugada, et al., A new approach to the differential diagnosis of a regular tachycardia with a wide QRS complex. *Circulation* 83:1651, 1991. Reprinted with permission.)

simultaneously. With bundle branch block or VT, the impulse activates one ventricle before the other, and consequently the spread of activation travels toward the second ventricle, producing an alteration in the normal axis. When activation originates in the ventricles and travels cephalad, the electrical axis is most likely to be in the upper quadrants, usually more negative than −30 degrees.

D. **P waves.** The presence of P waves may make the diagnosis clear but also can be deceiving. Often P waves may not even be apparent. Please note that a **1:1 relationship of P to QRS does not indicate the origin of the rhythm.**

For example, a 72-year-old woman with acute myocardial infarction was hypotensive with a rapid wide-complex tachycardia at a rate of 150 beats/minute. Among the prime concerns were ventricular or junctional tachycardia with retrograde conduction to the atria, atrial flutter with aberrancy, atrial tachycardia with block, atypical AV nodal reentry, and sinus tachycardia with bundle branch block. Since P waves were not seen, an intracardiac electrogram was recorded from the atria, demonstrating a 1:1 relationship of P to QRS. This finding excluded atrial flutter and atrial tachycardia with block but not the other two diagnoses. A 5-second burst of rapid atrial pacing produced a temporary increase in the tachycardia rate but maintenance of the 1:1 relationship and QRS configuration, excluding VT, one would have expected the QRS configuration to change if atrial overdrive was possible, or no change in the QRS configuration and rate with failure to capture the ventricles. With AV nodal reentry, termination of the arrhythmia or no change would have been expected. Thus, this patient had sinus tachycardia and bundle branch block, an ominous sign of severe left ventricular damage in acute myocardial infarction. The diagnosis may be established beyond doubt with advancement of the pacemaker electrode into the His position; however, this may be difficult in the coro-

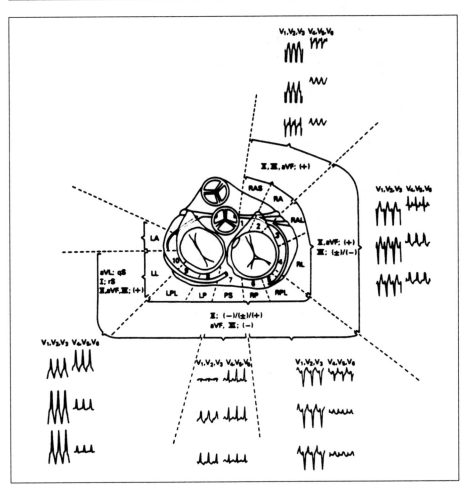

Fig. 4-13. Diagrammatic representation of 10 epicardial single accessory pathway sites mapped at surgery and six anatomic areas with distinctive electrocardiographic patterns during maximal preexcitation. (RAS/RA = right anteroseptal or right anterior accessory pathways; RAL/RL = right anterolateral or right lateral accessory pathways; RP/RPL = right posterior or right posterolateral accessory pathways; PS = posteroseptal accessory pathways; LPL/LP = left posterolateral or left posterior accessory pathways; LL = left lateral accessory pathways; + = positive delta wave; − = negative delta wave; ± = isoelectric delta wave.) (From L. Fananapazir et al., Importance of preexcited QRS morphology during induced atrial fibrillation to the diagnosis and localization of multiple accessory pathways. *Circulation* 81:580, 1990. Reprinted with permission.)

nary care unit if the procedure is done without fluoroscopy. Adequate recording instrumentation must also be available.

The clinician should always seek the **presence of P waves.** They may be hidden in the QRS complexes or ST segments. With certain arrhythmias, there may be a **characteristic pattern.** In atrial flutter there may be a sawtooth appearance to the P waves, seen best in limb leads II, III, aVF, and occasionally V$_1$ (Fig. 4-15). Often maneuvers may be necessary to establish the diagnosis. Carotid sinus massage and the Valsalva maneuver will increase vagal tone, slowing conduction at the AV node and thus decreasing the number of impulses conducted to the ventricles if the arrhythmia is not terminated. In atrial flutter, one may see a higher degree of block, sometimes varying, and the demonstration of identifiable P waves (Fig. 4-16). Often an atrial tachycardia will be abruptly interrupted.

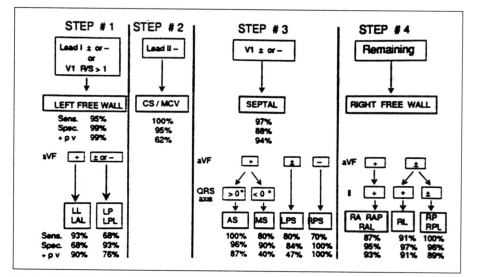

Fig. 4-14. ECG algorithm for localization of accessory pathway site. (R/S = R–S wave ratio; + = positive delta; ± = isoelectric delta; − = negative delta wave, sens = sensitivity; spec = specificity; +pv = positive predictive value; LL = left (L) lateral; LAL = L anterolateral; LP = L posterior; LPL = L posterolateral; LPS = L posteroseptal; RA = right (R) anterior; RAP = R anterior paraseptal; RAL = R anterolateral; RL = R lateral; RPL = R posterolateral; RP = R posterior; AS = R anteroseptal; MS = midseptal; RPS = R posteroseptal; CS/MCV = coronary sinus/middle cardiac vein.) (From M Arruda et al., ECG algorithm for predicting sites of successful radiofrequency ablation of accessory pathways. *PACE* 16:865, 1993. Reprinted with permission.)

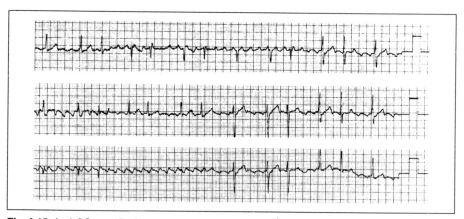

Fig. 4-15. Atrial flutter. In this case, the sawtooth pattern of flutter waves is observed in V_1 as well as II, III, and aVF. In addition, there are varying degrees of block from 2:1 to 4:1.

The **P wave axis** may be useful in determining the direction of atrial activation, but it will not always indicate the chamber of origin. For example, if a rhythm demonstrates inverted P waves in leads II, III, and aVF, it may represent a junctional or ventricular tachycardia with retrograde conduction to the atria but also may indicate an ectopic atrial focus with the origin still in the atria. The next **relationship** to evaluate is the one **between the P wave and the QRS complex**. Is it fixed, or does it vary? In some cases, careful measurement will reveal that what was thought to be a P wave was actually a T wave with a constant QRS–T interval. If in fact a P wave is present, what is the relationship to the QRS? Does it precede or follow it? With variation in the heart rate, this may become apparent. The clinician must dif-

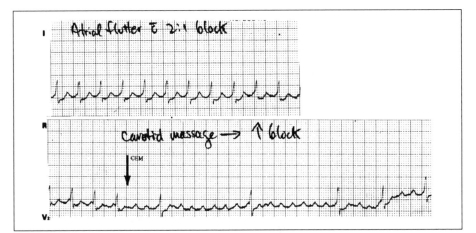

Fig. 4-16. Effect of carotid sinus massage on atrial flutter. Note increased vagal tone increasing the degree of block, clearly making the diagnosis of atrial flutter.

ferentiate between atrial activation of the lower conduction system and retrograde conduction to the atria. If the P wave seems to follow the QRS but varies in a regular fashion, is the problem a junctional tachycardia with retrograde Wenckebach block conducted to the atria? If there is an inconstant P–R interval and varying P wave morphologies, the problem may be a multifocal atrial tachycardia or chaotic atrial rhythm. Commonly, this is associated with severe lung disease. In the absence of a tachycardia, morphologically different P waves and varying P–R intervals may be related to a wandering atrial pacemaker.

E. **Atrioventricular dissociation.** Atrioventricular dissociation indicates that the rhythm controlling the ventricles does not originate in the atria. It is very important to distinguish AV dissociation from heart block. With complete heart block, the supraventricular impulses cannot penetrate into the ventricles because of conduction system disease. The ventricles then utilize a safety mechanism, an idioventricular rhythm, and there is AV dissociation. However, AV dissociation may also occur when a lower pacemaker usurps control of the heart from the atria by discharging at a faster rate. It thus becomes the dominant pacemaker of the heart, but there is no heart block. Occasionally a supraventricular impulse will find the ventricles repolarized and capture them. This impulse will be conducted with a narrow QRS (unless the patient has bundle branch block) in comparison to a wide QRS resulting from the VT. Occasionally the activation of the ventricles may occur simultaneously from a conducted supraventricular impulse and the ectopic ventricular focus to produce a **fusion beat** (Fig. 4-17). Depending on the timing, varying degrees of fusion may be observed. Thus, fusion beats are another sign of AV dissociation.

V. **Diagnosis of narrow-complex tachycardias.** Clues from the ECG become particularly important in dealing with supraventricular tachycardia since these arrhythmias most often have a prognosis that is benign in comparison to VT. The goal is to avoid invasive electrophysiologic study if possible. A group of Dutch researchers described their experience with narrow-complex tachycardias based on correlation of ECG data with electrophysiologic findings in patients referred for invasive evaluation [6].

A clinician faced with a narrow-complex tachycardia must differentiate among sinus tachycardia, ectopic atrial tachycardia, atrial flutter or fibrillation, AV nodal tachycardia, and a reciprocating tachycardia using an accessory pathway as the retrograde limb. Using five criteria (Table 4-8) in a decision-making tree analysis (Fig. 4-18), the authors were able to assess correctly 84% of arrhythmias in 57 patients by the ECG. Looking at the relationship between P and QRS, the authors found that 88% of reciprocating tachycardias had the P wave following the QRS, and 96% of AV nodal tachycardias had the P in the QRS (the majority of these had unidentifiable P waves on the surface ECG). For these two arrhythmias, the **location of the P wave** was most helpful. Analysis of the **P wave axis** showed that 100% of AV nodal tachycardias with a P wave within or behind the QRS had an inferior-superior axis (negative P in II and III). All cases of incessant atrial tachycardias using a retrograde accessory pathway had an

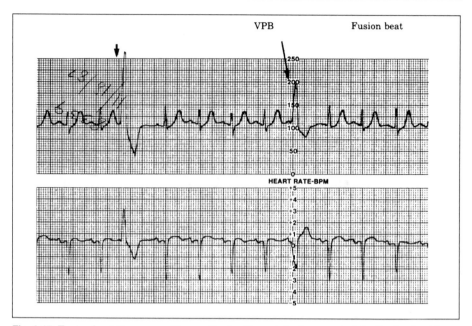

Fig. 4-17. Fusion beat (*long arrow*) in a patient with ventricular parasystole. Fusion beat has an intermediate morphology between a sinus beat and a ventricular ectopic beat.

inferior-superior axis. An intermediate axis (positive or biphasic P in II, biphasic or negative P in III) suggests circus movement tachycardia. A superior-inferior axis (positive P in II and III) suggests atrial tachycardia. **Mean atrial rate** varied: reciprocating tachycardia averaged 169 beats/minute (range 115–231); AV nodal tachycardia, 167 beats/minute (range 118–231); atrial flutter, 299 beats/minute (range 250–400); atrial tachycardia, 170 beats/minute (range 115–230); and incessant tachycardia, 146 beats/minute (range 118–194). Thus only atrial flutter can be reliably distinguished by rate. **Alternation of the QRS complex** was most common in reciprocating tachycardia (22%). **Relationship of the P to the QRS** was 1:1 in all patients with reciprocating tachycardia, AV nodal tachycardia, and incessant tachycardia; 100% of patients with atrial flutter and 30% of those with atrial tachycardia had second-degree AV block.

VI. History. Frequently, the physician examines the patient after the arrhythmia has terminated. If the arrhythmia was not documented by ECG or rhythm strip, history may be suggestive. It is important to determine the **circumstances that preceded the arrhythmia:** exercise, stress, emotion, caffeine intake, angina, hypoxia, ethanol intake, or metabolic abnormality. The answers to the following questions may aid in the diagnosis of the arrhythmia as well as the underlying cause:

Is this the **first episode?**
How often do the episodes occur?
Are the episodes paroxysmal?
How long do the episodes last?

Table 4-8. Criteria for evaluating narrow-complex tachycardia

P wave location in relation to QRS complex
Electrical axis of P wave
Atrial rate
Presence or absence of alternating changes of QRS complex
Relationship between atrial and ventricular rhythm

Source: From FW Bar et al., Differential diagnosis of tachycardia with narrow QRS complex (shorter than 0.12 second). *Am J Cardiol* 54:555–560, 1984.

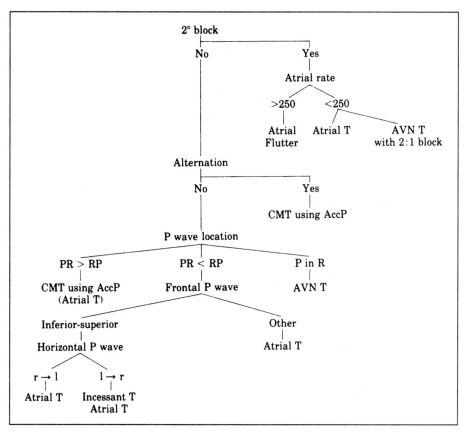

Fig. 4-18. Decision tree analysis of supraventricular narrow-complex tachycardia. (T = tachycardia; AVN = atrioventricular nodal; CMT = circus movement tachycardia; AccP = accessory pathway.) (From FW Bar et al., Differential diagnosis of tachycardia with narrow QRS complex (shorter than 0.12 second). *Am J Cardiol* 54:555–560, 1984.)

Is the patient aware of the heartbeat? Is it fast or slow, regular or irregular, or associated with "skipped beats"?

Did the episode cause palpitations, dizziness, presyncope ("brownout"), or syncope?

Was the episode witnessed? Did anyone check the patient's pulse?

How long did the period of unconsciousness last?

Did the patient note any sensation of choking, flushing, or throbbing in the neck before losing consciousness?

Did an observer note the patient's eyes to roll upward?

How was the arrhythmia terminated? Spontaneously?

Is the patient able to terminate the arrhythmia by specific maneuvers?

In addition it may be helpful to tap out a variety of rhythms and ask the patient to try to identify the most likely one involved. That only half of the patients will be aware of their heartbeat during an arrhythmia is a two-edged sword. While they may not be bothered by uncomfortable sensation, they may not be warned to seek medical attention. On the other hand, fear and anxiety over isolated premature beats (in the absence of serious heart disease) may be incapacitating.

In all patients, it is imperative to determine whether there is any serious underlying heart disease (see Chap. 8), since treatment must be directed at both arrhythmia and the cause.

VII. Physical examination. There are three particularly helpful parts of the cardiovascular examination when evaluating an arrhythmia: the intensity of the first heart sound (S1), the splitting of the second heart sound (S2), and the jugular venous pulse.

Just as with clues from the history, ECG, and arterial pulse, none is absolutely diagnostic. However, as more information is gathered, it may be possible to arrive at a probable diagnosis. It is unfortunate that a careful physical examination is quite often neglected today in favor of more sophisticated instrumentation and technology. It is quite amazing that Wenckebach in 1899 was able to describe type I second-degree AV block on the basis of the jugular venous pulsations, years before the ECG was available.

A. **Intensity of the first heart sound (S1).** The first heart sound corresponds to the closure of the AV valves, with the more intense mitral valve closure sound (M1) preceding the softer tricuspid valve closure sound (T1). The intensity of S1 depends primarily on the position of the valve at the onset of ventricular systole, as well as the rate of rise of pressure and tension in the ventricle. Certainly rheumatic scarring or other diseases may affect the mobility of the valvular leaflets and thus the intensity of S1.

If ventricular systole occurs after a short P–R interval, when the valves are still widely open, S1 will be loud as the valves snap back. With marked prolongation of the P–R interval, as occurs in first-degree AV block, the valves have time to float back to their closed position before the onset of ventricular systole, resulting in a soft S1. The compliance of the ventricle must also be accounted for, with a stiff noncompliant ventricle causing earlier closure of the AV valve.

Thus, if the P–R interval is constantly changing, as occurs in complete heart block, Wenckebach-type second-degree AV block, and junctional or ventricular tachycardia with AV dissociation, the intensity of S1 will vary. Other arrhythmias with varying times of activation between the atria and ventricles include atrial fibrillation, atrial flutter with varying block, and atrial tachycardia with varying block. Obviously, premature beats also cause variation of S1.

If the junctional or ventricular tachycardia is associated with constant retrograde conduction to the atria, the intensity of S1 will remain constant. Since the ability to appreciate how loud or soft S1 is may depend on the habitus and the presence of associated lung disease or pulmonary edema, the most useful part of this examination is to listen for **variation** in intensity.

B. **Splitting of the second heart sound (S2).** The second heart sound corresponds to closure of the semilunar valves with aortic valve closure (A2) preceding pulmonary valve closure (P2). Splitting of these two sounds corresponds to the slight asynchrony between the ventricles, as a result of slightly increased filling of the right ventricle (with longer right ventricular contraction) during inspiration.

Slow activation of the right ventricle because of RBBB or a pressure-volume overload of the right ventricle will accentuate the delay between A2 and P2, with a wider split. Shortened left ventricular ejection (as seen in wide-open mitral regurgitation) may move A2 earlier, another way to widen the split. If the right ventricle is activated before the left ventricle, as in patients with an artificial pacemaker in the right ventricle or in patients with LBBB, splitting of the second heart sound will be paradoxical, with P2 preceding A2.

Thus, activation of one ventricle before the other will cause a difference in the splitting of S2. This may occur with ventricular extrasystoles, VT, and earlier activation of one ventricle owing to aberrant conduction.

C. **Jugular venous pulse.** Examination of the jugular venous pulse allows evaluation of the mechanical activity in the right atrium. Normally right atrial systole causes an a wave with relaxation starting the x descent. As isovolumetric right ventricular contraction displaces the tricuspid valve upward, the x descent is interrupted by the c wave. As the right atrium fills during right ventricular contraction, the v wave is seen. After right ventricular systole and opening of the tricuspid valve, the v wave collapses with the y descent. Hemodynamic alterations such as tricuspid stenosis, pulmonic stenosis, and pulmonary hypertension will all transmit high pressures to the atrium, resulting in a **giant a wave.** Tricuspid regurgitation causes large, dominant v waves. Constrictive pericarditis displays a sharp, deep x descent and shorter y descent.

In atrial fibrillation, there will be no a wave because of the absence of atrial systole. **Cannon a waves** result from atrial contraction against a closed tricuspid valve and may be seen with AV dissociation. If there is retrograde conduction to the atria with junctional or ventricular tachycardia (ventricular contraction preceding atrial contraction), the cannon a waves will be constant. Otherwise the cannon a waves will be intermittent and a normal a wave seen if atrial contraction fortuitously precedes ventricular contraction. Commonly, cannon a waves are seen with ventricular extrasystoles, ventricular pacing, and complete heart block.

In atrial flutter, **flutter waves** may be seen in the jugular pulse, occurring at a rate of 300/minute and corresponding to the flutter waves on the ECG. In AV nodal tachycardia and reciprocating tachycardia using an accessory pathway, constant cannon a waves may be seen when atrial contraction occurs before the completion of the previous ventricular contraction.

Examination of the jugular pulse is difficult and impossible to interpret correctly if not performed with adequate lighting and proper positioning. Carotid pulsations must not be misinterpreted for venous pulsation. The jugular venous pulse is most useful in arrhythmias for detecting AV dissociation and noting atrial flutter.

D. **Cardiac maneuvers.** A number of cardiac maneuvers use vagal stimulation to produce slowing or termination of arrhythmias. In fact, many patients with paroxysmal AV nodal tachycardia volunteer the fact that they themselves have discovered methods to terminate their arrhythmias. Many of these are variations of the Valsalva maneuver or other ways to increase vagal tone.

1. **Valsalva maneuver.** The Valsalva maneuver is performed by expiration against a closed glottis. The patient inspires deeply, closes the mouth, and bears down. The Valsalva maneuver has four phases with specific physiologic effects. **Phase 1,** lasting 2–3 seconds, consists of an increase in intrathoracic pressure and emptying of the pulmonary veins with increased left ventricular filling. Left ventricular stroke work and systolic blood pressure increase. **Phase 2,** lasting as long as expiration continues, is associated with a reduction in systolic blood pressure and pulse pressure since there is a reduction in blood return to the heart. With the release of forced expiration, **phase 3** begins as the flow of blood into the right side of the heart is augmented. Finally, in **phase 4,** there is an overshoot as systolic blood pressure rises above the baseline value and a reflex sinus bradycardia occurs.

   The arrhythmia that most commonly terminates with the vagal stimulation of the Valsalva maneuver is paroxysmal AV nodal tachycardia. The termination is abrupt. However, additional measures often may be required before sinus rhythm is restored. Orthodromic reciprocating tachycardia may also block with increased vagal tone. Sinus tachycardia may slow during the vagal stimulation but will resume when the maneuver is finished. Ventricular tachycardia will show no response. In patients with atrial flutter or atrial tachycardia with block, vagal stimulation increases the amount of block, sometimes quite dramatically, but does not terminate the arrhythmia. Quite often, this maneuver establishes the diagnosis as the flutter waves or P waves become apparent. With atrial fibrillation, the Valsalva maneuver may slow the ventricular response, but it returns to the prior rate after the maneuver is completed. Finally, as noted above, in some reciprocating tachycardias, vagal stimulation may also terminate the arrhythmia or have no effect.

2. **Carotid sinus massage.** Stimulation of the carotid sinus will also result in vagal stimulation but is not without hazard, particularly in older individuals with carotid artery and cerebrovascular disease. Manipulation of the carotid artery and carotid sinus may dislodge atherosclerotic debris, with distal embolization and stroke.

   The right carotid sinus should always be stimulated first since the left cerebral hemisphere is usually dominant. In addition, some believe that right carotid stimulation is generally more effective. The other major complication of carotid massage is prolonged high-degree block, asystole, and death. Thus this is not a maneuver that one performs without caution and certainly not one to be recommended as self-therapy by the patient.

   After auscultation to exclude carotid bruits, the right carotid artery is palpated at its bifurcation just under the angle of the jaw. Gentle pressure is applied initially to make certain the patient does not have a hypersensitive carotid sinus. Pressure is then applied firmly with the index and middle fingers (sometimes also the fourth finger) with a massaging action for no longer than 4 seconds while simultaneously assessing the response of the arrhythmia. The stimulation may have to be repeated five or six times before abrupt conversion of the arrhythmia. Often simultaneous Valsalva maneuver with carotid sinus massage may be more effective than either alone.

   Again, the most likely maneuver to respond to carotid sinus massage is an AV nodal tachycardia. Sinus tachycardia and atrial fibrillation may temporarily have a slower ventricular response. Atrial flutter and atrial tachycardia with block will have a higher degree of block (see Fig. 4-16). VT will not respond.

3. **Other vagal maneuvers.** A number of other vagal maneuvers may also terminate arrhythmias. Eyeball pressure has been described but should be discouraged because of a possibility of injury to the eye, and other more effective measures are available. Less drastic measures that patients may describe as effective include drinking ice water, facial immersion in ice water, inducing gagging or vomiting by inserting a finger in the throat, or coughing.

The caveat regarding potential life-threatening complications of vagal stimulation deserves repetition. Since high-degree AV block and asystole may occur, precautions should be taken before performing the maneuvers. These precautions include intravenous (IV) access to administer medications such as atropine, lidocaine, or epinephrine; availability of a crash cart (including defibrillator, temporary pacemaker, and drugs as necessary); and continuous ECG monitoring.

VIII. **Response to specific drugs.** Specific pharmacologic therapy for specific arrhythmias is discussed separately. Nevertheless, here I discuss the response to verapamil and adenosine in patients with supraventricular tachycardias, as this may allow differentiation.

Verapamil, a calcium antagonist with a negative dromotropic effect, acts at the AV node (and the sinoatrial node) since it consists of calcium-channel-dependent pacemaker cells. Adenosine is an endogenous nucleoside that slows conduction time through the AV node. Since IV adenosine has become available, it has become the drug of choice for atrioventricular nodal tachycardia, replacing verapamil, propranolol, digoxin, edrophonium, or sympathomimetic infusion as first-line therapy. If the arrhythmia is indeed AV nodal tachycardia, 6–12 mg of IV adenosine will restore sinus rhythm in the majority of cases. If the rhythm is atrial fibrillation, adenosine will slow the ventricular response, but the rhythm almost always will remain atrial fibrillation. If the rhythm is atrial flutter, adenosine will increase the AV block. With both of these arrhythmias, the underlying fibrillatory or flutter waves will become more apparent as the ventricular response slows. Intravenous adenosine, as with IV verapamil, should be administered only in a setting that has the capability for temporary pacing, as asystole has been rarely observed.

Short-acting beta blockers such as propranolol will slow the ventricular response in atrial fibrillation and atrial flutter but do not have as potent an effect at the AV node as adenosine or verapamil. Propranolol may terminate some cases of AVnodal tachycardia. Digoxin quite often converts atrial flutter to sinus rhythm; however, this is a therapeutic maneuver and not a diagnostic one. Atrial fibrillation may revert to sinus rhythm after digoxin has slowed the ventricular response. Lidocaine is used to suppress VT. In the situation of atrial fibrillation with a wide-complex tachycardia and rapid rate (>250 beats/minute), restoration of normal conduction by IV lidocaine is good evidence for an accessory pathway (Wolff-Parkinson-White syndrome).

IX. **Additional electrocardiographic diagnostic tests**
   A. **Lewis leads.** When P waves are not apparent with the 12 standard ECG leads, exploring electrodes on the chest may allow distinction in certain cases. Although this technique does not always produce definitive results, it is noninvasive, is easy to perform, and takes less than 10 minutes. Since an ECG is performed anyway, it is simple to take two bipolar leads (for example, the left arm electrode and the right arm electrode, both of which result in limb lead I) and explore the precordium. The two electrodes are moved to different positions on the chest, and lead I is monitored for the appearance of P waves. If they appear, further manipulation may increase their size. If this technique is successful, it may aid in the diagnosis of supraventricular arrhythmias.
   B. **Esophageal electrodes.** Placement of an electrode in the esophagus behind the heart may permit the recording of P waves because of the proximity to the atria. Its disadvantage is that of the placement of a nasogastric tube. Optimal atrial recordings are obtained 40–50 cm from the nares. Special esophageal electrodes are available. When the electrode is in position and the ECG is being recorded, the electrode may be withdrawn to find the largest P waves (Fig. 4-19). With current technology, it is also possible to pace the atria through the esophagus and terminate arrhythmias.
   C. **Intraatrial electrode.** Direct recording from inside the atrium is one of the most accurate ways to record atrial activity, but it has the disadvantage of being invasive. It requires insertion of a temporary pacing electrode into a peripheral or central vein with advancement to the right atrium. If insertion is not being performed under fluoroscopy, the electrode should be connected to the ECG and constantly monitored for the appearance of a large atrial deflection. Connection of the electrode to the V lead of the ECG will provide a unipolar tracing. A better recording is obtained with a

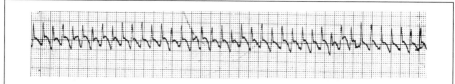

Fig. 4-19. Bipolar atrial electrogram recorded from an esophageal electrode revealing atrial flutter with a flutter rate of 300 beats/minute.

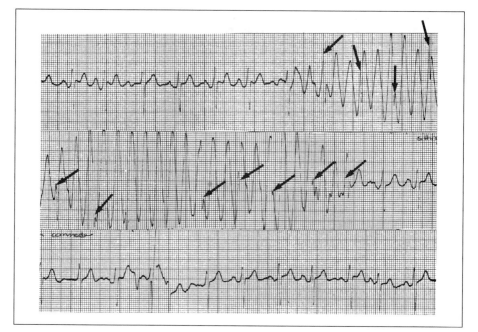

Fig. 4-20. Artifact simulating ventricular tachycardia. While at first glance the rhythm appears to be ventricular tachycardia, careful examination of the ECG reveals the remnants of the QRS complex (*arrows*) within the wide-complex tachycardia. The wide complexes are artifactual, and were caused by mechanical interference.

bipolar connection. This can easily be accomplished by connecting the two electrodes on the pacemaker to the right and left arm electrodes with alligator clips and monitoring standard lead I. After the diagnosis is made, the pacemaker may be used to terminate the arrhythmia, if possible and when appropriate. Care must be taken to avoid misplacing the pacing electrode into the ventricle and attempting overdrive pacing of the atrium.

In the electrophysiology laboratory, the pacing electrode may be advanced across the tricuspid valve to record the His potential. However, this requires specialized instrumentation for amplification and modification of the signal, as is discussed subsequently.

D. **Direct atrial recording.** The patient who has undergone open heart surgery almost always has pacing electrodes in both the atria and the ventricles that protrude through the chest wall. These epicardial wire electrodes are easily applied at the time of surgery and easily removed before discharge. They provide a safety factor for the patient if pacing is required and diagnostic ease if an arrhythmia develops.

As with the intraatrial electrogram, bipolar recordings provide a better image because they record the activity of a small area with electrodes close to each other; the unipolar electrogram encompasses a large area with electrodes far apart. Thus, when recording a bipolar atrial electrogram, it is easier to distinguish atrial activity from ventricular activity (see Chap. 6).

The connections to the ECG are as described previously. The right arm and left arm electrodes are connected to the atrial wires with alligator clips. (The leg electrodes are as usual.) Standard lead I is recorded in a bipolar fashion. If a unipolar electrogram is desired, lead II or III can be recorded without changing the leads. Once the diagnosis has been made, overdrive pacing may be performed through the same electrodes when appropriate.

X. Summary. The clinician must utilize all the clues available to make the diagnosis of the arrhythmia. He or she must:

1. Determine if the patient is hemodynamically compromised and whether the arrhythmia is responsible.
2. Review the ECG with attention to rate; regularity; QRS axis, width, and morphology; AV dissociation; and P waves (Fig. 4-20).
3. Review the history and physical examination.
4. Examine the response to cardiac maneuvers and drugs and the use of specialized electrode techniques to confirm the diagnosis.

Although none of these steps alone may be diagnostic, all of them together should allow narrowing the differential diagnosis to one or two possibilities. For the enigmatic case, invasive electrophysiologic evaluation may be necessary.

References

1. Marriott HJL. *Workshop in Electrocardiography* (1st ed). Oldsmar, FL: Tampa Tracings, 1972.
2. Wellens HJJ, Bar FWHM, Lie KI. The value of the electrocardiogram in the differential diagnosis of a tachycardia with a widened QRS complex. *Am J Med* 64:27–33, 1978.
3. Brugada P, et al. A new approach to the differential diagnosis of a regular tachycardia with a wide QRS Complex. *Circulation* 83:1649–1659, 1991.
4. Fananapazir L, et al. Importance of preexcited QRS morphology during induced atrial fibrillation to the diagnosis and localization of multiple accessory pathways. *Circulation* 81:578–585, 1990.
5. Arruda M, et al. ECG algorithm for predicting sites of successful radiofrequency ablation of accessory pathways. *PACE* 16:865, 1993.
6. Bar FW, et al. Differential diagnosis of tachycardia with narrow QRS complex (shorter than 0.12 second). *Am J Cardiol* 54:555–560, 1984.

Bibliography

Constant J. *Bedside Cardiology* (4th ed). Boston: Little, Brown, 1993.

Harvey WP, Ronan JA. Bedside diagnosis of arrhythmias. *Prog Cardiovasc Dis* 8:419–445, 1966.

Ronan JA, Gordon MS. Jugular venous pulse. *Cardiol Pract* 1:103–112, 1984.

Strobeck JE. Approach to the patient with cardiac disease: The physical examination. *Cardiovasc Rev Rep* 1:70–84, 1980.

Tavel ME. *Clinical Phonocardiography and External Pulse Recording* (4th ed). Chicago: Year Book, 1985.

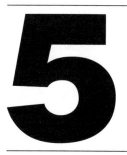

Syncope

Stephen C. Vlay

The evaluation of syncope is a common referral to the internist or cardiologist. A vast variety of conditions may result in syncope. Table 5-1 delineates the most common causes, starting with the noncardiac etiologies, for it is these that the physician must first exclude before referring the patient to the electrophysiologist. This chapter briefly describes the noncardiac causes of syncope and reviews the indications for evaluation of cardiac causes.

I. Noncardiac causes
A. Cerebrovascular disorders.
Altered consciousness may be seen with a wide variety of cerebrovascular conditions. Perhaps the most common is a seizure, which may result from a variety of disorders. Seizure disorders are documented by their appearance, their sequelae, and their characteristic appearance on electroencephalogram.

Interruption of cerebral blood flow, resulting in a cerebrovascular accident or transient ischemic attack (if the signs and symptoms resolve within 24 hours), is usually accompanied by classic neurologic signs including hemiplegia, hemiparesis, abnormal reflexes, and visual disturbances but not usually syncope. The diagnosis is confirmed by radiographic findings on CT or MRI scans. Vertebrobasilar insufficiency usually results in dizziness and rarely may result in syncope.
B. Carotid disease.
Carotid disease usually involves atherosclerotic narrowing of the carotid arteries, sometimes associated with an ulcerated plaque, which can serve as the nidus for platelet and fibrin clot. As a result of progressive stenosis or thromboembolus, cerebrovascular blood flow is impaired, and the patient may suffer transient loss of consciousness (usually severe disease of both carotid arteries).
C. Hemorrhagic.
Acute blood loss results in loss of both volume and the oxygen-carrying capacity of hemoglobin and may cause syncope or near syncope. Chronic blood loss is most likely to cause fatigue but may also result in syncope if the patient performs strenuous activity. The syncopal patient must be evaluated for any source of blood loss.
D. Metabolic.
A variety of metabolic conditions may result in syncope. In patients with diabetes, insulin shock due to hypoglycemia most commonly results from alteration in baseline condition and a dose of insulin higher than necessary. Diabetic ketoacidosis resulting in loss of consciousness is often associated with an intercurrent illness or stress that dramatically increases insulin requirements.

Other endocrine disturbances may also cause varying degrees of weakness, fatigue, and sometimes loss of consciousness. Adrenal insufficiency and severe hypothyroidism have characteristic findings.

Hypoxia due to a variety of pathophysiologic states may result in altered mental status. Massive pulmonary embolus may result in hemodynamic embarrassment in addition to hypoxia and cause syncope.
E. Drug induced.
The most common drugs involved with syncope are alcohol and recreational pharmaceuticals. Use of these drugs can result in accidents, permanent injuries, and death, particularly if the user is operating a motor vehicle or machinery. The signs and symptoms are known only too well.

Among prescribed medications, insulin has already been mentioned, with an excess causing hypoglycemia. Vasodilators and other antihypertensive agents may lower blood pressure sufficiently to cause loss of consciousness. Similarly, drugs with negative chronotropic or dromotropic effects may cause bradyarrhythmias. Certain antiarrhythmic drugs may actually cause arrhythmias (a proarrhythmic effect) and lead to loss of consciousness.

Table 5-1. Differential diagnosis of syncope

Noncardiac causes
Cerebrovascular
    Seizure disorder
    Rarely cerebrovascular accident or transient ischemic attack
    Narcolepsy
    Other neurologic disorder, including hydrocephalus
Carotid disease (usually bilateral and severe)
    Stenosis
    Ulceration plus thrombus
Hemorrhagic
Metabolic
    Diabetes mellitus
    Adrenal insufficiency
    Hypoxic (e.g., pulmonary embolus)
Drug induced
    Ethanol
    Recreational drugs
    Insulin
    Vasodilators
    Proarrhythmic effects of cardiovascular drugs
    Bradyarrhythmias due to cardiovascular drugs
Psychogenic
    Hyperventilation (hypocapnia)
    Hysteria and panic attacks
Reflex related
    Vasovagal
    Cardioneurogenic
    Carotid sinus hypersensitivity
    Micturition and defecation syncope
    Postural hypotension
    Tussive syncope
Orthostatic hypotension
    Dysautonomic syndromes (e.g., Shy-Drager)
    Drug induced
Pulmonary hypertension

Cardiac causes
Arrhythmia
    Tachyarrhythmia
    Bradyarrhythmia
    Conduction disturbance
    Pacemaker malfunction
Mechanical
    Valvular
        Aortic stenosis
        Mitral stenosis
    Hypertrophic obstructive cardiomyopathy
    Myxoma
    Pericardial tamponade

A careful history is essential. Furthermore, it is wise to save an extra tube of blood when evaluating a patient brought to the emergency room for evaluation of syncope since recognition of drug use or abuse may not always be immediately apparent.

F. Psychogenic. There are a multitude of behavioral and recognized psychiatric disturbances in which the patient will feign loss of consciousness. It is imperative to make the correct diagnosis so that an extensive medical evaluation is not undertaken.

Hyperventilation syndromes may also result in syncope, and these may be easier to deal with than major psychiatric problems since these patients are able to recognize the preceding signs of hyperventilation (e.g., circumoral hyperesthesias, rapid breathing) and modify their behavior.

G. Reflex related. A variety of reflexes may result in syncope. Most are related to peripheral vasodilation and/or bradyarrhythmias. The most common is vasovagal syncope, in which the patient may experience fear or pain resulting in stimulation of the vagus nerve, causing venous pooling and bradyarrhythmias, resulting in loss of consciousness.

Cardioneurogenic syncope is a term that characterizes the physiologic triggers and events that result in syncope. The subject has recently been extensively reviewed by Rubin et al. [1]. Triggers may be emotional, mechanical, painful, or thermal stimuli that activate the afferent limb of a reflex arc. The site of central input is the nucleus tractus solitarius in the medulla, but other higher cortical centers may also contribute. The efferent limb results from the imbalance of sympathetic and parasympathetic neural tone.

Normally when an individual stands, venous pooling occurs, reducing preload and cardiac output, with less distention of the aortic arch and carotid sinus baroreceptors. As a result, vagal afferent tone diminishes, allowing sympathetic efferent signals to predominate. Systemic vascular resistance, heart rate, and inotropy increase. Diastolic blood pressure increases, systolic decreases slightly, and mean arterial blood pressure is unchanged.

In patients with cardioneurogenic syncope, the reduction in preload is followed by a dramatically increased catecholamine response and hypercontractile state. As a result, mechanoreceptor C fibers located in the inferoposterior wall of the left ventricle receive excess stimulation and produce an excessive afferent response carried over the vagus and glossopharyngeal nerves. The sympathetic efferent neural traffic is overwhelmed. Clinically, inappropriate vasodilatation occurs and causes a fall in blood pressure. Accompanying physical symptoms include nausea, diaphoresis, pallor, and blurred vision. Tilt-table testing (see **III**) may be particularly helpful for the diagnosis of this condition (Fig. 5-1). Drugs that have demonstrated the most utility for the treatment of neurocardiogenic syncope include **beta blockers** (block catecholamine effects, which decrease stimulation of C fibers) and **disopyramide** (anticholinergic and negative inotropic effects). Some other agents that have been used with varying degrees of success include **scopolamine** (vagolytic activity), **theophylline** (potential inhibition of adenosine-mediated hypotension and bradyarrhythmia), **ephedrine** (alpha agonist), and rarely **hydrofluorocortisone** (mineralocorticoid properties). The other direct and indirect effects of these agents limit their application and tolerability in the majority of patients. An antidepressant, **fluoxetine,** may help some patients, but most physicians would hesitate to use this drug unless the patient had a specific indication for treatment of depression.

Nonpharmacologic measures include adequate hydration, support stockings, and rarely cardiac pacing. Pacing may prevent the profound bradycardia but will not correct the fall in blood pressure. If pacing is to be used, a dual chamber pacemaker is the best choice.

Carotid sinus hypersensitivity is a condition in which there is extreme sensitivity of the carotid baroreceptors. Even mild pressure (e.g., caused by a tight necktie or turning the neck suddenly) may cause reflex activity, pooling venous blood and decreasing the return to heart.

Micturition syncope is not uncommon in older men. Some of these patients may also have postural hypotension. It is the result of reflex stimulation (possibly even a cardioinhibitive reflux related to bladder tone) as well as hypovolemia.

Tussive syncope is similar in that vigorous coughing results in multiple stimuli (including increased intracranial pressure during coughing resulting in reduced cerebral blood flow and reflex cardiac slowing). Many of these patients have chronic lung disease.

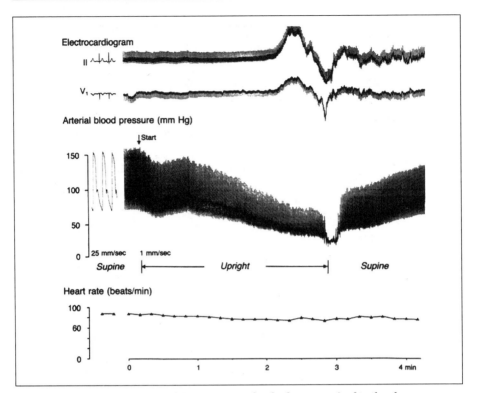

Fig. 5-1. A 72-year-old woman with breast cancer that had metastasized to the glosso-pharyngeal region had recurrent episodes of sudden lightheadedness, diaphoresis, and syncope. A dual-chamber pacemaker was implanted, but syncope recurred, always preceded by severe neck pain. During the tilt-table test with the pacemaker inactivated, the results of which are shown here, the patient's usual symptoms developed. She lost consciousness and had a seizure but regained consciousness immediately after she was returned to the supine position. The study shows a profound vasodepressor reaction with minimal slowing of the sinus rhythm. Treatment with disopyramide (150 mg 3 tid) eliminated the syncopal episodes over 5 months of follow-up. (From S Oswald, TG Trouton, *N Engl J Med* 329:30, 1993. Reprinted with permission.)

    H. Orthostatic hypotension. Postural hypotension and orthostatic hypotension refer to abrupt change in position, affecting the venous return to the heart. When the individual arises quickly, the blood pools and the patient feels lightheaded or faints. Vasodilator drugs exacerbate this type of response.

    I. Pulmonary hypertension. Pulmonary hypertension occasionally is associated with syncope. With exertion, the pulmonary artery may dilate, causing a vagally medi-ated bradycardia and fall in peripheral vascular tone.

II. Cardiac causes. The two major causes of cardiac syncope are mechanical and arrhyth-mia.

    A. Mechanical causes. Mechanical obstruction to forward cardiac flow is a problem that cannot be treated medically. Aortic stenosis, mitral stenosis, and atrial myxo-ma require definitive surgical therapy. Hypertrophic cardiomyopathy is sometimes treated surgically but more often responds to medical management with negative inotropic, chronotropic, and lusiotropic (effect on relaxation) drugs, as well as per-manent pacing (right ventricle activated first, paradoxical septal motion).

    B. Arrhythmias. Arrhythmias are the main focus of this book. If noncardiac causes have been excluded in the evaluation of syncope, the physician must consider tachy-arrhythmia, bradyarrhythmia, conduction disturbance (and permanent pacemaker malfunction if implanted). The process of evaluation is described in the appropriate chapters.

III. **Tilt-table testing.** An important tool in the diagnosis of syncope is tilt-table testing. In patients who have cardioneurogenic syncope, the head-up tilt test may provoke syncope and reproduce the patient's symptoms. The test is noninvasive, widely available, and reproducible. In patients with an abnormal test, medications can be administered and the test repeated. Medications that have been found useful act by interfering with the reflex stimulation described in **I.G.** Four protocols from different centers are provided (Tables 5-2 through 5-5).

Table 5-2. Tilt-table testing protocol 1

Multistage
1. 4–8-hour fast
2. Preparation
    Comfortable table with support for patient
    Intravenous access
    BP and HR monitoring
3. Administration of fluids and drugs
    Stage I: IV D5W: 5 min supine, 10 min 80 degree head up; terminate test if syncope
    Stage II: Isoproterenol 2 μg/min for 5 min while supine; isoproterenol 2 μg/min for 5 min at 80 degree head up; terminate test if syncope, continue for 10 min if only presyncope
    Stage III: Isoproterenol 5 μg/min for 5 min while supine; isoproterenol 5 μg/min for 10 min at 80 degree head-up tilt
4. Record HR, BP, and symptoms

Single stage
1. Steps 1–3 as for multistage protocol
2. Administration of fluids and drugs: isoproterenol 5 μg/min for 5 min while supine, isoproterenol 5 μg/min for 10 min at 80 degree head-up tilt; terminate test if syncope

Criteria for a positive test
1. Symptoms of syncope or presyncope
2. HR − BP product criteria: HR × BP ≤ 9000 mm Hg/min

HR = heart rate; IV = intravenous; D5W = 5% dextrose in water.
Source: Adapted from R Sheldon, Evaluation of a single-stage isoproterenol tilt-table test in patients with syncope. *JACC* 22:114–118, 1993.

Table 5-3. Tilt-table testing protocol 2

Protocol
Part I
    Overnight fast
    Supine for 5 min, obtain ECG
    Head-up tilt at 60–80 degrees for 10–60 min (positive yield is lower if the tilt angle is < 60 degrees)
    Measure HR and BP q2 min
Part II: Drug administration
    Isoproterenol, 1 μg/min with baseline measurements; isoproterenol 5 μg/min with head-up tilt

Interpretation of responses
Normal response
    HR increase 10–15 beats
    Diastolic BP increase of 5–10 mm Hg
    No change in systolic BP
Asymptomatic but abnormal response
    Heart rate increase 20 beats
    Absent chronotropic response
    Autonomic dysfunction
        Diastolic BP decrease
        No change in HR

Table 5-3 (continued)

Symptomatic and abnormal
   HR decrease
   BP decrease
   Hypotension precedes bradycardia, *or* hypotension without bradycardia, *or*
      autonomic dysfunction (diastolic BP decrease followed by systolic BP decrease)
Specificity
   Abnormal head-up tilt in asymptomatic patient: 6%
   Abnormal head-up tilt with isoproterenol: 11%
   Reproducibility

HR = heart rate.
Source: Adapted from AM Rubin, et al., The head-up tilt table test and cardiovascular neurogenic syncope. *Am Heart J* 125:476–482, 1993.

Table 5-4. Tilt-table testing protocol 3

Baseline measurements

Procedure
1. Head-up tilt (HUT) at 80 degrees for 30 min, with no medications
2. If nondiagnostic, administer isoproterenol until response: Isoproterenol 1 µg/min for 10 min at 80 degree HUT; isoproterenol 3 µg/min for 10 min at 80 degree HUT; isoproterenol 5 µg/min for 10 min at 80 degree HUT

Interpretation

Source: Adapted from DG Benditt, et al., Tilt table testing for evaluation of neurally-mediated (cardioneurogenic) syncope: Rationale and proposed protocols. *PACE* 14:1528–1537, 1991.

Table 5-5. Tilt-table testing protocol at University Hospital at Stony Brook

Preparation
4–8-hr fast
Intravenous (IV) access
Cardiac monitoring
BP monitoring

Procedure
Stage I
   IV D5W
   5 min supine
   10 min 80 degree head-up tilt
   Terminate test if syncope; if not go to stage II
Stage II
   Isoproterenol 5 µg/min
   5 min supine
   10 min 80 degree head-up tilt
   Terminate test if syncope or after 10 min

Criteria for a positive test
Syncope or near syncope
HR − BP product ≤ 9000 mm Hg/min
HR and/or BP decrease

Criteria for autonomic dysfunction
Decrease in diastolic BP (+/− decrease in systolic BP)
Absence of change in HR

Other abnormal responses
Absent heart response
Marked increase in HR

HR = heart rate.

Reference

1. Rubin AM, et al. The head-up tilt table test and cardiovascular neurogenic syncope. *Am Heart J* 125:476–482, 1993.

Bibliography

Almquist A, et al. Provocation of bradycardia and hypotension by isoproterenol and upright position in patients with unexplained syncope. *N Engl J Med* 320:346–351, 1989.

Bachinsky WB, et al. Usefulness of clinical characteristics in predicting the outcome of electrophysiologic studies in unexplained syncope. *Am J Cardiol* 69:1044–1049, 1992.

Barron SA, Rogovski Z, Hemli Y. Vagal cardiovascular reflexes in young persons with syncope. *Ann Intern Med* 118:943–946, 1993.

Benditt DG, et al. Tilt table testing for evaluation of neurally-mediated (cardioneurogenic) syncope: Rationale and proposed protocols. *PACE* 14:1528–1537, 1991.

Benditt DG, et al. Syncope: Causes, clinical evaluation, and current therapy. *Annu Rev Med* 43:283–300, 1992.

Brignole M, et al. A controlled trial of acute and long-term medical therapy in tilt-induced neurally mediated syncope. *Am J Cardiol* 70:339–342, 1992.

Brooks R, et al. Prospective evaluation of day-to-day reproducibility of upright tilt-table testing in unexplained syncope. *Am J Cardiol* 71:1289–1292, 1993.

Fitzpatrick AP, et al. Methodology of head-up tilt testing in patients with unexplained syncope. *JACC* 17:125–130, 1991.

Goldstein DS, et al. Circulatory control mechanisms in vasodepressor syncope. *Am Heart J* 104:1071–1075, 1982.

Grubb BP, et al. Head-upright tilt-table testing in evaluation and management of the malignant vasovagal syndrome. *Am J Cardiol* 69:904–908, 1992.

Krol RB, et al. Electrophysiologic testing in patients with unexplained syncope: Clinical and noninvasive predictors of outcome. *JACC* 10:358–363, 1987.

Lipsitz LA. Syncope in the elderly. *Ann Intern Med* 99:92–105, 1983.

Middlekauff HR, Stevenson WG, Saxon LA. Prognosis after syncope: Impact of left ventricular function. *Am Heart J* 125:121–127, 1993.

Milstein S, et al. Usefulness of disopyramide for prevention of upright tilt-induced hypotension-bradycardia. *Am J Cardiol* 65:1339–1344, 1990.

Patel A, Maloney A, Damato AN. On the frequency and reproducibility of orthostatic blood pressure changes in healthy community-dwelling elderly during 60-degree head-up tilt. *Am Heart J* 126:184–188, 1993.

Raviele A, et al. Usefulness of head-up tilt test in evaluating patients with syncope of unknown origin and negative electrophysiologic study. *Am J Cardiol* 65:1322–1327, 1990.

Sheldon R. Evaluation of a single-stage isoproterenol tilt-table test in patients with syncope. *JACC* 22:114–118, 1993.

Sra JA, et al. Unexplained syncope evaluated by electrophysiologic studies and head-up tilt testing. *Ann Intern Med* 114:1013–1019, 1991.

Sra JS, et al. Comparison of cardiac pacing with drug therapy in the treatment of neurocardiogenic (vasovagal) syncope with bradycardia or asystole. *N Engl J Med* 328:1085–1090, 1993.

Sra JS, et al. Use of intravenous esmolol to predict efficacy of oral beta-adrenergic blocker therapy in patients with neurocardiogenic syncope. *JACC* 19:402–408, 1992.

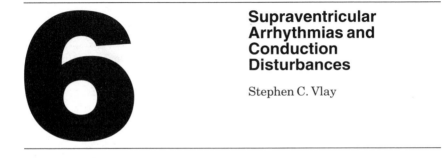

6

Supraventricular Arrhythmias and Conduction Disturbances

Stephen C. Vlay

This chapter deals with the supraventricular arrhythmias and conduction disturbances individually. It discusses diagnosis, etiology, and treatment, beginning with management of the acute arrhythmia. Note that the management reflects common practice, although not all antiarrhythmic agents have a specific indication by the Food and Drug Administration (FDA) for supraventricular arrhythmias. Among the type 1 drugs, only quinidine and flecainide have this indication with special precautions (see Chap. 14). Prevention of recurrent arrhythmias has been dramatically changed by the development of radiofrequency catheter ablation as a therapeutic option of choice once the initial arrhythmia is controlled. Finally the role of electrophysiologic testing in these cases is evaluated.

I. Supraventricular arrhythmias
A. Sinus bradycardia
1. **Features.** Sinus bradycardia is defined as a sinus rhythm with a rate below 60 beats/minute (Fig. 6-1). This rhythm is normal in the majority of cases and often reflects good cardiovascular conditioning. Drugs with a negative chronotropic effect such as beta blockers cause sinus bradycardia and represent the reason for bradycardia in many cardiac patients, for whom this is the desired effect. Thus, this finding requires no therapy, and the medication should not be discontinued merely for a slow rate.

   Table 6-1 presents the leading causes of sinus bradycardia. As with any other arrhythmia, it is imperative to determine the underlying cause. If the patient has hemodynamic compromise owing to a slow heart rate and poor cardiac output, therapy must be directed at the bradycardia as well.

2. **Treatment**
   a. **Intravenous atropine.** Atropine 0.5 mg intravenous (IV) is the initial treatment for symptomatic sinus bradycardia. In this dose range, one may occasionally observe further slowing caused by stimulation of the medullary vagal nuclei. Larger doses increase the heart rate by blocking vagal effects on the sinoatrial (SA) note. The dose may be repeated as necessary at a rate of 0.5 mg IV q5min but total dosage should not exceed 1.5–2.0 mg. Remember that atropine may result in a profound tachycardia that may be detrimental, particularly in the patient with acute myocardial infarction (MI). Consequently, these patients may be better treated with temporary atrial pacing. It is the exception, however, rather than the rule, that sinus bradycardia in acute MI requires specific therapy, either atropine or pacing. It is not unreasonable to try atropine first.
   b. **Isoproterenol.** Isoproterenol, a pure beta-adrenergic agonist with potent positive chronotropic effects, is the next drug to use. It is given by infusion, 1–2 mg of isoproterenol mixed in 500 ml 5% dextrose in water (D5W) (2–4 µg/ml), and is regulated by infusion pump to produce the desired heart rate. The infusion should start at 1–2 µg/minute, although doses up to 20 µg/minute may occasionally be required.
   c. **Electrical pacing.** Electrical pacing is the third option. In an emergency, external electrical pacemakers may obviate the need for IV pacemaker insertion. If the patient cannot tolerate the associated twitching sensation, transvenous pacing may become necessary. If the only problem is a sinus bradycardia with intact atrioventricular (AV) conduction, **atrial pacing** may suffice if a stable position can be found in the right atrium. If there is a problem with atrial capture or if the patient has disease of the distal conduction system, ven-

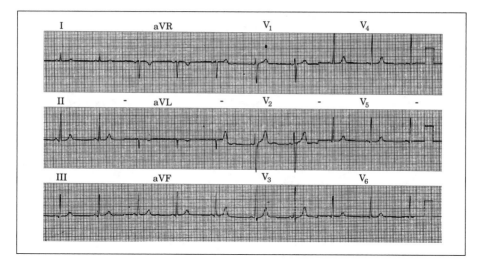

Fig. 6-1. Sinus bradycardia, rate 59 beats/minute, with an otherwise normal ECG.

Table 6-1. Causes of sinus bradycardia

1. Normal, especially during sleep
2. Cardiovascular conditioning in athlete
3. Cardiac drugs
    Beta blockers
    Calcium antagonists: Verapamil, diltiazem
    Amiodarone
4. Vagal stimulation owing to maneuvers or parasympathomimetic drugs
5. Sick sinus (tachycardia-bradycardia) syndrome
6. Myxedema (hypothyroidism)
7. Hypothermia
8. Central nervous system
    Eye surgery
    Meningitis
    Intracranial tumors
    Increased intracranial pressure
    Mental depression
9. Gram-negative sepsis
10. Neoplastic disorders
    Cervical tumors
    Mediastinal tumors
11. Vomiting
12. Myocardial infarction (MI)
13. Clonidine
14. Cimetidine
15. Reperfusion of posterior descending artery during thrombolytic therapy for acute MI

tricular pacing may be required. This has the disadvantage of the loss of atrial systole, which may contribute 15–20% of the cardiac output. Should permanent pacing become necessary, most of these patients may be candidates for dual chamber pacing.

   d. **Other drugs.** Other drugs that may cause sympathetic stimulation and reflex tachycardia, such as hydralazine, ephedrine, and nifedipine, may have some benefit in the patient who requires them as primary therapy for an associated problem. One becomes concerned, however, if the patient would be unable to take the medications in an emergency and might better be treated by pacing. Other individuals might have too rapid a heart rate with them.

   e. **Oral atropine.** Oral atropine or similar drugs such as methscopolamine bromide (2.5 mg PO q8h) have been given to some patients with bradycardia, but the effect on the heart is much less than with atropine. Again the considerations in **I.A.d** apply.

B. **Sinus tachycardia.** Sinus tachycardia is defined as a sinus rhythm with a heart rate faster than 100 beats/minute. Sinus tachycardia is a response to a stimulus, not a cause. It is imperative to determine, and direct therapy at, the underlying cause (Table 6-2). Attempts to slow the heart rate may be detrimental since the sinus tachycardia may be a physiologic response to maintain adequate cardiac output and tissue oxygenation. In fact, trials of digitalis or beta blockers may cause a greater imbalance between supply and demand at the tissue level. Digitalis may be useful, however, for the patient with congestive heart failure. Propranolol may be useful for the patient with thyrotoxicosis as specific measures for hyperthyroidism are considered.

   Often cardiology consultation for sinus tachycardia is requested. All of the causes in Table 6-2 are commonly seen by the clinician. The primary physician should exclude these possibilities first. However, when the rate of the tachycardia ranges between 150 and 180 beats/minute, other diagnoses must also be considered: atrial flutter with block, AV nodal tachycardia, ectopic atrial tachycardia, reciprocating tachycardia using an accessory bypass tract, and, in some cases, accelerated junctional or ventricular tachycardia. In these cases, cardiology consultation may be indicated.

C. **Sinus arrhythmia.** Sinus arrhythmia, one of the most common and most benign forms of arrhythmia, can be recognized by phasic variation in sinus cycle length and is usually related to changes in vagal tone. Most often the patients are young or elderly. It is frequently noted during respiration, with slow heart rates, or following an increase in vagal tone. Both drugs that enhance vagal tone (e.g., morphine, digitalis) and vagal stimulation of other organs, particularly the GI tract, may cause sinus arrhythmia.

Table 6-2. Causes of sinus tachycardia

1. Normal in infancy and early childhood
2. Sympathetic stimulation caused by emotional, exertional, or other physiologic stress
3. Anemia or hemorrhage
4. Hypoxia caused by pneumonia, pulmonary emboli, or other acute lung problem
5. Hyperthyroidism
6. Fever
7. Hypovolemia
8. Myocardial ischemia or infarction
9. Congestive heart failure
10. Shock
11. Drugs
      Sympathomimetic amines and other adrenergic agonists
      Atropine and other anticholinergic drugs
      Alcohol
      Caffeine (coffee, tea, cocoa, chocolate)
      Nicotine
12. Enhanced automaticity of sinus node

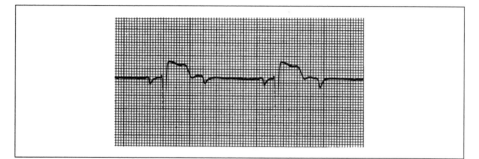

Fig. 6-2. Ventriculophasic sinus arrhythmia in the presence of complete heart block. Note that the P–QRS–P interval is shorter than the P–P interval.

Respiration may be accompanied by changes in vagal tone; with inspiration there is reflex inhibition. Thus, in sinus arrhythmia, the sinus rate increases (P–P interval shortens) with inspiration and slows (P–P interval lengthens) with expiration.

The **nonrespiratory** form of sinus arrhythmia (phasic variation unrelated to respiration) occurs most often with vagal stimulation of the GI tract and occasionally with digitalis toxicity. In some cases, an underlying cause will not be clear.

Sinus arrhythmia is benign and requires no treatment. As the heart rate increases, the phasic variation in sinus cycle length usually disappears. Rarely, some individuals may be symptomatic with sinus bradycardia and sinus arrhythmia. Here the treatment is that of symptomatic sinus bradycardia.

Finally, sinus arrhythmia may also occur in complete heart block. It is recognized by the fact that P–P intervals without an intervening QRS complex are longer than P–QRS–P intervals. This rhythm, called **ventriculophasic sinus arrhythmia,** may be related to changes in autonomic tone affected by changes in stroke volume (Fig. 6-2).

D. **Atrial fibrillation**
  1. **Features.** Atrial fibrillation is perhaps one of the most frequent arrhythmias the cardiologist and internist are asked to evaluate. The causes are listed in Table 6-3. The three main categories are (1) paroxysmal atrial fibrillation without disease of the heart or other organs, (2) paroxysmal atrial fibrillation with underlying heart disease, and (3) atrial fibrillation related to specific systemic problems. Again, as with any other arrhythmia, it is important to examine the patient for the precipitating factor and consider it in the treatment as well.

Table 6-3. Causes of atrial fibrillation and atrial flutter

1. Paroxysmal and unrelated to underlying heart or other organ disease
2. Related to underlying heart disease
   Valvular heart disease, particularly mitral stenosis and mitral regurgitation
   Hypertensive heart disease
   Cardiomyopathy, particularly dilated congestive and hypertrophic cardiomyopathies
   Acute myocardial ischemia or infarction
   Myocarditis
   Pericarditis, particularly viral, postcardiotomy, postinfarction, Dressler's syndrome, associated with acute myocardial infarction, neoplastic, and radiation associated
   Congenital heart disease, particularly atrial septal defect
3. Related to underlying systemic disorders
   Hypoxia owing to pneumonia, pulmonary emboli, or other acute or chronic lung disorder
   Hyperthyroidism
   Electrolyte imbalance
   Administration of sympathomimetic amines, e.g., aminophylline
   Other drugs such as alcohol, caffeine, amphetamines
   Hypotension and shock

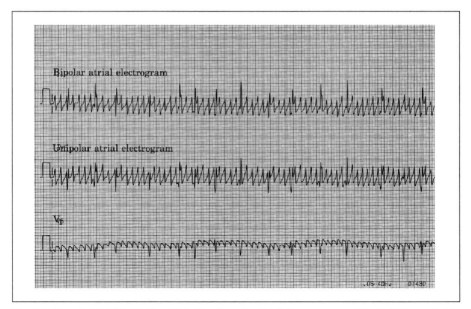

Fig. 6-3. Type I atrial fibrillation. Note the discrete atrial electrograms with slight irregularity in morphology as well as timing separated by discrete isoelectric baseline intervals.

The most difficult problems to deal with are those of underlying heart disease in which pressure-volume overloads of the atria have resulted in very large chambers. If the left atrial size on the echocardiogram is 4 cm or less, there is a good chance that sinus rhythm may be restored. When the left atrium is larger than 5 cm, the chances of restoring and maintaining sinus rhythm are small. Between 4 and 5 cm, the chances are diminished, but it is still worth a try, since the heart is hemodynamically more efficient in sinus rhythm and there is less chance of thromboembolism. Atrial systole contributes 15–20% of the cardiac output. In atrial fibrillation there is no effective atrial contraction, and the appearance of the atria has been described as a "bag of worms." The atrial rate may be 400–600 beats/minute.

On the ECG, atrial fibrillation is recognized as an irregularly irregular rhythm with absent P waves. Fibrillatory activity may be either coarse or fine. Waldo, Wells and colleagues have further described additional characteristics that permit a breakdown into four categories (Table 6-4) based on the appearance of the electrogram recorded directly from the atrium in patients after heart surgery [1]. The benefit of this categorization is primarily in distinguishing type I or II atrial fibrillation from atrial flutter since the treatment is different (Figs. 6-3 through 6-5). When the ventricular response to atrial fibrillation is rapid and there is some regularization, extra care should be taken to measure carefully the R–R intervals on the ECG.

Atrial fibrillation is thought to be due to reentry. The proposed mechanisms of atrial fibrillation include multiple wavelets from the atria, a single standing

Table 6-4. Characteristics of atrial fibrillation

Type I	Discrete atrial electrograms separated by discrete isoelectric intervals
Type II	Discrete atrial electrograms not separated by discrete isoelectric intervals
Type III	Absence of both discrete atrial electrograms and isoelectric intervals of any sort
Type IV	Electrogram varies among types I–III

Source: Adapted from JL Wells et al., Characterization of atrial fibrillation in man: Studies following open heart surgery. *PACE* 1:426–438, 1978.

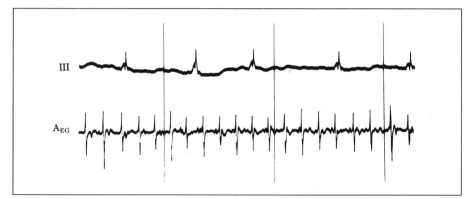

Fig. 6-4. Type II atrial fibrillation. Simultaneous recording of lead III and bipolar atrial electrogram (A_{EG}). Note the perturbations of the baseline between the otherwise discrete atrial complexes. The relatively discrete nature of the atrial complexes resembles atrial flutter, but the variability of morphology, polarity, amplitude, and cycle length indicates this is atrial fibrillation. (From JL Wells et al., Characterization of atrial fibrillation in man: Studies following open heart surgery. *PACE* 1:426–438, 1978.)

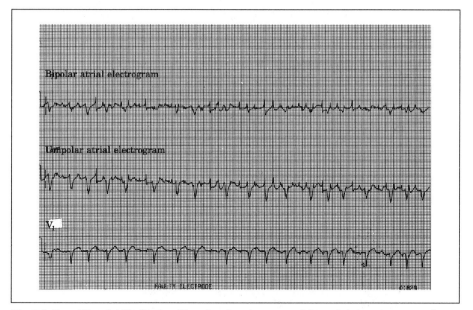

Fig. 6-5. Type III atrial fibrillation. Note the chaotic nature of the atrial electrograms and absence of an isoelectric baseline.

wave with fibrillatory conduction, an ectopic focus with fibrillatory conduction, and degeneration of paroxysmal supraventricular tachycardia or atrial flutter. It may be paroxysmal or chronic. The history is very important since cardioversion should not be attempted if the process is chronic and the patient's blood has not been anticoagulated. Similarly, if an underlying systemic disorder such as thyrotoxicosis or hypoxia has not been corrected, the chances of maintaining a regular rhythm are diminished. One must also ascertain what medications the patient is taking. Is the patient already taking a digitalis preparation? If so, when was the last dose? If there are signs of regularization on the ECG, suggesting a junctional rhythm, could the patient be suffering from digitalis toxicity? Control of the ventricular response in atrial fibrillation is the first goal of treatment. Usually the rate is controlled by decremental conduction at the level of the AV node. However, with intense sympathetic stimulation, this may be quite rapid—in the range of 160–180 beats/minute. If there is antegrade conduction down an accessory pathway, it may be as rapid as 300 beats/minute. If the ventricular response is very slow, and the patient is not receiving digitalis or beta blockers, the clinician must be concerned about disease of the AV node, as in the sick sinus or tachycardia-bradycardia syndrome.

2. **Treatment**

   a. **Electrical cardioversion.** If the atrial fibrillation is of known acute onset and the patient is hemodynamically embarrassed or having angina pectoris, electrical cardioversion may be necessary.

   b. **Digoxin.** Digoxin is the drug of choice for controlling the ventricular response in atrial fibrillation. Initially 0.5 mg is given IV. Although this dose is tolerated as a single bolus by the majority of individuals, it may be safer to administer 0.25 mg IV initially, wait 5 minutes, and then give the second 0.25 mg IV. It is always easier to give a second dose in a short period of time than to wish that the first larger dose had not been given. A total of 1.00–1.25 mg of digoxin may be given orally (PO) or IV over the first 24 hours as the loading or digitalizing dose. After the first 0.5 mg, the additional digoxin is given in increments of 0.25 mg q2–3h, but not any faster. The goal is to control the ventricular response in the range of 60–80 beats/minute. The maintenance dosage for the normal individual is 0.25 mg PO daily; for the patient in renal failure, it is 0.125 mg PO daily or every other day (see Chap. 14). Therapy must be individualized. Rare patients with chronic atrial fibrillation may require as much as 0.25 mg digoxin bid for adequate control and not experience toxicity. Others may have serious adverse effects at half that dose. **Caution:** Never give digitalis to a patient with an accessory pathway, since the drug may increase the effective refractory period of the AV node, shorten the refractory period of the bypass tract, and speed conduction down the bundle of Kent.

   c. **Propranolol hydrochloride, esmolol hydrochloride, and other beta blockers.** When the initial dose of digoxin fails to control the ventricular response, the addition of propranolol in small quantities often is beneficial. Even if the patient has borderline congestive heart failure, doses as low as 5 mg propranolol PO q6h may control the ventricular response. The dosage may be increased as needed and as tolerated. Usually in this situation, the propranolol can be given PO with efficacy; however, the IV route is also possible if given with caution. Generally, IV propranolol is given by slow IV push in 1-mg increments. Most individuals respond to 1 or 2 mg, and the maximum acute dose of 0.15 mg/kg must not be exceeded.

   In a cardiac care unit, another option is IV esmolol 500 µg/kg/minute over 1 minute, followed by a 4-minute maintenance infusion of 50 µg/kg/minute, with further dose adjustment as necessary.

   Long-term combined therapy may be indicated, and the physician may wish to consider a longer-acting beta blocker (see Chap. 14), although some of these drugs are not approved by the FDA for cardiac arrhythmias. Therapy could certainly be justified if there was another indication for the drug, such as hypertension. The patient with hypertrophic cardiomyopathy and atrial fibrillation is a special case. Digitalis is usually contraindicated in this disease, with beta blockers as one of the treatments of choice. However, the profound decompensation with loss of atrial systole makes the combination of digitalis and a beta blocker reasonable and necessary when the patient has atrial fibrillation. Similarly, patients with mitral stenosis benefit from remaining in sinus rhythm and fare poorly in atrial fibrillation when the ventricular response is rapid.

   d. **Diltiazem and verapamil.** Another way to control the ventricular response when digoxin alone is insufficient is with diltiazem or verapamil. In fact, some physicians consider intravenous diltiazem as first-line therapy. These drugs have a negative dromotropic effect (slows conduction) at the AV node and decrease the number of impulses reaching the ventricle. The initial dose of **IV diltiazem** is 0.25 mg/kg over 2 minutes. If the response is inadequate, a second dose, 15 minutes later, of 0.35 mg/kg may be given over 2 minutes. A continuous infusion of IV diltiazem at rates of 5–15 mg/hour may continue for 24 hours.

Alternatively, **IV verapamil** may be given with an initial bolus of 5 mg. This dose may be repeated and a maximal dosage of 0.075–0.150 mg/kg not exceeded. Verapamil is given slowly over a period of 2–3 minutes, since high-degree AV block or asystole may occur. The physician must be prepared to deal with these possible adverse outcomes.

Diltiazem and verapamil may be more useful than propranolol in patients with asthma, but both of these drugs and beta blockers share the property of negative inotropism, which may lead to overt congestive heart failure. Verapamil has a short half-life after IV administration, and another dose may be required after 30 minutes. Depending on the clinical situation, this may be an advantage or a disadvantage. Rarely, patients with paroxysmal atrial fibrillation revert to sinus rhythm after IV verapamil. The patients who respond usually have normal-sized atria and no underlying heart disease.

e. **Types 1 and 3 antiarrhythmic agents.** Therapy with **type 1 antiarrhythmic agents** may help restore sinus rhythm as well as provide some control of the heart rate. Since drugs such as quinidine may have a vagolytic effect at the AV node, promoting a fast ventricular response, it is imperative to block the AV node with digitalis before considering quinidine or procainamide therapy.

Many patients with an episode of paroxysmal atrial fibrillation convert to sinus rhythm after receiving the full loading dose of digoxin, although it may not be a direct effect of the drug. (See Chap. 14.) At this point, the clinician must determine the need for long-term therapy. If this is just one episode related to a specific precipitating factor that will not recur, chronic therapy may not be indicated. Similarly, the patient with infrequent paroxysmal episodes (perhaps the next one will be 2 years later) may not wish the inconvenience of daily medication and follow-up. The patient with recurrent episodes, some perhaps even asymptomatic, may be at a greater risk of thromboembolism and a candidate for maintenance antiarrhythmic therapy. Some of these individuals may also be candidates for chronic anticoagulation if the antiarrhythmic drugs fail to maintain sinus rhythm.

If sinus rhythm has not been restored and the physician elects for a trial of type 1 antiarrhythmic drugs or electrical cardioversion, prior anticoagulation should be performed for the patient with chronic atrial fibrillation and atrial fibrillation of uncertain or recent onset. Anticoagulation should be performed for 3 weeks before the attempt at cardioversion and continued for 2 weeks after cardioversion; although sinus rhythm may be restored, effective mechanical atrial contraction may be delayed. Some patients tolerate chronic atrial fibrillation well, particularly if ventricular contractility is good. If there is a serious contraindication to full anticoagulation, they are candidates for antiplatelet drug therapy.

An attempt at **chemical cardioversion** may be performed before electrical cardioversion. **Procainamide** may be given IV loading, with 1000 mg IV administered at a rate of 100 mg q5 minutes and watching for hypotension or orally with **procainamide 500–750 mg PO q6h.** Formerly very large doses of quinidine were given until sinus rhythm was restored. Because of the associated hazard, this method can no longer be justified. **Quinidine sulfate 300–400 mg PO q6h** or **quinidine gluconate 324–648 mg PO q8h** is given for 24–48 hours with attention paid to digoxin and quinidine levels. If quinidine is not desired, **disopyramide 100–200 mg PO q6h** may be substituted. Alternative oral drugs include **propafenone, flecainide, sotalol** (type 3), and **amiodarone** (type 3), each with appropriate monitoring and awareness of their toxicities and half-lives (some of these drugs may not be reasonable in individual cases and some do not have an FDA indication).

If chemical cardioversion is not successful, electrical cardioversion can be performed after withholding one digoxin dose. Some physicians do not attempt an initial trial of chemical cardioversion and proceed with electrical cardioversion. If the antiarrhythmic drug is not given before restoration of sinus rhythm, it may be started immediately after. Occasionally the physician may wish to try digoxin therapy alone rather than the combination of digoxin and a type 1 or type 3 drug, since all may have adverse effects, in addition to requiring frequent administration. This approach may be attempted, with the realization that recurrence of atrial fibrillation may require a second cardioversion.

Electrical cardioversion (see Chap. 2) carries a discrete risk of embolization (1–2%) despite anticoagulation therapy; however, the incidence is
greater when there is no anticoagulation. In addition, small emboli in organs
other than the brain or coronary arteries may go unnoticed. The physician
should remember the multitude of drug interactions possible when the
patient is taking digoxin, quinidine, and warfarin sodium (Coumadin).
Quinidine increases the digoxin level and the prothrombin time. Some physicians advocate transesophageal echocardiography before cardioversion to
identify thrombi, but even with this technique minute thrombi may not be
seen.

If chronic suppressive therapy with the type 1A antiarrhythmic drugs is
ineffective or tolerated, some of the newer drugs, such as propafenone (type
1C), flecainide (type 1C), or sotalol (type 3), may be more beneficial. For the
patient with refractory paroxysmal atrial fibrillation whose chances of maintaining a sinus rhythm are not hampered by a severely enlarged left atrium or
other scarring, **amiodarone** has been shown to be of value. Amiodarone therapy may be effective for this group of patients with refractory atrial arrhythmias in up to 85% of cases. After initial loading over a 3-week period (see
Chap. 14), electrical cardioversion will restore sinus rhythm, and it may be
maintained by low doses (amiodarone 200 mg PO daily). Since low-dose therapy is usually successful, there is a decreased risk of amiodarone toxicity. However, the long-term effects of amiodarone even in low doses still raise concern.
Therefore, this type of therapy in a young individual should be undertaken
only after conventional therapy has been exhausted, and the potential benefits outweigh the risks.

f. **Catheter ablation of the atrioventricular node and permanent pacing.**
Antiarrhythmic agents have undesirable adverse effects, particularly if the
need for drug therapy is chronic. Many electrophysiologists today consider the
safest therapy of paroxysmal or chronic atrial fibrillation to be control of
the ventricular response and anticoagulation, avoiding the use of the types 1
and 3 antiarrhythmic drugs. If the ventricular response cannot be easily controlled by digoxin, a beta blocker, or an appropriate calcium blocker, catheter
ablation of the AV node, creating complete heart block, is another consideration. This therapeutic avenue also requires the implantation of a permanent
pacemaker. For an active person, a pacemaker with rate responsiveness is
indicated. For an inactive patient, this feature may not be as critical.

Many patients obtain significant relief of symptoms with modification or
ablation of the AV node (many symptoms are related to the onset or termination of atrial fibrillation as well as the rapidity of the ventricular response),
but it is obtained by the creation of complete heart block and reliance on a permanent pacemaker. These decisions have to be made on an individual basis.
At the time this text goes to press, there are initial reports of restoring sinus
rhythm by catheter ablation techniques even in patients with chronic atrial
fibrillation.

g. **Anticoagulation.** In all the arrhythmias considered in this book, the assumption is that therapy will be successful and the patient will revert to sinus
rhythm. The one common situation in which the patient remains in the
arrhythmia is chronic atrial fibrillation. Usually there is chronic underlying
heart disease and an enlarged left atrium. The key to managing the arrhythmia is controlling the ventricular response and deciding on anticoagulation.
The ventricular response is usually controlled with digoxin, but occasionally
with a beta blocker or calcium antagonist (verapamil or diltiazem). Catheter
ablation of the AV node and permanent pacing is another option.

The major concern in chronic atrial fibrillation is the development of thrombi and subsequent embolization. More than half of all patients with systemic
embolization are found to have atrial fibrillation. If the site of embolization is
the middle cerebral artery, the results may be devastating and permanent.
This possibility must be considered whenever a decision not to anticoagulate
is made.

Chronic anticoagulation with warfarin sodium is recommended if atrial fibrillation occurs in the presence of systemic embolism or serious underlying
heart disease (valvular, thyrotoxic, coronary, or congenital) with congestive
heart failure. The value of anticoagulation in nonrheumatic atrial fibrillation
has been addressed in a number of recent studies. The American College of

Chest Physicians has held three conferences on antithrombotic therapy since the first edition of this book [2].

The Copenhagen AFASAK study was the first to demonstrate that the benefits of anticoagulation outweigh the risks [3]. The rate of stroke was 2.0% in those who received Coumadin and 5.5% in those who did not. Aspirin at a dose of 75 mg daily was ineffective for preventing stroke in atrial fibrillation.

The Boston Area Anticoagulation Trial for Atrial Fibrillation studied the effect of low-dose warfarin (prothrombin time 1.2–1.5 × control) on the risk of stroke in patients with nonrheumatic atrial fibrillation [4]. It followed 420 patients for an average of 2.2 years. The incidence of stroke and death was lower (0.41%/year, 2.25%/year, respectively) in the group receiving warfarin as compared to the control group (2.98%/year, 5.97%/year, respectively), 46% of whom were taking aspirin.

The Stroke Prevention in Atrial Fibrillation (SPAF) study followed 1130 patients with constant or intermittent atrial fibrillation for 1.3 years [5]. The patients were randomized to aspirin 325 mg, warfarin (prothrombin time 1.3–1.8 × control), or placebo. The rate of primary events (stroke or systemic embolus) was 6.3%/year for placebo versus 3.6%/year for aspirin. In the analysis with warfarin, the risk of primary events was 7.4%/year for placebo and 2.3%/year for warfarin. Primary events or death was reduced 58% by warfarin and 32% by aspirin.

Predictors for thromboembolism in atrial fibrillation in the SPAF study included recent onset of congestive heart failure, history of hypertension, and previous arterial thromboembolism [6]. Echocardiographic predictors included left ventricular dysfunction and left atrial size. The number of thromboembolic events was minimal if the left atrial size (cm/m²) was less than 2.0 cm/m², and increased as the size increased to 2.0–2.5 cm/m², and was highest at more than 2.5 cm/m².

The design of the Canadian Atrial Fibrillation Anticoagulation (CAFA) study was similar to other trials (AFASAK, SPAF) [7]. It was terminated early when results from these trials demonstrated a benefit from anticoagulation. The rates of nonlacunar stroke, noncentral nervous systemic embolism, and fatal or intracranial hemorrhage were 3.5% in warfarin-treated and 5.2% in control patients.

The Veterans Affairs Stroke Prevention in Nonrheumatic Atrial Fibrillation study studied the risk of cerebral infarction in patients with nonrheumatic atrial fibrillation treated with warfarin (prothrombin time 1.2–1.5 × control) as compared to control [8]. The incidence of cerebral infarction was 4.3%/year in the controls and 0.9%/year in warfarin-treated patients. The risk of major hemorrhage was low, and the benefit of anticoagulation extended to patients older than 70 years.

These trials indicate that the risk of stroke in patients with nonvalvular atrial fibrillation is approximately 5%/year and that warfarin can substantially reduce this risk with only a minimal risk of significant hemorrhage in properly chosen and monitored patients [9]. In fact, the risk of stroke is reduced by at least 59% by warfarin, and there is also a favorable trend in the reduction of vascular and all-cause mortality [10]. The risk of stroke for young patients with lone atrial fibrillation (without cardiovascular disease) is very low; the benefit from anticoagulation with warfarin may not be justified. It is not unreasonable to consider therapy with aspirin 325 mg daily. Lower-dose aspirin as in the AFASAK study did not have benefit. As patients age, the underlying substrate may change (hypertensive or ischemic heart disease, reduced left ventricular function), and the benefit from therapy may increase. Obviously as factors change, the patient must be reassessed.

In patients undergoing elective cardioversion for atrial flutter or atrial fibrillation, a study from the Cleveland Clinic indicated that anticoagulation was important for atrial fibrillation even if the duration was less than 1 week. It was not necessary for atrial flutter [11]. One must remember that some patients have both atrial flutter and atrial fibrillation or that type I atrial fibrillation may be confused with flutter; therefore, clinicians should be sure of the diagnosis before cardioverting without anticoagulation.

In summary, the bias is to anticoagulate in all cases of chronic atrial fibrillation unless there is a contraindication. For patients on Coumadin, the prothrombin time is maintained at 1.3–1.8 times control, as in the published studies. I hesitate to consider full anticoagulation in the frail, the elderly, and those with a known bleeding disorder or peptic ulcer disease. For these patients, therapy with an antiplatelet agent such as aspirin (if no ulcer) is recommended.

E. Atrial flutter

1. **Features.** Although not as common as atrial fibrillation, atrial flutter is more often associated with underlying heart disease. The major causes are listed in Table 6-3. It is important to direct therapy at the underlying problem. Atrial flutter is a more organized rhythm than atrial fibrillation and responds to different measures. The atria beat at a rate of 250–350/minute unless modified by type 1 antiarrhythmic drugs, which can slow the rate to 200/minute. If the jugular pulse is appropriately positioned, flutter waves may be appreciated. Unless an accessory pathway is present, atrial flutter usually occurs with 2:1 AV block and a ventricular response of approximately 150 beats/minute. When the flutter rate is slowed by type 1 drugs, there is a greater possibility of 1:1 AV conduction and aberration.

On the ECG, atrial flutter should always be suspected in any regular tachycardia of 140–180 beats/minute, even if the classic sawtooth flutter waves are not appreciated in leads II, III, aVF, and V_1. Since the atrial focus is usually low, in the vicinity of the AV junction, the sawtooth flutter waves have an inverted appearance. However, occasionally they may be upright, indicating a higher atrial focus. If there is varying block, one may see the flutter waves better, and they may be accentuated by carotid sinus massage (see Chap. 4). With alternation between 4:1 and 2:1 block, two levels of block have been hypothesized.

Waldo and MacLean have classified atrial flutter into two categories, based on the atrial rate and response to atrial pacing (Table 6-5) [12]. This classification has more clinical utility than the four types of atrial fibrillation. Type I atrial flutter has a slower atrial rate and can be interrupted by overdrive pacing (Fig. 6-6). Type II atrial flutter is resistant to pacing and requires aggressive treatment with drugs to slow the ventricular response (Fig. 6-7).

The important clinical point to remember is that atrial flutter must be considered in the differential diagnosis of a tachycardia of 150 beats/minute even if classic flutter waves are not present. The diagnosis can be made with the aid of vagal maneuvers, Lewis leads, esophageal electrodes, and intraatrial or direct atrial recordings (see Chap. 4). Once the diagnosis has been made, one of three main options of therapy can be selected, depending on the individual patient: electrical cardioversion, drug therapy, or overdrive pacing. Recommendations regarding anticoagulation in patients with atrial flutter are not as strict as for atrial fibrillation, since there is more effective atrial contraction in atrial flutter, which may explain the decreased incidence of systemic thromboembolism. The clinician must be certain that the rhythm is not alternating between atrial flutter and atrial fibrillation since the risk of thrombus would increase. As with atrial fibrillation, atrial flutter can be chronic in some cases and relatively well tolerated. Nevertheless, restoration of sinus rhythm with efficient atrial contribution to the cardiac output is desirable.

2. **Treatment**
   a. **Electrical cardioversion.** Electrical cardioversion is the treatment of choice if the patient is hemodynamically compromised. If the patient is hemodynamically stable, electrical cardioversion remains an alternative. Most often, it is possible to restore sinus rhythm with low-energy cardioversion (20–50 joules). Infrequently, atrial flutter is converted to atrial fibrillation, requiring a second cardioversion at higher energy. It is important to note that it is easier

Table 6-5. Characteristics of atrial flutter

Type	Atrial rate (beats/min)	Response to rapid atrial pacing
I	230–350	Can be interrupted with restoration of normal sinus rhythm
II	340–430	Unresponsive to pacing

Source: Adapted from AL Waldo, WAH MacLean, *Diagnosis and Treatment of Cardiac Arrhythmias Following Open Heart Surgery.* Mt. Kisco, N.Y.: Futura, 1980.

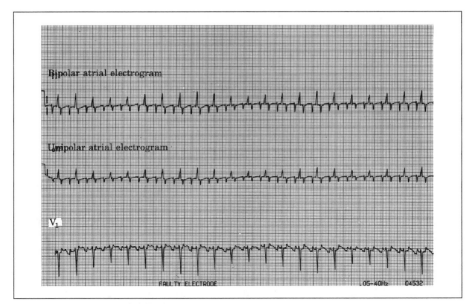

Fig. 6-6. Type I atrial flutter. In this tracing, the relationship of the atrial activity to the ventricular activity is easily demonstrated on the bipolar tracing since each deflection is an opposite direction.

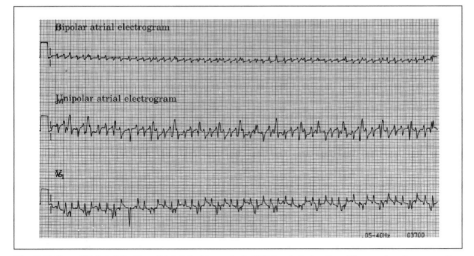

Fig. 6-7. Type II atrial flutter. Atrial flutter rate is 375 beats/minute with varying degrees of block limiting the ventricular response.

to control the ventricular response to atrial fibrillation than to atrial flutter. Thus, for the rare patient who will not remain in sinus rhythm, it may be better to be in atrial fibrillation than atrial flutter. In the acute management, some patients refuse electrical cardioversion and must be offered one of the other therapies.

b. **Overdrive pacing.** Overdrive pacing using rapid atrial pacing is a relatively easy way to convert atrial flutter to sinus rhythm. It has the advantage of avoiding electrical cardioversion or acute drug therapy (although maintenance antiarrhythmic regimens may be necessary for some). It is useful when there is concern about cardioversion in patients who have received large amounts of digitalis. It has the disadvantage of requiring an electrode in the atrium, which is not a problem for the patient immediately after open heart surgery who already has electrodes in position. Alternatively, transesophageal pacing can be performed, avoiding the necessity for intravascular access. Once the electrode is in position, the entire procedure usually can be accomplished in less than 5 minutes. Using the criteria for type I atrial flutter (and also including patients with rates borderline between types I and II) will provide for the highest success rate for this technique.

(1) Both poles of the electrode are connected to the special atrial pacemaker generator (bipolar pacing).

(2) The stimulus strength is set at 10–20 mA, since the atria require higher energies for capture.

(3) The ECG should be constantly monitored; the atrial wire must not be allowed to slip into the ventricle if using a transvenous electrode.

(4) Pacing must be performed at a critical rate (usually 125% of the spontaneous flutter rate) for a critical time (usually 10–20 seconds) to interrupt the type I atrial flutter and restore sinus rhythm. Otherwise the atrial flutter may be transiently "entrained," but flutter resumes as soon as the pacing ceases.

(5) Pacing is usually initiated at a rate slightly faster than the flutter rate and increased until the morphology of the P waves changes (usually 20–30% faster than the spontaneous rate). After demonstrating capture, pacing can be terminated abruptly or the rate slowed gradually to 100 beats/minute and stopped. The latter technique provides complete control of the atrial rate and may avoid a profound bradycardia that is occasionally seen in patients after termination of an atrial tachyarrhythmia. Certainly, if this situation should occur after abrupt termination, resuming pacing at a low rate will correct the temporary problem.

(6) Other techniques for pacing include constant pacing for intervals of 30 seconds and then terminating or slowing the pacing, as well as starting at a higher atrial rate rather than gradually increasing the rate. In some instances atrial pacing will precipitate atrial fibrillation, which has a good chance of spontaneously converting back to sinus rhythm, particularly after drug therapy. Atrial fibrillation may be more desirable than atrial flutter in terms of ability to control the ventricular response. For patients whose atrial flutter cannot be terminated by atrial pacing, it may be better to precipitate atrial fibrillation by short bursts of atrial pacing faster than 400–500 beats/minute. The ventricular rate must be controlled by digitalis.

c. Drug therapy. Drug therapy for atrial flutter consists of several agents.

Adenosine or verapamil can be administered to slow the ventricular response and assist in diagnosis by making the flutter waves more apparent as AV block increases. Occasionally verapamil 5–10 mg IV terminates the atrial flutter and restores sinus rhythm. If there is no contraindication to verapamil and it is administered in an appropriate setting, there is no harm in administering 5–10 mg IV and monitoring the response. In the majority of cases, the drug slows the ventricular response but does not restore sinus rhythm.

Digitalis is the drug of choice for atrial flutter. Particularly if the patient has no hemodynamic compromise, digitalis may restore sinus rhythm within the first 24 hours, avoiding electrical cardioversion or insertion of a temporary pacing electrode. Digoxin may be given IV or PO for the first dose, which is 0.5 mg (safer in two doses of 0.25 mg), and then PO for the next three doses of 0.25 mg q4–6h (total, 1.25 mg). If sinus rhythm is restored, the physician will have to decide whether chronic maintenance therapy is desirable. In the patient with underlying heart disease, chronic therapy may be necessary. In an acute situation, as after open heart surgery, the physician may elect to continue the digoxin for 1–2 months and then discontinue it once the precipitating factors are resolved.

If the ventricular response is not controlled by digoxin alone and the patient remains in atrial flutter, the addition of a beta blocker, **propranolol,** will slow the ventricular (but not atrial) rate. For patients who remain refractory to all of these maneuvers, it may be necessary to add a type 1 antiarrhythmic drug. Since some of these drugs have a vagolytic action at the AV node, the ventricular response must be controlled by digitalis, verapamil, or propranolol before adding quinidine, procainamide, or disopyramide.

Quinidine sulfate 300–400 mg PO q6h, quinidine gluconate 324–648 mg PO q8h, slow-release procainamide 500–750 mg PO q6h, or **disopyramide 100–200 mg PO q6h** may be given in addition to digitalis, verapamil, or propranolol with restoration of sinus rhythm in many cases. If the atrial flutter persists, there is no reason to continue the type 1 drug after an adequate trial. Quinidine and procainamide are generally better tolerated than disopyramide, and thus it would be reasonable to start with either of the former. Propafenone (type 1C), flecainide (type 1C), and sotalol (type 3) are additional considerations, but only flecainide is approved by the FDA for this indication. Once sinus rhythm is restored, the physician must decide whether maintenance therapy is appropriate, a decision that depends on the likelihood of recurrence. For the patient with refractory atrial flutter, as in atrial fibrillation, **amiodarone** (type 3) may be effective in up to 85% of refractory atrial tachyarrhythmias. After a 3-week loading period, sinus rhythm may be restored by electrical cardioversion and maintained by low-dose amiodarone (200 mg PO daily) (see Chap. 14). Amiodarone is a last-resort therapy for this arrhythmia and may be less desirable than nonpharmacologic therapy. The risk-benefit ratio must be carefully examined since the long-term effects in young patients may be inadequately understood, and there are potentially serious adverse reactions. Chronic drug therapy for refractory cases may involve greater risk than newer modalities, as discussed for atrial fibrillation. Creation of complete heart block by **radiofrequency catheter ablation** and implantation of a **permanent pacemaker** provides rate control and avoids antiarrhythmic drug toxicity. Recently, radiofrequency ablation techniques have been expanded to create lesions in the atria that prevent reentrant atrial flutter and maintain sinus rhythm.

F. Paroxysmal supraventricular tachycardia. When one hears the term *paroxysmal supraventricular tachycardia* (PSVT), one immediately thinks of PAT (paroxysmal atrial tachycardia) or AV nodal reentrant tachycardia, and in fact this is the most common variety (50%), but not the only one. Today paroxysmal supraventricular tachycardia is a general term referring to a number of arrhythmias with different electrophysiologic mechanisms (Table 6-6).

Atrioventricular nodal reentry is due to longitudinal dissociation into two pathways. One pathway (designated alpha) has a shorter refractory period but conducts more slowly than the other pathway (designated beta), which has a longer refractory period. Antegrade conduction usually occurs down the faster beta pathway during sinus rhythm, but an atrial premature beat may find this pathway refractory and travel down the alpha pathway. If the beta pathway has time to repolarize by the time this impulse reaches the end of the common pathway, it can travel retrograde, cause an atrial echo, and reexcite the alpha pathway (if that has recovered). If the time relationships are correct, a sustained reentrant tachycardia (**slow-fast**) (usually confined to the AV node) results. Alternatively the tachycardia may travel the other way (**fast-slow**), resulting in a long R–P tachycardia. These issues are discussed further in the section on electrophysiologic testing and in Chap. 13, on radiofrequency catheter ablation.

The presence of a **concealed AV bypass tract** is the second most common mechanism (Fig. 6-8). In these cases, the impulse travels antegrade down the AV node and retrograde up the accessory pathway. Since antegrade conduction does not occur in the accessory pathway, it is not readily apparent and may require demonstration by

---

Table 6-6. Paroxysmal supraventricular tachycardia

1. Atrioventricular nodal reentry (50%)
2. Concealed atrioventricular bypass tract (30–40%)
3. Sinus node reentry (3%)
4. Intraatrial reentry (<5%)
5. Automatic atrial tachycardia (<5%)

Source: Adapted from ME Josephson, SF Seides, *Clinical Cardiac Electrophysiology*. Philadelphia: Lea & Febiger, 1979. Pp. 147–190.

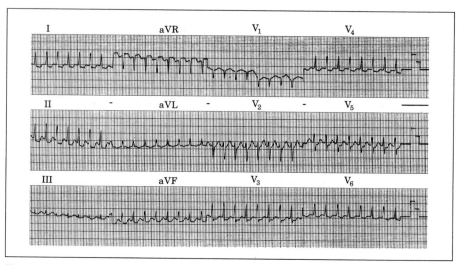

Fig. 6-8. Paroxysmal supraventricular tachycardia. The fast rate (200 beats/minute) suggested the possibility of a concealed bypass, later demonstrated by electrophysiologic study.

electrophysiologic evaluation. Thus, it is "concealed." Time relationships are important. For this macroreentrant circuit to be able to sustain a tachycardia, the total AV conduction time must be delayed long enough to allow first the ventricular end and then the atrial end of the accessory pathway to be capable of retrograde excitation.

Since the sinus node is an anatomic structure similar in certain respects to the AV node, it is not unexpected that reentry could also occur here as well. **Sinus node reentry** is localized to the sinus node and is not affected by the distal conduction system. An analogous situation occurs when the reentrant circuit is localized to another part of the atrium and is designated **intraatrial reentry.**

Finally, **automatic atrial tachycardia** is due to enhanced automaticity of a single focus within the atrium. It is caused by a different electrophysiologic mechanism than reentry and is resistant to programmed stimulation and physiologic or pharmacologic maneuvers. It often occurs as an incessant tachycardia.

1. **Atrioventricular nodal reentrant tachycardia**
   a. **Features.** Atrioventricular nodal reentrant tachycardia is a commonly seen arrhythmia and quite often is not associated with any underlying heart disease. Precipitating factors often include caffeine, alcohol, or sympathomimetic amines. In addition, it may be associated with the same underlying conditions that may cause atrial fibrillation or atrial flutter (see Table 6-3). This arrhythmia is characterized by a sudden onset and sudden termination. The rate range is 150–200 beats/minute but most often 180–200 beats/minute. Because of the mechanism described above, reentry within the AV node along the two pathways results in almost simultaneous excitation of the atria and ventricles. Thus, the P waves occur at the same time as the QRS complexes and are difficult to appreciate on the ECG. Occasionally part of the P wave may be seen in the terminal part of the QRS. During an electrophysiology study, it is easier to see the atrial and ventricular activity as discrete electrograms on the atrial and ventricular channels. Atrial and ventricular activity occurring simultaneously is definite evidence against the participation of an accessory bypass tract in the reentrant tachycardia (Fig. 6-9).
   b. **Treatment**
      (1) **Hemodynamic stability.** The cardinal rule regarding hemodynamic stability always applies. If there is hemodynamic embarrassment, electrical cardioversion should be promptly performed. As with atrial flutter, relatively low energies (20–25 joules) are usually sufficient to restore normal sinus rhythm. With AV nodal reentrant tachycardia, marked hypotension, angina, or congestive heart failure is unusual unless the patient has

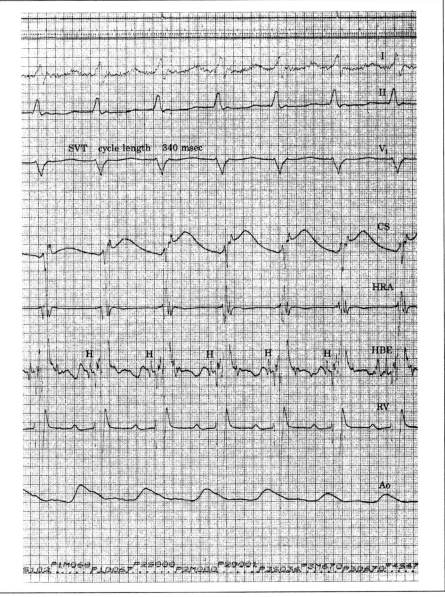

Fig. 6-9. Paroxysmal supraventricular tachycardia (PSVT). Electrophysiologic study with the following leads: I, II, V_1 (surface), coronary sinus (CS), high right atrium (HRA), His bundle electrogram (HBE), ventricular electrogram (endocardial) (RV), and aortic pressure (Ao). The rate of the tachycardia is 182 beats/minute. Note that the earliest activity occurs in the His bundle followed by ventricular activation and, 35 msec later, activity in the atria. HRA activation occurs 5 msec before CS. Atrial activation begins at the end of the QRS complex and is observed there in 30% of cases of PSVT caused by AV nodal reentry. The R–P interval is less than 50% of the R–R interval. The ratio PR/RP is greater than 1.

serious underlying heart disease. In fact, some patients spontaneously convert to sinus rhythm with sedation and relaxation.

(2) **Vagal maneuvers.** Performance of vagal maneuvers is the initial **treatment of choice** for AV nodal reentrant tachycardia. The **Valsalva maneuver** (see page 73) is easily learned by the patient and may result in a prompt termination of the arrhythmia. **Müller's maneuver** (deep inspiration against a closed glottis, performed by pinching the nose shut and attempting inspiration with the mouth closed at the end of a forced expiration) may also be effective. Gagging or other vagal stimuli (see page 74) may be used but are less pleasant. Should these maneuvers be unsuccessful, **carotid sinus massage** (see page 73) may be utilized if appropriate and safe for the individual patient. If the maneuvers do not terminate the arrhythmia, the rate may temporarily slow while the maneuver is being performed and again accelerate after completion. Frequently, though, the patient is able to terminate the arrhythmia without other assistance.

(3) **Adenosine.** If vagal maneuvers are ineffective, adenosine is the drug of choice for AV nodal reentrant tachycardia. It is extremely effective, has a very short half-life (less than 10 seconds), and is associated with few adverse effects. Occasionally after conversion, an initial bradycardia or atrial or ventricular ectopy is seen. Flushing, nausea, or vomiting is also possible. Side effects are self-limited due to the short half-life. Adenosine is successful in 60% of cases after the 6-mg IV dose and in 92% after the 12-mg IV dose.

(4) **Verapamil.** Verapamil is an alternative drug for AV nodal reentrant tachycardia. Owing to its negative dromotropic effect on the AV node, it is successful in terminating more than 90–95% of occurrences of this arrhythmia. Verapamil is given IV with an initial bolus of 5 mg. It may be repeated, with a maximal dosage of 0.075–0.150 mg/kg. Since high-degree AV block or asystole may result, the drug should be administered slowly over a period of 2–3 minutes. The physician must be capable of dealing with any adverse reactions. If the arrhythmia does not cease after the first 5 mg, vagal maneuvers should be repeated because they now may be successful in terminating the arrhythmia. Infrequently, the combination of vagal maneuvers and verapamil will not be effective in terminating the arrhythmia. At this time, the physician should reassess the clinical status of the patient before considering other drug therapy. If there are any signs of decompensation from prolonged tachycardia, it may be better to consider definitive therapy with electrical cardioversion. If not, the clinician may resort to alternative drugs for supraventricular tachycardia.

(5) **Propranolol.** Propranolol may be effective in terminating AV nodal reentrant tachycardia or may slow the ventricular response if it does not restore sinus rhythm. Propranolol is given cautiously at the rate of 0.5–1.0 mg/minute. The total dosage must not exceed 0.15 mg/kg, but 1–3 mg is generally sufficient. One must be aware of the potential problems of beta blockers (e.g., precipitation of bronchospasm, congestive heart failure).

(6) **Digitalis.** Digitalis slows AV conduction and may terminate AV nodal tachycardia. There may be differing opinions regarding whether to use propranolol or digitalis first after vagal maneuvers and verapamil fail. Today this problem is faced infrequently. One may use either, depending on the individual patient. Digoxin is given IV, starting with two 0.25-mg boluses (total 0.5 mg). Thereafter, additional 0.25-mg boluses may be given q2–4h, with the total dosage not exceeding 1.25 mg.

(7) **Edrophonium.** Edrophonium, a short-acting cholinesterase inhibitor, may be effective in terminating AV nodal reentrant tachycardia but is associated with nausea in some patients. It is given in an initial test dose of 1–3 mg IV and in a 10-mg dose over a period of 30 seconds. A history of asthma or the presence of hypotension is a contraindication to the use of this drug. It is rarely used today for this purpose and does not have an FDA indication for PSVT.

(8) **Vasopressors.** Vasopressors cause an elevation in BP, which results in reflex stimulation of the vagus mediated through baroreceptors in the carotid sinus and aorta. The BP is acutely increased to approximately 180

mg Hg, and vagal stimulation usually occurs at this point. Obviously this pharmacologic intervention carries the risk of inducing myocardial ischemia or infarction or a severe hypertensive episode with its sequelae. Therefore, it is contraindicated in patients at risk of these events.

Because of the efficacy of adenosine or verapamil, this section is included more for historic perspective. In the rare instances in which this method is utilized, the vasopressors are diluted in 10 ml of D5W and infused over 2–3 minutes. The vasopressors used include **phenylephrine** (0.5–1.0 mg), **metaraminol bitartrate** (0.5–1.0 mg), and **methoxamine hydrochloride** (3–5 mg).

(9) **Type 1 antiarrhythmic drugs.** Type 1 agents may depress conduction in one of the limbs of the reentry circuit. Usually these agents are used as prophylactic therapy rather than for acute termination. The drugs that may be of benefit are **quinidine sulfate 300–400 mg PO q6h, quinidine gluconate 324–628 mg PO q8h,** slow-release **procainamide 500–750 mg PO q6h,** and **disopyramide phosphate 100–200 mg PO q6h.**

(10) **Pacing.** Finally, if all of these other maneuvers and drugs fail, atrial or ventricular pacing may be able to terminate the arrhythmia by penetrating the AV node and breaking the reentry circuit.

(11) **Long-term therapy.** After the acute episode has been terminated, the physician must determine the desirability of long-term suppressive therapy. If the episodes occur infrequently, are well tolerated, and are easily terminated (particularly if they do not require a visit to the emergency room), chronic therapy may be unnecessary. With frequent interference with activities of daily living, however, definitive therapy is indicated. **For the patient with frequent episodes of AV nodal reentrant tachycardia, radiofrequency catheter ablation is the treatment of choice, avoiding chronic drug administration and toxicity.** (See Chap. 13.)

Alternatively, three drugs may be considered. Digitalis has the advantage of being quite effective, well tolerated, and convenient. **Digoxin 0.25 mg PO daily** is the usual maintenance dose for patients with normal renal function. **Propranolol** is another drug to consider (particularly the long-acting preparation for convenience). Generally a beta-blocking dose will suppress the majority of arrhythmias. Some patients may not tolerate the fatigue and CNS depression that can occur with propranolol and may tolerate a hydrophilic beta blocker better (see Chap. 14); however, not all of these drugs may be specifically indicated by the FDA for use in the treatment of arrhythmias. The third drug is a calcium blocker—either **diltiazem 60 mg PO q8h or verapamil hydrochloride 80–120 mg PO q8h** (or the longer-acting preparations)—but it may be less effective than the other choices. Rarely, combination drug therapy may be necessary, with the specific combination determined empirically.

2. **Tachycardia caused by a concealed atrioventricular bypass tract**
   a. **Features.** Tachycardia caused by a concealed AV bypass tract is often unrecognized rather than uncommon. Since the incidence of this arrhythmia is 30–40% of all paroxysmal supraventricular tachycardias, the physician is likely to encounter it in practice and must remember to consider this mechanism in the differential diagnosis.

   Triggering factors are the same as for AV nodal reentrant tachycardia. The clinician should consider the presence of a concealed AV bypass tract, particularly when the tachycardia is rapid (faster than 200 beats/minute) and when the P wave is seen to follow the QRS complex. If the P wave is negative in ECG lead I during PSVT, one should suspect a concealed bypass tract.

   b. **Treatment**
      (1) **Vagal maneuvers.** As in AV nodal reentrant tachycardia, vagal maneuvers are the first therapy to utilize. In contrast to AV nodal reentry, which requires only that the refractory period of the reentrant circuit be longer than the conduction time, termination of tachycardia resulting from a concealed AV bypass tract requires transient AV block. The **Valsalva maneuver** and **carotid sinus massage** (if appropriate for the individual patient) may be successful.
      (2) **Drug therapy.** Drug therapy may be necessary. The drugs to consider are **adenosine, verapamil, propranolol,** and **digoxin;** all may cause block to some degree at the AV node. It is important for the physician to be aware

that this is the only situation in which verapamil or digoxin may be given with relative safety to a patient with an accessory bypass tract. Adenosine is the safest to use because of its short half-life. If the patient conducts antegrade down the accessory pathway (antidromic conduction), particularly in atrial fibrillation, digoxin and verapamil may further block the AV node and favor accessory pathway conduction. This situation may lead to ventricular fibrillation.

(3) **Antiarrhythmic drugs.** Type 1 antiarrhythmic drugs, specifically **procainamide**, are useful to terminate the acute arrhythmia in patients with an accessory pathway. Chronic suppressive therapy can be successful with procainamide, quinidine, disopyramide, flecainide, propafenone, or sotalol. Ventricular preexcitation and associated tachyarrhythmias (the Wolff-Parkinson-White syndrome) are addressed separately in Chap. 7.

(4) **Radiofrequency catheter ablation.** As for recurrent symptomatic AV nodal reentrant tachycardia, radiofrequency catheter ablation for AV reentry has become the treatment of choice when the patient continues to have frequent arrhythmias that disrupt the patient's life. (See Chap. 13.)

3. **Sinus node reentry and supraventricular tachycardia**
   a. **Features.** Sinus node reentry is an uncommon cause of supraventricular tachycardia. There is no age or sex predilection, although most patients are older and have underlying heart disease. The usual rate of the tachycardia is 130–140 beats/minute (range 80–200). Recognition of sinus node reentry may be difficult. The P wave morphology is similar or identical to that of the sinus P wave. The P–R interval is usually short, but its length is related to the rate of the tachycardia. Since neither the AV node nor the ventricles are involved in the reentry circuit, AV block does not terminate the arrhythmia. AV Wenckebach block is often seen with the tachycardia.
   b. **Treatment**
      (1) **Carotid sinus massage** may slow and then terminate sinus node reentry. Other vagal maneuvers may be attempted.
      (2) **Propranolol** is one of the first drugs to try in sinus node reentry, although **verapamil** and occasionally **digitalis** may also be effective. All of these drugs may be effective as prophylactic therapy.
      (3) **Radiofrequency catheter ablation** is successful in selected patients who have frequent episodes.

4. **Intraatrial reentry and supraventricular tachycardia**
   a. **Features.** Intraatrial reentry is another uncommon cause of supraventricular tachycardia. Usually the patients have some underlying heart disease. On the ECG, the P wave morphology is usually different from that of the sinus P wave (Fig. 6-10). The usual rate is 130–140 beats/minute. The P–R interval is related to the tachycardia rate. As with sinus node reentry, the AV node and ventricles are not part of the reentry circuit.
   b. **Treatment.** It is difficult to recommend any standard treatment for intraatrial reentrant supraventricular tachycardia since it is incompletely understood. Type 1 antiarrhythmic drugs may be useful since they prolong atrial conduction and refractoriness. Propranolol may slow the ventricular response. Vagal maneuvers may produce block at the AV node but do not terminate the tachycardia. Endocardial mapping and radiofrequency catheter ablation can be successful in certain patients in whom the ectopic focus can be localized. (See Chap. 13.)

5. **Automatic atrial tachycardia**
   a. **Features.** Automatic atrial tachycardia is the last arrhythmia considered in the category of paroxysmal supraventricular tachycardia. Like sinus node reentry and intraatrial reentry, it accounts for only 5% of cases. The mechanism is enhanced automaticity rather than reentry. Automatic atrial tachycardia is frequently associated with severe underlying disease (Table 6-7) or digitalis toxicity.
   On the ECG, P waves are seen but differ from the sinus P wave. Since the focus is in the atria and subatrial structures do not participate, the development of AV block or bundle branch block does not affect the atrial rate or P–R interval. Unlike reentrant arrhythmias, automatic atrial tachycardia cannot be initiated or terminated by programmed atrial stimulation, although penetration of an atrial premature beat may reset the timing. Interestingly, this tachycardia may "warm up" after its initiation. The rate

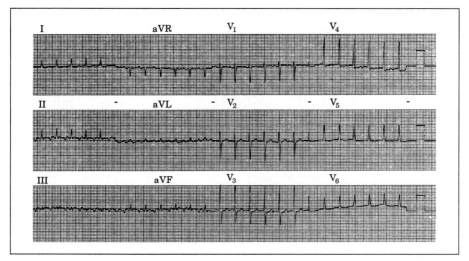

Fig. 6-10. Paroxysmal supraventricular tachycardia, rate 150 beats/minute. The inverted P waves (indicated by *arrows*) seen best in II, III, and aVF suggest an ectopic atrial focus.

of discharge of the automatic focus increases for a few beats until its final rate is achieved.

b. Treatment. Automatic atrial tachycardia is notoriously difficult to treat and is generally quite resistant to any intervention. Vagal maneuvers are usually ineffective. Therapy should be directed at the precipitating factor, if that is possible. Should the patient be hemodynamically compromised by the automatic atrial tachycardia, even electrical cardioversion may not be able to restore sinus rhythm, and treatment with vasopressors may be necessary. If digitalis is implicated, the drug must be discontinued and the potassium level corrected if the patient is hypokalemic. A digitalis level should be obtained and the patient monitored. If the patient has ventricular tachycardia as well with the digitalis toxicity, lidocaine may be necessary. In this situation, the use of digitalis antibodies may be considered. Most often, however, the patient with digitalis toxicity improves with the cessation of digitalis administration and monitoring alone.

If the patient with automatic atrial tachycardia is not taking digitalis and the ventricular response is rapid, digitalis or propranolol may be utilized to slow the ventricular rate, although success is not always possible. **Radiofrequency catheter ablation** may offer success for this difficult-to-manage arrhythmia.

G. Atrial tachycardia with block

1. Features. Atrial tachycardia with block is considered next, since an automatic atrial tachycardia may be the primary arrhythmia in a large percentage of cases. The other mechanism may be reentry. The majority of patients will have digitalis toxicity (Fig. 6-11). Atrial tachycardia with block may also occur in patients with

Table 6-7. Causes of automatic atrial tachycardia

1. Underlying heart disease: Acute myocardial infarction
2. Digitalis toxicity (particularly atrial tachycardia with block)
3. Chronic lung disease (especially with acute infectious process)
4. Alcohol ingestion
5. Amphetamine ingestion
6. Metabolic and physiologic derangements
   Hypokalemia
   Hypoxia
   Catecholamine release

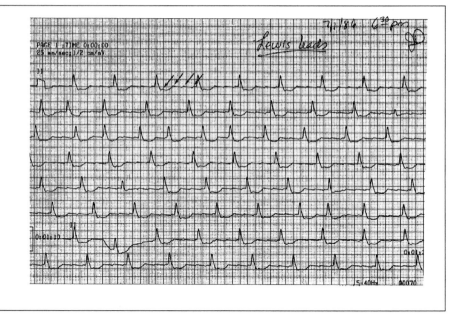

Fig. 6-11. Paroxysmal atrial tachycardia with 4:1 atrioventricular block in a patient with digitalis toxicity. The atrial rate is 228 beats/minute; the ventricular response is 57 beats/minute. The P waves (*arrows*) were demonstrated by Lewis leads (see Chap. 4).

chronic lung disease or in patients with coronary artery disease but not necessarily taking digitalis.

Electrocardiographically, the atrial rate is usually 150–200 beats/minute and the ventricular response governed by block at the AV node (usually Mobitz type I or Wenckebach block). This arrhythmia may be nonparoxysmal or paroxysmal. In the nonparoxysmal case, there may be a "warm-up" phenomenon, as seen in automatic rhythms.

2. **Treatment**
   a. **Digitalis-induced atrial tachycardia with block.** Monitor the patient. **Stop the digitalis.** Correct the potassium if the patient is hypokalemic. If there is associated ventricular tachycardia, consider lidocaine and the use of digitalis antibodies.
   b. **Atrial tachycardia with block in the absence of digitalis.** Treat the patient as with any other atrial tachycardia, using **vagal maneuvers** first and then considering **digitalis** to control the ventricular response. With persistence of atrial tachycardia with block, a type 1 antiarrhythmic drug such as **quinidine, procainamide,** or **disopyramide** should be added.

H. **Wandering atrial pacemaker**
   1. **Features.** A wandering atrial pacemaker occurs not uncommonly and is most likely to be observed in athletes, the young, and the elderly. In patients with this condition, the rhythm of the heart is not controlled exclusively by the sinus node as dominant pacemaker. Other foci in the atrium, or occasionally the AV junction, occasionally fire and conduct to the ventricles. On the ECG, different P wave morphologies (usually at least three) and different P–R intervals are noted. There may be a rhythmicity to the different P waves, which in some cases may be influenced by vagal tone (Fig. 6-12).
   2. **Treatment.** Treatment of wandering atrial pacemaker is unnecessary unless there is an associated symptomatic bradycardia.

I. **Multifocal atrial tachycardia or chaotic atrial rhythm**
   1. **Features.** The electrophysiologic findings in multifocal or chaotic atrial tachycardia are similar to those in wandering atrial pacemaker. There are at least three different atrial pacing sites (three distinct P waves) and varying P–R intervals. The rate of the tachycardia is usually 100–130 beats/minute. In the majori-

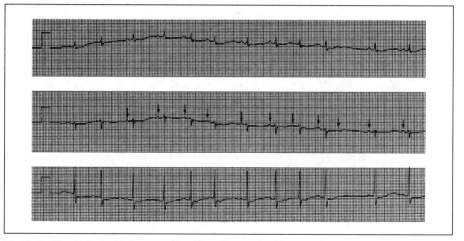

Fig. 6-12. Wandering atrial pacemaker. Note the varying P wave morphologies (*arrows*) and P–R intervals.

ty of cases, there is severe underlying pulmonary disease accompanied by some degree of hypoxia. Usually the problem is exacerbated by infection, administration of aminophylline drugs, or metabolic imbalance. It is unusual for digitalis to cause this arrhythmia.

2. **Treatment.** Treatment must be directed at the underlying cause. Administration of oxygen to the acutely hypoxic patient may be beneficial. Attempts must be made to optimize the ventilatory status. The urge to administer digitalis should be avoided, since digitalis is unlikely to be helpful and may even worsen the situation. If the ventricular response is very rapid, slowing its rate may be beneficial. However, the majority of patients with this arrhythmia cannot tolerate beta blockade because of the potential bronchospastic effects. Verapamil may be of some help; however, treatment of the underlying cause is most effective. For refractory cases, creation of complete heart block by **radiofrequency catheter ablation** and implantation of a **permanent pacemaker** provides control of the rate and avoid drug toxicity.

J. **Atrial premature beats**

1. **Features.** Atrial premature depolarizations, or beats, usually represent a discharge from another focus in the atria before the next sinus node discharge. If the premature beat is extremely early, it may find the AV node still refractory and not result in conduction to the ventricles. This phenomenon may be observed on the ECG as an early P wave (sometimes noted in the preceding T wave) that is not followed by a QRS complex. Commonly, this finding is referred to as **blocked atrial premature beat (APB).** Often the P wave is difficult to appreciate, particularly when it falls in the middle of the preceding T wave and may be recognized only by a minor deformity. In some leads, it may not even be apparent, and careful examination of all 12 leads is important before labeling the pause as a sinus arrest, sinus pause, or sinus exit block.

   If the APB arrives somewhat later, when the AV node is able to propagate an impulse but the distal conduction system has not fully recovered, the impulse may take a different route down to the ventricles, usually exhibiting bundle branch block. This phenomenon is called aberration (see Chap. 3). The earlier the conducted APB is, the more likely there will be aberration. The later the conducted APB is, the more likely it is that the QRS will appear normal.

   If the APB does not depolarize the sinus node and reset its timing (because the tissue is still refractory), there will be a **full compensatory pause.** Thus, the interval between the previous sinus beat and the sinus beat subsequent to the APB will be twice the normal P–P interval. If the APB can penetrate the sinus node, the next sinus beat will appear one sinus cycle length from that point in time. On the ECG, the subsequent sinus beat will occur earlier than expected (had there not been an APB) and result in a noncompensatory pause.

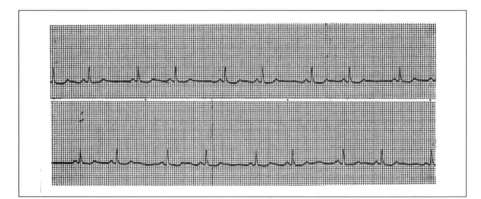

Fig. 6-13. Atrial premature beats in the pattern of atrial bigeminy.

Atrial premature beats may occur in specific patterns, or they may be random. If they occur every other beat, the pattern is described as **atrial bigeminy** (Fig. 6-13); if every third beat, **atrial trigeminy.** If there is a protected focus in the atria that rhythmically discharges and competes with the sinus node pacemaker, one may be dealing with **atrial parasystole.** The term *protected focus* refers to the fact that a sinus beat or other ectopic beat cannot alter the rhythmicity of the **parasystolic focus,** which is a form of **entrance block.** Parasystole may be suspected when the following criteria are present:

1. Nonfixed coupling (i.e., a varying interval between the sinus beat and atrial ectopic beat).
2. Fixed intervals or multiples of fixed intervals between the atrial ectopic beats.
3. Occasional fusion beats.
4. Capture of the atria by the ectopic focus when the atria are not refractory from a sinus node discharge.

The fact that parasystole is not always present and that occasionally an ectopic beat is absent when expected suggests the concept of **exit block.** Atrial parasystole may occasionally be manifest as atrial bigeminy.
   2. **Treatment.** In general, treatment of APBs is unnecessary since they cause no serious hemodynamic compromise and rarely are noted by the patient. The same factors that cause atrial fibrillation and atrial flutter may cause APBs (see Table 6-3). Atrial parasystole similarly requires no treatment.
      Atrial premature beats often result in or are associated with the development of atrial fibrillation, atrial flutter, and other sustained atrial tachyarrhythmias. In this situation, the clinician is dealing with suppression of the individual arrhythmia, and therapy is as described above. In general, **digitalis** is one of the first drugs to consider and is often quite effective as a single agent. If digitalis alone is ineffective, the addition or substitution of a type 1 antiarrhythmic drug such as **quinidine, procainamide, disopyramide, flecainide, propafenone,** or **sotalol** is a consideration. Occasionally propranolol may be useful. However, if the atrial premature beats are related to a specific cause such as alcohol, caffeine, or stress, these precipitating stressors should be avoided.
K. **Atrioventricular junctional rhythm and tachycardia**
   1. **Features.** The conduction system is a cascade of pacemakers at different levels (see Chap. 3). If the upper pacemaker fails to discharge and suppress the lower pacemakers within a certain period of time, one of the latter will fire and become the dominant pacemaker. When this occurs, an **escape rhythm** is present (Fig. 6-14). The lower pacemaker may also become dominant when it develops a more rapid discharge than the higher focus and usurps control (Fig. 6-15).
      Both of these mechanisms may occur in the region of the AV junction. If the escape mechanism occurs for one beat, it is described as a **junctional escape beat.** Electrocardiographically it is recognized as a narrow complex similar to the usual supraventricular conducted beat and occurring after a delay. There is no sinus P wave (that is conducted, although it may still be seen on the ECG),

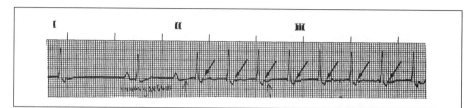

Fig. 6-14. Increasing atrioventricular block with escape by an accelerated junctional rhythm at a rate of 90 beats/minute. Note the retrograde P waves (*arrows*) following the junctional beats.

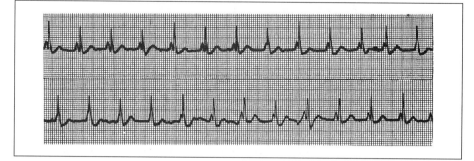

Fig. 6-15. Usurpation by a junctional pacemaker. Observe how the junctional focus competes with the sinus and gradually assumes dominance before slowing.

and quite often a retrograde P wave will be seen. In this situation, the AV junction excites the atria in a retrograde fashion and the ventricles in the usual antegrade manner. If the junctional beat occurs early, it is termed a **junctional premature beat.** It appears similar on the ECG, but there is no preceding delay. P waves may be before, during, and after the QRS complex. The longer the interval is between the QRS and the retrograde P wave (R–P interval), the more likely the beat is to originate distally or to be associated with retrograde conduction block. In fact, junctional rhythms may be associated with retrograde Wenckebach conduction to the atria. If the QRS complex is wide, differentiation of aberration from ventricular origin may be impossible without an endocardial electrogram.

Sustained junctional beats result in a **junctional escape rhythm,** which occurs when there is sinus bradycardia, sinus arrest, or heart block, or a **junctional tachycardia,** which occurs because of acceleration of the automatic focus in the AV junctional tissue (Fig. 6-16). The most common cause of junctional tachycardia is **digitalis toxicity.** Other causes are similar to those for automatic atrial tachycardia (see Table 6-7). In a patient not taking digitalis, myocardial infarction and myocarditis are prime underlying causes. Rarely, junctional tachycardia may present in patients without underlying systemic disease. It is important to distinguish this type of junctional tachycardia, which is **nonparoxysmal,** from the paroxysmal supraventricular tachycardias discussed earlier.

2. **Treatment**
   a. No treatment is usually necessary for junctional escape beats or junctional premature beats.
   b. If the patient has a junctional escape rhythm, the clinician must be concerned about conduction system disease in the upper pacemaker if the event is not related to a reversible cause. Often disease in both the sinus node and the AV node requires a permanent pacemaker (see below).
   c. Treatment of nonparoxysmal junctional tachycardia depends on the underlying cause. If the patient is taking digitalis, digitalis toxicity should be presumed to be present, particularly if the rhythm being treated with digitalis was chronic atrial fibrillation. Digitalis should be withheld, the patient monitored, a digitalis level obtained, and the potassium corrected if hypokalemia is

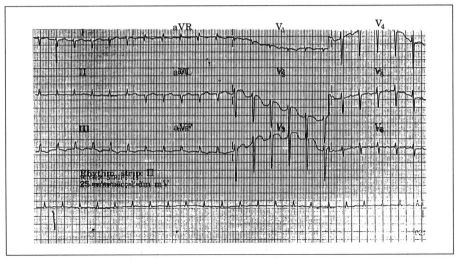

Fig. 6-16. Accelerated junctional rhythm in a patient with underlying chronic atrial fibrillation and right ventricular hypertrophy. This rhythm should always suggest enhanced automaticity caused by digitalis toxicity.

present. If ventricular tachycardia develops, treatment with lidocaine, propranolol, or digitalis antibodies may be necessary.

If the cause of the nonparoxysmal junctional tachycardia is myocardial infarction, myocarditis, or other systemic disorder, treatment is directed toward that specific problem and the arrhythmia treated supportively. If the underlying process does not resolve, treatment of the junctional tachycardia is not likely to be successful. With resolution of the underlying problem, the junctional tachycardia usually ceases.

  L. **Permanent form of junctional tachycardia** is an incessant tachycardia related to a posteroseptal bypass tract in the vicinity of the os of the coronary sinus. Reciprocating tachycardia can be eliminated by radiofrequency ablation close to the site that the slow pathway in AVNRT is encountered.

 II. **Conduction system disturbances.** Delay in conduction may occur at any level in the conduction system. Clinically, block will be most serious when it involves the AV node or His-Purkinje system. If the disease is severe enough, it may result in failure to conduct the impulse down to the lower chamber. Unless a subsequent impulse is able to conduct within a given period of time, it will be necessary for a lower pacemaker to take over with an escape rhythm. The major causes of conduction system problems are fibrosis of the conduction system or surrounding tissue, scarring owing to MI, severe vagal stimulation, and the effect of certain drugs.

  A. **Sinus arrest.** Sinus arrest occurs when there is failure of the rhythmic sinus node discharge, resulting in failure to depolarize the atrium (Table 6-8). It is important to distinguish sinus arrest from a blocked atrial premature beat (hidden in the preceding T wave) and from sinus arrhythmia (Fig. 6-17). If other (lower) pacemakers do not escape (indicating widespread conduction system problems), asystole may result (Fig. 6-18). Fortunately this event is infrequent; most often sinus arrest may

Table 6-8. Causes of sinus arrest and sinoatrial exit block

1. Acute myocardial infarction
2. Myocarditis
3. Degenerative fibrotic changes of sinoatrial node and atrium
4. Excessive vagal tone
5. Digitalis
6. Type 1 antiarrhythmic drugs

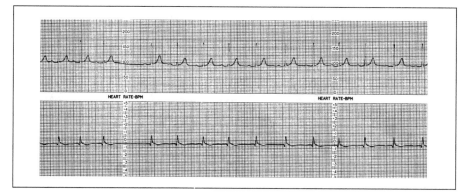

Fig. 6-17. Sinus arrest. There is no evidence of a blocked atrial premature beat in the preceding T wave.

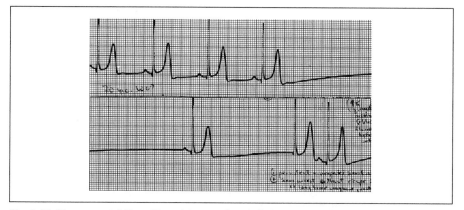

Fig. 6-18. Sinus arrest followed by a 4.8-second period of asystole, indicating disease of the distal conduction system. This patient required a permanent pacemaker.

not even be apparent. The patient who is symptomatic may require a permanent pacemaker. The necessity of pacing both the atrium and the ventricle must be assessed.

B. Sinoatrial block. Sinoatrial block is thought to differ from sinus arrest in that sinoatrial block is a form of exit block rather than impulse formation. Table 6-8 describes the conditions under which SA block may occur. Just as with block in the AV node, there may be several degrees of block.

  1. First-degree sinoatrial block. There is delay in impulse transmission from the SA node to the surrounding atrium. Conduction, however, is successful, and there are no dropped beats. For every impulse propagated from the SA node, there is a resulting P wave and atrial depolarization. Consequently, first-degree SA block cannot be appreciated on the ECG.

  2. Second-degree sinoatrial block. There is not only delay in impulse transmission but also failure to conduct, with loss of P waves. Further classification depends on the presence or absence of fixed block.

   a. Wenckebach (type I) second-degree sinoatrial block. The P–P intervals gradually shorten while the P–R interval remains constant. At the end of the cycle, there is a pause, resulting from a blocked impulse (no P wave). The duration of the pause is less than twice the shortest P–P interval. The following P–P cycle is longer than the P–P cycle before the pause (Fig. 6-19).

   b. Type II second-degree sinoatrial block. There is a fixed degree of block. One or more sinus impulses fail to reach the atria and occur in a fixed ratio (2:1, 3:1).

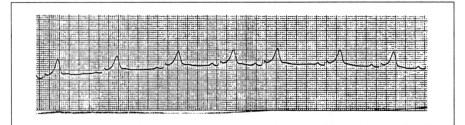

Fig. 6-19. Sinoatrial Wenckebach block. Note the constant P–R interval, shortening of the P–P interval, and dropping of a P wave.

3. **Third-degree sinoatrial block.** There is complete block of impulses from the SA node, resulting in absence of P waves and failure to depolarize the atria unless there is an ectopic focus.
4. **Treatment.** Transient SA block is usually asymptomatic and often unnoticed. It requires no therapy. If the patient is symptomatic with bradyarrhythmias, drugs such as atropine or sympathetic stimulants may be of short-term benefit. However, chronic problems with heart block resulting in a decreased cardiac output usually require a permanent pacemaker. Since disease may be present in the lower conducting system as well, the need to pace both the atria and the ventricles must be addressed (see Chap. 17).

C. **Sick sinus and tachycardia-bradycardia syndromes**
1. **Features.** The **sick sinus syndrome** and **tachycardia-bradycardia syndrome** refer to a constellation of conditions that may include clinical symptoms, sinus node dysfunction, and problems of conduction in the AV node as well. Not all clinicians consider these two syndromes to be the same; nevertheless, their many overlapping features make it best to consider them together in one section.

   Sinus node dysfunction is characterized by inappropriate bradycardia in the absence of drugs and the presence of SA block or sinus arrest. There may be rapid atrial tachyarrhythmias that occur paroxysmally and on termination are followed by severe bradyarrhythmias. Occasionally rescue by a lower pacemaker (junctional or idioventricular) may be necessary. Absence of an appropriate escape rhythm indicates AV conduction dysfunction. Short periods of asystole may be followed by ventricular tachycardia. This condition is not benign and may lead to asystole or life-threatening arrhythmias.

   Although the majority of patients with sick sinus syndrome or tachycardia-bradycardia syndrome have ischemic heart disease, a large number (particularly younger patients) have no other cardiac abnormalities. Pathologically, degenerative changes in the conduction system (both the SA and the AV node) and scarring of the surrounding tissues are seen.
2. **Treatment.** When the patient becomes symptomatic with bradyarrhythmias or has associated tachyarrhythmias requiring treatment with digitalis or other drugs (which may themselves cause severe bradycardia), it is time to insert a permanent pacemaker. The choice of pacemaker—atrial, ventricular, or dual chamber—will depend on the patient and his or her hemodynamic status (see Chap. 17). After implantation of the permanent pacemaker, drugs (as appropriate) to control the tachyarrhythmia may be given safely.

D. **Atrioventricular block.** Atrioventricular block occurs when atrial impulses fail to reach the ventricles. It may be complete or partial, with different implications for therapy. Block may occur anywhere in the lower conduction system; however, the more distal the block is, the more serious are the clinical implications.
1. **First-degree atrioventricular block.** Transmission of the impulse to the ventricles is delayed, but the impulse ultimately arrives. On the ECG, first-degree AV block is recognized by a P–R interval that exceeds 200 msec (Fig. 6-20). The site of delay with first-degree AV block is most often in the AV node but occasionally may be in the bundle of His, in the bundle branch–His-Purkinje system, or in multiple sites. If the delay is in the AV node, the A–H interval on the intracardiac electrogram will be prolonged. If the delay is lower, the H–V interval will be prolonged. The underlying process in first-degree AV block may be increased vagal tone, inferior wall myocardial infarction, myocarditis, degenerative disease, or

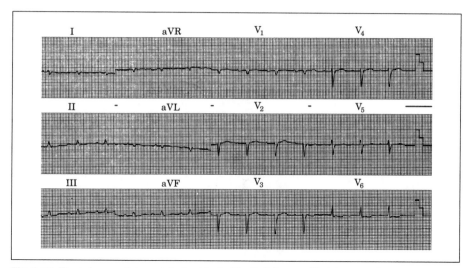

Fig. 6-20. First-degree atrioventricular block. The P–R interval is 0.24 second.

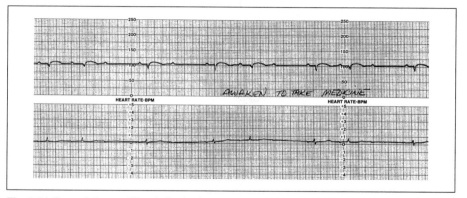

Fig. 6-21. Second-degree (Wenckebach) AV block. The P–R increases until the P wave no longer elicits a ventricular response. The longest increment in P–R interval occurs between the first and second cycles. The cycle containing the dropped beat is less than two of the shortest cycles, since the P–R in the first beat is the shortest.

drug effect (digitalis, beta-adrenergic blockers, calcium antagonists). First-degree AV block requires no specific treatment, only an awareness of the underlying problem, particularly when treatment with drugs that depress conduction is necessary.

  2. **Second-degree atrioventricular block.** Second-degree AV block exists when some of the atrial impulses fail to be conducted to the ventricles. Electrophysiologically, the site of delay may be predominantly in the AV node or predominantly in the lower conduction system. Consequently there may be different manifestations on the ECG and different prognostic implications. Second-degree AV block is classified as type I or type II. Often the types are named after the Viennese cardiologists who first described them. Type I is referred to as Wenckebach or Mobitz type I block. Type II is referred to as Mobitz type II block.

   a. **Wenckebach (Mobitz type I) second-degree atrioventricular block.** Type I block most often represents delay in the AV node (Fig. 6-21). Delay is less common in the distal conduction system and uncommon in the bundle of His. The underlying cardiac problems are the same as with first-degree AV block. Usually no treatment is necessary. The block resolves as the underlying process improves. A temporary pacemaker is not indicated.

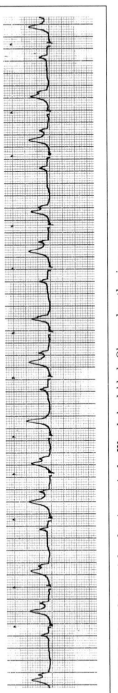

Fig. 6-22. Combined sinoatrial and atrioventricular Wenckebach block. Observe lengthening of the P–R, shortening of the P–P. In this tracing the AV Wenckebach block is predominant since no evidence of dropped P waves is seen.

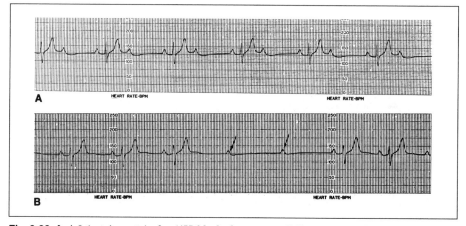

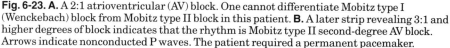

Fig. 6-23. A. A 2:1 atrioventricular (AV) block. One cannot differentiate Mobitz type I (Wenckebach) block from Mobitz type II block in this patient. **B.** A later strip revealing 3:1 and higher degrees of block indicates that the rhythm is Mobitz type II second-degree AV block. Arrows indicate nonconducted P waves. The patient required a permanent pacemaker.

Occasionally athletes with excellent cardiovascular conditioning may manifest Wenckebach block classically on the ECG. The P–P interval remains fairly constant, the P–R interval gradually increases, the R–R interval shortens, and then a P wave fails to conduct to the ventricles. The P–R interval increases because every beat conducted to the ventricles becomes progressively longer. The longest delay in the P–R interval occurs between the first and second cycles. Each subsequent increment in the P–R interval becomes less. The R–R interval tends to decrease after the dropped beat. The cycle containing the dropped beat (R–P–P–R) is less than two of the shortest cycles, since the P–R interval in the first beat of the cycle is the shortest. However, in clinical practice, classic Wenckebach periodicity is not always observed.

Wenckebach periodicity may be apparent on the ECG commonly as 4:3-, 3:2-, or 2:1-conducted intervals. Occasionally one can see Wenckebach block simultaneously in both the SA and AV nodes (Fig. 6-22). One important **caution:** If conduction is always 2:1, Wenckebach block (type I) cannot be distinguished from Mobitz type II block (Fig. 6-23). The clinician must find other intervals (e.g., 4:3, 5:4) to make the diagnosis of Wenckebach block.

It is also important to note that rapid atrial pacing will cause Wenckebach-type AV block in many people. This type of block is usually a physiologic finding. It is usually pathologic, however, when it occurs at normal heart rates. With rapid atrial pacing, "latency" of the AV node is encountered. Refractoriness (see Chap. 3) of the AV node increases, and the relative refractory period is encountered.

b. **Mobitz type II second-degree atrioventricular block.** Type II block is always pathologic and indicates disease of the distal conduction system. Most often patients have severe degenerative disease of the conduction system, myocardial infarction with extensive scarring, or drug effect. On the intracardiac electrogram, a prolonged H–V interval is observed (Fig. 6-24), and in some cases the His potential may be split. When a beat is dropped (P wave but no QRS complex), an atrial deflection will be observed to conduct to the His bundle, but there will be no ventricular electrogram.

On the ECG, the P–R interval remains constant, and conduction to the ventricles is in a ratio of 2:1, 3:1, 4:1, or occasionally higher. In contrast to the patient with Wenckebach type I block, the patient with Mobitz type II block and severe underlying heart disease may require a temporary and then a permanent pacemaker. Not infrequently, patients with extensive disease of the conduction system have conduction delay at multiple levels, rendering specific and distinct classification difficult. Nevertheless, the treatment must be directed at the degree of block.

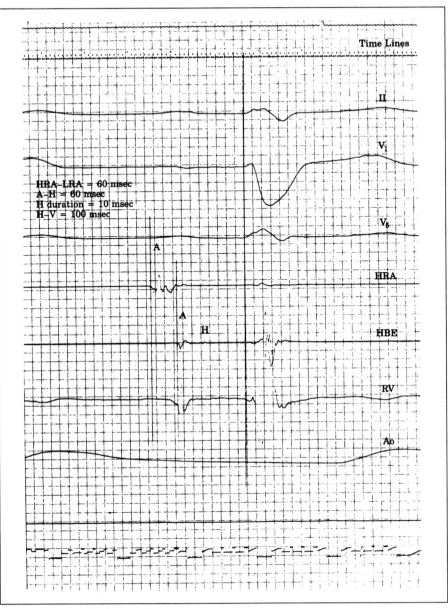

Fig. 6-24. Intracardiac intervals measured at the time of electrophysiologic study (surface leads II, V$_1$, and V$_5$; intracardiac leads high-right atrium [HRA], His bundle electrogram [HBE], right ventricular electrogram [RV], aortic pressure [Ao]) revealed a prolonged H–V interval of 100 msec. The H–V interval is measured from the His deflection to the earliest ventricular deflection.

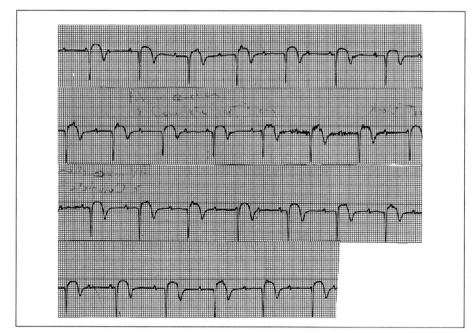

Fig. 6-25. Complete heart block with an escape rhythm of 58 beats/minute. The rate and the narrow QRS complexes suggest a high escape focus, possibly in the region of the bundle of His.

3. **Third-degree atrioventricular block.** When no supraventricular impulse can penetrate to excite the ventricles, third-degree or complete heart block is present. For the patient to survive, there must be an escape rhythm in the ventricles (usually an idioventricular rhythm at a rate of 30–40 beats/minute) to avoid asystole. The higher the anatomic location of the block is, the higher is the location of the escape pacemaker (usually) and the faster the escape rhythm. Anatomically block can occur at the AV node, the bundle of His, or below. Rates of 40–60 beats/minute may result if escape focus is in the region of the bundle of His (Fig. 6-25). In addition, the lower the site of the escape focus is, the wider is the QRS complex.

   In the electrophysiology laboratory, the site of the block may be detected by recording the His bundle electrogram. If every atrial deflection is conducted to the His bundle but there is no ventricular deflection, block is present in the distal conduction system. If atrial activation bears no relationship to the His spike but every His spike precedes ventricular activation, then block is present in the AV node. On the ECG, complete heart block is diagnosed by the failure to conduct any supraventricular impulses to the ventricle. If any do conduct, the condition cannot be considered complete heart block, only high-degree AV block. There is AV dissociation and an escape rhythm.

   There are many causes of complete heart block (Table 6-9), but in the majority of cases in adults, the cardiologist can attribute it to degenerative disease of the conduction system or to ischemic heart disease. Drug toxicity, sometimes owing to type 1 antiarrhythmic drugs or digitalis, is not infrequent. The pediatric cardiologist is more likely to see complete heart block that is congenital or related to surgery for a congenital defect. Treatment for the child with congenital heart block will depend on the presence of symptoms as well as the heart rate. If the escape focus rate is faster than 50 beats/minute, the incidence of symptomatic bradyarrhythmias and syncope is lower.

4. **Treatment.** Treatment is partially dependent on the presence of symptoms. For example, some older individuals with complete heart block may be totally asymptomatic, have no mental impairment, and be able to participate in sports or other exertional activity. This situation is much more likely when the escape heart rate is 45–60 beats/minute than when it is 30–45 beats/minute. It is not

unreasonable to follow these patients very carefully and intervene if they become symptomatic.

Conversely, the symptomatic patient with hemodynamic compromise requires prompt attention. Temporary pacing should be instituted as soon as possible (see Chap. 2). This can be accomplished in a variety of ways, depending on the clinical setting and availability of a physician skilled in transvenous pacemaker insertion. The ability to perform external pacing may obviate the need for emergency invasive procedures. If an external pacemaker is unavailable and preparations for transvenous pacing are being made, interim drug therapy should be utilized. **Atropine 0.5 mg IV** may be helpful if the block is at the AV node; however, this is infrequent. If the block is distal to the AV node, atropine treatment will not be successful, although no great harm will have been done. For patients with distal block, isoproterenol, starting at 1–2 μg/minute (1–2 mg isoproterenol in 500 ml D5W), should be infused. Unfortunately, isoproterenol may be detrimental in the patient with acute myocardial ischemia or infarction and must be given cautiously. If the patient is asystolic, the situation is worse. Therefore, the clinician must institute pacing as soon as possible and then withdraw the isoproterenol.

The need for permanent pacing depends on the underlying problem (see Chap. 17). If the heart block is due to drugs, there will be resolution after the offending drug is withdrawn. In some cases, however, the drug cannot be discontinued; for example, a patient whose symptomatic ventricular tachycardia is suppressed with a type 1 antiarrhythmic drug requires a permanent pacemaker and the drug.

E. **Bundle branch block.** Bundle branch block is frequently seen in the patient population and usually does not result in any serious impairment of AV conduction as long as one of the fascicles remains intact (see Chap. 3). Delay in one fascicle results in altered activation of the ventricle. The impulse travels down the functioning fascicle and activates the contralateral ventricle in a retrograde manner. Thus, the delay in activation is reflected in an increase in the QRS duration (which by definition in bundle branch block is ≧120 msec).

Right bundle branch block is recognized on the ECG by an rSR' configuration in lead V_1 and deep S waves in leads I and V_6 (Fig. 6-26). **Left bundle branch block** is observed to have a wide QS pattern in leads V_1 through V_3 (Fig. 6-27). When one of the divisions of the left bundle is blocked, the condition is described as **left anterior**

Table 6-9. Causes of heart block

1. Degeneration of the conduction system (Lev's disease and Lenègre's disease)
2. Ischemic heart disease
3. Drugs
4. Cardiomyopathy (particularly infiltrative)
5. Traumatic (penetrating or nonpenetrating) or surgical
6. Aortic stenosis (calcific)
7. Uncommon causes
    Diphtheria
    Syphilis
    Sarcoidosis
    Tumors
    Hemochromatosis
    Hyperthyroidism
    Myxedema
    Paget's disease
    Gout
    Lead poisoning
    Thrombotic thrombocytopenic purpura
    Polymyositis
    Amyloidosis
    Endocarditis
    Chagas' disease
    Rheumatoid nodules
    Lyme disease

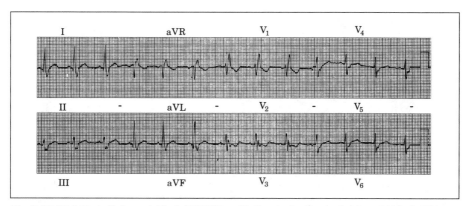

Fig. 6-26. Right bundle branch block (RBBB) and left anterior fascicular (hemi-) block. Note the rSR′ in V_1 and the deep S waves in I and V_6 characteristic of RBBB.

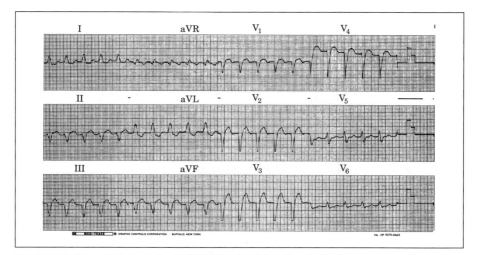

Fig. 6-27. Left bundle branch block. Note the wide QS pattern in V_1–V_3.

fascicular block (**left anterior hemiblock**) or **left posterior fascicular block (left posterior hemiblock).** In left anterior fascicular block, the QRS duration is normal, the QRS axis is markedly leftward (greater than -45 to -60 degrees) and morphologically there is a small q in I, a small r in III, and an r in aVR. In left posterior fascicular block, the QRS duration is normal, the QRS axis is greater than $+120$ degrees, and morphologically there is a small r in I and a small q in III. When left posterior fascicular block occurs as a result of MI, it represents compromise of blood flow in both the anterior descending and posterior descending arteries. It implies extensive myocardial scarring and a poor prognosis. Left posterior hemiblock is otherwise uncommon.

Block may occur at multiple levels and in multiple areas of one level. If there is complete block in all of the fascicles (the right bundle and left bundle; or the right bundle, left anterior fascicle, and left posterior fascicle), there will be complete heart block. If the block is only partial in all of the fascicles, only PR prolongation may be apparent. If one fascicle is completely blocked and the others partially blocked, the ECG may demonstrate bundle branch block plus first- or second-degree AV block (depending on the degree of block in the partially blocked branches). Block at the AV node and bundle of His may also produce these findings on the ECG; however, if the ECG demonstrates left bundle branch block at times, and right bundle branch block at other times, disease of both bundle branches is present.

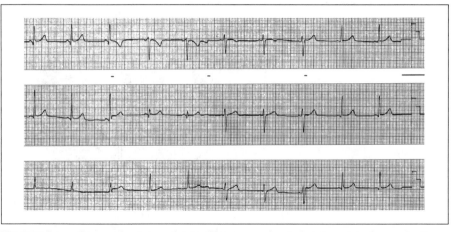

Fig. 6-28. Lown-Ganong-Levine syndrome. Observe accelerated atrioventricular conduction with a short P–R interval (0.10 second). This patient had a history of symptomatic palpitations.

Bifascicular block is frequently seen on the ECG. The most common combination is right bundle branch block and left anterior fascicular block. Right bundle branch block and left posterior fascicular block is less frequent. When both divisions of the left bundle are blocked, bifascicular block also exists. Although many patients may have bifascicular block, it is of minor importance in the majority of them. It is not an indication that progression to complete heart block will occur. No treatment is necessary, only routine follow-up (see Chap. 9).

III. **Electrophysiologic testing in the evaluation of supraventricular arrhythmias and conduction disturbances.** Electrophysiologic studies are performed to evaluate supraventricular arrhythmias and patients with preexcitation syndromes (Figs. 6-28 and 6-29) prior to radiofrequency catheter ablation. (These are discussed individually in Chaps. 7, 12, and 13.) Occasionally, there will be a case of refractory supraventricular tachycardia, sick sinus syndrome, or syncope of uncertain etiology that will derive major benefit from invasive electrophysiologic evaluation. Chapter 12 describes the protocols and methods. This discussion deals with the utility of clinical electrophysiology in supraventricular arrhythmias and conduction disturbances.

A. **Supraventricular arrhythmias**

Paroxysmal supraventricular tachycardia is a general term for a set of arrhythmias with varying electrophysiologic mechanisms (see Table 6-6). In cases that are refractory to empiric therapy, the electrophysiologic study may be valuable in specifically localizing the reentrant loop or detecting abnormal automaticity. The study allows therapeutic trials and assesses the response to drugs. Table 6-10 summarizes some of the responses to stimulation, the diagnostic value of activation sequence, and the effect of bundle branch block during supraventricular tachycardia. It is beyond the scope of this book to describe all of the details involved in differentiating one electrophysiologic mechanism from another. Nevertheless, the important points are discussed.

Atrial activation sequence and morphology of the P wave are the first items to assess. Normally with sinus rhythm, the activation occurs first in the high-right atrium, followed by atrial depolarization in the low-right atrium, as seen on the His bundle electrogram. In sinus node reentry, morphology and activation remain normal. The same holds true for a concealed bypass tract, but only if the tract is in the septum. Otherwise activation is eccentric. If there is reentry within the atria, activation is similarly abnormal. With an automatic atrial tachycardia, a different P wave will be observed, or there may be retrograde activation. If the tachycardia is AV nodal reentrant, the earliest activation will be seen on the His bundle electrogram.

The relationship of the atrial deflection to the QRS is also of value. Atrial activation occurs just before or at the onset of the QRS in two-thirds of AV nodal reentry cases and is at the end of or immediately after the QRS in one-third. Only rarely does it occur late after the QRS, presumably because of antegrade conduction down the faster pathway and retrograde conduction up the slow pathway. In contrast, atrial activation always follows the QRS (R–P <50% R–R) in the presence of a concealed bypass tract. With sinus node reentry, intraatrial reentry, and automatic atrial tachycardia, the R–P exceeds 50% of the R–R.

The response to programmed stimulation is most useful in assessing an automatic mechanism. Premature beats or pacing from the atria or ventricles will neither initiate nor terminate an automatic tachycardia. With penetration into the tissue, however, the timing of the automatic focus may be reset. With the reentrant mechanisms, the arrhythmia may be initiated or terminated by appropriately timed atrial or ventricular premature beats or by burst pacing. With AV nodal reentry or AV reentry via a concealed bypass tract, the earlier the atrial premature beat is, the more likely termination will occur. How timing affects the arrhythmia varies in each situation. In AV nodal reentry, the premature beat finds the alpha pathway refractory and collides with the circulating wave front in the beta pathway, extinguishing the reentry loop. If the premature beat is somewhat later and can conduct down both pathways, it collides again with the impulse in the beta pathway but resets the tachycardia because the impulse also went down the alpha pathway. A late atrial premature beat finds the reentrant circuit refractory, resulting in a full compensatory pause. Thus timing is critical and is influenced by tachycardia rate, distance of pacing site from reentrant loop, refractory period of the myocardium, and conduction velocity.

When there is a concealed bypass tract, the premature atrial depolarization renders the atria refractory to depolarization by the circulating wave front returning via the accessory pathway, blocks the returning impulse in the bypass tract, and may produce block in the AV node or His-Purkinje system. The effect of bundle branch block on the tachycardia produces characteristic changes in patients with a free-wall bypass tract. The key point is that the ventricles are part of the reentry loop. Ipsilateral bundle branch block (on the same side as the bypass tract) slows the tachycardia because the ventricle must be activated in retrograde fashion (producing a longer circuit). If the tachycardia cycle length is prolonged more than 25 msec, the diagnosis of a free-wall bypass tract is justified. With a septal bypass tract, prolongation is not as dramatic. It is important to ascertain that the increase in cycle length is related to prolonged ventriculoatrial (VA) conduction and not to H-V prolongation. With the other types of PSVT, there is no major effect of bundle branch block on tachycardia cycle length unless the H-V interval also increases.

VA conduction is usually present in patients with PSVT. Single ventricular premature beats document the presence of a bypass tract by demonstrating capture of the atria when the His-Purkinje system is refractory to stimuli or by capturing the atria earlier than expected with normal conduction. If VA conduction does not occur, or if VA block develops with pacing, a concealed bypass tract is unlikely. If AV block or VA block is present in the face of a continued paroxysmal supraventricular tachycardia, a concealed bypass tract is not participating since both atria and ventricles are part of the macroreentrant loop. Attention may then be directed to other mechanisms. VA conduction may occur via retrograde conduction over a bypass tract or via retrograde conduction in a pathway in the AV node. For a sustained tachycardia, the retrograde limb must be capable of repetitive stimulation at short cycle lengths.

Activation sequence during retrograde conduction provides further clues. If conduction occurs through the AV node, the earliest site of atrial activation is seen on the His bundle electrogram in the area of the low-right atrium or the os of the coronary sinus. If conduction occurs through the bypass tract, activation of the atria is different unless the bypass tract is in the septum.

Analysis of supraventricular arrhythmias should include plotting AV nodal conduction curves (Table 6-11). If discontinuous, they suggest dual pathways and a diagnosis of AV nodal reentry. (They are also valuable in determining the sites of atrioventricular block.) AV nodal reentry is dependent on a critical A–H interval. If conduction to the ventricles is required for PSVT, however, AV nodal reentry is not the mechanism. Similarly, if conduction to the His bundle is required for PSVT, sinus node or atrial reentry cannot be the mechanism. Sinus node or atrial reentry may be induced by an atrial premature beat that blocks above the bundle of His.

Once a diagnosis of automatic atrial tachycardia is made, mapping is a consideration for refractory cases. As previously described, automatic atrial tachycardia is notoriously drug resistant. If mapping can define the earliest site of activation, radiofrequency catheter ablation may be able to abolish this arrhythmia.

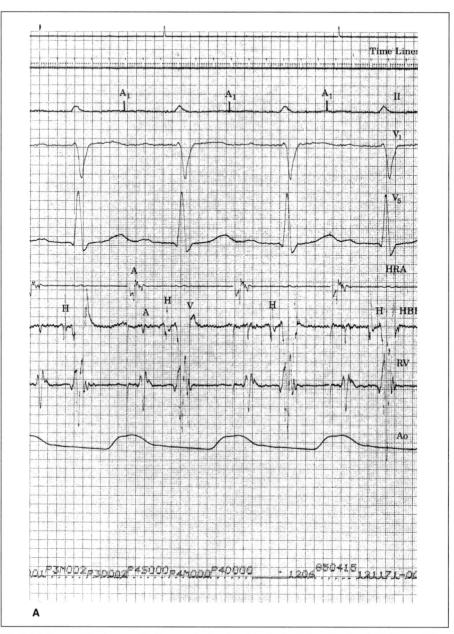

Fig. 6-29. Intermittent preexcitation on electrophysiologic study (surface leads II, V_1, and V_5; endocardial leads high-right atrium [HRA], His bundle electrogram [HBE], right ventricular electrogram [RV], and aortic pressure [Ao]). **A.** Atrial pacing at cycle length of 600 msec. Note the normal relationship of the A, His, and V deflections on the His bundle electrogram.
B. Same patient, same atrial pacing cycle length. The patient now exhibits preexcitation with simultaneous activation of the ventricle down the accessory pathway. Preexcitation is observed on the surface tracing by a widened QRS and on the HBE channel by the appearance of the His deflection in the ventricular electrogram.

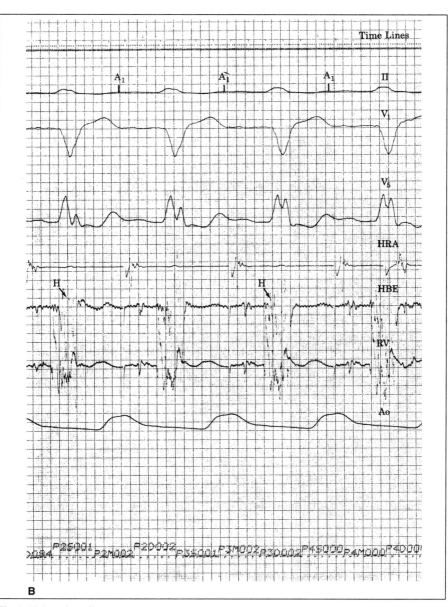

Fig. 6-29 (continued)

Diagnosis of PSVT may be complex and involves the analysis of a number of different parameters (see Table 6-10). In some cases, atrial mapping techniques must be employed to ascertain the atrial activation sequence. The electrophysiologist must be able to recognize various mechanisms and apply a comprehensive examination to differentiate them.

Finally, it is appropriate to discuss the role of electrophysiologic evaluation in patients with atrial fibrillation and atrial flutter. Direct atrial recording may be able to distinguish types I and II atrial flutter. When atrial fibrillation is very organized (type I atrial fibrillation), electrophysiologic study may help distinguish it from atrial flutter. Atrial overdrive pacing is quite effective for type I atrial flutter. Electrophysiologic evaluation may allow assessment of drug efficacy. However, it is usually unnecessary to evaluate the majority of cases with invasive studies. Such studies

Table 6-10. Electrophysiologic clues[a] in paroxysmal supraventricular tachycardia (PSVT)

Type of PSVT	Atrial activation sequence	P–QRS relationship during PSVT	Atrial programmed stimulation	Initiation and termination of PSVT				Effect of functional BBB during PSVT	Ventriculoatrial conduction
				APB	Atrial pacing	VPB	Ventricular pacing		
AV nodal reentry	Earliest site in HBE, followed by os of coronary sinus	A before or at onset of QRS (⅓) (R–P < 50% R–R) (PR/R–P > 1) A at end of or just after QRS (⅓) A well after QRS (rare) (long R–P, short P–R) (P–R/R–P < 0.75)	Very early APB: terminates PSVT Early APB: resets PSVT Late APB: full compensatory pause	Yes[b]	Yes	Yes	Yes	None	As V_1–V_2 shortens, V_2–A_2 prolongs directly as V_2–H_2
SVT with concealed bypass tract (CBT)	Eccentric if CBT in free wall of RV or LV Normal if CBT in septum	A follows QRS (R–P < 50% R–R)	Very early APB: terminates or may reset PSVT	Yes[c]	Yes	Yes[d]	Yes	Ipsilateral BBB slows PSVT owing to lengthening of reentry circuit[e]	If absent, or if present with block, favors other diagnosis V_2–A_2 constant as V_1–V_2 decreases V_2–A_2 constant as V_2–H_2 increases

Sinus node reentry	Normal	P–R directly related to tachycardia rate (R–P > 50% R–R)	Terminates PSVT	Yes	Yes	Yes[f]	Yes[f]	None[g]
Intraatrial reentry	Abnormal	P–R directly related to tachycardia rate (R–P > 50% R–R)	APB during refractory period of atrium produces IACD to initiate PSVT	Yes	Yes			None
Automatic atrial tachycardia	Different P or retrograde activation	P–R and A–H directly related to tachycardia rate (R–P > 50% R–R)	APB may reset automatic focus	No[h]	No	No	No	None[g]

APB = atrial premature beats; VPB = ventricular premature beats; BBB = bundle branch block; AV = atrioventricular; HBE = His bundle electrogram; SVT = supraventricular tachycardia; RV = right ventricle; LV = left ventricle; IACD = intraatrial conduction delay.

[a] These are electrophysiologic **clues** to the diagnosis of the type of PSVT, but may not always be present.

[b] Initiation is dependent on AV nodal conduction delay (critical A–H interval) but not coupling interval of APB.

[c] Initiation is dependent on total AV conduction time.

[d] Capture of atria by VPB when the His-Purkinje system is refractory is diagnostic of CBT.

[e] Lengthening of SVT cycle length >25 msec is diagnostic of free-wall bypass tract.

[f] If ventriculoatrial conduction is present.

[g] If H–V interval increases, first cycle after BBB is prolonged, and subsequent cycles are the same length as before BBB.

[h] Independent of intraatrial conduction or atrioventricular nodal delay.

should be restricted to patients with refractory arrhythmias. Certainly if a patient already has atrial wires in position after open heart surgery, I recommend direct atrial recording to make the diagnosis, if unclear from the ECG, and overdrive pacing of type I atrial flutter.

B. **Conduction disturbances.** The most common supraventricular conduction disturbance requiring pacemaker therapy is sinus node dysfunction. Most often, the diagnosis is apparent on the Holter monitor with long pauses (SA block or sinus arrest), paroxysmal atrial tachy- and bradyarrhythmias, and evidence of distal conduction disease. If the patient is symptomatic in the presence of these findings, further evaluation is unnecessary. For the symptomatic patient without documentation of sinus node dysfunction, electrophysiologic evaluation may be warranted. The sinus node may be evaluated with the sinus node recovery time (SNRT), primarily an evaluation of sinus node automaticity and SA conduction time (SACT), which measures conduction from the sinus node to the atria. Both tests, however, are limited in sensitivity and specificity. Basically the studies are useful when their results are markedly abnormal.

The symptomatic patient with prolonged SNRT or SACT will probably benefit from pacemaker insertion. The symptomatic patient with normal SNRT or SACT may have symptoms related to a noncardiac disorder. These generalizations have exceptions. Thus, there may be rare patients who remain symptomatic despite normal SNRT and normal SACT and have relief of their symptoms when a permanent pacemaker is implanted.

The electrophysiologic site of block in AV conduction disturbances has been described, and the role of electrophysiology testing before pacemaker insertion is discussed subsequently (Chap. 17). Measurement of the H–V interval is helpful in certain cases when it is uncertain whether symptoms are related to a cardiac rhythm disturbance. Programmed atrial stimulation may demonstrate prolongation of the H–V interval with atrial premature beats. Recording of a split His potential suggests intra-His block. It is important to remember that the incidence of H–V interval prolongation is much higher than the incidence of progression to complete heart block. Therefore, in the absence of symptoms, prolongation of the H–V interval alone is not an indication for a permanent pacemaker. (See Chap. 3 for a discussion of intracardiac intervals.)

Table 6-11. Factors favoring AV nodal reentry as mechanism of PSVT

1. Discontinuous AV nodal conduction curves demonstrating dual AV nodal pathways (A_1–A_2 versus H_1–H_2, A_1–A_2 versus A_2–H_2)
2. Induction facilitated by functional bundle branch block or prolongation of H–V interval
3. Initiation of PSVT dependent on critical A–H interval (also seen with AV reentry)

AV = atrioventricular; PSVT = paroxysmal supraventricular tachycardia.

References

1. Wells JL, et al. Characterization of atrial flutter: Studies in man after open heart surgery using fixed atrial electrodes. *Circulation* 60:665–673, 1979.
2. American College of Chest Physicians. *Chest* 102(Suppl)303–549S, 1992.
3. Petersen P, et al. Placebo-controlled, randomised trial of warfarin and aspirin for prevention of thromboembolic complications in chronic atrial fibrillation: The Copenhagen AFASAK Study. *Lancet* 1989 1:175–179.
4. Boston Area Anticoagulation Trial for Atrial Fibrillation Investigators. The effect of low-dose warfarin on the risk of stroke in patients with nonrheumatic atrial fibrillation. *N Engl J Med* 323:1505–1511, 1990.
5. Stroke Prevention in Atrial Fibrillation Investigators. Stroke prevention in atrial fibrillation study: Final results. *Circulation* 84:527–539, 1991.
6. Stroke Prevention in Atrial Fibrillation Investigators. Predictors of thromboembolism in atrial fibrillation: Clinical features of patients at risk. *Ann Intern Med* 116:1–5, 1992.
7. Connolly SJ, et al. Canadian atrial fibrillation anticoagulation (CAFA) study. *J Am Coll Cardiol* 18:349–355, 1991.

8. Ezekowitz MD, et al. Warfarin in the prevention of stroke associated with nonrheumatic atrial fibrillation. *N Engl J Med* 327:1406–1412, 1992.
9. Albers GW, et al. Stroke prevention in nonvalvular atrial fibrillation. *Ann Intern Med* 115:727–736, 1991.
10. Cairns JA, Connolly SJ. Nonrheumatic atrial fibrillation: Risk of stroke and role for antithrombotic therapy. *Circulation* 84:469–481, 1991.
11. Arnold AZ, et al. Role of direct current cardioversion in patients with atrial fibrillation or atrial flutter. *J Am Coll Cardiol* 19:851–855, 1992.
12. Waldo AL, MacLean WAH. *Diagnosis and Treatment of Cardiac Arrhythmias Following Open Heart Surgery: Emphasis on the Use of Atrial and Ventricular Epicardial Wire Electrodes*. Mt. Kisco, NY: Futura, 1980.

Bibliography

Most of the recent developments in the diagnosis and treatment of supraventricular arrhythmias are related to the development of catheter ablation techniques. Consult the numerous references in Chap. 13.

Akhtar M. Supraventricular Tachycardias: Electrophysiologic Mechanisms, Diagnosis and Pharmacologic Therapy. In ME Josephson, HJJ Wellens (eds), *Tachycardias: Mechanisms, Diagnosis, Treatment*. Philadelphia: Lea & Febiger, 1984. Pp 137–169.

Akhtar M. *Cardiac Arrhythmias and Related Syndromes*. Cardiology Clinics series. Philadelphia: Saunders, 1993.

Atkins JM, et al. Ventricular conduction blocks and sudden death in acute myocardial infarction: Potential indications for pacing. *N Engl J Med* 288:281–284, 1973.

Bauernfeind RA, Gallastegui J. Role of Electrophysiologic Studies in the Diagnosis of Paroxysmal Supraventricular Tachycardias. In B Surawicz, CP Reddy, EN Prystowsky (eds), *Tachycardias*. Boston: Martinus Nijhoff, 1984. Pp 185–197.

Belhassen B, Pelleg A. Acute management of paroxysmal supraventricular tachycardia: Verapamil, adenosine triphosphate or adenosine? *Am J Cardiol* 54:225–227, 1984.

Berne RM, DiMarco JP, Belardinelli L. Dromotropic effects of adenosine and adenosine antagonists in the treatment of cardiac arrhythmias involving the atrioventricular node. *Circulation* 69:1195–1197, 1984.

Bigger JT. Management of Arrhythmias. In E Braunwald (ed), *Heart Disease: A Textbook of Cardiovascular Medicine* (4th ed). Philadelphia: Saunders, 1992.

Bigger JT. Mechanisms and Diagnosis of Arrhythmias. In E Braunwald (ed), *Heart Disease: A Textbook of Cardiovascular Medicine*. (4th ed). Philadelphia: Saunders, 1992.

Bigger JT. Supraventricular tachycardia. *Hosp Pract* August 1980. Pp 45–55.

Boineau JP. Atrial flutter: A synthesis of concepts. *Circulation* 72:249–257, 1985.

Brugada P, Wellens HJJ. Electrophysiology, Mechanisms, Diagnosis and Treatment of Paroxysmal Recurrent Atrioventricular Nodal Reentrant Tachycardia. In B Surawicz, CP Reddy, EN Prystowsky (eds), *Tachycardias*. Boston: Martinus Nijhoff, 1984. Pp 131–157.

Cabin HS, et al. Risk for systemic embolization of atrial fibrillation without mitral stenosis. *Am J Cardiol* 65:1112–1116, 1990.

Chesebro JH, et al. Anticoagulant and antiplatelet therapy in acute coronary syndromes and atrial fibrillation. *Cardiol Rev* 1:167–176, 1993.

Chung EK. *Principles of Cardiac Arrhythmias*. Baltimore: Williams & Wilkins, 1983.

Coumel P. Atrial Fibrillation. In B Surawicz, CP Reddy, EN Prystowsky (eds), *Tachycardias*. Boston: Martinus Nijhoff, 1984. Pp 231–244.

Das G, Anand KM, Ankineedu K. Atrial pacing for cardioversion of atrial flutter in digitalized patients. *Am J Cardiol* 41:308–312, 1978.

Dhingra RC, et al. Significance of left axis deviation in patients with chronic left bundle branch block. *Am J Cardiol* 42:551–556, 1978.

Dhingra RC, et al. Significance of block distal to the His bundle induced by atrial pacing in patients with chronic bifascicular block. *Circulation* 60:1455–1463, 1979.

Dhingra RC, et al. Significance of HV interval in 517 patients with chronic bifascicular block. *Circulation* 64:1265–1271, 1981.

Dhingra RC, et al. Significance of chronic bifascicular block without apparent organic heart disease. *Circulation* 60:33–42, 1979.

DiMarco JP, et al. Adenosine: Electrophysiologic effects and therapeutic use for terminating paroxysmal supraventricular tachycardia. *Circulation* 68:1254–1263, 1983.

DiMarco JP, et al. Diagnostic and therapeutic use of adenosine in patients with supraventricular tachyarrhythmias. *J Am Coll Cardiol* 6:417–425, 1985.

Dreifus LS, Michelson EL. Supraventricular Tachycardia: Its Pathophysiology, Diagnosis, and Treatment. *College of Medicine Cardiology Series. Ser.* Vol 7, no 1. 1984.

Falk RH, Podrid P. *Atrial Fibrillation: Mechanisms and Management.* New York: Raven Press, 1992.

Fisch C, Surawicz B. *Cardiac Electrophysiology and Arrhythmias.* New York: Elsevier, 1991.

Fisch GR, Zipes DP, Fisch C. Bundle branch block and sudden death. *Prog Cardiovasc Dis* 23:187–224, 1980.

Fleg JL, Das DN, LaKatta EG. Right bundle branch block: Long term prognosis in apparently healthy men. *J Am Coll Cardiol* 1:887–892, 1983.

Goldberg RJ, et al. Impact of atrial fibrillation on the in-hospital and long-term survival of patients with acute myocardial infarction: A community-wide perspective. *Am Heart J* 119:996–1001, 1990.

Gomes JA, et al. Sustained symptomatic sinus node reentrant tachycardia: Incidence, clinical significance, electrophysiologic observations and the effects of antiarrhythmic agents. *J Am Coll Cardiol* 5:45–57, 1985.

Greenspahn BR, et al. Chronic bifascicular block: Evaluation of familial factors. *Ann Intern Med* 84:521–525, 1976.

Grogan EW, Waxman HL. Management of Supraventricular Tachycardias. In LS Dreifus (ed), *Cardiac Arrhythmias: Electrophysiologic Techniques and Management.* Philadelphia: Davis, 1985. Pp 261–278.

Guarnieri T, et al. The nonpharmacologic management of the permanent form of junctional reciprocating tachycardia. *Circulation* 69:269–277, 1984.

Hauer RNW, et al. Long-term prognosis in patients with bundle branch block complicating acute anteroseptal infarction. *Am J Cardiol* 49:1581–1585, 1982.

Hindman MC, et al. The clinical significance of bundle branch block complicating acute myocardial infarction: 1. Clinical characteristics, hospital mortality and one year followup; 2. Indications for temporary and permanent pacemaker insertion. *Circulation* 58:679–688, 689–699, 1978.

Hollander G, et al. Bundle branch block in acute myocardial infarction. *Am Heart J* 105:738–743, 1983.

Horowitz LN. *Current Management of Cardiac Arrhythmias.* Philadelphia: Decker, 1991.

Horowitz LN, Alexander JA, Edmunds LH. Postoperative right bundle block: Identification of three levels of block. *Circulation* 62:319–328, 1980.

Josephson ME. Paroxysmal supraventricular tachycardia: An electrophysiologic approach. *Am J Cardiol* 41:1123–1126, 1978.

Josephson ME, Kastor JA. Supraventricular tachycardia: Mechanisms and management. *Ann Intern Med* 87:346–358, 1977.

Josephson ME (ed). Atrial Flutter and Fibrillation. In *Clinical Cardiac Electrophysiology: Techniques and Interpretations.* Philadelphia: Lea & Febiger, 1979. Pp 191–210.

Josephson ME (ed). Supraventricular Tachycardias. In *Clinical Cardiac Electrophysiology: Techniques and Interpretations.* Philadelphia: Lea & Febiger, 1979. Pp 147–190.

Karpawich PP, et al. Congenital complete atrioventricular block: Clinical and electrophysiologic predictors of need for pacemaker insertion. *Am J Cardiol* 48:1098–1102, 1981.

Kastor JA. Atrioventricular block. *N Engl J Med* 292:462–465, 572–574, 1975.

Klein GJ, et al. Cryosurgical ablation of the atrioventricular node–His bundle: Long-term follow-up and properties of the junctional pacemaker. *Circulation* 61:8–15, 1980.

Klein RC, Vera Z, Mason DT. Intraventricular conduction defects in acute myocardial infarction: Incidence, prognosis, and therapy. *Am Heart J* 108:1007–1013, 1984.

Lee WK. Clinical approach to atrial fibrillation. *Cardiovasc Rev Rep* 6:958–964, 1986.

Levine JH, Michael JR, Guarnieri T. Treatment of multifocal atrial tachycardia with verapamil. *N Engl J Med* 312:21–25, 1985.

McAnulty JH, et al. A prospective study of sudden death in "high risk" bundle branch block. *N Engl J Med* 299:209–215, 1978.

McAnulty JH, et al. Natural history of "high risk" bundle branch block: Final report of a prospective study. *N Engl J Med* 307:137–143, 1982.

Manani GBJ, Goldberger AL. Cardioversion of atrial fibrillation: Consideration of embolization, anticoagulation, prophylactic pacemaker, and long term success. *Am Heart J* 104:617–621, 1982.

Mandel WJ. *Cardiac Arrhythmias* (2nd ed). Philadelphia: Lippincott, 1986.

Mannino MM, Mehta D, Gomes JA. Current treatment options for paroxysmal supraventricular tachycardia. *Am Heart J* 127:475–480, 1994.

Meyers DG, Gonzalez ER, Nelson WP. The role of prophylactic anticoagulation in cardioversion of atrial fibrillation. *Cardiovasc Rev Rep* 6:647–660, 1985.

Morady F, Scheinman MM. Paroxysmal supraventricular tachycardia: I. Diagnosis, II. Treatment. *Mod Concepts Cardiovasc Dis* 51:107–112, 113–117, 1982.

Myerburg RJ, Kessler KM, Castellanos A. Recognition, Clinical Assessment and Management of Arrhythmias and Conduction Diseases. In RC Schlant et al (eds), *Hurst's The Heart: Arteries and Veins* (8th ed). New York: McGraw-Hill, 1994. Pp 705–758.

NHBLI Working Group on Atrial Fibrillation. Current understanding and research imperatives. *J Am Coll Cardiol* 22:1830–1834, 1993.

Ohkawa S, et al. Electrophysiologic and histologic correlations in chronic complete atrioventricular block. *Circulation* 64:215–231, 1981.

Pastore JO, et al. The risk of advanced heart block in surgical patients with right bundle branch block and left axis deviation. *Circulation* 57:677–680, 1978.

Perloff JK, Roberts NK, Cabeen WR. Left axis deviation: A reassessment. *Circulation* 60:12–21, 1979.

Peters RW, et al. Serial electrophysiologic studies in patients with chronic bundle branch block. *Circulation* 65:1480–1485, 1982.

Pine MB, et al. Excess mortality and morbidity associated with right bundle branch block and left anterior fascicular block. *J Am Coll Cardiol* 1:1207–1212, 1983.

Portillo B, Zaman L, Castellanos A. Tachycardias in Which the Reentry Circuit Includes Atrioventricular Bypass Tracts. In B Surawicz, CP Reddy, EN Prystowsky (eds), *Tachycardias*. Boston: Martinus Nijhoff, 1984. Pp 159–172.

Rabkin SW, Mathewson FAL, Tate RB. Natural history of marked left axis deviation (left anterior hemiblock). *Am J Cardiol* 43:605–610, 1979.

Rahimtoola SH, McAnulty JH. High risk bundle branch block. *Hosp Pract* January 1981. Pp 73–92.

Reddy CP. Supraventricular Ectopic Tachycardias Due to Mechanisms Other Than Reentry. In B Surawicz, CP Reddy, EN Prystowsky (eds), *Tachycardias*. Boston: Martinus Nijhoff, 1984. Pp 173–183.

Reddy CP, McAllister RG. Effect of verapamil on retrograde conduction in atrioventricular nodal reentrant tachycardia. *Am J Cardiol* 54:535–543, 1984.

Reiffel JA, et al. Electrophysiologic Studies of the Sinus Node and Atria. In LS Dreifus (ed), *Cardiac Arrhythmias: Electrophysiologic Techniques and Management.* Philadelphia: Davis, 1985. Pp 37–59.

Saichin A, Dreifus LS, Michelson EL. Electrophysiologic Studies of the AV Conduction System and AV Nodal Arrhythmias. In LS Dreifus (ed), *Cardiac Arrhythmias: Electrophysiologic Techniques and Management.* Philadelphia: Davis, 1985. Pp 61–82.

Schamroth L. *The Disorders of Cardiac Rhythm.* Oxford, England: Blackwell, 1980.

Schneider JF, et al. Newly acquired right bundle branch block. *Ann Intern Med* 92:37–44, 1980.

Schneider JF, et al. Newly acquired left bundle branch block: The Framingham study. *Ann Intern Med* 90:303–310, 1979.

Schneider JF, et al. Comparative features of newly acquired left and right bundle branch block in the general population: The Framingham study. *Am J Cardiol* 47:931–940, 1981.

Smith WM, Gallagher JJ. Management of Arrhythmias and Conduction Abnormalities. In JW Hurst (ed), *The Heart: Arteries and Veins* (5th ed). New York: McGraw-Hill, 1982. Pp 557–575.

Strasberg B, et al. Natural history of chronic second-degree atrioventricular nodal block. *Circulation* 63:1043–1049, 1981.

Stroke Prevention in Atrial Fibrillation Investigators. Predictors of thromboembolism in atrial fibrillation: Echocardiographic features of patients at risk. *Ann Intern Med* 116:6–12, 1992.

Surawicz B, Reddy CP. Tachycardia-Bradycardia Syndrome. In B Surawicz, CP Reddy, EN Prystowsky (eds), *Tachycardias.* Boston: Martinus Nijhoff, 1984. Pp 199–211.

Touboul P, Waldo AL. *Atrial Arrhythmias.* St. Louis: Mosby Year Book, 1990.

Vassallo JA, et al. Endocardial activation of left bundle branch block. *Circulation* 69:914–923, 1984.

Waldo AL, Plumb VJ, Henthorn RW. Observations on the Mechanism of Atrial Flutter. In B Surawicz, CP Reddy, EN Prystowsky (eds), *Tachycardias.* Boston: Martinus Nijhoff, 1984. Pp 213–229.

Watson RDS, et al. The Birmingham Trial of permanent pacing in intraventricular conduction disorders after myocardial infarction. *Am Heart J* 108:496–501, 1984.

Watson RM, Josephson ME. Atrial flutter: 1. Electrophysiologic substrates and modes of initiation and termination. *Am J Cardiol* 45:732–741, 1980.

Waxman MB, et al. Vagal techniques for termination of paroxysmal supraventricular tachycardia. *Am J Cardiol* 46:655–664, 1980.

White HD, et al. Efficacy and safety of timolol for prevention of supraventricular tachyarrhythmias after coronary artery bypass surgery. *Circulation* 70:479–484, 1984.

Yeh SJ, et al. Termination of paroxysmal supraventricular tachycardia with a single oral dose of diltiazem and propranolol. *Circulation* 71:104–109, 1985.

Zipes DP. Second-degree atrioventricular block. *Circulation* 60:465–472, 1979.

Zipes DP. Specific Arrhythmias: Diagnosis and Treatment. In E Braunwald (ed), *Heart Disease: A Textbook of Cardiovascular Medicine* (4th ed). Philadelphia: Saunders, 1992. Pp 667–726.

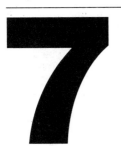

The Preexcitation Syndromes

G. Lee Dolack and Gust H. Bardy

Preexcitation is defined as an early depolarization of ventricular parenchymal myocardium using an alternate conduction pathway from atrium to ventricle other than the usual pathway of the atrioventricular (AV) node–His bundle–Purkinje system. The most common form of preexcitation is the Wolff-Parkinson-White (WPW) syndrome, which is due to accessory AV pathways or Kent bundles [1]. This chapter reviews the basic electrophysiology and wide range of clinical issues related to the WPW syndrome.

I. **The electrocardiogram and accessory pathway anatomy.** The original clinical descriptions of WPW syndrome referred to otherwise healthy individuals who had palpitations and tachycardia [2–6]. Electrocardiographically, WPW syndrome is characterized by a delta wave, or slurred initial upstroke of the QRS, that is associated with a P–R interval of 0.12 second or less (Figs. 7-1 through 7-3) [1]. It is ventricular preexcitation that yields the delta wave and aberrant QRS that superficially resemble those of bundle branch block.

Accessory AV pathways can occur anywhere along the AV groove with the exception of the area between the aortic valve and the mitral valve. In the past, WPW syndrome was categorized electrocardiographically into type A and type B patterns [7]. The type A pattern referred to a predominantly upright QRS morphology in lead V_1 associated with left-sided accessory pathways. The type B pattern referred to a negative QRS morphology in V_1 due to right-sided accessory pathways. This classification, however, is not clinically useful and is of limited accuracy, in particular when considering posterior septal accessory pathways. In general, accessory pathways are considered in terms of four general anatomic locations: left free wall, posterior septum, right free wall, or anterior septum [1]. The majority of accessory pathways (47%) are located in the left free-wall position. The next most common location is in the posterior septum (27%), followed by the right free-wall position (17%), and the anterior septum (9%) (Fig. 7-4).

The anatomic understanding of WPW syndrome is incomplete. Histologically, accessory AV pathways consist of parenchymal myocardium rather than specialized conduction tissue [8, 9]. From isolated postmortem studies, we have learned that most left-sided accessory AV pathways skirt the epicardial side of the anulus fibrosis [9–11]. Right-sided pathways, on the other hand, appear to traverse the AV groove through an area where the tricuspid anulus is structurally deficient [10]. It is not clear whether most accessory AV pathways are discrete bands of tissue only a few microns wide or are broad bands of tissue extending over 1 cm or more. Some histologic evidence suggests that AV pathways may be quite discrete [10]. Clinical experience, however, indicates that accessory AV pathways are not usually pinpoint but rather more broadly based. Surgical results, for example, are better when the dissection extends more than 1 cm on either side of the site of earliest epicardial activation [11].

The ECG findings of a patient with WPW syndrome can be confused with other electrocardiographic abnormalities, including ischemic heart disease, conduction system disease, and right ventricular hypertrophy. Figures 7-1 through 7-3 show ECGs of patients with WPW syndrome that have various delta wave and QRS morphologies that might mimic the ECG findings in other forms of cardiac disease. In order to appreciate the ECG diagnosis of WPW syndrome, it is pertinent to review the surface ECG of the patient without WPW syndrome as it relates to events occurring in the conduction system of the heart. As noted in Fig. 7-5 (left), the P–R interval comprises a series of events including atrial, AV nodal, His bundle, bundle branch, and Purkinje fiber conduction. In the absence of preexcitation, the surface QRS begins only after parenchymal ventricular myocardium has been depolarized, that is, after AV nodal, His bundle, and Purkinje fiber depolarization (Fig. 7-5, left). In the case of WPW syndrome (Fig. 7-5, right), depo-

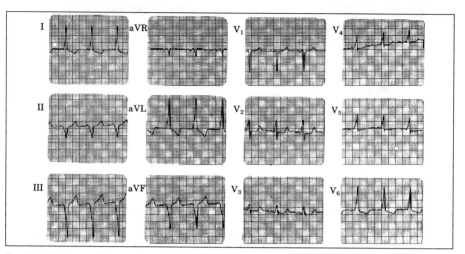

Fig. 7-1. Electrocardiogram from a Wolff-Parkinson-White syndrome patient with a posterior septal accessory atrioventricular pathway with typically negative delta waves in limb leads II, III, aVF, and aVR and an isoelectric delta wave in V_1. This QRS pattern is sometimes mistaken for that of an inferior wall myocardial infarction.

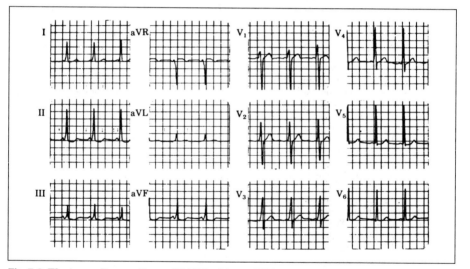

Fig. 7-2. Electrocardiogram from a Wolff-Parkinson-White syndrome patient with an anterior septal, parahisian accessory pathway. The delta wave is positive in I, II, III, and aVF and in the right precordial leads. This ECG could be misread as consistent with left ventricular hypertrophy.

larization of ventricular myocardium via the accessory AV pathway results in a delta wave and an "aberrant" QRS. The degree of preexcitation (i.e., the extent of aberration of the initial part of the surface QRS) depends on the balance between accessory pathway and AV node–His bundle–Purkinje system depolarization. In patients with far-left-sided accessory pathways, who also have relatively rapid conduction via the AV node–His–Purkinje system, the delta wave may be very slight or even absent. On the other hand, patients with right-sided accessory AV pathways may have a markedly aberrant QRS with a pronounced delta wave because of rapid impulse propagation from the sinus node to the nearby accessory pathway.

Anatomic location is not the only factor accounting for the degree of preexcitation. The rapidity with which the accessory pathway conducts, its refractory period, and the

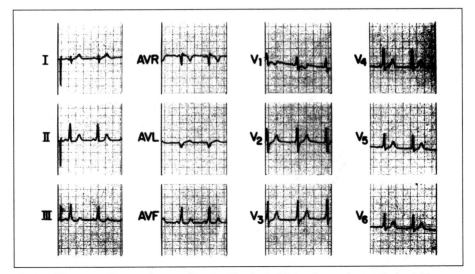

Fig. 7-3. Electrocardiogram from a patient with a far left lateral accessory pathway with typically negative delta waves in I and aVL and positive delta waves in V_1–V_6. This ECG could be misinterpreted as consistent with a lateral or posterior myocardial infarction.

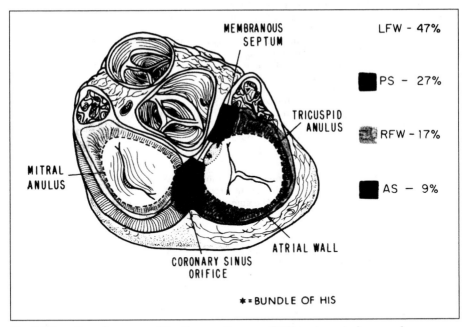

Fig. 7-4. Location of accessory AV pathways. Because of different surgical approaches, accessory pathway location has been divided into four basic areas along the atrioventricular groove: left free wall (LFW), posterior septum (PS), right free wall (RFW), and anterior septum (AS).

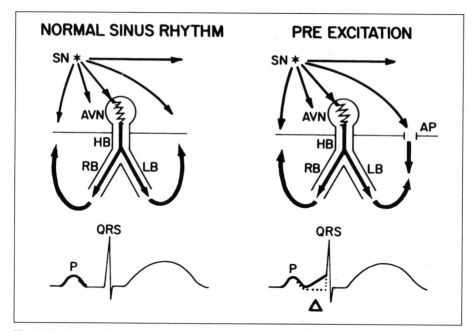

Fig. 7-5. *Left:* Correlation between surface ECG and intracardiac activation sequence in the absence of preexcitation. Cardiac activation proceeds from the sinus node (SN) through parenchymal atrial tissue to the atrioventricular node (AVN), His bundle (HB), and Purkinje system and then to the parenchymal ventricular myocardium. Note that the PR segment is a composite of atrial, AV nodal, His bundle, bundle branch, and Purkinje depolarization. The QRS correlates with parenchymal ventricular depolarization. *Right:* Correlation between preexcited ECG and intracardiac events. The prominence of the delta wave on the surface ECG depends on the amount of parenchymal myocardium depolarized via the accessory pathway (AP) instead of via the normal conduction system. The delta wave (or degree of preexcitation) will vary depending on accessory pathway conduction characteristics, accessory pathway location, and the relative rapidity of conduction through the AV node and His-Purkinje system. (RB = right bundle; LB = left bundle.)

autonomic tone influencing AV nodal conduction all have an effect on the amount of ventricular myocardium depolarized via the accessory pathway. For example, in patients with fluctuating autonomic tone, the amount of preexcitation may vary from marked to none, depending on whether the AV node is conducting slowly (e.g., high vagal tone, as in sleep) or rapidly (e.g., in a vagolytic, adrenergic state, as during exercise).

Intracardiac electrograms provide more direct information as to whether ventricular depolarization occurs predominantly over the accessory pathway or over the normal AV node–His bundle–Purkinje system. One of the electrophysiologic hallmarks of preexcitation is the presence of a short His-ventricular (H–V) interval. The normal H–V interval ranges between 30 and 60 msec. Fig. 7-6A shows a standard intracardiac recording from the region of the AV node–His bundle in a patient with a normal conduction system and no accessory AV pathway. It is measured from the onset of the His bundle electrogram to the first evidence of ventricular depolarization, as noted on the surface ECG. The first ventricular depolarization on the surface ECG correlates with the earliest parenchymal ventricular activity.

In patients with WPW, the H–V interval is abnormally short because parenchymal ventricular activation occurs early. Fig. 7-6B, from a patient with WPW, demonstrates the characteristically short H–V interval. In this patient, parenchymal ventricular depolarization occurred partially via the accessory AV pathway and partially via the His–Purkinje system. Typically, in fully preexcited states, the His bundle deflection is not visible, either because ventricular depolarization occurs entirely via the accessory AV pathway or because His bundle activation is so delayed relative to the ventricles that the His bundle deflection is not discernible in the much larger ventricular electro-

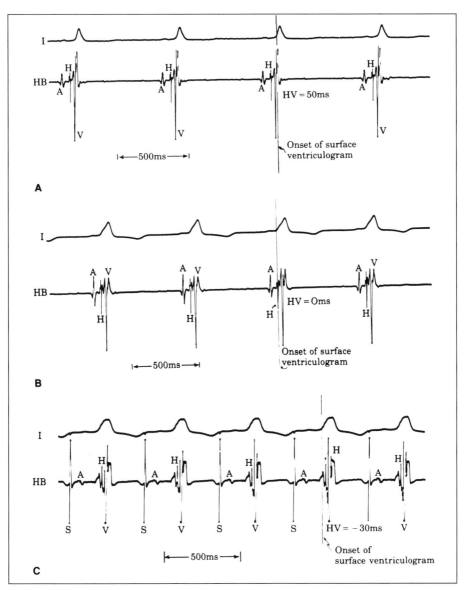

Fig. 7-6. A. Sinus rhythm recording of surface and intracardiac electrograms in a patient with no Wolff-Parkinson-White syndrome and normal atrioventricular conduction. The first electrogram is limb lead I; the second, a His bundle (HB) recording. Note the normal His–ventricular (H–V) interval of 50 msec that is characteristic of normal (i.e., orthodromic) ventricular depolarization. The vertical line marks the onset of ventricular depolarization as determined from the surface QRS. The H–V interval is measured from the onset of the His deflection to the onset of the surface QRS. **B.** Sinus rhythm recording of surface and intracardiac electrograms in a patient with an accessory AV pathway showing the characteristically short (0 msec) H–V interval that is one of the electrophysiologic hallmarks of preexcitation. The His bundle is activated orthodromically, but the ventricle is activated by both the His-Purkinje system and the accessory pathway. The early activation of the ventricle via the accessory AV pathway accounts for the shortened H–V interval. **C.** ECG from same patient as in *B*. A paced atrial rhythm results in more marked preexcitation with a shorter H–V interval (-30 msec). This increase in preexcitation is a consequence of AV node delay. Because of AV nodal decremental properties, more of the ventricle is depolarized via the accessory pathway, which results in a more aberrant QRS and an even shorter H–V interval.

gram. This finding is commonly observed during rapid atrial pacing, when AV node conduction may be too slow to accommodate a rapid atrial rate. Ventricular activation in this instance may occur entirely via the accessory AV pathway (Fig. 7-6C). Table 7-1 describes maneuvers performed during electrophysiologic testing to evaluate characteristics of accessory pathway syndromes.

II. **Demographic data and associated clinical conditions.** The prevalence of WPW syndrome ranges between 0.1 and 0.4% [12]. The incidence of newly diagnosed cases has been estimated at 3.96/100,000 persons per year [13]. Usually the patient is male [12].

Table 7-1. Maneuvers performed during electrophysiologic evaluation of accessory pathway characteristics in the Wolff-Parkinson-White syndrome

Maneuver	Reason
Mapping of atrial activation sequence during orthodromic reciprocating tachycardia	To determine where along the AV groove the shortest ventriculoatrial interval is located. This point corresponds to the accessory pathway location and helps document the tachycardia mechanism
Antegrade pacing at multiple locations along the atrioventricular groove at a set pacing cycle length (usually 400–450 msec)	To determine where along the AV groove maximal preexcitation occurs during atrial pacing. This is another way to determine accessory pathway location
Antegrade and retrograde decremental pacing and refractory period determinations	To determine antegrade and retrograde conduction characteristics of the accessory pathway and the AV node
Insertion of interpolated PVCs from the right ventricular apex during orthodromic reciprocating tachycardia when the His bundle is refractory	By inserting a PVC into tachycardia simultaneous with or just before the His bundle deflection, the presence of an accessory pathway can be definitively documented by demonstrating advancement of the subsequent atrial depolarization. If the atrial activation sequence can be advanced following a PVC, when that premature impulse could not have entered the atrium via the His bundle and AV node, then an accessory pathway must be present
Induction of bundle branch block during orthodromic reciprocating tachycardia	Helps differentiate septal from free-wall accessory pathways by demonstrating major ventriculoatrial interval changes. An increase in the shortest ventriculoatrial interval of 35 msec or more indicates the presence of a free-wall rather than a septal accessory pathway
Induction of atrial fibrillation	To confirm rapidity of the ventricular response during atrial fibrillation and determine the shortest R–R interval occurring via the accessory pathway. If the shortest R–R interval is less than 250 msec, the patient is at higher risk of having ventricular fibrillation. The induction of atrial fibrillation also allows one to determine whether multiple accessory pathways are present by observing changes in the delta wave morphology

AV = atrioventricular; PVC = premature ventricular complex.

The syndrome can become manifest at any age, although it typically presents in infancy or the second or third decade of life [13]. Though considered a sporadic congenital abnormality, an increased prevalence of preexcitation among first-degree relatives of individuals with preexcitation compared with the general population has been described (0.35% versus 0.15%) [14].

WPW syndrome has been associated with other forms of heart disease. Ebstein's anomaly is the most common concomitant abnormality and is associated with WPW syndrome in 5–26% of cases [1, 15–17]. The second most common associated congenital heart disease is an atrial septal defect, but this occurs predominantly in patients who also have Ebstein's anomaly [17]. A host of other abnormalities occur sporadically (<1%), including persistent left-sided superior vena cava [18] and ventricular septal defect [1, 19].

The number of asymptomatic patients with ECG findings consistent with preexcitation has ranged widely from series to series (between 12 and 82%) [13, 20]. In a recent community-based study of the inhabitants of Olmstead County, Minnesota [13], 47% of patients were asymptomatic at the time of diagnosis. Of these individuals, 21% subsequently developed symptoms.

III. **Mechanisms of tachycardia in WPW syndrome.** A variety of tachycardias can occur in patients with the WPW syndrome [1, 21]. The most common arrhythmia is orthodromic reciprocating tachycardia (also called paroxysmal atrial tachycardia, paroxysmal supraventricular tachycardia, circus movement tachycardia, macroreentrant tachycardia, or AV reentrant tachycardia) [1, 21].The second most common arrhythmia is atrial fibrillation [1, 21–24], which is followed in frequency of occurrence by antidromic (preexcited) reciprocating tachycardias [25] and ventricular fibrillation [1, 26]. The incidence of orthodromic reciprocating tachycardia in symptomatic patients with WPW syndrome is approximately 84% [21]. Atrial fibrillation is seen in up to 51% of patients with symptomatic WPW [21]. Orthodromic reciprocating tachycardia and atrial fibrillation occur concurrently in 38% of patients [21]. Antidromic or preexcited reciprocating tachycardia is less common and occurs in 10% of patients [25]. The incidence of ventricular fibrillation in patients with WPW is unknown. In one large series of high-risk patients referred for surgical treatment of their WPW syndrome, 14% had suffered ventricular fibrillation before their referral [26]. In a community-based study, however, the incidence of ventricular fibrillation in symptomatic WPW syndrome is estimated at only 0.25% per year [13].

IV. **Electrocardiography and electrophysiology of tachycardia.** Orthodromic reciprocating tachycardia is most commonly manifested on the surface ECG as a narrow QRS tachycardia with evidence of retrograde P waves in the ST–T segment (Fig. 7-7A) [1]. On occasion, however, orthodromic reciprocating tachycardia can manifest as a wide-complex tachycardia with either right bundle branch block or left bundle branch block morphology owing to functional delay in one of the bundle branches [27, 28].

Electrophysiologically, orthodromic reciprocating tachycardia is characterized by a macroreentrant circuit in which the His-Purkinje system and ventricular myocardium are depolarized antegradely while the accessory pathway and atria are depolarized retrogradely [1]. The retrograde atrial impulse then reenters the AV node and perpetuates the circuit. An electrophysiologic hallmark of reciprocating tachycardia is an eccentric retrograde atrial activation sequence in which the earliest atrial depolarization occurs near the accessory pathway (Fig. 7-7B).

There are several mechanisms by which orthodromic reciprocating tachycardia can arise [1, 29]. One common triggering event is a premature ventricular impulse that blocks retrogradely in the AV node and depolarizes the atria via the accessory pathway (Fig. 7-8). This atrial depolarization leads, in turn, to AV node–His-Purkinje activation with establishment of a macroreentrant circuit. In certain patients with WPW syndrome, orthodromic reciprocating tachycardia may be initiated by a premature atrial depolarization (Fig. 7-9). For this to occur, the effective refractory period of the accessory AV connection must be longer than the effective refractory period of the AV node. A premature atrial depolarization may occur early enough so that it is not conducted antegradely to the ventricle via the accessory pathway but rather is conducted over the AV node in such a way that the ventricle is depolarized entirely via the His–Purkinje system, which results in a normal QRS morphology. In this circumstance, the ventricular depolarization wave front may subsequently reach the base of the heart in the vicinity of the accessory pathway's ventricular insertion site at a time when the accessory pathway has repolarized. If the accessory pathway is now receptive to retrograde depo-

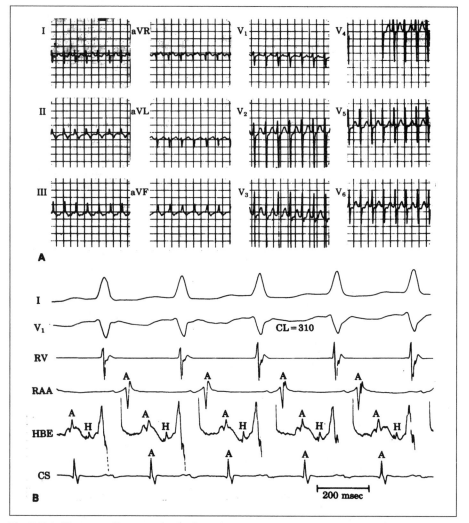

Fig. 7-7. A. Electrocardiogram of orthodromic reciprocating tachycardia utilizing a posterior septal accessory pathway. This macroreentrant tachycardia is characterized by antegrade conduction over the AV node–His bundle–Purkinje system (thus the normal QRS) with retrograde atrial depolarization via the accessory pathway. The retrograde atrial depolarization is manifested on the surface ECG as a retrograde P wave evident in the T wave of leads II, III, aVF, and V_1. Clearly discernible retrograde P waves in the ST–T wave help establish the diagnosis of orthodromic reciprocating tachycardia and eliminate the typical form of AV node reentrant tachycardia from the differential diagnosis. **B.** Surface and intracardiac electrocardiograms during orthodromic reciprocating tachycardia in a patient with an anterior septal accessory AV pathway showing an eccentric retrograde atrial activation sequence. The earliest atrial activity is recorded from right atrial appendage tissue (RAA) adjacent to the accessory pathway. The atrial signal from the His bundle electrogram (HBE) activates next, followed by left atrial tissue as recorded from the coronary sinus (CS). (Other electrograms shown: surface leads I and V_1; right ventricle [RV]. CL = cycle length.)

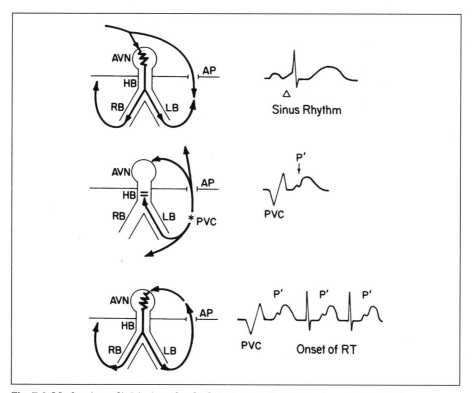

Fig. 7-8. Mechanism of initiation of orthodromic reciprocating tachycardia (RT) after a premature ventricular contraction (PVC). The PVC blocks retrogradely in the atrioventricular node (AVN) but activates the atria via the accessory pathway (AP). This dissociation of the AV node and the AP, together with unidirectional block in the AV node, is the typical setting for reentry. After retrograde depolarization of the atria, the impulse reenters the AV node antegradely and reactivates the ventricles orthodromically, thus leading to the onset of orthodromic reciprocating tachycardia. (HB = His bundle, LB = left bundle, P' = retrograde P wave, RB = right bundle.)

larization, the wave front can retrogradely enter the atrium, reenter the AV node, and establish a macroreentrant circuit.

In some instances, orthodromic reciprocating tachycardia may result during sinus rhythm without an antecedent premature impulse (Fig. 7-10). In such cases, fluctuation in autonomic tone may serve to dissociate AV node and accessory pathway conduction in such a manner as to establish reentry. For example, many patients with the WPW syndrome develop tachycardia during exercise. It is possible that in this circumstance AV nodal conduction is facilitated by an increase in circulating catecholamines and a concomitant decrease in vagal tone. This mechanism may be particularly likely to occur in patients with far-left lateral accessory pathways.

In whatever manner orthodromic reciprocating tachycardia is initiated, it persists until the reentrant circuit is blocked in one of its main limbs: the AV node, the His-Purkinje system, or the accessory pathway [1, 30, 31]. Most commonly, tachycardia terminates with block in the AV node. This is represented electrocardiographically by the last tachycardia QRS being followed by a retrograde P wave.

Another form of AV macroreentrant reciprocating tachycardia in the WPW syndrome is antidromic reciprocating tachycardia, a form of preexcited reciprocating tachycardia. This is characterized electrocardiographically by a wide QRS (fully preexcited) morphology that can be difficult to differentiate from that of ventricular tachycardia (Fig. 7-11) [25]. Antidromic reciprocating tachycardia is a consequence of antegrade activation of the ventricle entirely via the accessory pathway, with the retrograde limb of the reentrant circuit consisting of the His bundle and AV node (Fig. 7-12A). In some patients

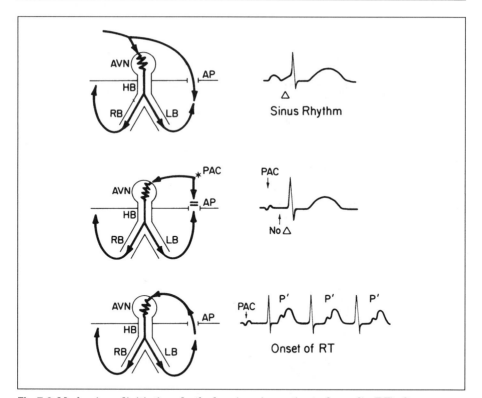

Fig. 7-9. Mechanism of initiation of orthodromic reciprocating tachycardia (RT) after a premature atrial contraction (PAC). A PAC may occur early enough that it is not conducted antegradely to the ventricle via the accessory pathway (AP) (perhaps because of the AP's long antegrade effective refractory period) but is conducted over the atrioventricular node (AVN). The ventricle thus is depolarized entirely via the His-Purkinje system, resulting in a normal QRS. In this circumstance, the ventricular depolarization wave front may reach the base of the heart at the atrioventricular groove in the vicinity of the AP's ventricular insertion when the AP has repolarized. If the AP is now receptive to retrograde depolarization, the impulse can retrogradely reenter the atrium and establish the macroreentrant circuit of orthodromic reciprocating tachycardia. (HB = His bundle; RB = right bundle; LB = left bundle; P' = retrograde P wave.)

with multiple accessory pathways, such preexcited reciprocating tachycardias may be more complicated, incorporating multiple simultaneous antegrade and retrograde pathways in the reentrant circuit (Fig. 7-12B–F). Electrophysiologically, antidromic reciprocating tachycardia is characterized by a retrograde atrial activation sequence that spreads from the AV node to the right and left atria in a symmetric fashion (Fig. 7-13). Typically, a retrograde His depolarization precedes the retrograde atrial deflection (Fig. 7-13). As with orthodromic reciprocating tachycardia, antidromic reciprocating tachycardia also usually terminates with block in the AV node [25].

The arrhythmia in the WPW syndrome with the most potential for triggering hemodynamic collapse or even ventricular fibrillation is atrial fibrillation [26]. Although atrial fibrillation in the general population occurs most commonly in the presence of underlying structural heart disease, atrial fibrillation in the WPW syndrome usually arises in the absence of underlying anatomic atrial abnormalities [22–24]. Electrocardiographically, atrial fibrillation in the WPW syndrome is characterized by a rapid, irregular, wide-complex tachycardia usually manifesting with completely preexcited QRS complexes (Fig. 7-14). However, the ECG may show occasional normal QRS complexes because of intermittent depolarization of the ventricle via the AV node–His-Purkinje system. In some instances, the QRS is typical of fusion of ventricular depolarization over both the AV node and the accessory pathway.

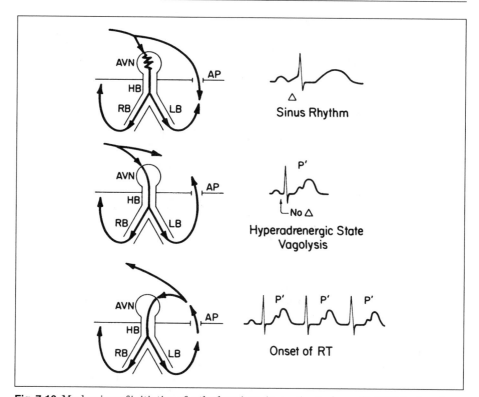

Fig. 7-10. Mechanism of initiation of orthodromic reciprocating tachycardia (RT) during sinus rhythm. In some instances, fluctuation in autonomic tone may serve to dissociate activation over the accessory pathway (AP) and the atrioventricular node (AVN) in a manner that establishes reentry. For example, during exercise, AV nodal conduction is facilitated by an increase in circulating catecholamines and a concomitant decrease in vagal tone. Exercise also shows transatrial conduction. While AV nodal conduction is facilitated, a sinus impulse may traverse the AV node–His–Purkinje system and reenter the atrium before an AP can be penetrated antegradely from the sinus impulse. This sequence of events may be particularly likely in patients with far left lateral APs. (HB = His bundle; RB = right bundle; LB = left bundle; P′ = retrograde P wave.)

The most likely mechanism for the development of atrial fibrillation is as a consequence of orthodromic reciprocating tachycardia [1, 24, 32, 33]. While in orthodromic reciprocating tachycardia, it is possible that atrial stretch, tissue hypoxia, or fragmentation of atrial conduction could lead to atrial destabilization with disruption of the macroreentrant orthodromic reciprocating tachycardia and with the development of atrial fibrillation [1, 32]. Support for this concept comes from the observation that after successful catheter ablation, most patients with clinical atrial fibrillation and WPW no longer experience this arrhythmia.

On occasion, atrial fibrillation can be of such rapidity that it can deteriorate to ventricular fibrillation [1, 26]. Ventricular fibrillation in patients with WPW syndrome has been observed principally in those who have multiple accessory pathways, reciprocating tachycardia, and rapid ventricular response to atrial fibrillation [1, 26]. The development of ventricular fibrillation is probably accounted for by rapid ventricular rates during atrial fibrillation that lead to hypotension with subsequent ventricular ischemia.

V. Therapy. The therapeutic approach to the patient with WPW syndrome should be based on a careful consideration of a variety of clinical factors such as age, severity of symptoms, underlying arrhythmia, lifestyle, and risk of sudden cardiac death. For example, in a patient whose primary arrhythmia is a rarely occurring, mildly disturbing, orthodromic reciprocating tachycardia, the most appropriate therapy may simply be instruction in the use of vagal maneuvers. If such an individual has a particular lifestyle con-

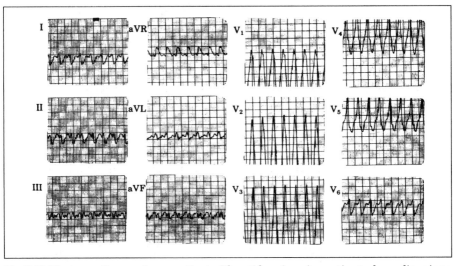

Fig. 7-11. Electrocardiogram from a patient with antidromic reciprocating tachycardia using a left lateral accessory pathway. This tracing superficially resembles that seen in ventricular tachycardia. It would be difficult to make the diagnosis of antidromic reciprocating tachycardia without an electrophysiologic study.

sideration such as competitive athletics or an avocation such as mountaineering, a recommendation for catheter ablation may be more reasonable, even for the mildly symptomatic patient. At the other end of the spectrum, a patient who has suffered hemodynamically significant, rapid, preexcited atrial fibrillation clearly should be urged to undergo definitive therapy with catheter ablation.

A. Acute management. The emergency control of tachycardia in the WPW syndrome depends on the type of tachycardia. If the patient is known to have WPW syndrome and a narrow QRS, regular tachycardia on 12-lead ECG (see Fig. 7-7A), it is reasonable to assume that this is an orthodromic reciprocating tachycardia, and emergency drug therapy can be directed toward interrupting the macroreentrant circuit in either the AV node or the accessory pathway. The most simple intervention is a vagal maneuver. If this maneuver fails, intravenous (IV) adenosine (6–12 mg) or verapamil (5–10 mg) is nearly uniformly successful in terminating tachycardia by blocking conduction in the AV node. Adenosine is particularly attractive because of its very short half-life and limited hemodynamic effects [34]. Intravenous diltiazem (0.25–0.35 mg/kg) has been shown to be similarly effective [35]. Procainamide, which exerts its effect primarily on the accessory pathway [1, 36], can be used in patients resistant to AV nodal blockade, in doses of 12–15 mg/kg administered at rates of 50 mg/minute. The principal side effect from IV procainamide is hypotension, which usually can be corrected by slowing the procainamide infusion rate and administering fluids.

The acute therapy for atrial fibrillation is more limited than that available for orthodromic reciprocating tachycardia. If the patient is hemodynamically stable and does not need emergent cardioversion, IV procainamide is the drug of choice because it slows antegrade conduction over the accessory pathway and facilitates the termination of atrial fibrillation [1, 36]. Several drugs can accelerate conduction over the accessory pathway and precipitate a more rapid ventricular response, leading to a worsened hemodynamic status and possible deterioration to ventricular fibrillation [37–39]. Digoxin [37], lidocaine [38], and particularly verapamil [39] can accelerate the ventricular response. The mechanisms by which verapamil may precipitate ventricular fibrillation are multiple. Verapamil may decrease the antegrade effective refractory period, thereby facilitating antegrade conduction. As a peripheral vasodilator and negative inotrope, verapamil can also promote hypotension and decrease cardiac output, resulting in coronary hypoperfusion and myocardial ischemia. In addition, because it has a negative dromotropic effect on the AV node [20, 40], verapamil may diminish the number of atrial impulses that traverse the AV

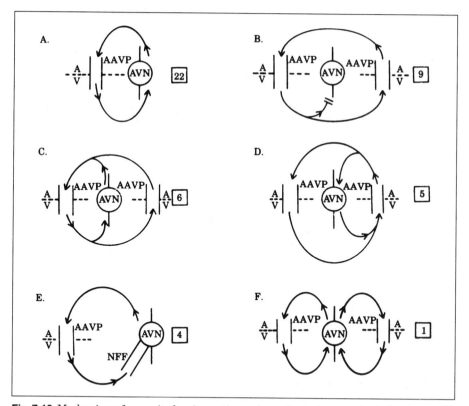

Fig. 7-12. Mechanism of preexcited reciprocating tachycardia in 47 cases. **A.** Mechanism of classic antidromic reciprocating tachycardia. **B–F.** A variety of other preexcited reciprocating tachycardia mechanisms in patients with multiple accessory pathways. The number of cases is shown in the squares. (A = atrium; V = ventricle; AAVP = accessory atrioventricular pathway; AVN = atrioventricular node; NFF = nodofascicular fiber.) (From GH Bardy et al., Preexcited reciprocating tachycardia in patients with Wolff-Parkinson-White syndrome: Incidence and mechanisms. *Circulation* 70:377–391, 1984. Reproduced with permission.)

node and, in turn, prevent concealed retrograde penetration of the accessory pathway [39, 41]. In this setting, the accessory pathway would function at a rate limited by its intrinsic refractoriness. Intravenous verapamil therefore should not be used in the emergent treatment of WPW patients with atrial fibrillation.

B. Chronic management. Chronic therapy for WPW syndrome should be based on severity of symptoms and lifestyle considerations. Radiofrequency catheter ablation has revolutionized the management of the WPW syndrome. As is discussed in Chap. 13, catheter ablation can be curative in over 90% of patients with minimal risk [42]. As opposed to surgery, which was previously performed in patients with life-threatening or drug-refractory arrhythmias [21], virtually any symptomatic patient with WPW can be considered a candidate for this procedure. If it is decided to manage a patient pharmacologically, the drug regimen chosen should not increase the risk of a rapid ventricular response during atrial fibrillation [37–39]. As a rule, chronic oral digoxin and verapamil should be avoided in all patients with WPW syndrome, even those without documented atrial fibrillation. Chronic therapy with type 1 antiarrhythmic agents, on the other hand, is often effective [36, 43]. Procainamide, quinidine, and disopyramide are effective in suppressing antegrade and retrograde accessory pathway conduction [36, 43]. Flecainide [44] and propafenone [45] can also be useful in suppressing both normal AV and accessory AV pathway conduction and are effective in controlling clinical arrhythmias. Amiodarone [46] is also very effective, but its toxicity profile limits its use in younger patients.

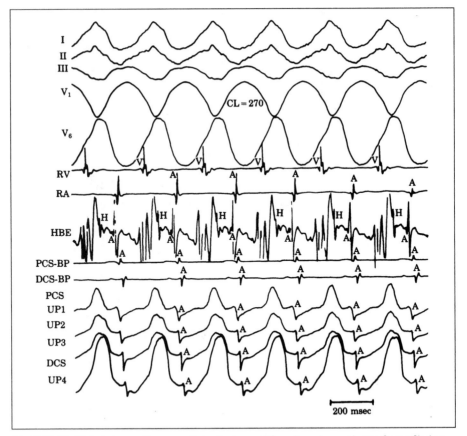

Fig. 7-13. Multiple intracardiac recordings during antidromic reciprocating tachycardia in a patient with an anterior septal accessory pathway. Electrograms from top to bottom are limb leads I, II, and III; precordial leads V_1 and V_6; intracardiac electrograms from the right ventricle (RV), right atrium (RA), His bundle (HBE), and coronary sinus (CS). The CS signals are proximal bipole (PCS-BP), distal bipole (DCS-BP), and CS unipoles (UP) 1–4, proximal to distal. Cycle length (CL) is 270 msec. Note the retrograde atrial activation sequence that spreads from the AV node (HBE) to the right atrium (RA) and to the left atrium (CS) in a symmetric fashion. A retrograde His deflection precedes the earliest retrograde atrial depolarization on the HBE, which provides further evidence of antidromic reciprocating tachycardia. (From GH Bardy et al., Preexcited reciprocating tachycardia in patients with Wolff-Parkinson-White syndrome: Incidence and mechanisms. *Circulation* 70:377–391, 1984. Reproduced with permission.)

Beta blockers can be useful in preventing or slowing orthodromic reciprocating tachycardia. Their effect of antegrade conduction, however, is generally believed to be small [47]. Nevertheless, we have noticed an occasional patient in whom conduction accelerates over the accessory pathway during atrial fibrillation because of AV node blockade. This may be due to decreased concealed retrograde penetration of the accessory pathway because of AV nodal blockade [41], as might be observed with digoxin and verapamil. Consequently, treatment of atrial fibrillation in patients with WPW syndrome with beta blockers alone is not recommended.

In patients with infrequent, mildly symptomatic orthodromic reciprocating tachycardia who favor pharmacologic therapy, cocktail therapy may be most appropriate [48]. Procainamide in a large, oral bolus (25 mg/kg) commonly terminates the tachycardia within 60 minutes and keeps the patient from having to go to an emergency room.

It is important to emphasize that patients suffering from chronically recurring tachycardia may be subjected to drug therapy for many years with the attendant

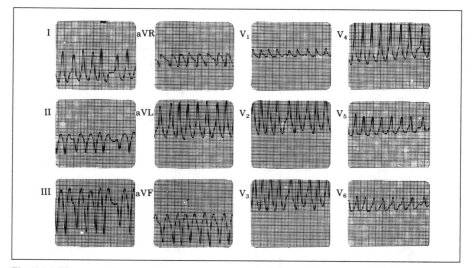

Fig. 7-14. Electrocardiogram from a patient with atrial fibrillation and ventricular activation over a posterior septal accessory pathway. Note the irregularity of the R–R intervals, which is a clue to the diagnosis and helps differentiate this rhythm from other forms of wide-complex tachycardia.

drug side effects, risks, and recurrent symptoms. In general, patients with life-threatening arrhythmias (atrial fibrillation with a rapid ventricular response) and patients with frequent tachycardia of any mechanism should be strongly considered for catheter ablation.

VI. **Approach to the patient with asymptomatic preexcitation.** The approach to the asymptomatic patient with a delta wave on the surface ECG has been controversial [1, 49]. In rare cases, patients can have ventricular fibrillation as the first clinical manifestation of the WPW syndrome [26]. Risk stratification for sudden cardiac death therefore has been a major concern in these usually otherwise healthy individuals. The clinical characteristic most closely associated with a history of ventricular fibrillation is the rate of antegrade conduction over an accessory pathway during atrial fibrillation [26]. In the original study from Duke University, all patients with WPW and a history of ventricular fibrillation had R–R intervals of 250 msec or less, measured during atrial fibrillation [26]. On the basis of this study, electrophysiologic testing to induce atrial fibrillation and document the ventricular response has been recommended as a means of risk-stratifying asymptomatic patients. The specificity of this test, however, is too low to be useful given the very low incidence of sudden death in this population [49].

The utility of electrophysiologic testing in asymptomatic patients was evaluated prospectively in a Canadian study of 75 asymptomatic patients followed for an average of 4.3 years [50]. Measured R–R intervals during induced atrial fibrillation of less than 250 msec were seen in 31% of patients. No patient died suddenly. Furthermore, only 8% of patients developed symptoms. In a recent long-term community-based study [13], there were no sudden deaths in 36 asymptomatic patients followed for over 10 years. Symptoms did, however, develop in 21% of these patients. On the basis of these studies, a clinical history of no symptoms is associated with an excellent prognosis, and electrophysiologic testing is not justified in these patients. An assessment of the antegrade properties of the accessory pathway occasionally can be obtained noninvasively. Spontaneous loss of preexcitation on ambulatory recording or during exercise testing is associated with a slower (>250 msec) ventricular response during atrial fibrillation [51, 52]. Also, loss of preexcitation with administration of procainamide (550 mg over 20 minutes) correlates well with R–R intervals more than 250 msec during atrial fibrillation [53].

VII. **Concealed accessory AV pathways.** A concealed accessory AV pathway conducts only in the retrograde direction and clinically gives rise to a single arrhythmia: orthodromic reciprocating tachycardia. The ECG does not manifest a delta wave because of the

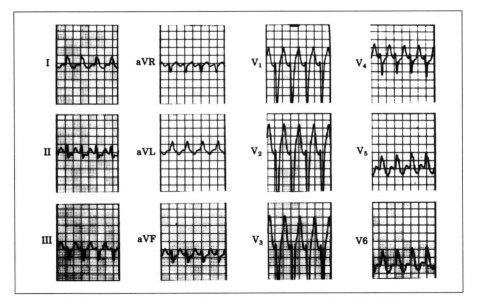

Fig. 7-15. Electrocardiogram from a patient with reciprocating tachycardia utilizing a nodoventricular Mahaim fiber in the antegrade direction. The typical QRS morphology is left bundle branch block with a left axis.

absence of antegrade conduction over the accessory AV pathway. There are no published data available defining the true incidence of concealed accessory pathways compared to manifest ones. Our experience in a referral institution, however, indicates that concealed and manifest accessory pathways occur about equally in our patient population.

VIII. Variants of the WPW syndrome. Several electrophysiologic substrates have been described that produce electrocardiographic variants of the WPW syndrome. The syndrome of a short P–R interval, normal QRS complex, and paroxysmal supraventricular tachycardia is commonly referred to as the Lown-Ganong-Levine (LGL) syndrome [1, 54]. An atriohisian tract or James fiber bypassing AV nodal delay has been proposed as the mechanism for the short P–R interval and the substrate for tachycardia. Though described anatomically [55], there is no evidence for the participation of such a pathway in clinical arrhythmias. In fact, there is no evidence for the existence of a distinct LGL syndrome. It is likely that such patients have AV nodal reentry or a concealed bypass tract and a variant of normal AV nodal conduction [1, 56].

Mahaim fibers are accessory AV connections thought originally to bridge the AV node to the right ventricular endocardium (nodoventricular fibers) or the right bundle branch (nodofascicular fibers) [1, 57]. More recent studies suggest that most of these pathways originate from the right atrial free wall rather than the AV node [58, 59]. This is a rare conduction abnormality, found in fewer than 3% of patients with the preexcitation syndrome [57, 60, 61]. Mahaim fibers are more commonly seen in patients who have Ebstein's anomaly [60]. In addition, they may be associated with accessory AV pathways [57, 60, 61]. On occasion, they occur in an isolated state in a normal heart [29, 60, 61].

Characteristic electrophysiologic features of Mahaim fibers include conduction in the antegrade direction only and decremental conduction (slowed conduction with faster rates). The typical tachycardia is antidromic using the Mahaim fiber as the antegrade limb and the normal conduction system as the retrograde limb (Fig. 7-15). Since the pathway inserts into the right ventricle or right bundle branch, Mahaim tachycardia will have left bundle branch block morphology because of preexcitation of the right ventricle [61]. A Mahaim fiber can also serve as a "bystander" to the more common arrhythmia of AV node reentrant tachycardia [29]. On occasion, a Mahaim fiber can serve as a limb of a macroreentrant circuit associated with an accessory pathway [25]. These pathways have recently been shown to be amenable to radiofrequency catheter ablation at their atrial insertion along the tricuspid anulus [62].

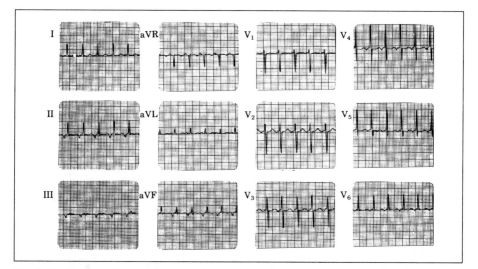

Fig. 7-16. Electrocardiogram from a patient with the permanent form of junctional reciprocating tachycardia owing to a decrementally conducting posterior septal accessory AV pathway. Note the long R–P′ interval and characteristically negative P waves in leads II, III, and aVF.

Fasciculoventricular connections are associated with a normal P–R interval and a fixed preexcited QRS complex [60]. They arise from the His bundle or more distal conduction system and insert in ventricular myocardium, shortening the H–V interval. They have not been shown to produce arrhythmias.

The "permanent" form of functional reciprocating tachycardia (PJRT) is another variant of the preexcitation syndromes characterized clinically by incessant or nearly incessant narrow QRS-complex tachycardia. Electrophysiologic, surgical, and anatomic data have confirmed that PJRT is a consequence of a retrograde-only posterior septal accessory AV pathway with nodal or decremental conducting properties [30, 63]. Electrocardiographically, PJRT manifests as a relatively slow tachycardia (rates 130–170 beats/minute) with a long R–P interval (i.e., the R–P interval is greater than the P–R interval) and with an inverted P wave in ECG leads II, III, and aVF (Fig. 7-16). It is treated in much the same way as standard concealed posterior septal accessory AV pathways.

References

1. Gallagher JJ, et al. The preexcitation syndromes. *Prog Cardiovasc Dis* 20:285–327, 1978.
2. Wilson FN. A case in which the vagus influenced the form of the ventricular complex of the electrocardiogram. *Arch Intern Med* 16:1008–1027, 1915.
3. Cohn AE, Fraser FR. Paroxysmal tachycardia and the effect of stimulation of the vagus nerves by pressure. *Heart* 5:93–105, 1913, 1914.
4. Bain CWC, Hamilton CK. Electrocardiographic changes in rheumatic carditis. *Lancet* 1:807–809, 1926.
5. Hamburger WW. Bundle branch block: Four cases of intraventricular block showing some interesting and unusual clinical features. *Med Clin North Am* 13:343–362, 1929.
6. Wolff L, Parkinson J, White PD. Bundle branch block with short P–R interval in healthy young people prone to paroxysmal tachycardia. *Am Heart J* 5:685–704, 1930.
7. Rosenbaum FF, et al. The potential variations of the thorax and the esophagus in anomalous atrioventricular excitation (Wolff-Parkinson-White syndrome). *Am Heart J* 29: 281–326, 1945.
8. Davies MJ, Anderson RH, Becker AE. *The Conduction System of the Heart.* London: Butterworth, 1983. Pp 189–190.
9. Lunel AAV. Significance of anulus fibrosus of heart in relation to AV conduction and

ventricular activation in cases of Wolff-Parkinson-White syndrome. *Br Heart J* 34: 1263–1271, 1972.

10. Becker AE, et al. The anatomical substrates of Wolff-Parkinson-White syndrome: A clinicopathologic correlation in 7 patients. *Circulation* 57:870–879, 1978.

11. Klein GJ, Hackel DB, Gallagher JJ. Anatomic substrate of impaired antegrade conduction over an accessory atrioventricular pathway in the Wolff-Parkinson-White syndrome. *Circulation* 61:1249–1256, 1980.

12. Sherf L. General Considerations. In L Sherf, HN Neufeld (eds), *The Preexcitation Syndrome: Facts and Theories*. New York: Yorke Medical Books, 1978. Pp 1–24.

13. Munger TM, et al. A population study of the natural history of Wolff-Parkinson-White syndrome in Olmstead County, Minnesota, 1953–1989. *Circulation* 87:866–873, 1993.

14. Vidallet HJ, et al. Familial occurrence of accessory atrioventricular pathways (preexcitation syndrome). *N Engl J Med* 317:65–69, 1987.

15. Watson H. Natural history of Ebstein's anomaly of tricuspid valve in childhood and adolescence: An international cooperative study of 505 cases. *Br Heart J* 36:417–427, 1974.

16. Giuliani ER, Fuster V, Brandenburg RO. Special review: Ebstein's anomaly: The clinical features and natural history of Ebstein's anomaly of the tricuspid valve. *Mayo Clin Proc* 54:163–173, 1979.

17. Smith WM, et al. The electrophysiologic basis and management of symptomatic recurrent tachycardia in patients with Ebstein's anomaly of the tricuspid valve. *Am J Cardiol* 49:1223–1234, 1982.

18. Davis D, et al. Persistent left superior vena cava in patients with congenital atrioventricular preexcitation conduction abnormalities. *Am Heart J* 101:677–679, 1981.

19. Sherf L. General Consideration. In L Sherf, HN Neufeld (eds), *The Preexcitation Syndrome: Facts and Theories*. New York: Yorke Medical Books, 1978. Pp 1–24.

20. Zipes DB, Fisher JC. Effects of agents which inhibit the slow channel on sinus node automaticity and atrioventricular conduction in the dog. *Circ Res* 34:184–192, 1974.

21. Gallagher JJ, et al. Results of Surgery for Preexcitation Caused by Accessory Atrioventricular Pathways in 267 Consecutive Cases. In ME Josephson, HJJ Wellens (eds), *Tachycardias: Mechanisms, Diagnosis and Treatment*. Philadelphia: Lea and Febiger, 1984. Pp 259–269.

22. Campbell RWF, et al. Atrial fibrillation in the preexcitation syndrome: *Am J Cardiol* 40:514–520, 1977.

23. Bauernfeind RA, et al. Paroxysmal atrial fibrillation the Wolff-Parkinson-White syndrome. *Am J Cardiol* 47:562–569, 1981.

24. Sharma A, et al. Atrial fibrillation in patients with Wolff-Parkinson-White syndrome: Incidence after surgical ablation of the accessory pathway. *Circulation* 72:161–169, 1985.

25. Bardy GH, et al. Preexcited reciprocating tachycardia in patients with Wolff-Parkinson-White syndrome: Incidence and mechanisms. *Circulation* 70:377–391, 1984.

26. Klein GJ, et al. Ventricular fibrillation in the Wolff-Parkinson-White syndrome. *N Engl J Med* 301:1080–1085, 1979.

27. Kerr CR, Gallagher JJ, German LD. Changes in ventriculoatrial intervals with bundle branch block aberration during reciprocating tachycardia in patients with accessory atrioventricular pathways. *Circulation* 66:196–201, 1982.

28. Pritchett ELL, et al. Ventriculoatrial conduction time during reciprocating tachycardia with intermittent bundle branch block in Wolff-Parkinson-White syndrome. *Br Heart J* 38:1058–1064, 1976.

29. Bardy GH, et al. Mechanisms of tachycardia utilizing a nodofascicular Mahaim fiber. *Am J Cardiol* 54:1140–1141, 1984.

30. Farre G, et al. Reciprocal tachycardia using accessory pathways with long conduction times. *Am J Cardiol* 44:1099–1109, 1979.

31. Bar FW, et al. Differential diagnosis of tachycardia with narrow QRS complex (shorter than 0.12 second). *Am J Cardiol* 54:555–560, 1984.

32. Sung RJ, et al. Mechanisms of spontaneous alternation between reciprocating tachycardia and atrial flutter/fibrillation in the Wolff-Parkinson-White syndrome. *Circulation* 56:409–416, 1977.

33. Roark SF, et al. Observations on the occurrence of atrial fibrillation in paroxysmal supraventricular tachycardia. *Am J Cardiol* 57:571–575, 1986.

34. Lerman B. Cardiac electrophysiology of adenosine. *Circulation* 83:827, 1991.

35. Huycke EC, et al. Intravenous diltiazem for termination of reentrant supraventricular tachycardia: A placebo controlled, randomized double blind, multicenter study. *J Am Coll Cardiol* 3:538, 1989.

36. Sellers TD, et al. Effects of procainamide and quinidine sulfate in the Wolff-Parkinson-

White syndrome. *Circulation* 55:15–22, 1977.

37. Sellers TD, Bashore TM, Gallagher JJ. Digitalis in the preexcitation syndrome: Analysis during atrial fibrillation. *Circulation* 56:260–267, 1977.

38. Akhtar M, Gilbert DJ, Shenasa M. Effect of lidocaine on atrioventricular response via the accessory pathway in patients with Wolff-Parkinson-White syndrome. *Circulation* 63:435–441, 1981.

39. Gulamhusein S, et al. Acceleration of the ventricular response during atrial fibrillation in the Wolff-Parkinson-White syndrome after verapamil. *Circulation* 65:348–354, 1982.

40. Wil AL, Cranefield PF. Effect of verapamil on the sinoatrial and atrioventricular nodes of the rabbit and the mechanism by which it arrests reentrant atrioventricular nodal tachycardia. *Circ Res* 35:413–425, 1974.

41. Klein GJ, Yee R, Sharma AD. Concealed conduction in accessory atrioventricular pathways: An important determinant of the expression of arrhythmias in patients with Wolff-Parkinson-White syndrome. *Circulation* 70:402–411, 1984.

42. Jackman WM, et al. Catheter ablation of accessory atrioventricular pathways (Wolff-Parkinson-White syndrome) by radiofrequency current. *N Engl J Med* 324:1605, 1991.

43. Kerr CR, et al. Electrophysiologic effects of disopyramide phosphate in patients with Wolff-Parkinson-White syndrome. *Circulation* 65:869–878, 1982.

44. Neuss H. Effects of flecainide on electrophysiologic properties of accessory pathways in the Wolff-Parkinson-White syndrome. *Circulation* 69:347–353, 1983.

45. Ludmer PL. Efficacy of propafenone in Wolff-Parkinson-White syndrome: Electrophysiologic findings and long term follow-up. *JACC* 9:1357–1363, 1987.

46. Feld GK, et al. Electrophysiologic basis for the suppression by amiodarone of orthodromic supraventricular tachycardia complicating preexcitation syndromes. *J Am Coll Cardiol* 3:1289–1307, 1984.

47. Denes P, et al. Effects of propranolol on anomalous pathway refractoriness and circus movement tachycardia in patients with preexcitation. *Am J Cardiol* 41:1061–1067, 1978.

48. Benson DW, et al. Periodic procainamide for paroxysmal tachycardia. *Circulation* 72:147–152, 1985.

49. Klein GJ, et al. Asymptomatic Wolff-Parkinson-White: Should we intervene? *Circulation* 80:1902–1905, 1989.

50. Leitch JW, et al. Prognostic value of electrophysiologic testing in asymptomatic patients with the Wolff-Parkinson-White pattern. *Circulation* 82:1718–1723, 1990.

51. Klein GJ, et al. Intermittent preexcitation in the Wolff-Parkinson-White syndrome. *Am J Cardiol* 52:292–296, 1983.

52. Sharma AD, et al. Sensitivity and specificity of invasive and noninvasive testing for risk of sudden death in Wolff-Parkinson-White syndrome. *J Am Coll Cardiol* 10:373–381, 1987.

53. Boahene KA, et al. Value of a revised procainamide test in the Wolff-Parkinson-White syndrome. *Am J Cardiol* 65:195–200, 1990.

54. Benditt DG, et al. Characteristics of atrioventricular conduction and the spectrum of arrhythmias in Lown-Ganong-Levine syndrome. *Circulation* 57:454–465, 1978.

55. Brechenmacher C. Atrio His bundle tracts. *Br Heart J* 37:853–855, 1975.

56. Jackman WM, et al. Reevaluation of enhanced atrioventricular nodal conduction: Evidence to suggest a continuum of normal atrioventricular physiology. *Circulation* 67:441–448, 1983.

57. Gallagher JJ, et al. Variants of the Preexcitation Syndrome. In MB Rosenbaum, MV Elizari (eds), *Frontiers of Cardiac Electrophysiology*. Boston: Martinus Nijhoff, 1983. Pp 724–772.

58. Tchou P, et al. Atriofascicular connection or a nodoventricular Mahaim fiber? Electrophysiologic elucidation of the pathway and associated reentry circuit. *Circulation* 77:837–848, 1988.

59. Klein GJ, et al. "Nodoventricular" accessory pathway: Evidence for a distinct accessory atrioventricular pathway with atrioventricular node like properties. *J Am Coll Cardiol* 11:1035–1040, 1988.

60. Gallagher JJ, et al. Role of Mahaim fibers in cardiac arrhythmias in man. *Circulation* 64:176–189, 1981.

61. Bardy GH, et al. Electrocardiographic clues suggesting the presence of a nodofascicular Mahaim fiber. *J Am Coll Cardiol* 3:1161–1168, 1984.

62. Klein LS, et al. Radiofrequency ablation of Mahaim fibers at the tricuspid annulus. *Circulation* 87:738–747, 1993.

63. Gallagher JJ, Sealy WC. The permanent form of junctional reciprocating tachycardia: Further elucidation of the underlying mechanism. *Eur J Cardiol* 8:413–430, 1978.

Ventricular Arrhythmias

Stephen C. Vlay

8

Treatment of ventricular arrhythmias is less controversial than it once was [1–7]. For patients with symptomatic ventricular tachycardia (VT), the indications for therapy are well established. The asymptomatic individual with nonsustained three-beat salvos on ambulatory monitoring deserves evaluation, but empiric therapy has potential hazard. CAST (Cardiac Arrhythmia Suppression Trial) substantiated the point that "no study has ever conclusively demonstrated improved survival if asymptomatic VT is treated with antiarrhythmic drugs. In fact, almost all antiarrhythmic drugs have arrhythmogenic potential and infrequently may exacerbate asymptomatic nonsustained VT into sustained symptomatic VT or ventricular fibrillation (VF)." Greater recognition of the potential of antiarrhythmic drugs for causing sudden cardiac death (SCD) changed the prescribing habits of physicians who at one time would have considered one of these drugs if isolated ventricular premature beats (VPBs) were observed on the ECG.

Initial attempts to assess the risk of VPBs led Lown and Wolf [8] to propose a grading system for ventricular ectopy (Table 8-1). Complex and frequent ectopy has been associated with an increased risk of sudden death, while low-grade ectopy has a benign prognosis. Objections to the original Lown classification include the fact that the patient is characterized by the highest grade, while characteristics of lower grades may also be present [9]. Thus, the individual with asymptomatic VT, multiform VPBs, and more than 30 uniform VPBs/hour may be different from the individual with asymptomatic VT alone, yet both are considered grade 4B. Additionally, the grading system does not take into account any underlying heart disease. When reporting the results of ambulatory monitoring, the clinician should note, in addition to the descriptive analysis, all the Lown grades the patient fits into, not only the highest. Frequent and complex ventricular ectopy usually reflects underlying heart disease of varying severity. The individual with asymptomatic VT and coronary artery disease may have a different prognosis from one with asymptomatic VT and mitral valve prolapse (MVP). Thus, it is important to know the underlying anatomic substrate. The R-on-T phenomenon may be most important in the presence of acute ischemia or a prolonged Q–T interval. Despite these criticisms, the Lown classification system remains an important tool in classifying arrhythmias.

With many variables to consider, it becomes imperative to evaluate each case individually and to determine which studies are indicated. Unnecessary studies must be avoided, but there are times when an aggressive approach is mandatory. Key points in treating patients with ventricular arrhythmias can be found in Table 8-2.

I. Approach to the patient with ventricular ectopy

A. History. In the clinical recognition of arrhythmias, historical details may provide clues to the nature of the arrhythmia. The most important determination is **whether the patient's symptoms are due to an arrhythmia** or to another cause, possibly of neurologic or vascular origin. The physician must assess the severity of the symptoms. Does the patient experience only the sensation of a "missed" or "skipped" beat? Is there a sense of throbbing, flushing, or rapid palpitations? Does the patient become syncopal or nearly syncopal, indicating hemodynamic compromise? The answers to these questions determine the classification of the patient into the **symptomatic** or **asymptomatic** ventricular ectopy group, a critical distinction because the treatment for each may be quite different.

B. Physical exam. Unless the arrhythmia is manifest at the time of examination, its value lies primarily in assessing the nature of the underlying heart disease. The special clues for differentiating arrhythmias are discussed in Chap. 4.

C. **Candidates for further study.** The extent of further evaluation depends on the complexity of the ventricular ectopy, the underlying heart disease, and how symptomatic the patient is.

1. **Asymptomatic patients.** The asymptomatic patient, in whom isolated, uniform VPBs are observed, will usually require only a careful history, identification of cardiac risk factors, and a physical examination. The ECG provides limited information unless the results are grossly abnormal. The laboratory examination indicates whether a transient electrolyte abnormality may have caused an arrhythmia. The chest x ray will be diagnostic of an underlying disorder only infrequently. Depending on the patient's age, risk profile, and physical findings, the physician may elect further tests, such as an echocardiogram or exercise test, to establish a specific diagnosis.

   If a patient has asymptomatic VT, a search for the underlying heart disease is in order. It is important to note that evaluation will not necessarily lead to treatment. In addition to echocardiography and stress testing, further definition of the underlying problem with radionuclide techniques (thallium or sestamibi, radionuclide angiography) may be necessary.

2. **Symptomatic patients.** One must be more aggressive with the symptomatic individual, particularly the patient who survives symptomatic sustained VT, out-of-hospital cardiac arrest, or VF. While noninvasive testing provides the initial diagnostic information, these life-threatening arrhythmias (when not associated with acute myocardial infarction [MI]) may recur if not adequately prevented and merit extensive evaluation. The patient may not be fortunate enough to be resuscitated during the second episode. Consequently cardiac catheterization and clinical electrophysiologic studies are recommended for these individuals. Very few physicians will disagree with this approach; however, those who do must bear the burden of incomplete information and perhaps therapy of unproved efficacy.

Table 8-1. Modified grading system for ventricular ectopy

1.	Fewer than 30 uniform VPBs/hour
	A. Fewer than 1/minute
	B. More than 1/minute
2.	More than 30 uniform VPBs/hour
3.	Multiform VPBs
4A.	Couplets (two consecutive VPBs)
4B.	Triplets (three or more consecutive VPBs)
5.	R-on-T phenomenon

VPBs = ventricular premature beats.
Source: Modified from B Lown and M Wolf, Grading system for ventricular ectopy. *Circulation* 44: 130–142, 1971.

Table 8-2. Key points in treating patients with ventricular arrhythmias

1. Is the arrhythmia symptomatic (associated with hemodynamic compromise) or asymptomatic?
2. Is there serious underlying heart disease?
3. Is the arrhythmia likely to recur, or was it due to a transient (and nonrecurrent) precipitating factor?
4. What is the risk of sudden cardiac death?
5. Does the case require evaluation by invasive procedures (cardiac catheterization, electrophysiologic study), or is noninvasive testing sufficient?
6. Is the risk of drug therapy greater than the risk of not treating the patient?
7. If drug therapy is necessary, which agent should be selected to maximize benefit and minimize risk?
8. Is drug therapy sufficient, or should additional measures such as internal cardioverter-defibrillator devices (with antitachycardia pacing, low-energy cardioversion, and high-energy defibrillation) or arrhythmia surgery be considered?

The patient who is symptomatic, that is, has "dizzy spells," and manifests complex ventricular ectopy but not VT, presents a more difficult situation. Noninvasive testing is necessary, but no one is eager to recommend invasive procedures without good reason, since they are not without potential morbidity and expense. Some of these individuals may be successfully treated with the noninvasive approach, particularly if their symptoms are frequent, reproducible, provoked by stress testing, and completely suppressed by empiric therapy. Nevertheless, if the patient remains symptomatic despite cardiac and noncardiac noninvasive testing and despite initial therapeutic trials, invasive studies may provide the final answer.

D. Noninvasive studies

1. **Holter monitoring.** Twenty-four-hour ECG recording provides evidence of supraventricular or ventricular ectopy or conduction disturbances that may cause dizziness or syncope (see Chap. 10). Because of the day-to-day variability of ectopy, at least 72 hours of monitoring is necessary before seeking another cause for the symptoms. Indeed there will be a number of patients whose symptoms occur as soon as the monitor has been removed. For this group, the availability of an event recorder that can be activated at the onset of the arrhythmia is useful. The event record is either stored and later retrieved or immediately transmitted to a central office by telephone.

    Electrocardiographic recording is not only a diagnostic tool but also provides a measure of efficacy of treatment. Patients in whom both symptoms and ventricular ectopy can be suppressed may benefit from the noninvasive approach and possibly avoid invasive studies.

    All patients with serious arrhythmias should undergo Holter monitoring before and after therapy to assess the response to specific drugs. Monitoring may also allow correlation between clinical outcome and the method used to guide therapy (empiric, noninvasive, or invasive).

    Signal-averaging techniques (see Chap. 11) may provide further, although somewhat limited, information to identify patients at higher risk of VT after MI or in patients with cardiomyopathy. Low-amplitude, high-frequency potentials at the end of the QRS complex have been correlated with delayed and fragmented ventricular activation noted during endocardial mapping.

2. **Exercise testing.** Patients suspected of having serious arrhythmias may benefit from exercise testing as part of the initial evaluation if it is physically possible and there are no contraindications. If the patient has known ischemia, exercise testing is unnecessary for diagnostic purposes but may provide physiologic data about the response of the arrhythmia to preceding ischemia or changes in heart rate (Fig. 8-1). Patients with ischemia as a triggering mechanism may benefit from beta-blocker therapy of the underlying heart disease. Exercise testing may reproduce the arrhythmia in patients with catecholamine-sensitive VT (see **VII. E**). These patients may respond to beta blockade, which blunts the effect of catecholamines on the heart. Conversely, patients with frequent ectopy at rest that is suppressed by increasing heart rate may have an exacerbation of the ectopy with drugs that slow the heart rate. The value of exercise testing is further described in Chap. 10.

3. **Echocardiography.** The value of the echocardiogram in the treatment of arrhythmias is in the identification of the underlying cardiac disorder, if any. The M-mode and two-dimensional echocardiograms are particularly useful in demonstrating MVP, hypertrophic or dilated cardiomyopathy, and asynergic areas or aneurysm in ischemic heart disease. These are the most common anatomic substrates. The pediatric cardiologist will use echocardiography to evaluate congenital heart disease, with a notably high incidence of arrhythmias in tetralogy of Fallot (particularly postoperatively). Occasionally the older adult who is examined for atrial arrhythmias may be discovered to have an undiagnosed atrial septal defect. The addition of Doppler techniques may further categorize valvular disease and even permit an estimation of valve area.

4. **Radionuclide techniques.** Radionuclide techniques enhance the sensitivity and specificity of exercise testing. Electrocardiographic changes cannot be used to evaluate the possibility of ischemia in a patient with left bundle branch block, left ventricular hypertrophy, Wolff-Parkinson-White syndrome, or baseline ST–T wave abnormalities that are nonspecific or associated with digitalis (or other drugs). Imaging with thallium 201 or sestamibi will indicate and localize areas of normal perfusion, temporary ischemia, or permanent scar. Gated blood

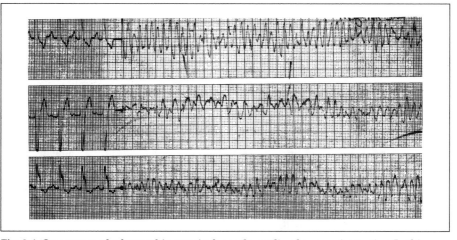

Fig. 8-1. Occurrence of polymorphic ventricular tachycardia after exercise testing. In this very unusual case, polymorphic ventricular tachycardia developed 3 minutes after the end of exercise. The patient had left bundle branch block but no other underlying heart disease. Interestingly, electrophysiologic testing (EPS) reproduced the same polymorphic ventricular tachycardia, which is often a nonclinical response during EPS.

pool imaging will assess ejection fraction as well as regional and global ventricular dysfunction. If the radionuclide ventriculogram is performed during the arrhythmia, computer analysis of time activity variations may allow phase mapping [10]. This technique, however, has not replaced endocardial mapping.

E. **Invasive studies.** The necessity for invasive studies depends on the severity of the arrhythmia. Patients with infrequent low-grade ectopy or even asymptomatic non-sustained VT usually do not require cardiac catheterization or electrophysiologic testing for management of the arrhythmia. In some of these cases, cardiac catheterization is performed to evaluate the underlying heart disease (e.g., in the patient with ischemia early in the exercise test).

The survivor of sudden cardiac arrest caused by sustained VT or VF, when not associated with acute MI, presents a different situation. If associated with acute MI, the arrhythmia usually is not a recurrent problem, owing to the transient nature of the precipitating event and the possibility that the irritable focus is extirpated in the scarring process. When VT or VF occurs in the absence of acute MI, the anatomic substrate remains unchanged, and the potential for recurrence remains high. Perhaps the patient will not be fortunate enough to be resuscitated during the next episode. Therefore, it is desirable to obtain as much data as possible about the anatomic substrate for VT or VF, in order to direct therapy against the underlying disorder as well as the arrhythmia. Consequently, I recommend that **all survivors of sudden cardiac arrest (not associated with acute MI) who are candidates for further evaluation and therapy undergo cardiac catheterization (including coronary arteriography and left ventriculography) when these tests are not contraindicated.** Similarly, **these patients are also candidates for electrophysiologic study (EPS) with therapy directed by the response to antiarrhythmic drugs** (i.e., suppression of inducibility).

There is little argument that the survivor of VT or VF requires EPS when ambulatory monitoring reveals little or no ventricular ectopy. The patient with frequent, symptomatic, complex ventricular ectopy presents a different situation. Arrhythmia experts favoring the noninvasive approach would argue that suppression of symptomatic complex ectopy with appropriate drug therapy indicates a good response and prognosis. The invasive electrophysiologist would disagree, saying that suppression during initial monitoring may not predict protection against recurrence of VT or VF once the patient leaves the hospital. A number of drugs may suppress ectopy, but the patient may remain at risk of VT or VF. As with any other disorder, therapy must be individualized. I prefer the electrophysiologic approach for survivors of VT or VF. For patients with mildly symptomatic, nonhypotensive sustained VT, the argument for the noninvasive approach may be stronger. This controversy is discussed in detail in Chaps. 15–16.

1. **Cardiac catheterization.** Cardiac catheterization remains the gold standard. It allows definitive assessment of hemodynamics, coronary anatomy, ventricular contractility, and valvular disorders. Important prognostic variables include the extent and severity of coronary artery disease and the amount of left ventricular dysfunction, as assessed by cardiac chamber size and wall thickness, global and regional contractility, ejection fraction, and left ventricular end-diastolic pressure (LVEDP). Some investigators have suggested that a narrowing of the left anterior descending artery before the first septal perforator is an independent predictor of outcome in patients who have survived sudden cardiac arrest caused by VT or VF [11, 12]. Other important variables include certain segmental contraction abnormalities, as well as variables of left ventricular function such as ejection fraction and LVEDP.

   Most patients with VT or VF who are referred to the catheterization lab will have underlying coronary artery disease (65–80% in most series). Cardiomyopathies, the next most common category (15–25%), may include dilated congestive (with normal coronary arteries), hypertrophic, or infiltrative myopathies. Valvular disease is discovered in another 5–10% of patients, possibly because of pressure-volume overload problems related to the stenotic or regurgitant valve, resulting in abnormalities of ventricular function. Mitral valve prolapse is an interesting underlying cause of atrial and ventricular ectopy. Rarely, it may be associated with SCD. However, it is uncertain whether MVP is responsible or coincidental; possibly some of these patients have another problem, such as primary electrical disease that precipitated VT or VF. Nevertheless, a recent study suggests that some patients with MVP who die suddenly tend to be relatively young women without mitral regurgitation [13].

   Uncommon underlying causes of ventricular tachyarrhythmias include arrhythmogenic right ventricular dysplasia, congenital heart disease, and the prolonged Q–T syndrome (perhaps more unrecognized than uncommon). Rarely, no anatomic abnormality will be found. There are three possible explanations for this: (1) The patient has primary electrical disease with an otherwise normal heart, (2) the disease is in a very early stage of development and is not yet grossly apparent, or (3) our diagnostic methods are not sufficiently sensitive to detect the problem. A study using myocardial biopsy in patients with VT and apparently normal hearts revealed inflammatory cell infiltration, suggesting a subclinical myocarditis in some patients [14] and fibrosis or other structural changes in others.

2. **Electrophysiologic studies.** The subject of EPS is covered in depth in Chap. 12. Briefly, EPS consist of the temporary placement of catheter electrodes into the heart to record intracardiac electrograms and to stimulate various sites. Conduction is assessed for abnormalities. Programmed electrical stimulation attempts to reproduce the arrhythmia and then suppress it with various antiarrhythmic agents (Fig. 8-2). Suppression usually predicts prevention of recurrence, although some drugs may have clinical benefit despite continued inducibility. Electrophysiologic testing provides an immediate method of diagnosing and treating the arrhythmia, avoiding discharge on empiric therapy that may be demonstrated to be ineffective weeks or months after the patient leaves the hospital.

   Electrophysiologic testing permits further evaluation of cases that are refractory to drugs. Endocardial mapping permits identification of the tachycardia zone, which may allow extirpation of the irritable focus by surgical techniques (endocardial resection, encircling ventriculotomy, cryoablation), or possibly by catheter techniques (still investigational for most types of VT except that originating from the right ventricular outflow tract [RVOT]). Other options include the consideration of a tiered therapy internal cardioverter-defibrillator (ICD).

II. Importance of ventricular ectopy

A. **Simple ectopy.** Simple ectopy, that is, uniform VPBs, occurs commonly and is not necessarily associated with serious underlying heart disease (Fig. 8-3). Probably almost everyone has had an isolated VPB, even if it was not noticed. Clinical studies over three decades have consistently shown that in the absence of symptoms and serious underlying heart disease, simple ventricular ectopy is benign and does not predispose to an increased risk of sudden death [15–25].

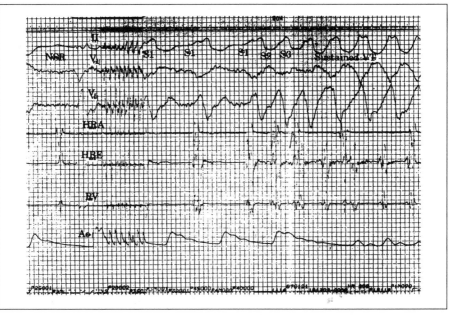

Fig. 8-2. Induction of sustained monomorphic ventricular tachycardia (VT) during electrophysiologic testing by the $V_1V_2V_3$ technique: eight paced ventricular stimuli at a constant cycle length (S1) followed by a premature ventricular couplet (S2S3). The leads recorded are II, V_1, V_5 (surface), high right atrium (HRA), His bundle electrogram (HBE), right ventricle (RV) (endocardial), and aortic pressure (Ao). (NSR = normal sinus rhythm.)

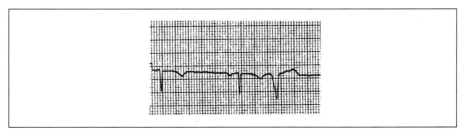

Fig. 8-3. Isolated ventricular premature beat.

B. **Complex ectopy including nonsustained ventricular tachycardia.** Frequent and complex ectopy is more likely to be associated with underlying heart disease and sometimes, but not always, an increased risk of sudden death (Figs. 8-4 and 8-5) [26–38]. Hinkle observed frequent and complex ectopy in middle-aged men with heart disease [26]. Although asymptomatic arrhythmias occurred in 93%, the number of coronary deaths in men with 10 or more VPBs/1000 complexes was greater than expected. Frequent VPBs increased the risk of death and sudden death **independent** of any other risk factor [27]. In this study, complexity did not add risk over that of frequency. It is important to note that the presence of ventricular ectopy did not increase the chance of death in those without coronary disease or major risk factors.

The studies by Ruberman et al. demonstrated the importance of complexity in 1739 male survivors of MI [28–31]. The 1-hour recording identified 25% of the population with an increased risk of sudden death. Complex ectopy (Lown grade 3 or higher) carried a threefold risk of sudden death over a 24-month period (as compared to simple ectopy) and was demonstrated to be an independent risk factor. The results were unchanged over a 66-month follow-up period. Runs of two or more consecutive VPBs and the R-on-T phenomenon each carried a higher risk for sudden

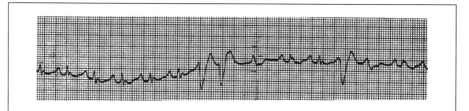

Fig. 8-4. Ventricular couplet. Two consecutive ventricular premature beats. Lown class 4A.

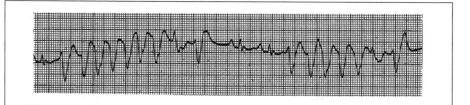

Fig. 8-5. Nonsustained ventricular tachycardia. Three or more consecutive ventricular premature beats lasting less than 30 seconds. Lown class 4B.

death than other complex ectopy (Fig. 8-6), although there was no difference for non-sudden death. With continued controversy over the importance of the R-on-T phenomenon, it would have been interesting if the analysis had been performed without the inclusion of R-on-T.

Other earlier studies in survivors of MI similarly noted increased risk with complexity. While the Coronary Drug Project found a twofold frequency of death when one or more VPBs were observed on the resting ECG [32], Kotler et al. noted that the majority of sudden deaths occurred with Lown grade 2 or higher [33]. The studies by Moss et al. again commented on the importance of Lown grade 2 or higher, with VT identifying individuals whose risk of cardiac death was doubled [34–38]. Complex VPBs made an independent contribution to the risk of sudden death.

It is obvious that a pattern is emerging. Complex ectopy in the absence of serious heart disease does not necessarily have a poor outcome, although complex ectopy is more likely to be associated with underlying problems. Complex ectopy after MI carries a higher risk of both cardiac death and SCD, with the highest risk noted in those with VT.

The time that ectopy is observed is important. Complex arrhythmias that occur in the convalescent phase of MI distinguish the group at risk for subsequent sudden death; early arrhythmias do not [39, 40]. Some patients may not have a problem with ectopy in the acute phase of MI but may demonstrate it the week before discharge.

Currently our patients are monitored on a telemetry floor prior to discharge. A signal-averaged ECG may provide further risk stratification, particularly if the patient has impaired left ventricular function and demonstrates nonsustained VT on telemetry. Most often, complex ventricular ectopy is associated with left ventricular dysfunction and ischemia. These patients are more likely to have lower mean ejection fraction, higher peak creatine kinase during the MI, a greater number of proximally narrowed major coronary arteries, a greater number of abnormally contracting left ventricular segments, and a higher incidence of prior MI [41–43].

Complex ectopy increased the risk of SCD in studies from the Johns Hopkins Hospital. Bigger et al. also noted the higher risk of cardiac death within 6 months if VT was noted in the 2-week period after MI [44, 45]. Note that these studies addressed increased risk but not treatment. An attempt to suppress asymptomatic complex ectopy in these survivors of MI may not necessarily result in improved survival.

A number of studies have focused on patients with complex ectopy, particularly nonsustained VT. Follansbee et al. studied 37 patients of 518 found to have nonsustained VT [46]. Nine of 19 with congestive cardiomyopathy died suddenly, as compared to only 1 of the 18 with other diagnoses. This study points out the risk in

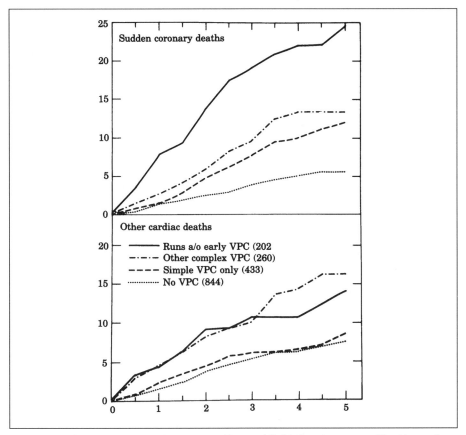

Fig. 8-6. Deaths among 1739 male survivors of myocardial infarction assessed by 1 hour of ambulatory monitoring. The 5-year follow-up using sudden and nonsudden cardiac deaths as end points indicates that two or more consecutive ventricular premature beats (VPB) and the R-on-T phenomenon placed the patient at highest risk for sudden cardiac death. (a/o = and/or.) (From W Ruberman et al., Ventricular premature complexes and sudden death after myocardial infarction. *Circulation* 64:298, 1981.)

patients with cardiomyopathy. Kennedy et al. noted that individuals with frequent ventricular ectopy and apparently normal coronary arteriograms were more likely to have subtle abnormalities of myocardial function, including increased left ventricular volume, increased LVEDP, and decreased mean velocity of circumferential fiber shortening [47].

Further studies again indicate an increased risk of sudden death with complex VPBs 4 weeks after MI [48]. Holmes et al. concluded that complex VPBs represent an independent mortality risk in both ischemic and nonischemic dilated cardiomyopathy [49]. In survivors of SCD, suppression of VT on ambulatory monitoring was associated with increased survival [50]. Patients who no longer were grade 4B had an annual mortality of 2.9%, compared with 37.5% for those with persistent VT. In a further study by the Johns Hopkins group, my colleagues and I noted that continued nonsustained VT on ambulatory monitoring predicts a higher risk of recurrence in survivors of SCD despite the fact that symptomatic episodes of VT had been abolished [51].

Fleg and Lakatta studied the importance of exercise-induced nonsustained VT (three to six beats) at peak exercise in 10 subjects without serious heart disease [52]. All continued to have a favorable prognosis over a 2-year period.

It is fitting to end this section with a careful analysis of the work by Kennedy et al., who evaluated the long-term follow-up of asymptomatic healthy individuals with frequent and complex ventricular ectopy [53]. Kennedy's group followed 73 asymptomatic, apparently healthy subjects with a mean of 566 VPBs/hour, including multiform in 63%, couplets in 60%, and nonsustained VT in 26%, over a 10-year period. A favorable outcome was noted in the absence of specific antiarrhythmic drug therapy. This study dramatically illustrates that antiarrhythmic drug therapy may not be necessary and that the prognosis is benign even if asymptomatic complex ectopy is present, as long as there is no serious underlying cardiac problem that merits attention.

Thus, it is important to note not only the frequency and complexity of VPBs but also the underlying anatomic substrate. Complex ectopy is usually associated with underlying heart disease; when it is not, the prognosis is more favorable. The higher degrees of complexity, particularly nonsustained VT, indicate a higher risk of SCD when associated with ischemic or nonischemic cardiomyopathy. Nevertheless, no large-scale study has conclusively demonstrated improved survival with antiarrhythmic drugs in the asymptomatic patient. Rather, the opposite is the case.

C. Specific substrate abnormalities and complex ectopy

  1. Coronary artery disease. Frequent ventricular ectopy has been related to the presence of abnormally contracting ventricular segments in patients with coronary disease [54, 55]. Vismara et al. related the frequency of complex forms to the extent of coronary atherosclerosis [40]. Calvert et al. noted that both the incidence and complexity of VPBs increased with multivessel disease, elevated LVEDP, or asynergy [56]. My associates and I studied a group of survivors of sudden cardiac arrest with recurrent VT refractory to conventional drugs and treated with investigational agents [57]. All had nonsustained VT on Holter monitoring. Disease in only one segment of coronary artery correlated with survival. As the degree of narrowing in the left anterior descending artery proximal to the first septal perforator increased, the percentage surviving decreased. This variable and the degree of dysfunction in certain segments of the left ventricle were significant independent predictors of survival in a multivariate analysis. These variables were independent predictors of survival in addition to ejection fraction and LVEDP.

  2. Cardiomyopathy. Complex ventricular ectopy is frequently associated with various cardiomyopathies [58]. In some cases complexity has more prognostic importance.

  Patients with dilated congestive cardiomyopathies frequently manifest complex ventricular ectopy and nonsustained VT [46]. These patients are at risk for sudden death. The importance of VT in congestive cardiomyopathy and the value of electrophysiologic testing are discussed in Chaps. 1 and 12. The most powerful indicators of outcome are left intraventricular conduction delay, pulmonary capillary wedge pressure, ventricular arrhythmias, mean right atrial pressure, ejection fraction, atrial fibrillation or flutter, and the presence of S3 gallop [59].

  One study indicated that while asymptomatic malignant ventricular arrhythmias occurred frequently, death usually resulted from worsening congestive heart failure [60]. Nevertheless, another group of authors from the same institution pointed out that sustained ventricular tachyarrhythmias could further destabilize compromised hemodynamics, leading to cardiovascular collapse and sudden death [61]. The incidence of sudden death in these patients may be as high as 25–30% in the first 2 years of the illness. In patients with nonsustained VT but without prior cardiac arrest or sustained VT, EPS is helpful when sustained VT is inducible. If VT is inducible and suppressed by drugs, the prognosis is favorable. If it is not suppressed, an ICD may be justified. Patients who have had a prior cardiac arrest fit into standard indications for ICD therapy. Unfortunately, the majority of patients with nonischemic cardiomyopathy initially may not have symptomatic arrhythmias and may be noninducible at EPS, resulting in a therapeutic dilemma.

  At this point, there are insufficient data to make a general recommendation about prophylactic ICD therapy for this population. To treat every patient with a device would cost billions of dollars for every life potentially saved (and for how long if overall left ventricular dysfunction deteriorates further and results in a congestive heart failure death?). Larsen et al. have raised these questions [62] and indicate that along with ICD therapy for selected patients, amiodarone is another potential option. A trial currently under way in Germany (AICD—Dilated Cardiomyopathy Trial) may provide answers. As with coronary disease, risk stratification algorithms may allow application of the most appropriate therapy (angiotensin converting enzyme [ACE] inhibitors, low-dose beta blockers, amiodarone, or ICD) for the individual patient.

Hypertrophic cardiomyopathy patients frequently have associated ventricular ectopy [63, 64], which seems to place them at higher risk of sudden death. In one of the studies from the National Institutes of Health (NIH), sudden cardiac catastrophe was more frequently observed in patients with asymptomatic VT on ambulatory monitoring (25%) than in patients without VT (3%) [65–67]. Survival of 75% of patients with VT indicated that additional variables were cofactors (a notion similar, perhaps, to the thoughts about destabilization of patients with congestive cardiomyopathy). Frank et al. noted variability over time of potentially lethal arrhythmias in this condition and suggested annual Holter monitoring for surveillance [68].

Other cardiomyopathies also have associated ventricular ectopy: infiltrative disorders such as sarcoidosis [69], arrhythmogenic right ventricular dysplasia [70, 71], muscular dystrophy [72], Chagas' disease, cardiomyopathy associated with human immunodeficiency virus (HIV), and a variety of others. The basic disorder is altered ventricular function, which occasionally begins as a myocarditis. Theoretically any disorder that causes myocardial injury has the potential to cause ventricular ectopy, with varying degrees of severity and influence on outcome.

3. **Mitral valve prolapse.** Mitral valve prolapse is associated with both supraventricular and ventricular ectopy. Potential explanations have included (1) increased tension on the papillary muscles owing to the floppy mitral valve, causing ventricular ectopy; (2) mitral regurgitation and jet effect to explain atrial ectopy; and (3) associated myocardial involvement.

It is uncertain whether the rare cases of sudden cardiac death in patients with MVP are related to the abnormal valve and syndrome or are the result of an unrelated problem, primary electrical disease. Dollar and Roberts [13] observed that the patients who died were younger, were more often women, and had a lower frequency of mitral regurgitation.

Winkle et al. observed that only half their patients with MVP had frequent and complex VPBs [73]. The correlation between symptoms and complex ectopy was poor. Other investigators similarly found it difficult to correlate arrhythmias, demographic variables, physical findings, or ECG changes [74]. Occasionally, however, symptomatic VT is observed in patients with MVP [75, 76]. Chesler et al. noted endocardial friction lesions in 11 of 14 patients with MVP who died suddenly because of arrhythmias [77]. In 5 of the patients, a thrombotic lesion containing fibrin and platelets was observed in the angle between the posterior leaflet and left atrial wall. Mitral valve prolapse may be associated with serious symptoms, even in the elderly [78]. In addition, arrhythmias may be more frequent when there is hemodynamically important mitral regurgitation [79].

4. **Other valvular disease.** Valvular disease may cause pressure-volume overload leading to altered myocardial function and ventricular ectopy. Mitral regurgitation unrelated to MVP or ischemic heart disease may be associated with arrhythmias [79]. The relationship between function and arrhythmias has been observed with aortic valvular disease, occasionally with reduction in arrhythmias as a result of improved ventricular function after valve replacement [80, 81]. However, one study of 102 patients failed to demonstrate a correlation between the grade of ventricular ectopy and the degree of aortic stenosis or regurgitation, ventricular hemodynamics, or the presence of coronary artery disease [82].

D. **Summary.** Analyzing the situation from the viewpoint of structural heart disease, the more severe the abnormality is, the more likely is the presence of associated ectopy. Uretz et al. noted that wall motion abnormalities, ejection fraction, category of disease, and age correlate with VPB severity [83]. This study examined a general population and did not observe a relationship between the number of diseased coronary arteries and ectopy. In studies of patients who had survived sustained VT, relationships were noted between coronary artery disease and wall motion abnormalities as well as ejection fraction [57, 84]. While indexes such as hemodynamic and angiographic variables contribute to the risk of sudden death, the presence of arrhythmias, such as VT, is an independent variable that increases the risk.

Remember that complex ventricular ectopy, especially VT, usually reflects serious underlying heart disease, which should be evaluated. Symptomatic arrhythmias resulting in cardiovascular collapse or hemodynamic compromise are most critical and require therapy of the acute event to prevent recurrence. The patient with simple ectopy who is completely asymptomatic or notes "skipped beats" has minimal risk in most cases.

III. Previous recommendations and current practice. It is of historic interest to review previous treatment recommendations because some have changed dramatically as a result of studies performed in the last ten years.

The following caveat cannot be repeated often enough: While **asymptomatic** complex ectopy increases the risk of SCD, no study has conclusively demonstrated improved survival with suppression of asymptomatic ectopy with antiarrhythmic drugs. In fact, these drugs can be harmful and cause exacerbation of arrhythmias. Treatment of patients with **symptomatic** (syncope, near-syncope) ventricular arrhythmias is necessary. Zipes recommended treatment of sustained VT regardless of whether underlying heart disease was present, nonsustained VT in the presence of structural heart disease, and symptomatic nonsustained VT in the absence of structural heart disease [1]. Patients with asymptomatic nonsustained VT or other ventricular ectopy in the absence of structural heart disease would be followed but not treated.

Lown recommended treatment of (1) survivors of sudden cardiac arrest not associated with acute MI, (2) exercise-induced VT, (3) high-grade ventricular ectopy (grade 4A, 4B, or 5) after MI or in the patient under stress, (4) prolonged Q–T syndrome and ectopy over grade 2, (5) VPBs in MVP, (6) VPBs in intermittent prolonged Q–T syndrome, and (7) VPBs in the presence of angina [2].

Bigger would treat frequent and complex VPBs during the acute phase of MI; in the 3–6 months after infarction; and in patients with chronic ischemia, cardiomyopathy, or MVP [3]. He would also treat survivors of VT or VF, symptomatic VPBs (hemodynamic compromise), and frequent VPBs (> 10/hour) but not asymptomatic ectopy in a young patient.

Smith and Gallagher recommended treatment of multiform and R-on-T VPBs in addition to VT [4]. Josephson would base treatment on the response to programmed electrical stimulation [5]. Vlay and Reid recommended treatment of survivors of sustained VT or VF (not associated with acute MI), patients with inducible VT or VF, and possibly those with more than three to five beats of nonsustained VT [6]. Nonsustained VT in the presence of severe underlying heart disease would be treated if no major adverse drug effects occurred. Lower grades such as couplets or multiform ectopy would be treated only if associated with hypotension, dizziness, syncope, or troublesome palpitations.

Except for sustained VT or VF, there is a lack of complete agreement even among these references. To assess how the cardiology community was treating patients, a survey of university cardiologists addressed the issue of treating completely asymptomatic patients with frequent VPBs, complex VPBs, or asymptomatic VT in the presence of varying anatomic substrates [7] (Fig. 8-7). As the degree of complexity increased, the number of physicians treating their patients increased for all categories. Physicians were also more likely to treat the patient if the underlying cardiac disorders were serious. In this same survey, 95% of physicians felt that ventricular ectopy should be treated and suppressed if it could be related to dizziness or syncope. Thus, the greatest controversy remained with the treatment of asymptomatic, nonsustained VT. Most cardiologists treated asymptomatic, nonsustained VT with ischemic heart disease, cardiomyopathy, or prolonged Q–T syndromes, although some did not treat it with MVP (33%) or no clinical evidence of coronary artery disease (36%). The differences of opinion among arrhythmia specialists make the issue of treatment confusing to the general cardiologist and internist. The result of this survey were not recommendations, only observations of current practice. Many physicians dealing with arrhythmias found themselves in the minority opinion. Nevertheless, although guidelines are useful, treatment should be individualized.

IV. Recent clinical investigations. Since the arrhythmogenic potential of antiarrhythmic drugs has become more widely recognized (see Chap. 14), physicians are becoming more reluctant to treat asymptomatic ventricular ectopy, particularly with an empiric selection of drugs. Some studies have attempted to determine whether prophylactic treatment confers the benefit of improved survival.

  A. Landmark studies on arrhythmia management

  1. **Timolol, Encainide, Sotalol Trial (TEST).** This study enrolled patients with potentially malignant arrhythmias in the presence of left ventricular dysfunction (ejection fraction <40%) after MI. Potentially malignant arrhythmias were defined as nonsustained VT, or an average of 10 or more VPBs/hour.

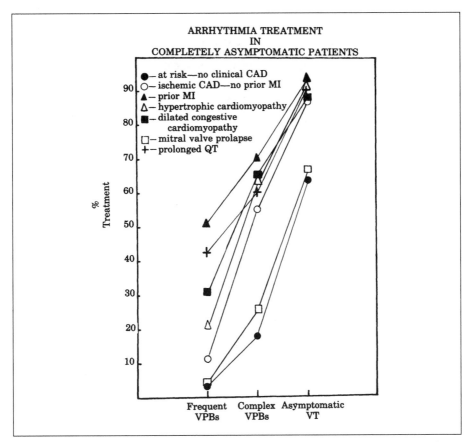

Fig. 8-7. Treatment of arrhythmias in completely asymptomatic patients. Three grades of ventricular ectopy are designated on the abscissa. The ordinate is the percentage of university cardiologists treating their patients for each grade of ectopy. As is apparent, general agreement was not achieved in this group of arrhythmia specialists except for the treatment of nonsustained ventricular tachycardia (VT) in patients with serious underlying heart disease. (CAD = coronary artery disease; MI = myocardial infarction; VPBs = ventricular premature beats.) (From SC Vlay, How the university cardiologist treats ventricular premature beats: A nationwide survey of 65 university medical centers. *Am Heart J* 110:907, 1985.)

Treatment began 6–28 days after the MI. The patients were randomized to treatment with timolol (10 mg bid), encainide (50 mg bid), or sotalol (320 mg bid). Thus, the trial compared a beta blocker, a type 1C antiarrhythmic agent, and a type 3 drug that has some beta-blocking properties.

Preliminary results were reported in November 1985 by the Hahnemann Cardiovascular Research Group. Timolol was not effective in suppressing ventricular arrhythmias; encainide suppressed ventricular arrhythmias and was well tolerated; and sotalol seemed to be associated with a statistically significant proarrhythmic effect. No statistically significant difference in total deaths was seen among the groups. Because of these findings and difficulty with enrollment (only 55 subjects), the study was concluded early. The increase in life-threatening arrhythmias in patients receiving sotalol was particularly disturbing [85].

2. **The aprindine-placebo trial.** A study from Johns Hopkins analyzed 142 patients after MI randomized in a double-blind fashion to treatment with aprindine or placebo. Patients were entered 9 days after MI and followed for 1 year. Sixty patients had ejection fractions less than 40%, 22 had ventricular ectopy that was Lown grade 3 or higher, and 60 had both criteria. Arrhythmias during Holter

monitoring were reduced in the aprindine-treated patients. There was no difference in mortality, either total death or sudden death, between the groups. The only difference noted in outcome was that median duration of survival before death was 82 days longer in the patients receiving aprindine. Thus, preliminary data suggested that mortality may have been delayed but not avoided [86].

3. **Multidrug study.** The only study that seemed to suggest an improvement in survival was a retrospective analysis of 50 subjects with chronic coronary artery disease [87]. An attempt was made to suppress frequent (>30 multiform VPBs) and complex (Lown grade $\geq$ 4A) ventricular ectopy on ambulatory monitoring with single or combined drugs, including quinidine, mexiletine, sotalol, oxprenolol, amiodarone, prajmaline, disopyramide, and phenytoin. There was a higher incidence of total death in the patients who failed to respond to empiric therapy; however, this was a nonrandomized, non-placebo-controlled study with only four SCDs in the entire population.

4. **CAPS and CAST trials.** These trials were designed to address the issue of whether empiric treatment of ventricular arrhythmias improves survival.

   a. **Cardiac Arrhythmia Pilot Study (CAPS).** This study enrolled 502 patients with more than 10 VPBs/hour on 24-hour ECG monitoring. The left ventricular ejection fraction was over 20%, and randomization occurred 6–60 days after MI. Drug therapy included encainide, flecainide, imipramine, moricizine, and placebo. Drug dosage was adjusted to achieve more than 70% reduction in VPB frequency and more than 90% suppression of VPB runs, except for placebo group patients. Suppression of ectopy was achieved as follows: encainide (79%), flecainide (83%), imipramine (52%), moricizine (66%), and placebo (37%). As a second drug for patients who failed to respond to imipramine or moricizine, encainide (68%) and flecainide (69%) were effective. Flecainide had the highest incidence of worsening heart failure. Imipramine was poorly tolerated and subsequently excluded from CAST. This pilot study indicated that a formal trial was possible [88].

   b. **Cardiac Arrhythmia Suppression Trial (CAST).** The results of this trial were reported in the *New England Journal of Medicine* [89]. Patients were eligible for enrolment 6 days to 2 years after MI if they had at least 6 VPBs/hour on ambulatory ECG and no runs of VT (>15 beats) at a rate of more than 120 beats/minute Left ventricular ejection fraction was required to be under 55% if the patient was recruited within 90 days of MI and under 40% if recruited 90 days after MI. Flecainide was not given to patients with left ventricular ejection fraction (LVEF) below 30%; instead they received encainide or moricizine as first drugs. The primary end point was death or cardiac arrest with resuscitation, both due to arrhythmia.

   Of 1498 patients, 857 were randomized to encainide (432 active drug, 425 placebo) and 641 to flecainide (323 active drug, 318 placebo). There were more deaths in the active drug group after a mean follow-up period of 10 months. Arrhythmia was the cause of death in 59 patients (43 on active drug, 16 on placebo). In 22 patients dying of nonarrhythmia cardiac causes (mostly cardiogenic shock associated with acute MI or chronic congestive heart failure), 17 were on active drug and 5 on placebo. For the 8 dying of noncardiac causes, 3 were on active drug and 5 on placebo. Nonlethal events were equally distributed between the active drug and placebo groups. Due to the increased mortality with encainide and flecainide, the trial with these two drugs was discontinued, but the effect of moricizine was further evaluated in CAST II.

   The entry criteria were modified for CAST II. Enrollment time was narrowed to 4–90 days after MI. Patients had to have a left ventricular ejection fraction below 40%. A higher dosage of moricizine was permitted, and the early titration was double blind with a placebo. The definition of disqualifying VT was modified to allow patients with more serious arrhythmias into the trial. This trial was also terminated early because the results indicated that patients treated with moricizine had an excessive cardiac mortality rate during the first 2 weeks of exposure to the drug. The chance of long-term survival benefit was considered unlikely [90, 91].

   CAST did not include quinidine, procainamide, or disopyramide (type 1A) due to the frequent necessity of discontinuation due to side effects, as well as the inability to achieve the degree of suppression necessary for the trial. Tocainide and mexiletine (type 1B) were excluded due to the high incidence of intolerable side effects and the only moderate suppression of ventricular ectopy. Propafenone seemed to be a reasonable choice, but long-term efficacy was not well defined at the time, and the drug does have beta-blocking activity, which might have confused the results. Amiodarone had complex pharmacokinetics and long-term toxicity, which was not justifiable in asymptomatic patients. Whether the inclusion of any of these drugs would have altered survival even though ventricular ectopy might not have been as effectively suppressed remains unknown.

The mortality rate in the placebo group may have contributed to the differences in survival. Many high-risk patients were excluded before randomization. Half the placebo patients in CAST had LVEF above 40%. These are some of the unavoidable pitfalls in clinical research. It is difficult to design a study that will not have unforeseen influences. The reader must realize that the results of this study apply to asymptomatic postinfarction patients who satisfied specific study entry criteria and may or should not be extrapolated to all patients with ventricular ectopy [92, 93].

5. **Cardiac Arrest Study Hamburg.** This was a randomized, controlled study of survivors of sudden cardiac arrest not related to acute MI. Patients were randomized to therapy with amiodarone, metoprolol, propafenone, or an ICD without antiarrhythmic drugs [94]. After 11 months of follow-up, there was a significantly higher incidence of total mortality in the propafenone arm, resulting in withdrawal of this agent from the study. This study provided more concern about type I drugs.

6. **Results of landmark studies.** These studies changed the practice of arrhythmia management, particularly for those who treated ventricular arrhythmias empirically. As some had previously warned, the empiric administration of antiarrhythmic drugs was demonstrated to contribute to early death due to proarrhythmia and worsened survival due to the cardiac depressant effects of specific agents.

B. **Studies of amiodarone.** Several studies evaluated the short- and long-term effects of amiodarone. The Basel Antiarrhythmic Study of Infarct Survival (BASIS) demonstrated improved 1-year survival in patients with frequent or complex ventricular ectopy after MI [95]. Patients either received low-dose amiodarone (200 mg daily after 5 days of loading with 1000 mg) or were assigned to a control group. The reduction in total and cardiac death was seen in the first year, with no significant mortality difference in subsequent years. This study was one of the first to show benefit from treating postinfarction arrhythmias with an antiarrhythmic drug.

The pilot of the Canadian Amiodarone Myocardial Infarction Arrhythmia Trial (CAMIAT) also demonstrated a favorable effect for amiodarone [96]. A Polish study suggested a significant reduction in cardiac mortality and ventricular arrhythmias with amiodarone [97]. Amiodarone was loaded with 800 mg daily for the first week and then maintained on 400 mg 6 days/week for 12 months. The dosage could be reduced for bradycardia or prolongation of the Q–T interval. The reduction in mortality was due to reduction in cardiac mortality and a reduction in sudden death.

The Cardiac Arrest in Seattle: Conventional Versus Amiodarone Drug Evaluation (CASCADE) study randomized survivors of out-of-hospital VF (not associated with acute MI) to either amiodarone or to EPS or Holter-guided therapy [98]. Survival was better with amiodarone than for conventional therapy in terms of cardiac death, resuscitation from VF, ICD shock, or arrhythmic events at 2, 4, and 6 years. This advantage was obtained at the cost of a higher incidence of serious drug side effects.

C. **General guidelines.** Other than with amiodarone [99], a drug with serious potential adverse effects, there is no firm evidence to support empiric and prophylactic antiarrhythmic drug treatment in asymptomatic patients. General recommendations are based on the current understanding of the substrate abnormality, the potential for SCD balanced against the risk and benefit of antiarrhythmic drugs or ICD devices.

V. Current recommendations
A. **Symptomatic patients.** If the **symptoms** are **manifest as cardiovascular collapse, treatment is imperative.** The acute episode must be dealt with immediately; chronic therapy is based on the risk of recurrence. When VT or VF is associated with the acute phase of MI, usually there is little risk of recurrence, and chronic therapy is often not necessary. In the absence of an acute precipitating factor such as MI, severe electrolyte disturbance, or drug toxicity, there is **high risk of recurrent VT or**

VF. These cases **need comprehensive evaluation** and **suppressive treatment** with antiarrhythmic drugs, arrhythmia surgery, or electronic devices, if necessary. The patient whose symptoms are milder may require less vigorous therapy. Nevertheless, if **symptoms** such as **dizziness or near-syncope** are **related** to **sustained or nonsustained VT, treatment is necessary.** The patient who experiences **palpitations** related to **ventricular couplets** or **multiform** or **uniform ventricular ectopy** but has **no symptoms of hemodynamic embarrassment** should be examined for the potential for sustained VT or VF. This assessment may be performed by the noninvasive or invasive approach, depending on the clinical situation. If there is **no reason to suspect the potential for SCD and the palpitations are intolerable, treatment can be administered to decrease the nuisance value of the VPBs.**

B. **Asymptomatic patients.** Patients with **nonsustained VT** noted fortuitously on ECG monitoring pose a more difficult problem, and the following recommendations reflect my bias.

First, a search for underlying heart disease should be performed. If the **nonsustained VT is truly asymptomatic** and there is **no evidence of underlying heart disease,** it is not unreasonable to **follow the patient without prescribing antiarrhythmic drug therapy.** If the patient has a **severe underlying heart disease,** it is not unreasonable to consider **antiarrhythmic drug therapy for nonsustained VT and perhaps recommend EPS-guided therapy.** However, antiarrhythmic drug therapy may have the potential to cause a proarrhythmic effect and possibly even SCD. Antiarrhythmic drugs have adverse effects and may not prolong survival. For these reasons **I do not recommend antiarrhythmic drug therapy for truly asymptomatic ventricular ectopy** (i.e., **couplets** or **multiform** or **uniform VPBs**). Remember that suppression of ventricular ectopy does not necessarily mean that SCD will be prevented. This recommendation applies to patients with or without underlying heart disease.

A survey of recent editions of comprehensive textbooks reveals general agreement. Zipes does not recommend treatment of asymptomatic VT and makes therapeutic decisions to prevent symptoms from sustained and nonsustained VT [100]. Myerburg, Kessler, and Castellanos divide ventricular arrhythmias into benign (no independent increase in risk), significant (independent increase in risk), and potentially lethal (untreated can lead to proximate fatality) to determine therapy [101]. Bigger recommends treatment of symptomatic arrhythmias [102]. Josephson, Buxton, and Marchlinski do not treat VT in the absence of organic heart disease (except prolonged QT syndrome) and favor EPS-guided therapy [103].

VI. Treatment of specific arrhythmias

A. **Invasive versus noninvasive approach.** Management of cardiovascular collapse as a result of sustained VT or VF is discussed in Chap. 2. These recommendations are standard. The issue of whether to use the noninvasive (Holter, exercise testing) or invasive (electrophysiologic) approach to guide therapy is briefly discussed here and in greater detail in Chaps. 15–16. Platia and Reid studied 44 survivors of VT or VF [104]. After treatment with antiarrhythmic drug therapy, the patients underwent EPS and ambulatory monitoring, with a mean of 18 months of follow-up. Of the 14 patients with inducible sustained VT and the 12 with nonsustained VT (3–13 beats), 23 of the 26 experienced recurrent, symptomatic, sustained VT or SCD. Only 1 patient of the 18 whose VT was noninducible died suddenly. Thus, the positive predictive value of EPS was 88%, and the negative predictive value was 94%. Of the 10 patients with nonsustained VT on Holter, 7 had an unfavorable outcome (70% positive predictive value). Of 34 patients without Lown grade 4B arrhythmias, 17 had an unfavorable outcome (negative predictive value = 50%). Thus, EPS provided a higher predictive accuracy than ambulatory monitoring in this population of survivors of SCD, which was a highly select group. This study has been criticized for the lack of baseline EPS in all patients, but this was due to hemodynamically unstable persistent VT.

Swerdlow and Peterson examined 32 survivors of VT or VF not associated with acute MI [105]. All had serious coronary artery disease. Electrophysiologic testing was performed in 90% and Holter monitoring in 71%. Drug efficacy was able to be assessed in 96% of those undergoing EPS but only in 70% evaluated by ambulatory monitoring. Again EPS was found to be more useful in guiding therapy than the noninvasive method.

In another study population, Graboys et al. were able to assess 94% (100 of 106) of the patients with ventricular tachyarrhythmias by ambulatory monitoring [106].

Perhaps the difference in study populations is the key to understanding the differences in approach:

1. The patient with symptomatic life-threatening arrhythmias who has only minimal ventricular ectopy while asymptomatic can be evaluated properly only with EPS.
2. The patient with less symptomatic arrhythmias (i.e., not causing cardiovascular collapse) who has frequent ectopy on ambulatory monitoring that can be correlated with the symptoms may be well evaluated and treated by noninvasive means.
3. There will be a number of patients with symptomatic VT and some ectopy on ambulatory monitoring who may be treated either way (EPS or Holter).

Certainly, the abolition of nonsustained VT may signal a good prognosis [50, 51]. Nevertheless, there will be additional patients who will die suddenly despite improvement on ambulatory monitoring. The problem is that it is not always easy to differentiate the patients who fall into each of these three categories. EPS may provide the most complete data but may be an unnecessary risk and expense for some patients. Ambulatory monitoring may be useful for a very select group of patients but may not be predictive for all. For the patients in the third category, EPS may offer increased safety at the price of some unnecessary testing and expense.

The debate over the optimal method for evaluating the response to antiarrhythmic drug therapy in patients with life-threatening ventricular arrhythmias continues. The Electrophysiologic Study versus the Electrocardiographic Monitoring Trial (ESVEM) was designed to answer this question. It was a multicenter randomized clinical study involving 486 subjects with a mean age of 65 years. Male gender (88%), coronary artery disease (84%), previous MI (82%), and LVEF of 32% were the other predominant characteristics. The presenting arrhythmias were sustained VT (73%), sudden death, resuscitated (22%), and syncope with subsequent EPS revealing inducible VT (5%) [107].

Patients were randomized to serial drug evaluation by Holter monitoring and exercise test or by EPS. Patients underwent testing in random order of up to six antiarrhythmic drugs (imipramine, mexiletine, procainamide, quinidine, sotalol, pirmenol, propafenone) until one or none was predicted to be effective. Efficacy criteria for the Holter arm included VPB suppression (100% runs of VT > 15 beats, 90% of shorter runs, 80% pairs, 70% all VPBs) and absence of exercise-induced VT. For the EPS arm, suppression of inducible VT over 5 beats was required.

Patients were followed until recurrence of arrhythmia or the end of the study. Prediction of drug efficacy was achieved in 77% of the Holter arm and in only 45% of the EPS arm. LVEF below 25% and the presence of coronary artery disease were negative correlates of efficacy in the EPS arm. Evaluation took longer in the EPS arm (25 days) than in the Holter arm (10 days).

As with similar clinical trials, this study has been criticized for the demographic characteristics of the population studied, the number of patients excluded after screening, and the criteria used to determine efficacy in both the Holter and EPS arms. Furthermore, with the availability of ICDs and the known adverse effects of chronic drug therapy, physicians are no longer routinely recommending serial drug testing but rather moving ahead quickly with an electronic device.

Nevertheless, the ESVEM study did indicate that for certain selected patients, the noninvasive approach was a possible option and had certain benefits. The next paper demonstrated that although Holter monitoring was more likely to result in a successful prediction of drug efficacy than EPS, there was no significant difference in the success of therapy as selected by the two methods [108].

Electrophysiologists remain reluctant to decide chronic therapy for cardiac arrest survivors on the basis of noninvasive testing alone. In a study of patients with symptomatic sustained VT/VF, Steinbeck et al. concluded that effective suppression of inducible arrhythmia by antiarrhythmic drugs was associated with a better outcome than was lack of suppression, consistent with previous reports on the validity of EPS-guided therapy [109].

A subsequent ESVEM paper analyzed the response to specific drugs [110]. Adverse drug effects and the actual probability of recurrent arrhythmia after prediction of efficacy by either Holter or EPS were lower for sotalol than for any other drug. Furthermore, risk of death from any cause, cardiac causes, and arrhythmia were lower with sotalol than any other drug. The superiority of sotalol in this study was an unexpected finding.

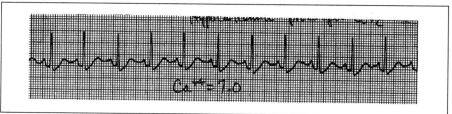

Fig. 8-8. Hypocalcemia with Q–T interval prolongation. The serum calcium was 7.0. Hypocalcemia usually is not associated with serious arrhythmias, but further prolongation of the Q–T interval is undesirable (see text).

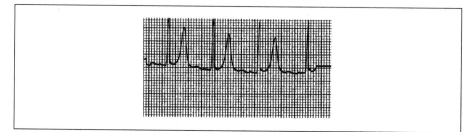

Fig. 8-9. Hyperkalemia. Note the peaked T waves. Severe hyperkalemia may result in a sinoventricular rhythm (see Chap. 3).

B. **Treatment of the substrate abnormality**
1. **The cardiac disorder.** After establishment of the underlying cardiac diagnosis, therapy is directed toward that particular problem in addition to the arrhythmia. Ischemia is treated as appropriate with nitrates, beta blockers, and calcium antagonists. Selected patients may require angioplasty or coronary artery bypass graft surgery. Heart failure is treated with digitalis, diuretics, vasodilators, ACE inhibitors, or other inotropic agents as appropriate for each patient. Hypertrophic cardiomyopathy is treated with beta blockers or calcium antagonists. In certain cardiomyopathies, treatment may be guided by the findings on myocardial biopsy. In coronary or valvular disease, cardiac surgery is often a consideration. Careful thought should be given not only to the specific procedure indicated (e.g., coronary artery bypass grafting) but also to the possibility of concurrent arrhythmia surgery or implantation of an electronic device such as a pacemaker or defibrillator.
2. **The rhythm disorder.** Next, attention is directed at definitive establishment of the arrhythmia diagnosis. Occasionally it may be necessary to utilize EPS to ascertain the nature of a wide-complex tachycardia (i.e., VT versus supraventricular tachycardia [SVT]) before deciding on specific antiarrhythmic therapy. It is also important to exclude certain extrinsic factors that may be arrhythmogenic. **Mechanical irritability** may result from temporary pacemakers or pulmonary artery monitoring catheters and may be remedied by repositioning. Laboratory evaluation allows identification and correction of **hypoxia, hypokalemia, hypomagnesemia,** or other electrolyte abnormalities (Figs. 8-8 and 8-9). Remember that many drugs, including digitalis and other antiarrhythmic agents, tricyclic antidepressants, and phenothiazines, may be arrhythmogenic.
   Once the arrhythmia is diagnosed, specific antiarrhythmic agents alone or in combination may be successful. Again one must remember that specific arrhythmias in different substrate abnormalities may respond differently. The clinician should have a good understanding of antiarrhythmic drugs before prescribing them and keep certain pharmacotherapeutic guidelines in mind (see Chap. 14). Just as the indications for treatment have been somewhat arbitrary, the choice of antiarrhythmic drug often is empiric and guided by experience. Other considerations include adverse effects, cost, and convenience. The ideal drug—inexpensive, effective, well tolerated, with infrequent and convenient dosing intervals—

has not yet been found. Occasionally an agent will serve more than one purpose; a beta blocker has antiarrhythmic, antihypertensive, and anti-ischemic effects; amiodarone has both antiarrhythmic and vasodilator properties.

Therapy must be individualized [7]. The response to therapy should be documented (by Holter monitoring and EPS). Blood levels of the drug or drugs may be helpful [111] once the patient is stable on the final regimen (may not be particularly useful with amiodarone). If the patient returns with recurrent arrhythmia, the blood level will help distinguish drug inefficacy (drug in therapeutic range), insufficient drug (low level), and drug toxicity (high level). It is essential to develop a plan for deciding which to use first.

C. Choice of drug

1. **Beta-adrenergic blocker drugs.** The goal is to use the least toxic drug to achieve effective therapy. One class of drug that is occasionally useful for arrhythmias is the beta-adrenergic blocker. Both propranolol and acebutolol have Food and Drug Administration (FDA) indications for the treatment of arrhythmias, but other members of the class are also effective. Sotalol is approved for life-threatening ventricular arrhythmias, but its type 3 activity and potential effect on the Q–T interval do not allow it to be generalized with other beta blockers. Beta blockers without intrinsic sympathomimetic activity raise the VF threshold. They also may be useful for preventing arrhythmias caused by ischemia. As single antiarrhythmic drug therapy for ventricular arrhythmias, they are particularly useful in two situations: MVP and catecholamine-sensitive ventricular tachyarrhythmias. In most other cases, beta blockers alone have limited efficacy for hypotensive sustained VT.

   In MVP, in addition to a direct antiarrhythmic effect, beta blockers may decrease tension on the papillary muscles by decreasing contractility, which in turn may decrease arrhythmias. Beta-blocker therapy should be a primary consideration in patients with ventricular (or atrial) arrhythmias related to MVP that require therapy.

   Patients with catecholamine-sensitive ventricular tachyarrhythmias (and this includes exercise-induced VT) respond very well to beta-blocker therapy, and this is one of the drugs of choice. By blunting the catecholamine effect on the end organ, the myocardium, the arrhythmia may be prevented. This mechanism may also explain the benefit of beta blockers in some dilated cardiomyopathies [112–115].

2. **Antiarrhythmic drugs.** Type 1 or type 3 antiarrhythmic agents, alone or in conjunction with an ICD, will be used for the majority of patients. In some patients with infrequent life-threatening VT/VF, the ICD alone without drugs is an alternative form of therapy. The modified Vaughn Williams classification and the new classification based on the Sicilian Gambit are discussed in further detail in Chap. 14.

   Some physicians may question the utility of the Vaughn Williams classification, but it does provide a basis for comparison of the effects on depolarization and repolarization, which is useful when considering the combination of agents.

   Currently, the following agents are FDA approved for the treatment of arrhythmias:

   Type 1A: quinidine, procainamide, disopyramide
   Type 1B: lidocaine, tocainide, mexiletine
   Type 1C: flecainide, propafenone
   Type 3: amiodarone, bretylium, sotalol

   The choice of agent is based on the individual patient, the underlying disease, the potential side effects, and other underlying conditions, such as arthritis or chronic diarrhea, which would make several choices unwise. Beta blockade should be considered when indicated. In my schema, five drugs should be considered as first-line agents: quinidine, procainamide, disopyramide, mexiletine, and sotalol. After the ESVEM trial, many utilize sotalol first. Quinidine, procainamide, and disopyramide have been used extensively, and their efficacy and toxicities are well recognized. Mexiletine (and tocainide) may be effective less often in patients with truly refractory VT. Type 1C drugs have a significant potential for proarrhythmia and are considered second-line therapy, after 1A agents alone or in combination with 1B agents. Of the 1C agents, propafenone, with its beta-blocking activity, may be less likely than flecainide to cause dangerous arrhythmias. Propafenone alone, if effective and if tolerated, may be easier for the patient than a combination such as quinidine and mexiletine. Amiodarone is the last choice.

a. **Type 1 drugs.** Since quinidine's major toxicity is gastrointestinal (GI), I avoid it **initially** in a patient with ulcer disease, chronic diarrhea, or other GI disturbance. Similarly, because procainamide may be associated with a lupuslike syndrome, it is a poor first choice in patients with arthritis or collagen vascular disease. In patients with a prolonged Q–T, quinidine, procainamide, disopyramide, and sotalol should **not** be used; all of them prolong repolarization and the Q–T interval and could make these patients more vulnerable to malignant ventricular arrhythmias. Both mexiletine and tocainide shorten repolarization (and the Q–T interval) and would be more favorable choices in this situation.

A decision to use the type 1B drugs must consider their toxicities, which are primarily related to the CNS and GI tract. Consequently, based on the individual patient, the anatomic substrate, the length of the Q–T interval, and the tendency toward particular adverse effects, I would choose one of these drugs for chronic therapy. Drug therapy, however, remains empiric. If the first failed or caused adverse effects, I would select another. By the time the patient fails two drug trials, the physician should start to consider the indication for amiodarone and/or an ICD.

A few words are necessary about the other type 1B drugs. Lidocaine is available only intravenously (IV). Phenytoin is not approved by the FDA for arrhythmias, although it is rarely useful, sometimes in combination with procainamide. At one time it was used for digitalis toxic arrhythmias, but the availability of Fab antibodies has made this unnecessary.

Second-choice drugs include disopyramide and flecainide, although many physicians (and pharmaceutical companies) may disagree with me in considering these agents as second-line drugs. Disopyramide has a number of side effects that contraindicate it often in the patient who needs it most: the middle-aged or older male who may have some heart failure. In this patient, its negative inotropic effect may exacerbate the heart failure, and its anticholinergic effects may result in urinary retention, constipation, or xerostomia. However, disopyramide may be a first-line drug in other selected patients, such as the young woman without heart failure who may need an antiarrhythmic drug or the patient with hypertrophic cardiomyopathy who may benefit from both the negative inotropic and antiarrhythmic effects. Flecainide also has negative inotropic effects. The reason for considering it as a second-line drug is its negative inotropy and the fact that selected patients with poor left ventricular function may develop intractable VT or VF (particularly at higher dosages). In patients without heart failure, flecainide may be a safe and effective drug but **must be used very cautiously.** There have been reports of VT/VF even with normal left ventricular function.

b. **Type 3 drugs.** Should all of these agents fail, one must have a third-line drug. Amiodarone is approved for treatment of refractory VT but has a number of serious potential adverse effects that make it wise to keep this drug in reserve. In fact, combination therapy or propafenone should be considered before resorting to amiodarone. I am particularly reluctant to use amiodarone in a young person, unless it is the only remaining choice. I am much less concerned about amiodarone side effects in the elderly patient. If side effects start to occur at 80 or 90 years, one can deal with them at that time. If pulmonary fibrosis occurs at age 40, the consequences can be devastating, particularly if another form of therapy was available. Nevertheless, of all the antiarrhythmic drugs, amiodarone is the drug that is most likely to be effective, for both supraventricular and ventricular tachyarrhythmias, once all others have failed. Its toxicity and potential toxicity are minimized by using the lowest effective dosage. Combination of amiodarone with another drug can minimize the toxicity of both. Often patients who fail initial therapy will benefit from ICD therapy. These comments are meant to serve as a caveat, to discourage inappropriate use of the drug, but also to observe that amiodarone may be a very effective and lifesaving drug when used correctly and when the benefits justify the risks. Newer drugs continue to be investigated, although there are no "wonder" drugs on the horizon. They should be considered when approved drugs are ineffective or contraindicated.

3. **Combinations of drugs.** Combinations of antiarrhythmic agents may be more effective than individual agents and associated with less toxicity. There are a

multitude of possible combinations. One must always account for the electro-physiologic effects and potential toxicities.

    a. Two type 1A drugs. A combination of two type 1A drugs is most useful when the therapeutic dose of one agent alone produces undesirable toxicity. Quinidine may control the arrhythmia but cause diarrhea; disopyramide may control the arrhythmia but result in constipation. A combination of quinidine and disopyramide, each at a lower dose, may control the arrhythmia and avoid either too frequent or infrequent bowel movement. It would be unwise to consider the combination of high-dose quinidine and high-dose procainamide or disopyramide because of additive effects on prolonging repolarization, thus causing an acquired prolonged Q–T syndrome.

    b. A type 1A and a type 1B drug. The combination of a 1A and a 1B drug has appeal from the viewpoint of repolarization. One drug (1A) prolongs it and the other (1B) shortens it, allowing for more (i.e., combined) depression of phase 0 depolarization but less of an effect on repolarization. The combination of quinidine and mexiletine has been described in the literature [116, 117] (Fig. 8-10). In the past, I have successfully combined quinidine and tocainide (unpublished observations). Rarely, I have observed efficacy of phenytoin with procainamide or phenytoin and a beta blocker, but these combinations are successful so infrequently that I usually do not even consider them as a possible alternative.

    c. Combinations with a type 1C drug. Few data are available on the efficacy of a type 1C drug with any other drug.

    d. Combination with a type 2 drug (beta-adrenergic blocker). Quite often a beta blocker and a type 1 drug have been used for supraventricular arrhythmias. Some data suggest some value of this combination for ventricular arrhythmias. Frequently patients may be taking this combination for treatment of ischemia (beta blocker) and arrhythmia (type 1 drug). Usually there is no harmful effect unless the type 1 drug has negative inotropic properties that are additive to those of the beta blocker.

    e. Digitalis and a type 1 drug. The combination of digitalis and a type 1 drug is most useful for supraventricular tachycardias. Digitalis is usually not effective for ventricular arrhythmias unless they are secondary to heart failure.

    f. Amiodarone (type 3) and a type 1 drug. There are two reasons to consider combining amiodarone with a type 1 drug: (1) to diminish the potential toxicity of amiodarone (with a lower dose) and (2) to increase the efficacy if the arrhythmia is refractory to amiodarone alone. The use of amiodarone alone and in combination with other drugs is considered in greater detail in Chap. 14.

4. Empiric nature of arrhythmia treatment. Arrhythmia therapy remains empiric. It is not possible to assess the patient and predict which drug will be successful. The physician must choose a drug based on experience, previous success rate, potential toxicity, and patient characteristics. If the first choice fails, another trial must be undertaken. This applies to both the noninvasive and invasive approaches to evaluation. Occasionally time may be saved by adding a compatible drug to one already being taken. In this situation, one would not have to wait for the washout before seeing the effect of the second drug. Certainly, however, it is preferable to have one drug rather than two. The utility of using the response to procainamide during EPS to guide therapy with other drugs is discussed in Chap. 12.

    The efficacy of drug therapy often is related to the skill and knowledge of the physician, for subtle alterations or combinations may render inadequate therapy effective.

VII. Specific arrhythmias

  A. Ventricular ectopy. The treatment of ventricular ectopy can be accomplished with the considerations listed above. It is very important for the physician to remember that the **primary goal of therapy is the prevention of symptomatic arrhythmias** (those causing dizziness, hypotension, syncope) and **sudden cardiac death.** The abolition of ventricular ectopy on the ECG may be an optimistic sign but does not necessarily indicate that the primary goal has been accomplished. In fact, if the primary goal is achieved, the presence of infrequent and simple ectopy on the ambulatory ECG is of minor concern.

    The physician must recall that different underlying substrates have different prognoses when associated with ventricular ectopy and may require more or less

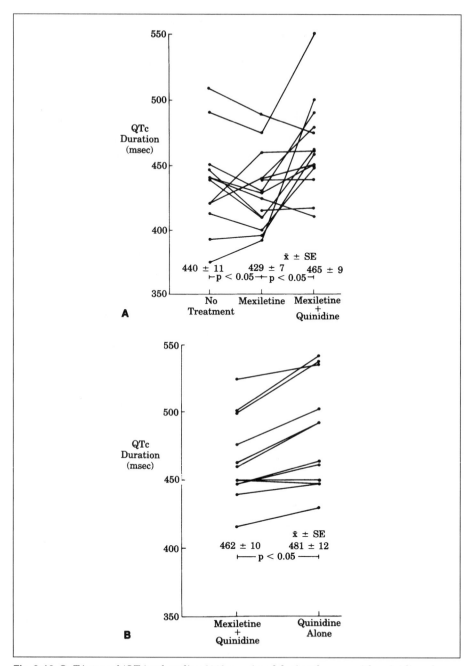

Fig. 8-10. Q–T interval (QTc) at baseline (440 msec) and during therapy with quinidine alone (481 msec), mexiletine alone (429 msec), and combined mexiletine and quinidine (465 msec). Mexiletine shortens the Q–T, quinidine prolongs it, and the combination decreases the prolonged Q–T seen with quinidine alone. (From HJ Duff et al., Mexiletine in the treatment of resistant ventricular arrhythmia: Enhancement of efficacy and reduction of dose-related side effects by combination with quinidine. *Circulation* 67:1127, 1983.)

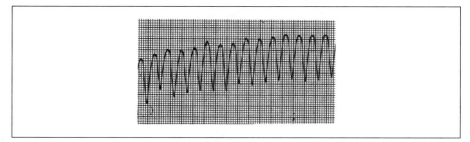

Fig. 8-11. Ventricular flutter. Rate, 272 beats/minute.

aggressive therapy. Often the refractory case may need further evaluation and treatment. The patient who continues to have recurrent symptomatic and life-threatening arrhythmias may require electrophysiologic testing if arrhythmia surgery, antitachycardia pacing, or an ICD is being considered. These modalities are discussed in Chaps. 12 (EPS), 17 (antitachycardia pacing), 18 (ICD), and 19 (surgery).

B. **Ventricular tachycardia and ventricular flutter.** In the acute setting, patients with symptoms of acute cardiovascular collapse, VT, and ventricular flutter are managed as described in Chap. 2, with electrical cardioversion the treatment of choice. Additional therapy with IV lidocaine, procainamide, or bretylium may assist in the restoration of sinus rhythm. Ventricular flutter is a very rapid form of VT that often has a sine wave appearance (Fig. 8-11). Accelerated idioventricular rhythm (AIVR) is a slow form of VT (60–110 beats/minute) that usually does not require treatment. Most often, AIVR is observed intermittently in patients with underlying heart disease. Abolishing AIVR with lidocaine in the absence of a pacemaker may cause asystole and death.

Chronic suppressive therapy for VT depends on the cause of the arrhythmia and the potential for recurrence.

C. **Ventricular fibrillation.** Ventricular fibrillation is discussed in Chap. 2 (Fig. 8-12). It results in severe impairment of the circulation and is invariably fatal unless CPR is instituted within minutes. It is useful to know that coughing creates pressure differences between the intrathoracic and extrathoracic veins, which can help maintain the circulation despite the absence of effective cardiac contraction [118, 119]. This maneuver sometimes may be used to advantage during a cardiac arrest.

Defibrillation is the treatment of choice for VF. It is accomplished by using 200–400 joules of electrical countershock, as described in Chap. 2. If sinus rhythm is not restored, acidosis, hypoxia, or hypokalemia may be contributory and must be corrected while CPR continues. Bretylium is one drug for VF as it has the potential for chemical defibrillation and may facilitate electrical defibrillation. (The probability of chemical defibrillation is extremely low.) Lidocaine may also be used during resuscitation from VF. The rationale for using lidocaine is that VF is preceded by VT in more than 80% of cases [120–122]. Once sinus rhythm is restored, lidocaine may prevent recurrent VT.

D. **Spasm-induced ventricular tachycardia.** Prinzmetal's angina is a relatively uncommon cause of ischemic heart disease. Rarely, these patients will have myocardial ischemia or myocardial injury that results in sustained and symptomatic VT. Treatment must be directed at the primary process—that is, the coronary spasm. The drugs of choice in this situation are the calcium antagonists, as discussed in Chap. 14, with potent vasodilators such as nifedipine and amlodipine in the dihydropyridine class and other drugs such as verapamil and diltiazem. Often nitrate therapy in addition to a calcium antagonist becomes necessary. Usually specific antiarrhythmic drug therapy is not necessary and also not likely to be successful. By preventing coronary spasm and myocardial ischemia and injury, the arrhythmia may be prevented.

E. **Catecholamine-sensitive ventricular tachycardia.** Some VTs may be exacerbated by stress or exercise [123–131]. Most of these patients are young and have **normal coronary arteries.** VT seems to be stimulated by the release of catecholamines. This problem has also been described as exercise-induced VT, but perhaps the term **catecholamine-sensitive VT** is better because there are a number of these patients

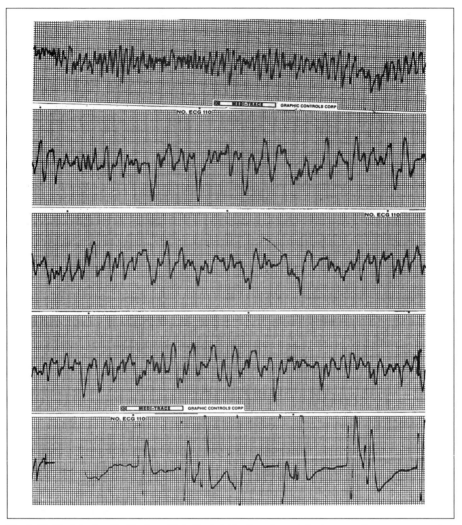

Fig. 8-12. Ventricular fibrillation. Note the totally chaotic ventricular complexes accompanied by loss of organized cardiac contraction. Normal sinus rhythm is restored after electrical defibrillation.

whose VT occurs at rest. As expected, catecholamine-sensitive VT responds to therapy with beta blockers. Some type 1 drugs have also been found to be effective in selected cases. Mapping studies have described both a right [131] and a left [129] ventricular origin of the irritable focus or tachycardia zone. Coumel has suggested that nadolol may be more beneficial than propranolol [125] (Fig. 8-13). A scheme for classifying catecholamine-sensitive VT was proposed in which type I included those with normal coronary arteries with either no detectable heart disease (IA) or those with cardiomyopathy (IB), and type II included those with ischemic heart disease [126]. Catecholamine-sensitive VT usually responds well to a relatively nontoxic type of drug (i.e., beta blocker) and may be refractory to most other antiarrhythmic drugs. Catecholamine-sensitive VT usually is not inducible at EPS, unless facilitated by isoproterenol. One of the keys to the diagnosis, after VT has been documented, is the presence of normal coronary arteries. Occasional patients with coronary disease may have ischemia-induced ventricular arrhythmias, which is a different situation.

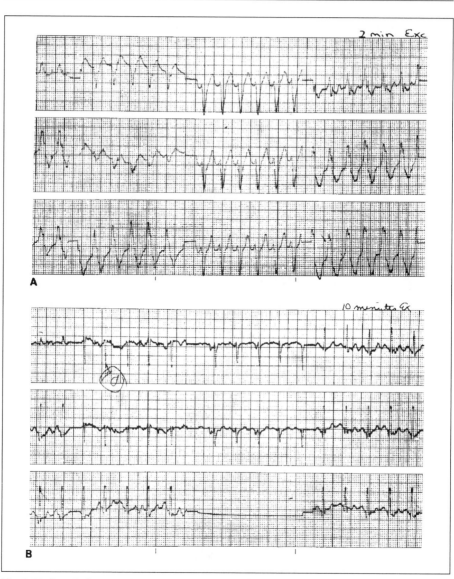

Fig. 8-13. Catecholamine-sensitive ventricular tachycardia (VT). **A.** Induction of nonhypotensive VT at 2 minutes of exercise. The patient was asymptomatic and stated she would continue her work if she were at home. **B.** Same patient after treatment with nadolol. Neither VT nor other ventricular ectopy could be induced at a high level of exercise (10 minutes on the Bruce protocol).

F. **Right ventricular outflow tract tachycardia.** Ventricular tachycardia originating from the RVOT may have more than one mechanism. In some cases, it may be catecholamine sensitive and inducible only by isoproterenol infusion. In many patients the mechanism may be related to **triggered activity** as atrial or ventricular pacing at certain cycle lengths induces the tachycardia, which then can be suppressed by verapamil [127, 128]. Some of these patients also respond to adenosine. If inducible by programmed extrastimuli but not suppressed by verapamil, then classic reentry is the mechanism. RVOT tachycardia usually has left bundle branch block morphology with an inferior axis. Mapping (particularly pace mapping) can identify the site of origin. Today, in addition to drug suppression, radiofrequency catheter ablation (see

Chap. 13) can provide an alternative therapy. **Left septal origin** of **ventricular tachy-cardia (Belhassen's VT)** has also been described and may be treated with ablation therapy.

G. **Reperfusion arrhythmias.** The era of thrombolysis has resulted in some salvage of myocardium and also created some associated problems. It became apparent that successful thrombolysis could be associated with both ventricular ectopy and brady-arrhythmias. Bradyarrhythmias were particularly noted when the artery reper-fused was the posterior descending coronary artery. When the anterior descending coronary artery was involved, ventricular ectopy and occasionally VT or VF were noted. These arrhythmias are treated in the usual manner and are a problem mostly in the acute reperfusion period. An accelerated idioventricular rhythm is also a fre-quently observed arrhythmia that usually requires no specific therapy. These arrhythmias may serve as a marker for reperfusion [132, 133].

H. **Ventricular arrhythmias in the pediatric population and those with congenital heart disease.** Ventricular tachycardia or VF is uncommon in childhood and, when it occurs, is usually associated with underlying heart disease. Pedersen et al. found a variety of heart disease in their 18 patients, ranging from MVP, cardiomyopathy, myocarditis, and prolonged Q-T syndrome to hypokalemia [134]. Bergdahl et al. reviewed 71 reported cases of VT not associated with heart disease or systemic dis-orders and noted only 4 deaths (5.6%) [135]. They called for a conservative approach to management.

Vetter et al. performed EPS in 7 pediatric patients with VT and found a high inci-dence of automatic mechanisms rather than reentry [136]. Rocchini et al. assessed prognosis in 38 patients aged 1–20 years [137]. Outcome was related to the presence of underlying disease (including MVP, myocarditis, prolonged Q–T syndrome, post-operative tetralogy of Fallot, other valvular disease, and total anomalous pul-monary venous return), the rate of the VT, and the results of treadmill testing (exac-erbation of arrhythmia with exercise).

Benson et al. noted the utility of EPS to reproduce the arrhythmia responsible for cardiac arrest [138]. Morady et al. advocated an aggressive approach toward young patients with VT or VF, since there was a 13% incidence of recurrent VT and a 10% mortality over an 18-month period, despite therapy in their series of 31 patients aged 16–40 years [139]. Garson et al. noted the applicability of arrhythmia surgery in infants with VT caused by primary cardiac tumors [140]. Fulton et al. perhaps summed up the matter of evaluation of VT in children without heart disease best by recommending that symptomatic patients be treated and studied by EPS if antiar-rhythmic therapy is inadequate [141]. Asymptomatic patients may not need thera-py but deserve careful follow-up.

In regard to specific disorders, much attention has been directed at patients who have undergone surgery for tetralogy of Fallot. Sustained VT postoperatively is related to reentry at the operative site in the right ventricular outflow tract [142] or due to widespread areas of right ventricular myocardial damage [143]. Exercise-induced arrhythmias and ambulatory monitoring identify some patients at risk of sudden death [144], but not all such patients [145]. Patients who suffered syncope were likely to have inducible nonsustained or sustained VT at EPS. Garson et al. correlated a favorable outcome (prevention of sudden cardiac death) with aggressive antiarrhythmic management of ventricular arrhythmias [146]. Ventricular ectopy noted on routine ECG was observed in all patients who died suddenly but only 12% of those who remained alive. Successful regimens in their population included phenytoin, propranolol, quinidine, disopyramide phosphate, mexiletine, and amio-darone. It is noteworthy that phenytoin achieved a success rate of 88% in these patients, which is quite different from the efficacy of this drug in treating adult arrhythmias.

I. **Ventricular tachycardia in pregnancy.** Pregnancy causes a number of physiologic changes, including an increased blood volume and cardiac output. If the patient has underlying heart disease such as cardiomyopathy, congenital disease, or valvular prob-lems (particularly mitral stenosis), serious hemodynamic stress may result and possi-bly cause or exacerbate rhythm disturbances. In some women, a peri- or postpartum cardiomyopathy may develop (starting in the last month of pregnancy or shortly after delivery), which must be differentiated from exacerbation of preexisting cardiomyop-athy.

If a patient has VT during pregnancy, there are multiple issues requiring attention: (1) diagnosis of the underlying cardiac disorder (realizing the limitations of diagnostic testing during this time period—avoiding unnecessary radiation in particular), (2) management of the altered hemodynamic state, (3) treatment of the cardiac disorder with attention to the problems of the fetus, (4) diagnosis and treatment of the VT (Is treatment really necessary?), and (5) effects of antiarrhythmic drugs on the fetus.

If the mother requires **digitalis** for heart failure or arrhythmia, it may be administered without undue concern; it has no teratogenic potential and can be given with relative safety. The dosage is identical to that in the nonpregnant patient [147, 148]. **Beta blockers** similarly have little teratogenic potential but may complicate delivery. At this point, the decision to treat with a beta-blocking drug must take into account the risk-benefit ratio. If the patient has catecholamine-sensitive VT, uncontrolled hyperthyroidism, or hypertrophic cardiomyopathy requiring beta blockade, the use of these agents is indicated. Beta blockers can be used with relative safety, provided that careful attention is provided during delivery and in the first few days of life. Bradycardia, spontaneous respiration, and hypoglycemia are of particular concern, but all of these can be managed by an alert obstetric and neonatal team. Therefore, if the patient requires therapy with beta blockers, treatment need not be avoided as long as the pregnancy is managed as one at potentially higher risk.

Quinidine and **procainamide** have been used during pregnancy without adverse effects to the mother or fetus. The major question always arises: Does the patient really require antiarrhythmic drug therapy? If the answer is yes, the clinician may use quinidine or procainamide, with attention to drug efficacy and blood level. Lidocaine similarly can be considered if IV infusion of an antiarrhythmic drug is necessary to control sustained VT. The possibility of fetal bradycardia should be remembered, but there is no documented teratogenic effect.

Phenytoin has the potential for causing fetal motor and mental retardation, particularly when taken during the first trimester. **It should be avoided.** Even in digitalis-toxic ventricular arrhythmias, it is preferable to treat the patient with lidocaine if necessary. With the availability of digitalis antibodies, there is little reason to consider phenytoin if lidocaine fails to control the VT.

At this time, there is insufficient evidence to recommend the use of any other type 1 or type 3 antiarrhythmic drugs during pregnancy. The safety data are not available. In fact, investigational protocols consider pregnancy one of the exclusion criteria. Fortunately, pregnant women rarely are included in the population requiring treatment for refractory VT or VF. If a woman requiring antiarrhythmic drug therapy with one of the newer agents because of refractory VT or VF (or even refractory SVT) becomes pregnant, the risk-benefit issues must again be addressed. What is the risk of the pregnancy to the mother? Is treatment with the current regimen absolutely necessary? If yes, are the unknown risks to the fetus acceptable? If no, can other drugs or modalities of treatment be substituted?

Verapamil, a calcium antagonist, is used primarily for SVT, although rare cases of VT have responded. The use of verapamil during pregnancy still has not been completely evaluated. There are concerns about its effects on conduction as well as its negative inotropic and vasodilative properties.

A recent chapter on the use of antiarrhythmic agents in pregnancy addressed the safety of some of the newer drugs [149]. The authors divided the drugs into three categories:

Safe: lidocaine, digoxin
Relatively safe: quinidine, procainamide, propranolol
Probably safe: mexiletine, disopyramide, verapamil, amiodarone

Thus the use of antiarrhythmic drugs during pregnancy depends on the necessity of treatment and the choice of the least toxic agent. In many cases, individual decisions must be made. I highly recommend careful reading of the three references cited in this section before embarking on antiarrhythmic drug therapy in this population.

J. **Drug-induced ventricular tachycardia.** One of the major achievements of the past 10 years, the recognition that antiarrhythmic drugs may not only suppress but also exacerbate ventricular arrhythmias, has resulted in more judicious prescribing habits. Nevertheless, drug toxicity still occurs, sometimes with recommended dosages and occasionally with excessive amounts (e.g., suicide attempts).

1. **Digitalis toxicity.** With digitalis, increased ventricular ectopy may be one of the first signs of toxicity, with sustained VT one of the most life-threatening. Bidirectional VT is particularly suggestive of digitalis toxicity. Fisch and Knoebel classify digitalis toxic arrhythmias as follows: (1) ectopic rhythms owing to reentry or enhanced automaticity or both, (2) depression of pacemakers, (3)

depression of conduction, (4) ectopic rhythms with simultaneous depression of conduction, (5) atrioventricular (AV) dissociation caused by suppression of the dominant pacemaker and escape of a subsidiary pacemaker versus inappropriate acceleration of a lower pacemaker, and possibly (6) triggered automaticity [150].

The treatment of digitalis toxicity begins with its recognition and stopping the digitalis preparation. Patients with VT must be monitored in the coronary care unit (CCU). Lidocaine is the first drug to use because of its availability and ease of administration. Electrical cardioversion should be avoided because of the extreme electrical instability and the potential for VF, but if the patient has no BP, there is no choice.

Phenytoin is another drug that was considered extremely useful at one time. In fact, digitalis toxicity was the situation in which phenytoin has the most utility as an antiarrhythmic agent (although the FDA does not approve this indication). Phenytoin was carefully given by IV infusion. The serum potassium should be corrected if the level is low.

In the majority of cases, discontinuation of digitalis and treatment with lidocaine will be sufficient. In cases of massive overdose, digoxin-specific antibody may be lifesaving. The theory is that glycoside-induced inhibition of myocardial sodium potassium adenosine triphosphatase and monovalent cation active transport may be reversed by high-affinity glycoside-specific antibodies [151]. Less immunogenic antibody fragments (Fab) distribute more rapidly and in a wider distribution volume than the whole antibody, resulting in a faster and more effective reversal of toxicity. Fragments can also be excreted by glomerular filtration rather than degraded by the reticuloendothelial system. In the series cited, Fab was effective in 95% of patients with life-threatening ventricular tachyarrhythmias.

2. **Type 1 antiarrhythmic agents.** When the use of an antiarrhythmic drug that may prolong repolarization (i.e., the Q–T interval as measured on the ECG) is considered, one must assess the baseline Q–T. If it is prolonged already, addition of a drug such as quinidine, procainamide, disopyramide, or a phenothiazine could cause serious toxicity. High dosages of these drugs with a normal Q–T interval can also increase the Q–T interval markedly. With an increased vulnerable period (and possibly more frequent VPBs), the possibility of induced polymorphic ventricular tachycardia in the form of torsades de pointes arises. The treatment of choice is CCU monitoring, discontinuation of the offending drug, and isoproterenol infusion (shortening repolarization and increasing the heart rate) as the initial steps. Atrial or ventricular pacing often will suppress the polymorphic VT. Infusion of magnesium sulfate as a bolus of 2 g IV, with a second bolus of 2–4 g 15 minutes later, followed by a continuous infusion of 3–30 mg/minute for up to 48 hours may be helpful [152].

All of the type 1 agents have a 5–10% incidence of proarrhythmic effects. Only one mechanism was presented above for the type 1A drugs, but multiple factors, including negative inotropic effects, may also be contributory. The recent experience with flecainide should make us particularly cautious [153, 154]. At dosages higher than currently recommended, some VT patients with severely impaired left ventricular function developed intractable VT or VF and could not be resuscitated. Discontinuation of any drug suspected of causing VT and measurement of the blood level are the two initial steps in treatment.

K. **Torsades de pointes.** Torsades de pointes (Fig. 8-14) has been described as polymorphic VT occurring in the presence (or rarely absence) of a prolonged Q–T interval [155]. The prolongation of the Q–T interval may be congenital or acquired. It may be difficult to reproduce the native arrhythmia with programmed electrical stimulation in the electrophysiology laboratory [156]. The treatment has already been described above. If polymorphic VT occurs in the absence of a prolonged Q–T, drugs such as quinidine or procainamide may be used. The true torsades de pointes syndrome should also be distinguished from polymorphic VT caused by triple or greater extrastimuli during EPS.

L. **Long Q–T syndrome.** Prolonged Q–T syndromes may be acquired as described above or may be congenital [157–166]. Two types of the latter have been described. Jervell and Lange-Nielsen's syndrome has an autosomal recessive inheritance and is associated with congenital deafness. The Romano-Ward syndrome, autosomal dominant, is associated with normal hearing. The heart is otherwise normal. The Romano-Ward long Q–T phenotype is linked to the Harvey ras-1 gene on chromo-

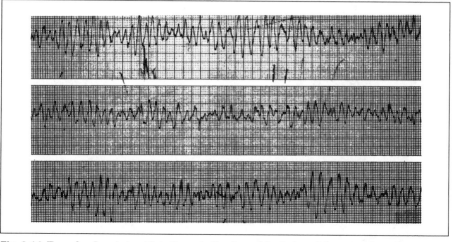

Fig. 8-14. Torsades de pointes. Note the spindle-shaped "twisting of the points" in a patient with a prolonged Q–T. This arrhythmia is treated by drugs that shorten the Q–T interval and by overdrive pacing or isoproterenol infusion during emergencies.

some 11 in many families. Mutation of the disease gene alters the G protein function of the gene and interferes with delayed rectifier potassium current and beta-receptor channel signaling [167]. In gene carriers, the amount of Q–Tc prolongation did not predict which individuals would experience ventricular arrhythmias, syncope, or sudden death [168]. Additional reports on families with the long Q–T syndrome did indicate that significant contributing variables for syncope or death before age 50 included prolongation of the Q–Tc (≥ 0.50 second), history of cardiac event (syncope or cardiac arrest), and heart rate (resting < 50 beats/minute) [169]. For patients without congenital syndromes, one study indicated that Q–Tc prolongation independently contributed to cardiovascular risk [170].

In addition to the drug-induced acquired form of the prolonged Q–T syndrome, a prolonged Q–T may be seen in patients with myocardial infarction, hypokalemia, hypocalcemia, hypomagnesemia, and some CNS problems [159, 161, 162]. When considering a diagnosis of the prolonged Q–T interval, one expects a corrected Q–T interval longer than 440–460 msec.

Schwartz has called attention to the importance of hypoactivity of right and hyperactivity of left cardiac sympathetic nerves and has studied the effects of left sympathectomy involving the first four or five thoracic ganglia. A recent worldwide report revealed that left cardiac sympathetic denervation significantly decreased the incidence of tachyarrhythmic syncope and sudden death [171].

Should all patients with congenital prolonged Q–T syndrome be treated? Certainly symptomatic patients require therapy. Beta blockers are the first drugs to consider because of their antiadrenergic effects. Furthermore, combination of a beta blocker with permanent pacing makes sense since pacing prevents bradyarrhythmias and pauses and contributes to more homogeneous repolarization [172]. The incidence of syncope is reduced but may not provide complete protection. If the patient continues to be symptomatic, left cardiac sympathectomy may be considered. Another option is the automatic ICD [160, 173]. For asymptomatic patients with the congenital prolonged Q–T syndrome, the physician must make a decision about the potential risk of death with the first episode of syncope. Possibly family history may be influential, if a sibling has died in this manner. Risk factors associated with syncope and death include congenital deafness, history of syncope, female gender, and history of VF or torsades de pointes [159].

In regard to the acquired prolonged Q–T syndrome, it is often difficult to decide when prolongation of the Q–T represents a therapeutic or a toxic effect [151]. If only minimal, it may just represent an antiarrhythmic effect, that is, reduction of dispersion of action potential duration or refractoriness. In fact, a drug with these effects, amiodarone, has been considered for some patients with the prolonged Q–T syndrome.

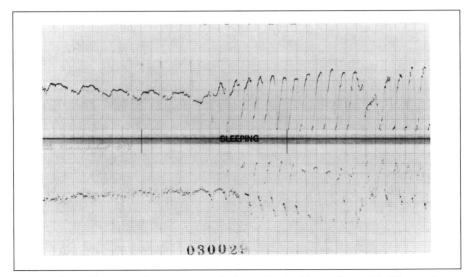

SLEEPING

030025

Fig. 8-15. Initiation of ventricular tachycardia in a patient with a prolonged Q–T interval. This arrhythmia resulted in sudden cardiac death. (From SC Vlay et al., Documented sudden cardiac death in prolonged Q–T syndrome. *Arch Intern Med* 144:833–835, 1984. Copyright 1984, American Medical Association.)

The physician must not allow the prolonged Q–T syndrome to go unrecognized (Fig. 8-15). The indication for treatment depends on the presence of symptoms, the length of the Q–T interval, risk factors, the potential for modifying contributory factors such as quinidine therapy, and the ability to tolerate therapy. Beta blockers are the drugs of choice and are usually well tolerated.

M. **"Electrical storm" or incessant VT or VF.** Occasionally a patient presents with severe electrical instability manifest as intractable VT or VF, resulting in SCD. Nothing—oxygen, lidocaine, procainamide, bretylium tosylate, correction of metabolic abnormalities—seems to help. This situation, described by some as electrical storm, may be the electrophysiologic equivalent of the patient with cardiogenic shock, with mortality just as high. It is quite frustrating since all efforts by the physician prove fruitless.

In 1985, the group from Hahnemann reported control of VT or VF by IV amiodarone in 76% of 21 patients with refractory VT or VF previously requiring multiple electrical cardioversions [174]. Nineteen of the 21 patients had previous MI—9 within the preceding 30 days. Amiodarone was given IV at 10 mg/kg for 24 hours, followed by oral amiodarone. Allowing these cases to be controlled in the early critical hours may permit further evaluation (such as EPS) and therapy (medical, surgical, electronic device).

No major trials have confirmed these data. Part of the problem with IV amiodarone was the associated hypotension. At this point we await further trials, as well as a new preparation of IV amiodarone expected to be approved by the FDA in the near future.

N. **Electromechanical dissociation.** Another problem with a dismal outcome is electromechanical dissociation (EMD), which signifies electrical activity in the absence of effective mechanical contraction. It is usually a terminal arrhythmia in end-stage heart disease. Nevertheless, there are some reversible causes that must be promptly recognized and corrected if the patient is to be saved. The most salvageable of the causes is pericardial tamponade, with emergency pericardiocentesis as the treatment of choice. If pericardial tamponade is due to myocardial rupture, the prognosis remains grim. Other possible causes of EMD are tension pneumothorax and hypovolemia.

O. **Ventricular parasystole.** Ventricular parasystole is a relatively benign rhythm. The cardiologist should not miss the diagnosis of parasystole, which is recognized by nonfixed coupling (of the premature ventricular beat to the preceding sinus beat), constant interectopic intervals, and fusion beats (Fig. 8-16). The reason that the

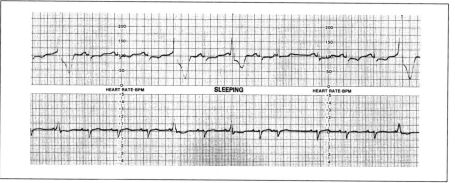

Fig. 8-16. Ventricular parasystole. This electrocardiogram reveals ventricular parasystole with nonfixed coupling, constant interectopic intervals, and a fusion beat. The rhythm usually is associated with a benign prognosis.

wide complex is not always seen is that the ventricle may be rendered refractory by the preceding sinus beat or there may be exit block within the parasystolic focus. Entrance block prevents the parasystolic focus from being depolarized by other electrical impulses. Parasystole may also occur in the atrium or AV node. Ventricular parasystole does not require treatment. However, rarely one may encounter a parasystolic ventricular tachycardia that requires further evaluation.

References

1. Zipes DP. Specific Arrhythmias: Diagnosis and Treatment. In E Braunwald (ed), *Heart Disease: A Textbook of Cardiovascular Medicine* (2nd ed). Philadelphia: Saunders, 1984. Pp 721–723.
2. Lown B. Cardiovascular Collapse and Sudden Cardiac Death. In E Braunwald (ed), *Heart Disease: A Textbook of Cardiovascular Medicine* (2nd ed). Philadelphia: Saunders, 1984. Pp 797–798.
3. Bigger JT. Management of Arrhythmias. In E Braunwald (ed), *Heart Disease: A Textbook of Cardiovascular Medicine* (1st ed). Philadelphia: Saunders, 1980. Pp 734–735.
4. Smith WM, Gallagher JJ. Management of Arrhythmias and Conduction Abnormalities. In JW Hurst (ed-in-chief), *The Heart* (5th ed). New York: McGraw-Hill, 1982. P 568.
5. Josephson ME, et al. Electrophysiologic and hemodynamic studies in patients resuscitated from cardiac arrest. *Am J Cardiol* 46:948, 1980.
6. Vlay SC, Reid PR. Ventricular ectopy: Etiology, evaluation, and therapy. *Am J Med* 73:899–913, 1982.
7. Vlay SC. How the university cardiologist treats ventricular premature beats: A nationwide survey of 65 university medical centers. *Am Heart J* 110:904–912, 1985.
8. Lown B, Wolf M. Approaches to sudden death from coronary heart disease. *Circulation* 44:130–142, 1971.
9. Bigger JT, Wenger TL, Heissenbuttel RH. Limitations of the Lown grading system for the study of human ventricular arrhythmias. *Am Heart J* 93:727–729, 1977.
10. Swiryn S, et al. Sequential regional phase mapping of radionuclide gated biventriculograms in patients with sustained ventricular tachycardia: Close correlation with electrophysiologic characters. *Am Heart J* 103:319–332, 1982.
11. Vlay SC, et al. Anatomic substrate and clinical outcome in survivors of sudden cardiac death: A multivariate analysis. *Cardiovasc Rev Rep* 7:861–875, 1986.
12. Vlay SC, et al. Prediction of sudden cardiac arrest: Risk stratification by anatomic substrate. *Am Heart J* 126:807–815, 1993.
13. Dollar AL, Roberts WC. Morphologic comparison of patients with mitral valve prolapse who died suddenly with patients who died from severe valvular dysfunction of other conditions. *J Am Coll Cardiol* 17:921–931, 1991.
14. Strain JE, et al. Results of endomyocardial biopsy in patients with spontaneous ventricular tachycardia but without apparent structural heart disease. *Circulation* 68:1171–1181, 1983.

15. Hiss RG, Averill KH, Lamb LE. Electrocardiographic findings in 67,375 asymptomatic subjects. *Am J Cardiol* 6:96–107, 1960.
16. Rodstein M, Wolloch L, Gubner RS. Mortality study of the significance of extrasystoles in an insured population. *Circulation* 44:617–625, 1971.
17. Fisher FD, Tyroler HA. Relationship between ventricular premature contractions on routine electrocardiography and subsequent sudden death from coronary heart disease. *Circulation* 47:712–719, 1973.
18. Chiang BN, et al. Relationship of premature systoles to coronary heart disease and sudden death in the Tecumseh Epidemiologic Study. *Ann Intern Med* 70:1159–1166, 1969.
19. Chiang BN, et al. Predisposing factors in sudden cardiac death in Tecumseh, Michigan. *Circulation* 41:31–37, 1970.
20. Kennedy HL, et al. Effectiveness of increasing hours of continuous ambulatory electrocardiography in detecting maximal ventricular ectopy. *Am J Cardiol* 42:925–930, 1978.
21. Morganroth J, et al. Limitations of routine long-term electrocardiographic monitoring to assess ventricular ectopic frequency. *Circulation* 58:408–414, 1978.
22. Glasser SP, Clark PE, Applebaum HJ. Occurrence of frequent complex arrhythmias detected by ambulatory monitoring. *Chest* 75:565–568, 1979.
23. Brodsky M, et al. Arrhythmias documented by 24-hour continuous electrocardiographic monitoring in 50 male medical students without apparent heart disease. *Am J Cardiol* 39:390–395, 1977.
24. Kennedy HL, Underhill SJ. Frequent or complex ventricular ectopy in apparently healthy subjects. *Am J Cardiol* 38:141–148, 1976.
25. Romhilt DW, et al. Arrhythmias on ambulatory electrocardiographic monitoring in women without apparent heart disease. *Am J Cardiol* 54:582–586, 1984.
26. Hinkle LE, Carver ST, Stevens M. The frequency of asymptomatic disturbances of cardiac rhythm and conduction in middle aged men. *Am J Cardiol* 24:629–650, 1969.
27. Hinkle LE, Carver ST, Argyros DC. The prognostic significance of ventricular premature contractions in healthy people and in people with coronary heart disease. *Acta Cardiol* 28(Suppl):5–53, 1974.
28. Ruberman W, et al. Ventricular premature beats and mortality after myocardial infarction. *N Engl J Med* 297:750–757, 1977.
29. Ruberman W, et al. Repeated one-hour electrocardiographic monitoring of survivors of myocardial infarction at six-month intervals: Arrhythmia detection and relation to prognosis. *Am J Cardiol* 47:1197–1204, 1981.
30. Ruberman W, et al. Ventricular premature complexes and sudden death after myocardial infarction. *Circulation* 64:297–305, 1981.
31. Ruberman W, et al. Ventricular premature beats and mortality of men with coronary heart disease. *Circulation* 52(Suppl III):199–203, 1975.
32. Tominaga S, Blackburn H. The Coronary Drug Project Research Group: Prognostic importance of premature beats following myocardial infarction. *JAMA* 223:1116–1124, 1973.
33. Kotler MN, et al. Prognostic significance of ventricular ectopic beats with respect to sudden death in the late postinfarction period. *Circulation* 47:959–966, 1973.
34. Moss AJ, et al. Ventricular arrhythmias 3 weeks after acute myocardial infarction. *Ann Intern Med* 75:837–841, 1971.
35. Moss AJ, et al. Prognostic grading and significance of ventricular premature beats after recovery from myocardial infarction. *Circulation* 52(Suppl III):204–210, 1975.
36. Moss AJ, et al. Clinical significance of ventricular ectopic beats in the early posthospital phase of myocardial infarction. *Am J Cardiol* 39:635–640, 1977.
37. Anderson KP, DeCamilla J, Moss AJ. Clinical significance of ventricular tachycardia (three beats or longer) detected during ambulatory monitoring after myocardial infarction. *Circulation* 57:890–897, 1978.
38. Moss AJ, et al. Ventricular ectopic beats and their relation to sudden and nonsudden cardiac death after myocardial infarction. *Circulation* 60:998–1003, 1979.
39. Vismara LA, Amsterdam EA, Mason DT. Relation of ventricular arrhythmias in the late hospital phase of acute myocardial infarction to sudden death after hospital discharge. *Am J Med* 59:6–12, 1975.
40. Vismara LA, et al. Identification of sudden death risk factors in acute and chronic coronary artery disease. *Am J Cardiol* 39:821–828, 1977.
41. Schulze RA, et al. Ventricular arrhythmias in the late hospital phase of acute myocardial infarction. *Circulation* 52:1006–1011, 1975.
42. Schulze RA, et al. Left ventricular and coronary angiographic anatomy: Relationship to ventricular irritability in the late hospital phase of acute myocardial infarction. *Circulation* 55:839–843, 1977.

43. Schulze RA, Strauss HW, Pitt B. Sudden death in the year following myocardial infarction. *Am J Med* 62:192–199, 1977.
44. Bigger JT, et al. Risk stratification after acute myocardial infarction. *Am J Cardiol* 42:202–210, 1978.
45. Bigger JT, Weld FM, Rolnitzky LM. Prevalence, characteristics and significance of ventricular tachycardia (three or more complexes) detected with ambulatory electrocardiographic recording in the late hospital phase of acute myocardial infarction. *Am J Cardiol* 48:815–823, 1981.
46. Follansbee WP, Michelson EL, Morganroth J. Nonsustained ventricular tachycardia in ambulatory patients: Characteristics and association with sudden cardiac death. *Ann Intern Med* 92:741–747, 1980.
47. Kennedy HL, et al. Objective evidence of occult myocardial dysfunction in patients with frequent ventricular ectopy without clinically apparent heart disease. *Am Heart J* 104:57–65, 1982.
48. Olson HG, et al. Prognostic implications of complicated ventricular arrhythmias early after hospital discharge in acute myocardial infarction: A serial ambulatory electrocardiography study. *Am Heart J* 108:1221–1228, 1984.
49. Holmes J, et al. Arrhythmias in ischemic and nonischemic dilated cardiomyopathy: Prediction of mortality by ambulatory electrocardiography. *Am J Cardiol* 55:146–151, 1985.
50. Lown B. Sudden cardiac death: The major challenge confronting contemporary cardiology. *Am J Cardiol* 43:313–328, 1979.
51. Vlay SC, Kallman CH, Reid PR. Prognostic assessment of survivors of ventricular tachycardia and ventricular fibrillation with ambulatory monitoring. *Am J Cardiol* 54:87–90, 1984.
52. Fleg JL, Lakatta EG. Prevalence and prognosis of exercise induced nonsustained ventricular tachycardia in apparently healthy volunteers. *Am J Cardiol* 54:762–764, 1984.
53. Kennedy HL, et al. Long term followup of asymptomatic healthy subjects with frequent and complex ventricular ectopy. *N Engl J Med* 312:193–197, 1985.
54. Califf RM, et al. Relationships among ventricular arrhythmias, coronary artery disease, and angiographic and electrocardiographic indicators of myocardial fibrosis. *Circulation* 57:725–732, 1978.
55. Sharma SD, Ballantyne F, Goldstein S. The relationship of ventricular asynergy in coronary artery disease to ventricular premature beats. *Chest* 66:358–362, 1974.
56. Calvert A, Lown B, Gorlin R. Ventricular premature beats and anatomically defined coronary heart disease. *Am J Cardiol* 39:627–634, 1977.
57. Vlay SC, et al. Relationship of specific coronary lesions and regional left ventricular dysfunction to prognosis in survivors of sudden cardiac death. *Am Heart J* 108:1212–1220, 1984.
58. Fowler NO. Differential diagnosis of cardiomyopathies. *Prog Cardiovasc Dis* 14:113–128, 1971.
59. Unverferth DV, et al. Factors influencing the one year mortality of dilated cardiomyopathy. *Am J Cardiol* 54:147–152, 1984.
60. Maskin CS, Siskind SJ, LeJemtel TH. High prevalence of nonsustained ventricular tachycardia in severe congestive heart failure. *Am Heart J* 107:896–901, 1984.
61. Miura DS, et al. The association of cardiomyopathies and ventricular tachycardia with sudden death. *Cardiovasc Rev Rep* 6:1127–1134, 1985.
62. Larsen L, Markham J, Haffajee CI. Sudden death in idiopathic dilated cardiomyopathy: Role of ventricular arrhythmias. *PACE* 16:1051–1059, 1993.
63. Savage DD, et al. Prevalence of arrhythmias during 24 hour electrocardiographic monitoring and exercise testing in patients with obstructive and nonobstructive hypertrophic cardiomyopathy. *Circulation* 59:866–875, 1979.
64. Frank MJ, et al. Long-term medical management of hypertrophic obstructive cardiomyopathy. *Am J Cardiol* 42:993–1000, 1978.
65. Maron BJ, et al. Prognostic significance of 24 hour ambulatory electrocardiographic monitoring in patients with hypertrophic cardiomyopathy. *Am J Cardiol* 48:252–257, 1981.
66. Maron BJ, et al. Sudden death in patients with hypertrophic cardiomyopathy: Characterization of 26 patients without functional limitation. *Am J Cardiol* 41:803–810, 1978.
67. Maron BJ, Roberts WC, Epstein SE. Sudden death in hypertrophic cardiomyopathy: A profile of 78 patients. *Circulation* 65:1388–1394, 1982.
68. Frank MJ, et al. Potentially lethal arrhythmias and their management in hypertrophic cardiomyopathy. *Am J Cardiol* 53:1608–1613, 1984.

69. Silverman KJ, Hutchins GM, Bulkley BH. Cardiac sarcoid: A clinicopathologic study of 84 unselected patients with systemic sarcoidosis. *Circulation* 58:1204–1211, 1978.
70. Marcus FI, et al. Right ventricular dysplasia: A report of 24 adult cases. *Circulation* 65:384–398, 1982.
71. Mayari DE, et al. Arrhythmogenic right ventricular dysplasia: A generalized cardiomyopathy. *Circulation* 68:251–257, 1983.
72. Perloff JK. Cardiac rhythm and conduction in Duchenne's muscular dystrophy: A prospective study of 20 patients. *J Am Coll Cardiol* 3:1263–1268, 1984.
73. Winkle RA, et al. Arrhythmias in patients with mitral valve prolapse. *Circulation* 52:73–81, 1975.
74. DeMaria AN, et al. Arrhythmias in the mitral valve prolapse syndrome. *Ann Intern Med* 84:656–660, 1976.
75. Campbell RWF, et al. Ventricular arrhythmias in syndrome of balloon deformity of mitral valve. *Br Heart J* 38:1053–1057, 1976.
76. Wei JW, et al. Mitral valve prolapse syndrome and recurrent ventricular tachyarrhythmias. *Ann Intern Med* 89:6–9, 1978.
77. Chesler E, King RA, Edwards JE. The myxomatous mitral valve and sudden death. *Circulation* 67:632–639, 1983.
78. Kolibash AJ, et al. Mitral valve prolapse syndrome: Analysis of 62 patients aged 60 years and older. *Am J Cardiol* 52:534–539, 1983.
79. Kligfield P, et al. Complex arrhythmias in mitral regurgitation with and without mitral valve prolapse: Contrast to arrhythmias in mitral valve prolapse without mitral regurgitation. *Am J Cardiol* 55:1545–1549, 1985.
80. v. Olshausen K, et al. Determinants of the incidence and severity of ventricular arrhythmias in aortic valve disease. *Am J Cardiol* 51:1103–1109, 1983.
81. v. Olshausen K, et al. Ventricular arrhythmias before and late after aortic valve replacement. *Am J Cardiol* 53:142–146, 1984.
82. Klein RC. Ventricular arrhythmias in aortic valve disease: Analysis of 102 patients. *Am J Cardiol* 53:1079–1083, 1984.
83. Uretz EF, Denes P, Ruggie N. Relation of ventricular premature beats to underlying heart disease. *Am J Cardiol* 53:774–780, 1984.
84. Lam W, et al. Angiographic correlates of recurrent sustained ventricular tachycardia in chronic ischemic heart disease. *Am Heart J* 105:928–933, 1983.
85. Spielman S, et al. Drug therapy in high risk patients following acute myocardial infarction: The results of the timolol, encainide, sotalol trial. *Circulation* 72:15, 1985.
86. Gottlieb S, et al. Prophylactic antiarrhythmic therapy of high risk postinfarction patients: Mortality is delayed but not reduced. *Circulation* 72:358, 1985.
87. Hoffmann A, et al. Suppression of high grade ventricular ectopic activity by antiarrhythmic drug treatment as a marker for survival in patients with chronic coronary artery disease. *Am Heart J* 107:1103–1108, 1984.
88. The CAPS investigators: Effects of encainide, flecainide, imipramine, and moricizine on ventricular arrhythmias during the year after myocardial infarction: The CAPS. *Am J Cardiol* 61:501–509, 1988.
89. Echt DS, et al. Mortality and morbidity in patients receiving encainide, flecainide, or placebo. The Cardiac Arrhythmia Suppression Trial. *N Engl J Med* 324:781–788, 1991.
90. The CAST II Investigators: Effect of the antiarrhythmic agent moricizine on survival after myocardial infarction. *N Engl J Med* 327:227–233, 1992.
91. Green HL, et al. The cardiac arrhythmia suppression trial: First CAST . . . then CAST II. *J Am Coll Cardiol* 19:894–898, 1992.
92. Akhtar M, et al. CAST and beyond: Implications of the Cardiac Arrhythmia Suppression Trial. *Circulation* 81:1123–1127, 1990.
93. Bigger JT. The events surrounding the removal of encainide and flecainide from the Cardiac Arrhythmia Suppression Trial (CAST) and why CAST is continuing with moricizine. *J Am Coll Cardiol* 15:243–245, 1990.
94. Siebels J, et al. ICD versus drugs in cardiac arrest survivors. *PACE* 16:552–558, 1993.
95. Burkhart F, et al. Effect of antiarrhythmic therapy on mortality in survivors of myocardial infarction with asymptomatic complex ventricular arrhythmias: Basel Antiarrhythmic Study of Infarct Survival (BASIS). *J Am Coll Cardiol* 16:1711–1718, 1990.
96. Cairns JA, et al. Post-myocardial infarction mortality in patients with ventricular premature depolarizations: Canadian Amiodarone Myocardial Infarction Arrhythmia Trial Pilot study. *Circulation* 84:550–557, 1991.
97. Ceremuzynski L, et al. Effect of amiodarone on mortality after myocardial infarction: A double-blind, placebo-controlled, pilot study. *J Am Coll Cardiol* 20:1056–1062, 1992.

98. The CASCADE Investigators: Randomized antiarrhythmic drug therapy in survivors of cardiac arrest. *Am J Cardiol* 72:280–287, 1993.
99. Pfisterer ME, et al. Long-term benefit of 1-year amiodarone treatment for persistent complex ventricular arrhythmias after myocardial infarction. *Circulation* 87:309–311, 1993.
100. Zipes DP. Specific Arrhythmias: Diagnosis and Treatment. In Braunwald E (ed), *Heart Disease* (4th ed). Philadelphia: Saunders, 1992. Pp 667–726.
101. Myerburg RJ, Kessler KM, Castellanos A. Recognition, Clinical Assessment and Management of Arrhythmias. In RC Schlant et al. (eds), *Hurst's The Heart, Arteries and Veins* (5th ed). New York: McGraw-Hill, 1994. Pp 705–758.
102. Bigger JT. Cardiac Arrhythmias. In JB Wyngaarden, LH Smith, JC Bennett (eds), *Cecil Textbook of Medicine* (19th ed). Philadelphia: Saunders, 1992. Pp 228–250.
103. Josephson ME, Buxton AE, Marchlinski FE. The Tachyarrhythmias. In KJ Isselbacher, et al. (eds), *Harrison's Principles of Internal Medicine* (13th ed). New York: McGraw-Hill, 1994. Pp 1019–1037.
104. Platia EV, Reid PR. Comparison of programmed electrical stimulation and ambulatory electrocardiographic (Holter) monitoring in the management of ventricular tachycardia and ventricular fibrillation. *J Am Coll Cardiol* 4:493–500, 1984.
105. Swerdlow CD, Peterson J. Prospective comparison of Holter monitoring and electrophysiologic study in patients with coronary artery disease and sustained ventricular tachyarrhythmias. *Am J Cardiol* 56:577–580, 1985.
106. Graboys TB, et al. Long term survival of patients with malignant ventricular arrhythmia treated with antiarrhythmic drugs. *Am J Cardiol* 50:437–443, 1982.
107. ESVEM Investigators: Determinants of predicted efficacy of antiarrhythmic drugs in the electrophysiologic study versus electrocardiographic monitoring trial. *Circulation* 87:323–329, 1993.
108. Mason JW (for the ESVEM Investigators). A comparison of electrophysiologic testing with Holter monitoring to predict antiarrhythmic-drug efficacy for ventricular tachyarrhythmias. *N Engl J Med* 329:445–451, 1993.
109. Steinbeck G, et al. A comparison of electrophysiologically guided antiarrhythmic drug therapy with beta-blocker therapy in patients with symptomatic, sustained ventricular tachyarrhythmias. *N Engl J Med* 327:987–992, 1992.
110. Mason JW (for the ESVEM Investigators). A comparison of seven antiarrhythmic drugs in patients with ventricular tachyarrhythmias. *N Engl J Med* 329:452–458, 1993.
111. Vlay SC, Kallman CH, Reid PR. The utility of aprindine levels in the management of ventricular arrhythmias. *J Am Coll Cardiol* 5:738–743, 1985.
112. Waagstein F, et al. Effect of chronic beta-adrenergic receptor blockade in congestive cardiomyopathy. *Br Heart J* 37:1022–1036, 1975.
113. Engelmeier RS, et al. Improvement in symptoms and exercise tolerance by metoprolol in patients with dilated cardiomyopathy: A double blind, randomized, placebo-controlled trial. *Circulation* 72:536–546, 1985.
114. Anderson JL, et al. A randomized trial of low-dose beta blockade therapy for idiopathic dilated cardiomyopathy. *Am J Cardiol* 55:471–475, 1985.
115. Alderman J, Grossman W. Are beta adrenergic–blocking drugs useful in the treatment of dilated cardiomyopathy? *Circulation* 71:854–857, 1985.
116. Duff HJ, et al. Mexiletine in the treatment of resistant ventricular arrhythmias: Enhancement of efficacy and reduction of dose-related side effects by combination with quinidine. *Circulation* 67:1124–1128, 1983.
117. Greenspan AM, et al. Efficacy of combination therapy with mexiletine and a type 1A agent for inducible ventricular tachyarrhythmias secondary to coronary artery disease. *Am J Cardiol* 56:277–284, 1985.
118. Criley JM, Blaufuss AH, Kissel GL. Cough induced cardiac compression: Self-administered form of cardiopulmonary resuscitation. *JAMA* 236:1246–1250, 1976.
119. Rudikoff MT, et al. Mechanisms of blood flow during cardiopulmonary resuscitation. *Circulation* 61:345–352, 1980.
120. Panidis IP, Morganroth J. Sudden death in hospitalized patients: Cardiac rhythm disturbances detected by ambulatory electrocardiographic monitoring. *J Am Coll Cardiol* 2:798–805, 1983.
121. Kempf FC, Josephson ME. Cardiac arrest recorded on ambulatory electrocardiograms. *Am J Cardiol* 53:1577–1582, 1984.
122. Milner PG, et al. Ambulatory electrocardiographic recordings at the time of fatal cardiac arrest. *Am J Cardiol* 56:588–592, 1985.
123. Wu D, Kou HC, Hung JS. Exercise triggered paroxysmal ventricular tachycardia. *Ann Intern Med* 95:410–414, 1981.

124. Palileo EV, et al. Exercise provocable right ventricular outflow tract tachycardia. *Am Heart J* 104:185–193, 1982.
125. Coumel P, et al. Role of the sympathetic nervous system in nonischaemic ventricular arrhythmias. *Br Heart J* 47:137–147, 1982.
126. Vlay SC. Catecholamine sensitive ventricular tachycardia. *Am Heart J* 114:455–461, 1987.
127. Lerman BB, et al. Adenosine sensitive ventricular tachycardia: Evidence suggesting cyclic AMP-mediated triggered activity. *Circulation* 74:270–278, 1986.
128. Gill JS, et al. Verapamil for the suppression of idiopathic ventricular tachycardia of left bundle branch block-like morphology. *Am Heart J* 126:1126–1133, 1993.
129. Rahilly GT, et al. Clinical and electrophysiologic findings in patients with repetitive monomorphic ventricular tachycardia and otherwise normal electrocardiogram. *Am J Cardiol* 50:459–468, 1982.
130. Pietras RJ, et al. Chronic recurrent right ventricular tachycardia in patients without ischemic heart disease: Clinical hemodynamic and angiographic findings. *Am Heart J* 105:357–366, 1983.
131. Buxton AE, et al. Right ventricular tachycardia: Clinical and electrophysiologic characteristics. *Circulation* 68:917–927, 1983.
132. Goldberg S, et al. Reperfusion arrhythmia: A marker of restoration of antegrade flow during intracoronary thrombolysis for acute myocardial infarction. *Am Heart J* 105:26–32, 1983.
133. Fujimoto T, et al. Electrophysiologic observations on ventricular tachyarrhythmias following reperfusion. *Am Heart J* 105:210–219, 1983.
134. Pederson DH, et al. Ventricular tachycardia and ventricular fibrillation in a young population. *Circulation* 60:988–997, 1979.
135. Bergdahl DM, et al. Prognosis in primary ventricular tachycardia in the pediatric patient. *Circulation* 62:897–901, 1980.
136. Vetter VL, Josephson ME, Horowitz LN. Idiopathic recurrent sustained ventricular tachycardia in children and adolescents. *Am J Cardiol* 47:315–322, 1981.
137. Rocchini AP, Chun PD, Dick M. Ventricular tachycardia in children. *Am J Cardiol* 47:1091–1097, 1981.
138. Benson DW, et al. Cardiac arrest in young ostensibly healthy patients: Clinical, hemodynamic, and electrophysiologic findings. *Am J Cardiol* 52:65–69, 1983.
139. Morady F, et al. Clinical characteristics and results of electrophysiologic testing in young adults with ventricular tachycardia or ventricular fibrillation. *Am Heart J* 106:1306–1314, 1983.
140. Garson A, et al. Surgical treatment of ventricular tachycardia in infants. *N Engl J Med* 310:1443–1445, 1984.
141. Fulton DR, et al. Ventricular tachycardia in children without heart disease. *Am J Cardiol* 55:1328–1331, 1985.
142. Horowitz LN, et al. Electrophysiologic characteristics of sustained ventricular tachycardia occurring after repair of tetralogy of Fallot. *Am J Cardiol* 46:446–452, 1980.
143. Deanfield J, McKenna W, Rowland E. Local abnormalities of right ventricular depolarization after repair of tetralogy of Fallot: A basis for ventricular arrhythmias. *Am J Cardiol* 55:522–525, 1985.
144. Kavey REW, Blackman MS, Sondheimer HM. Incidence and severity of chronic ventricular dysrhythmias after repair of tetralogy of Fallot. *Am Heart J* 103:342–350, 1982.
145. Garson A, et al. Induction of ventricular tachycardia during electrophysiologic study after repair of tetralogy of Fallot. *J Am Coll Cardiol* 1:1493–1502, 1983.
146. Garson A, et al. Prevention of sudden death after repair of tetralogy of Fallot: Treatment of ventricular arrhythmias. *J Am Coll Cardiol* 6:221–227, 1985.
147. Tamari I, et al. Medical treatment of cardiovascular disorders during pregnancy. *Am Heart J* 104:1357–1362, 1982.
148. Rotmensch HH, Elkayam U, Frishman W. Antiarrhythmic drug therapy during pregnancy. *Ann Intern Med* 98:487–497, 1983.
149. Rotmensch HH, Pines A, Donchin Y. Antiarrhythmic Drugs in Pregnancy. In U Elkayam, N Gleicher (eds), *Cardiac Problems in Pregnancy*. New York: Alan R. Liss, 1990. Pp 361–379.
150. Fisch C, Knoebel SB. Digitalis cardiotoxicity. *J Am Coll Cardiol* 5:91A–98A, 1985.
151. Wenger TL, et al. Treatment of 63 severely digitalis-toxic patients with digoxin-specific antibody fragments. *J Am Coll Cardiol* 5:118A–123A, 1985.
152. Tzivoni D, Keren A. Suppression of ventricular arrhythmias by magnesium. *Am Heart J* 65:1397–1399, 1990.

153. Reid PR, et al. Evaluation of flecainide acetate in the management of patients at high risk of sudden cardiac death. *Am J Cardiol* 53:1088–1118, 1984.
154. Oetgen W, et al. Clinical and electrophysiologic assessment of oral flecainide acetate for recurrent ventricular tachycardia: evidence for exacerbation of electrical instability. *Am J Cardiol* 52:746–750, 1984.
155. Horowitz LN, et al. Torsade de pointes: Electrophysiologic studies in patients without transient pharmacologic or metabolic abnormalities. *Circulation* 63:1120–1128, 1981.
156. Bhandari AK, et al. Electrophysiologic testing in patients with the long QT syndrome. *Circulation* 71:63–71, 1985.
157. Somberg JC, Singh BN (eds). Proceedings of the symposium on QT prolongation: Antiarrhythmic and arrhythmogenic effects. *Am Heart J* 109:395–430, 1985.
158. Schwartz PJ, Stone HL. Left stellectomy in the prevention of ventricular fibrillation caused by acute myocardial ischemia in conscious dogs with anterior myocardial infarction. *Circulation* 62:1256–1265, 1980.
159. Moss AJ, et al. The long QT syndrome: A prospective international study. *Circulation* 71:17–21, 1985.
160. Bhandari AK, et al. Efficacy of left cardiac sympathectomy in the treatment of patients with the long QT syndrome. *Circulation* 70:1018–1023, 1984.
161. Surawicz B, Knoebel SB. Long QT: Good, bad or indifferent? *J Am Coll Cardiol* 4:398–413, 1984.
162. Ahnve S, et al. Prognostic importance of QT interval at discharge after acute myocardial infarction: A multicenter study of 865 patients. *Am Heart J* 108:395–400, 1984.
163. Packer DL, et al. Sudden death after left stellectomy in the long QT syndrome. *Am J Cardiol* 54:1365–1366, 1984.
164. Lewis BH, Antman EM, Graboys TB. Detailed analysis of 24 hour ambulatory electrocardiographic recordings during ventricular fibrillation or torsade de pointes. *J Am Coll Cardiol* 2:426–436, 1983.
165. Kay GN, et al. Torsade de pointes: The long short initiating sequence and other clinical features: Observations in 32 patients. *J Am Coll Cardiol* 2:806–817, 1983.
166. Vlay SC, et al. Documented sudden cardiac death in prolonged QT syndrome. *Arch Intern Med* 144:833–835, 1984.
167. Vincent GM. Hypothesis for the molecular physiology of the Romano-Ward long QT syndrome. *J Am Coll Cardiol* 20:500–503, 1992.
168. Vincent GM, et al. The spectrum of symptoms and QT intervals in carriers of the gene for the long QT syndrome. *N Engl J Med* 327:846–852, 1992.
169. Moss AJ, et al. The long QT syndrome. *Circulation* 84:1136–1144, 1991.
170. Schouten EG, et al. QT interval prolongation predicts cardiovascular mortality in an apparently healthy population. *Circulation* 84:1516–1523, 1991.
171. Schwartz PJ, et al. Left cardiac sympathetic denervation in the therapy of congenital long QT syndrome. *Circulation* 84:503–511, 1991.
172. Moss AJ, et al. Efficacy of permanent pacing in the management of high-risk patients with the long QT syndrome. *Circulation* 84:1524–1529, 1991.
173. Eldar M, et al. Combined use of long-term cardiac pacing for patients with the long QT syndrome. *J Am Coll Cardiol* 20:830–837, 1992.
174. Kutalek SP, et al. Emergent use of intravenous amiodarone for refractory ventricular tachycardia (abstract no. 1094). *Circulation* 72(Suppl III):274, 1985.

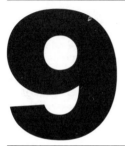

Arrhythmias and Conduction Disturbances in the Acute Phase of Myocardial Infarction

Stephen C. Vlay

Arrhythmias that occur during the acute phase of myocardial infarction (MI) may have a devastating effect on the mortality of patients for whom medical assistance is not readily available. In fact, ventricular fibrillation (VF) is much more common during the first 4 hours of acute MI than in the subsequent 48 hours. This mechanism explains why 30–40% of individuals suffering acute MI may die of VF before they reach the hospital. The proliferation of paramedic teams and public education programs about CPR has resulted in salvage of lives, but the losses remain alarmingly high. Since life-threatening arrhythmias often occur without warning, the efficacy and desirability of prophylactic treatment has been a hotly debated issue.

I. Prognostic implications of arrhythmias

A. **Ventricular arrhythmias occurring early in the myocardial infarction.** Ventricular tachycardia (VT) or VF occurring in the presence of acute MI has a different prognosis from VT or VF in the absence of acute MI. In the latter situation, the anatomic substrate remains unchanged and the patient remains at risk of recurrent cardiac arrest unless a successful intervention is found. In acute MI, the irritable focus or tachycardia zone may be involved in the scarring process related to the infarction. Thus, the anatomic substrate is altered and the irritable focus possibly extirpated. Consequently the teaching has been that patients who survive VT or VF in the first 24–72 hours of MI have no greater risk of recurrent malignant tachyarrhythmias than those who do not manifest those arrhythmias during this period. One study suggested that patients with anterior wall MI who suffered VT or VF in the first 72 hours had a higher risk of sudden cardiac arrest within the next year than patients with this event in inferior wall MI [1]. It is unclear whether the poorer prognosis is related to the initial arrhythmias or due to extensive substrate damage, which results in greater vulnerability.

Another point that requires differentiation is whether VF resulted **from** or resulted **in** acute MI, as the two may have different prognostic importance. Consider the situation in which ventricular irritability is the initiating factor. Associated hypotension may cause extensive myocardial necrosis, possibly in a distribution far from the irritable focus. This patient may remain at high risk of recurrence. Clearly this is a different situation from myocardial injury resulting in irritability in the infarct zone, which results in eventual scarring of the irritable focus. These distinctions may be difficult to make and may partially explain differences in survival data. Generalizations may not be applicable to individual patients.

A distinction must also be made between primary and secondary VF. **Secondary ventricular fibrillation** refers to the situation in which the arrhythmia occurs secondary to another event or precipitating factor such as cardiogenic shock or possibly metabolic or electrolyte disturbance. **Primary ventricular fibrillation** occurs in the absence of these causes.

B. **Ventricular arrhythmias occurring in the convalescent phase of myocardial infarction.** In contrast to arrhythmias occurring in the initial phase of MI, complex and frequent ventricular ectopy occurring in the convalescent phase of MI is associated with a less favorable prognosis. The Ruberman studies analyzed the clinical outcomes of 1739 male survivors of acute MI by a 5-year follow-up [2]. Patients with runs of two or more consecutive ventricular premature beats or the R-on-T phenomenon had a higher risk of sudden cardiac death (SCD) than those with other complex ectopy. All forms of complex ectopy had a higher incidence of nonsudden cardiac death than simple or no ectopy. A number of other studies have also documented the higher risk of SCD in survivors of MI with complex ectopy on the ECG. In Vismara's study, complex arrhythmias noted after discharge from the coronary care unit (CCU) distinguished the group at high risk for SCD, while early arrhythmias did not [3]. In addition, the absence of ectopy in the acute phase did not exclude its appearance during convalescence. The work of Schulze et al. indicated that survivors of MI with complex arrhythmias in the convalescent phase had more extensive cardiac dysfunction, manifest by lower ejection fraction, high creatine kinase levels, a greater number of proximally narrowed major coronary arteries, more prior MIs, and more abnormalities of regional left ventricular contraction [4]. Bigger et al. described a higher incidence of SCD in patients with VT 2 weeks after MI [5].

Thus, complex ventricular ectopy, particularly VT, in the convalescent phase of MI places the survivor at higher risk of subsequent SCD. Nevertheless, no study has yet demonstrated improvement in survival with antiarrhythmic drug treatment of patients with asymptomatic complex ectopy. The Cardiac Arrhythmia Suppression Trial study has validated this statement.

C. **Supraventricular arrhythmias after myocardial infarction.** Supraventricular arrhythmias that occur after MI are usually not life threatening. Certainly the overall efficiency of cardiac function may be impaired, and occasionally there may be hemodynamic embarrassment. The majority of supraventricular tachyarrhythmias are tolerated. Nevertheless, they usually reflect serious cardiac dysfunction and an impaired cardiovascular reserve.

The arrhythmias most commonly seen are sinus tachycardia, atrial fibrillation, and atrial flutter. Treatment must be directed not only at the arrhythmia but also at improving cardiac efficiency. Usually these patients have impaired ventricular contractility and manifest congestive heart failure. Depending on the individual situation, diuretics, vasodilators, angiotensin converting enzyme (ACE) inhibitors, or inotropic agents may be necessary.

II. Prophylaxis and treatment of arrhythmias
A. Ventricular tachycardia and ventricular fibrillation
1. **Prophylactic therapy.** Of the variety of studies performed regarding the efficacy of prophylactic therapy, only a few have demonstrated benefit. The first question asked is, Why treat if the patient is in sinus rhythm and asymptomatic [6]? Quite often patients with acute MI may suddenly demonstrate VT or VF without warning arrhythmias. A warning arrhythmia might be described as a low-grade or complex ventricular ectopy that is nonsustained and presages a malignant ventricular tachyarrhythmia that results in cardiovascular collapse. Not all warning arrhythmias may be observed, even in the CCU. Ventricular tachycardia or VF that occurs in the CCU usually can be successfully treated, but it often requires formal resuscitative efforts. It would be preferable if this situation could be avoided, thus reducing the morbidity, although the mortality is unchanged. Prophylaxis may be more important in terms of mortality in the prehospital setting, when the facilities and personnel available may be more limited. The risk-benefit ratio of prophylactic intervention must be weighed.

The study of Lie et al. indicated a benefit when patients received lidocaine prophylactically outside the hospital [7]. Similar conclusions were drawn by the Valentine et al. study [8]; however, it was somewhat clouded by design flaws. A number of other studies, however, failed to demonstrate benefit and asserted that prophylactic administration could be associated with hypotension and other side effects [9, 10]. The Netherlands study [11] and editorial commentary by Lown [12] shed new light on the controversy. Not only did the group receiving prophylactic lidocaine have improved outcome with fewer episodes of VF, but the benefit started after the administration of the drug. Before the drug, the incidence of VF was the same in each group, indicating that no bias entered by patient selection.

The effects of prophylactic antiarrhythmic drug therapy in acute MI were assessed by meta analysis from 138 trials on 98,000 patients [13]. The routine use of type 1 agents was associated with increased mortality. Mortality was reduced by type 2 agents (beta blockers). Amiodarone seemed to have a favorable effect, but the analysis was limited by the number of subjects. The data from calcium blockers did not appear to be promising [13].

If there is any benefit at all from the prophylactic administration of lidocaine to patients with suspected MI, it occurs in the first 2 hours of MI, the period of greatest vulnerability, and requires administration by paramedic personnel before transportation to the hospital. If this therapy is adopted, drugs are administered **most safely** in the **presence of cardiac monitoring.** The recommended dose is lidocaine 50–100 mg intravenously (IV), depending on the body weight.

After the first 4 hours, the incidence of VF diminishes, and the clinician must again consider the risk-benefit ratio. Lidocaine can be a toxic drug, particularly in elderly patients and those with heart failure or liver dysfunction. Antman and Berlin noted a decrease in the incidence of VF during acute MI [14]. Patients with acute MI are now likely to receive beta blockers and have aggressive correction of hypokalemia. Statistically, Antman and Berlin calculated that 400 patients would have to be treated prophylactically to prevent one episode of VF. These authors proposed the reduction of prophylactic lidocaine for patients with acute MI and also for those admitted as "rule-out" MI. When lidocaine is used, it should be for limited duration, since the majority of ventricular arrhythmias occur in the first 6–12 hours. In fact, this last point may explain differences in survival studies. Patients with acute MI who are admitted are already survivors. Many of the patients with early VF die before reaching the emergency room, presenting a preselection bias. Those who make it to the hospital are less likely to have malignant ventricular arrhythmias.

Part of the decision regarding the institution of prophylactic lidocaine therapy for the first 6–24 hours reflects a personal bias on the part of the physician. At University Hospital at Stony Brook, we have changed our bias. We no longer recommend prophylactic lidocaine due to the low risk of VF, the potential toxicity of lidocaine, and the unfavorable risk-benefit ratio. If a patient has a cardiac arrest, resuscitation from VT or VF in the CCU is usually successful, although morbidity from CPR, intubation, and electrical countershock is possible.

2. **Active therapy.** When a patient actively manifests complex symptomatic or asymptomatic arrhythmias, the treatment is the same as described for VT and VF (Chaps. 2 and 8). If the patient is hemodynamically compromised, cardioversion or defibrillation is the treatment of choice. Lidocaine is the drug of first choice for VT. A committee of the American College of Cardiology (ACC) and American Heart Association (AHA) provided recommendations for the use of lidocaine in acute MI [15]:

   Type I (general agreement that it is usually indicated, always acceptable, and considered useful/effective). Indications for lidocaine include patients with acute myocardial ischemia or infarction, or both, with frequent ventricular premature beats that are greater than 6/minute, R-on-T, multiform, or occurring in salvos of three or more; sustained VT or VF.
   Type IIa (controversial but acceptable, weight of evidence in favor of usefulness/efficacy). Indications for lidocaine include the arrhythmias described for type I in patients with suspected myocardial infarction or ischemia or both.
   Type IIb (controversial but acceptable, not well established by evidence, can be helpful and probably not harmful). Indications include prophylactic administration in the presence of uncomplicated acute myocardial ischemia or infarction or both, without ventricular ectopy in patients less than 70 years old and within the first 6 hours of onset of symptoms.
   Type III (not indicated, may be harmful). Indications include patients with proven allergy or hypersensitivity to lidocaine.

These recommendations were made in 1990. There would be little disagreement among cardiologists about administering lidocaine for nonsustained VT in acute MI, but many might disagree about lidocaine for 6 VPBs/hour in acute myocardial ischemia. Therapy should be individualized.

The usual dose recommendations [16] are an initial bolus of 50–100 mg, followed 15 minutes later with a second bolus of 50 mg [17, 18] to maintain blood levels, and then continuing with a 2-mg/minute constant infusion with titration upward to 4 mg/minute as necessary to treat symptomatic episodes. The ACC/AHA Task Force Committee was more specific:

   Initial IV bolus: 1 mg/kg, not to exceed 100 mg.
   Additional boluses: Administer 0.5 mg/kg q8–10min if necessary, to a maximal dose of 4 mg/kg.
   Maintenance dose: 20–50 µg/kg/minute.

Treatment of patients at higher risk of complications from lidocaine must be individualized and may require a lower-dose infusion.

Note that doses of 4 mg/minute are probably necessary for antifibrillatory effects but are associated with a higher risk of toxicity. When discontinuing lidocaine, there is no necessity to taper the rate of infusion [19]. Discontinuation of the infusion results in an automatic tapering of the plasma level due to tissue levels of the drug. The levels decrease exponentially, obeying first-order kinetics. Minimum effective levels are reached after 4½ hours. The use of beta blockers such as metoprolol in the acute phase of MI may elevate the VF threshold and further decrease the chance of VF.

If lidocaine is unsuccessful, procainamide should be added. An alternative drug is bretylium, particularly if the patient has VF. However, the potential hypotensive effects must be appreciated and dealt with. An additional infusion of phenylephrine may be necessary to maintain the BP while the bretylium administration continues.

The treatment of patients with intractable VT and VF, described by some as "electrical storm," presents the most severe challenge to the cardiologist. Treatment often is unsuccessful despite the administration of multiple antiarrhythmic drugs, electrical cardioversions or defibrillations, overdrive pacing, or even more invasive modalities. The administration of additional investigational antiarrhythmic drugs in this situation requires considerable thought and extreme caution. Of major concern is the potential proarrhythmic effect of multiple drugs in combination. An unfavorable outcome may also be unfairly attributed to the investigational agent even though multiple factors may be contributory. Until a clear course of action can be recommended with more certainty for this unfortunate complication of electrical storm, the care of the individual patient must be guided by clinical judgment. There is some suggestive evidence that IV amiodarone may have some utility in this situation, but as yet this still remains investigational.

3. **The use of magnesium in acute myocardial infarction.** While the importance of abnormalities of serum potassium has long been appreciated, the role of magnesium in arrhythmias has only recently been recognized [20–32]. The value of magnesium therapy for torsades de pointes and polymorphic VT is well documented. While hypomagnesemia is detrimental in acute MI, the value of prophylactic administration of magnesium for all patients remains uncertain.

Hypomagnesemia occurs with nutritional deficiency (including alcoholism), malabsorption, renal disease, drug therapy (particularly diuretics, some antimicrobials, cyclosporine, antineoplastic agents), and metabolic disorders.

Magnesium slows sinus node recovery time (SNRT) and prolongs atrioventricular (AV) nodal conduction. It does not interact with the fast sodium–mediated channel or the slow calcium–mediated channel but instead has a direct effect on potassium channels [20]. It may be effective for supraventricular tachycardia (SVT) [21]. Magnesium also has effects on contractility (influencing intracellular calcium influx through the sarcolemma, competing with calcium binding, and modulating cyclic adenosine monophosphate) [28].

Epidemiologic studies have demonstrated a relationship between magnesium deficiency and sudden death [22]. Magnesium deficiency may result in this outcome, particularly when the patient is hypokalemic [25, 30].

Some individual and metaanalyses have suggested a benefit from the prophylactic administration of magnesium to patients admitted with acute MI [24, 28, 32]. Nevertheless, Ott and Fenster [26] observed that although the incidence of arrhythmias was reduced, it was not associated with decreased morbidity or mortality. They warned that routine use of magnesium supplementation for patients with acute MI was safe but of unproved value. Preliminary reports of ISIS-4 did not find a benefit from 24 hours of IV magnesium [33].

Consequently, it is recommended that magnesium deficiency be identified and corrected. However, routine prophylactic use of magnesium may not be beneficial.

B. **Supraventricular tachycardia.** Prophylactic therapy for supraventricular tachyarrhythmias is not recommended. Quite often a patient will have received a beta blocker for the acute phase of MI, which is standard therapy in many hospitals if there are no specific contraindications. The presence of beta blockade may decrease the incidence of atrial arrhythmias.

If a patient develops any of the supraventricular arrhythmias during acute MI, he or she should be treated as described in Chap. 6. If the patient is hemodynamically compromised, prompt electrical cardioversion is indicated. Digoxin is one of the drugs of choice for atrial fibrillation and atrial flutter. Adenosine is now the drug of choice for paroxysmal supraventricular tachycardia resulting from AV nodal reentry. In some cases, overdrive pacing may be preferable to drug therapy or if cardioversion is not desirable because of excessive digoxin loading.

III. **Treatment of conduction disturbances in acute myocardial infarction.** Conduction disturbances may occur in acute MI. They may be divided into three categories: those not requiring intervention, those definitely requiring pacemaker therapy, and those in which pacemaker insertion remains controversial (Table 9-1). A task force of the ACC and AHA on Assessment of Diagnostic and Therapeutic Cardiovascular Procedures provided guidelines for the early management of patients with acute MI [15], in which they addressed the issue of temporary pacing. Indications were graded as follows:

Type I: Usually indicated, always acceptable, and considered useful/effective.
Type II: Acceptable, of uncertain efficacy, and may be controversial. *a* = weight of evidence in favor of usefulness/efficacy, *b* = not well established by evidence, can be helpful and probably not harmful.
Type III: Not indicated, may be harmful.

A. **Historical overview.** Atkins et al. reviewed the outcome of 77 cases of ventricular conduction defects in the presence of acute MI [34]. Complete heart block developed in 43% with right bundle branch block (RBBB). Late sudden death occurred in five of six with RBBB and left axis deviation with transient complete heart block during MI, whereas eight similar patients with complete heart block and permanent pacing were alive.

The Duke study pooled data from five centers [35]. In 432 patients, the most common conduction disturbances were left bundle branch block (LBBB) (38%) and RBBB with left anterior fascicular block (LAFB) (34%). Progression to second- or third-degree AV block occurred in 22%. Both the hospital and first-year mortality rates were 28%. Increased hospital mortality was observed in patients who progressed to high-degree AV block (47%).

After discharge, patients not continuously paced had a higher incidence of sudden death or recurrent high-degree AV block (65%) than patients continuously paced. It was recommended that patients at high risk of high-degree AV block receive prophylactic temporary pacing. These groups include those with RBBB and LAFB, RBBB

Table 9-1. Treatment of conduction disturbances during acute myocardial infarction

Pacemaker therapy not required
Asymptomatic bradycardia
First-degree AV block
Second-degree AV block (Wenckebach, Mobitz type I)
Preexistent bifascicular block
Accelerated idioventricular rhythm causing AV dissociation

Pacemaker therapy required
Asystole
Symptomatic bradyarrhythmias without escape rhythm
Second-degree AV Block (Mobitz type II)
Third-degree (complete) AV block
New RBBB + LAFB
New RBBB + LPFB
New LBBB
Alternating bundle branch block

Pacemaker therapy controversial
Second-degree AV Block (Wenckebach, Mobitz type I) with hypotension not responsive to atropine
Sinus bradycardia or sinus pauses not responsive to atropine
Atrial or ventricular overdrive pacing for incessant ventricular tachycardia
Bifascicular block of unknown duration
LBBB + first-degree AV block of unknown duration

AV = atrioventricular; RBBB = right bundle branch block; LAFB = left anterior fascicular block; LPFB = left posterior fascicular block; LBBB = left bundle branch block.

and left posterior fascicular block (LPFB), or alternating bundle branch block. Patients with isolated RBBB or LBBB are thought to be at lower risk. P–R prolongation in some studies seems to increase the risk of high-degree AV block.

It is important to note that the high mortality is related to left ventricular pump failure, with temporary pacing not affecting survival. Sudden cardiac death may be due to VT or VF. Nevertheless, patients who survive high-degree AV block should receive permanent pacemakers. Patients with conduction disturbances but without high-degree AV block do not benefit from permanent pacing. There is some suggestion that some of these patients with extensive anterior wall myocardial necrosis may benefit from permanent pacing, but this was not conclusively demonstrated.

Fisch et al. reviewed the literature extensively [36]. They recommended prophylactic pacing in acute MI with bifascicular conduction disturbances in those with alternating RBBB and LBBB, RBBB and LAFB, RBBB and LPFB, and LBBB and P–R prolongation. They also considered acute anterior wall MI with either RBBB or LBBB as an indication for prophylactic pacing, although they admitted it was controversial. The risk of pacemaker insertion must be accounted for. Preexistent RBBB or LBBB was not an indication for prophylactic pacing.

Hollander et al. studied 47 patients who were admitted with bundle branch block and acute MI [37]. They noted a high risk of progression to high-degree AV block if the patient had compromise of the left anterior descending artery (resulting in anterior wall MI) and preexisting bifascicular block or LBBB. Prophylactic pacing was recommended. Hauer et al. found that prophylactic pacing did not affect prognosis in patients with bundle branch block complicating acute anteroseptal MI [38].

Klein et al. reviewed the incidence of progression to complete heart block in patients with acute MI and bifascicular block: isolated RBBB, 23%; RBBB and LAFB, 31%; LBBB, 16% [39]. In addition, the presence of Mobitz type II AV block almost guarantees the ultimate development of complete heart block. Mortality varied: isolated RBBB, 44%; RBBB and LAFB, 38%; RBBB and LPFB, 48%; LBBB, 29%. To some extent these mortality data are dependent on the coronary blood supply to the conduction system. Klein et al. recommended temporary pacing for patients with acute MI and acute onset of RBBB and LAFB, RBBB and LPFB, or alternating bundle branch block, regardless of the P–R interval. Pacing was not recommended for first-degree AV block, new RBBB or LBBB, or preexistent bifascicular block with a normal P–R interval.

Permanent pacing was recommended for patients with bifascicular block with transient high-grade (Mobitz type II or complete) heart block, and possibly bifascicular block with prolonged H–V intervals. Watson et al. reported the Birmingham experience of permanent pacing after MI [40]. There was no significant difference in those paced and those followed medically. Progression of the conduction disorder was not observed, and the H–V interval did not predict outcome. Ventricular tachycardia or VF was an important cause of death.

B. **Current recommendations. (See Table 9-1.)**
   1. **Pacemaker therapy not required.** Patients with inferior wall MI are more likely to have bradycardia than those with anterior wall MI. If beta-blocker therapy is administered in the acute phase of MI, bradycardia may be present regardless of the location of the infarct. If the patient is hemodynamically stable—no evidence of hypotension, diminished perfusion of vital organs, or heart failure owing to bradycardia—no therapy is necessary. If the patient is symptomatic, the physician may elect to try atropine sulfate first. However, this means of therapy provides only a temporary solution and may lead to an unwanted tachycardia. Certainly, in severe compromise, atropine sulfate should be administered and pacing instituted later. If time permits, temporary pacing should be accomplished relatively rapidly, by an external or an invasive mode.

   If the patient is stable and the rhythm is sinus bradycardia of more than 40–45 beats/minute, no therapy is necessary, and the patient should be monitored. Certain logistic considerations also apply. If the patient is in a university hospital where assistance from residents and fellows is rapidly available, or if a temporary external pacemaker is present in the CCU, the patient can be observed. If the patient is in a smaller community hospital, if ancillary personnel and devices are unavailable, or if the physician resides a considerable distance from the hospital, it may not be unreasonable to insert a temporary transvenous pacemaker if the patient has a heart rate lower than 40–45 beats/minute. Certainly the ability to pace with an external pacemaker may limit the need for invasive procedures and their potential complications.

First-degree AV block and second-degree AV block of the Wenckebach variety usually represent a problem at the AV node but not the distal conduction system (see Chap. 6). Unless the patient is symptomatic, treatment is unnecessary. Patients with anterior wall MI and Wenckebach block should be carefully monitored for progression.

The ACC/AHA Task Force Committee recognizes **type III indications** as first-degree AV block; type I second-degree (Wenckebach) AV block with normal hemodynamics; accelerated idioventricular rhythm causing AV dissociation; and pre-existing bundle branch block.

2. **Pacemaker therapy required.** Any symptomatic bradyarrhythmias causing hemodynamic compromise require temporary pacing. High-degree AV block, either Mobitz type II second-degree AV block or complete heart block (third-degree AV block), requires temporary pacing, particularly if associated with anterior wall MI. It is not mandatory to pace these conduction disturbances in an asymptomatic patient with inferior wall MI. Logistic considerations as described for asymptomatic bradyarrhythmias apply nevertheless. With Mobitz type II, there is a very high chance of progressing to complete heart block, and disease of the distal conduction system must be suspected. Patients with new impairment of the fascicular system (i.e., the bundle branches) deserve temporary pacing if certain conditions are met. There is no need to insert a pacemaker if the bundle branch block is preexistent. There is complete agreement that temporary pacing is indicated if the patient has a new RBBB and either LAFB or left posterior fascicular block. In fact, left posterior fascicular block, if caused by coronary artery disease, implies worse disease and a poorer prognosis since its dual blood supply, derived from both the anterior and posterior descending arteries, is compromised (see Chaps. 2 and 6). Patients with LBBB and first-degree AV block are similarly at high risk and deserve pacing.

The ACC/AHA Task Force Committee recognizes the following as **type I** indications: asystole; complete heart block; new RBBB plus LAFB or LPFB; new LBBB; type II second-degree (Mobitz II) AV block; and symptomatic bradycardia not responsive to atropine.

3. **Pacemaker therapy controversial.** Whereas prophylactic pacemaker therapy for bifascicular block is accepted, temporary pacing if the patient has an LBBB with first-degree AV block of unknown duration is controversial. Some physicians wish to be cautious. A major point should be considered with LBBB. Insertion of a temporary pacemaker or Swan-Ganz pulmonary artery monitoring catheter may cause a transient RBBB by mechanical trauma. In the presence of LBBB, complete heart block may occur. Although creation of new RBBB is more likely to occur with the novice operator, it can nevertheless occur when performed by an experienced clinician. He or she should be able to deal with consequences quickly, manipulating the pacing electrode to a position of capture and avoiding hemodynamic embarrassment.

The ACC/AHA Task Force Committee recognizes the following as **type IIa** indications: type I second-degree AV block with hypotension not responsive to atropine; sinus bradycardia not responsive to atropine; recurrent sinus pauses not responsive to atropine; and atrial or ventricular overdrive pacing for incessant ventricular tachycardia. **Type IIb** indications include: LBBB plus first-degree AV block of unknown duration; and bifascicular block of unknown duration.

C. **Indications for permanent pacemaker insertion after myocardial infarction.** Indications for inserting permanent pacemakers are covered in detail in Chap. 17. Guidelines for permanent pacing after MI have been set by a Task Force on Assessment of Diagnostic and Therapeutic Cardiovascular Procedures (Committee on Pacemaker Implantation) of the ACC and the AHA [41]. A requirement for temporary pacing during acute MI is no longer considered to constitute an indication for permanent pacing. Mortality is related to the extent of myocardial necrosis as well as the specific nature of the conduction disturbance. **Type I** (general agreement that implantation should be performed) indications include persistent high-degree AV block or complete heart block with block in the His-Purkinje system. Transient advanced AV block and associated bundle branch block also merit permanent pacing. **Type II** (implantation is frequently performed, but divergence of opinion exists regarding the necessity) indications include patients with persistent advanced block at the AV node. (Certainly the presence or absence of symptoms at the heart rate will be important in this decision.) **Type III** (general agreement that a permanent pacemaker is unnecessary) indications include transient AV conduction disturbances in the absence of intraventricular conduction defects; transient AV block in the presence of isolated LAFB; acquired LAFB in the absence of AV block; and persistent first-degree AV block in the presence of bundle branch block not demonstrated previously. It is important to remember that permanent pacing may not prevent sudden cardiac arrest, since these patients may die from VT and VF, not from progression to complete heart block.

References

1. Schwartz PJ, Zaza A, Grazi S. Effect of ventricular fibrillation complicating acute myocardial infarction on long term prognosis: Importance of the site of infarction. *Am J Cardiol* 56:384–389, 1985.
2. Ruberman W, et al. Repeated one-hour electrocardiographic monitoring of survivors of myocardial infarction at six-month intervals: Arrhythmia detection and relation to prognosis. *Am J Cardiol* 47:1197–1204, 1981.
3. Vismara LA, Amsterdam EA, Mason DT. Relation of ventricular arrhythmias in the late hospital phase of acute myocardial infarction to sudden death after hospital discharge. *Am J Med* 59:6–12, 1975.
4. Schulze RA, Strauss HW, Pitt B. Sudden death in the year following myocardial infarction. *Am J Med* 62:192–199, 1977.
5. Bigger JT, Weld FM, Rolnitzky LM. Prevalence, characteristics and significance of ventricular tachycardia (three or more complexes) detected with ambulatory electrocardiographic recording in the late hospital phase of acute myocardial infarction. *Am J Cardiol* 48:815–823, 1981.
6. Harrison DC. Should lidocaine be administered routinely to all patients after acute myocardial infarction? *Circulation* 58:581–584, 1978.
7. Lie KI, et al. Lidocaine in the prevention of primary ventricular fibrillation. *N Engl J Med* 291:1324–1326, 1974.
8. Valentine PA, et al. Lidocaine in the prevention of sudden death in the pre-hospital phase of acute infarction: A double blind study. *N Engl J Med* 291:1327–1331, 1974.
9. Lie KI, et al. Efficacy of lidocaine in preventing primary ventricular fibrillation within one hour after a 300 mg intramuscular injection. *Am J Cardiol* 42:486–488, 1978.
10. Dunn HM, et al. Prophylactic lidocaine in the early stage of suspected myocardial infarction. *Am Heart J* 110:353–362, 1985.
11. Koster RW, Dunning AJ. Intramuscular lidocaine for prevention of lethal arrhythmias in the prehospitalization phase of acute myocardial infarction. *N Engl J Med* 313:1105–1110, 1985.
12. Lown B. Lidocaine to prevent ventricular fibrillation. *N Engl J Med* 313:1154–1155, 1985.
13. Teo KK, Yusuf S, Furberg CD. Effects of prophylactic antiarrhythmic drug therapy in acute myocardial infarction. *JAMA* 270:1589–1595, 1993.
14. Antman EM, Berlin JA. Declining incidence of ventricular fibrillation in myocardial infarction. *Circulation* 86:764–773, 1992.
15. Gunnar RM, et al. Guideline for the early management of patients with acute myocardial infarction. *J Am Coll Cardiol* 16:249–292, 1990.
16. Ribner HS, Frishman WH. Prophylactic lidocaine therapy in acute myocardial infarction. *Cardiovasc Rev Rep* 2:395–401, 1981.
17. Wyman MG, et al. Multiple bolus technique for lidocaine administration during the first hours of an acute myocardial infarction. *Am J Cardiol* 41:313–317, 1978.
18. Wyman MG, et al. Multiple bolus technique for lidocaine administration in acute ischemic heart disease. *JACC* 2:764–769, 1983.
19. Reid PR. Lidocaine: To taper or not to taper. *J Clin Pharmacol* 16:162–164, 1976.
20. DiCarlo LA, et al. Effects of magnesium sulfate on cardiac conduction and refractoriness in humans. *J Am Coll Cardiol* 7:1356–1362, 1986.
21. Gullestad L, et al. The effect of magnesium versus verapamil on supraventricular arrhythmias. *Clin Cardiol* 16:429–434, 1993.
22. Eisenberg MJ. Magnesium deficiency and sudden death. *Am Heart J* 124:544–549, 1992.
23. Hilton TC, et al. Electrophysiologic and antiarrhythmic effects of magnesium in patients with inducible ventricular tachyarrhythmia. *Clin Cardiol* 15:176–180, 1992.
24. Horner SM. Efficacy of intravenous magnesium in acute myocardial infarction in reducing arrhythmias and mortality. *Circulation* 86:774–779, 1992.

25. Millane TA, Ward DE, Camm AJ. Is hypomagnesemia arrhythmogenic? *Clin Cardiol* 15:103–108, 1992.
26. Ott P, Fenster P. Should magnesium be part of the routine therapy for acute myocardial infarction? *Am Heart J* 124:1113–1118, 1992.
27. Perticone F, Adinolfi L, Bonaduce D. Efficacy of magnesium sulfate in the treatment of torsade de pointes. *Am Heart J* 112:847–849, 1986.
28. Reinhart RA. Clinical correlates of the molecular and cellular actions of magnesium on the cardiovascular system. *Am Heart J* 121:1513–1522, 1991.
29. Schecter M, et al. Beneficial effect of magnesium sulfate in acute myocardial infarction. *Am J Cardiol* 66:271–274, 1990.
30. Surawicz B. Is hypomagnesemia or magnesium deficiency arrhythmogenic? *J Am Coll Cardiol* 14:1093–1096, 1989.
31. Tzivoni D, Keren A. Suppression of ventricular arrhythmias by magnesium. *Am J Cardiol* 65:1397–1399, 1990.
32. Yusuf S, Teo K, Woods K. Intravenous magnesium in acute myocardial infarction: An effective, safe, simple, and inexpensive intervention. *Circulation* 87:2043–2046, 1993.
33. ISIS-4 (Fourth International Study of Infarct Survival Collaborative Group). ISIS-4: A randomized factorial trial assessing early oral captopril, oral mononitrate, and intravenous magnesium sulphate in 58,050 patients with suspected acute myocardial infarction. *Lancet* 345: 669–685, 1995.
34. Atkins JM, et al. Ventricular conduction blocks and sudden death in acute myocardial infarction: Potential indications for pacing. *N Engl J Med* 288:281–284, 1973.
35. Hindman MC, et al. The clinical significance of bundle branch block complicating acute myocardial infarction: 1. Clinical characteristics, hospital mortality and one year follow-up. 2. Indications for temporary and permanent pacemaker insertion. *Circulation* 58:679–699, 1978.
36. Fisch GR, Zipes DP, Fisch C. Bundle branch block and sudden death. *Prog Cardiovasc Dis* 23:187–224, 1980.
37. Hollander G, et al. Bundle branch block in acute myocardial infarction. *Am Heart J* 105:738–743, 1983.
38. Hauer RNW, et al. Long term prognosis in patients with bundle branch block complicating acute anteroseptal infarction. *Am J Cardiol* 49:1581–1585, 1982.
39. Klein RC, Vera Z, Mason DT. Intraventricular conduction defects in acute myocardial infarction: Incidence, prognosis and therapy. *Am Heart J* 108:1007–1013, 1984.
40. Watson RDS, Glover DR, Page AJF. The Birmingham trial of permanent pacing in patients with intraventricular conduction disorders after acute myocardial infarction. *Am Heart J* 108:496–501, 1984.
41. Committee on Pacemaker Implantation of the ACC and AHA. Task force on assessment of diagnostic and therapeutic cardiovascular procedures. Dreifus LS, et al. Guidelines for implantation of cardiac pacemakers and antiarrhythmia devices. *J Am Coll Cardiol* 18:1–13, 1991.

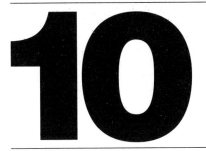

Noninvasive Evaluation of the Patient with Cardiac Arrhythmia

Anne H. Dougherty and
Gerald V. Naccarelli

Pretreatment evaluation of patients with known or suspected arrhythmias is aimed at identification of the specific clinical arrhythmia, evaluation of underlying cardiovascular disease, and risk stratification. Electrocardiographic documentation of the arrhythmia is essential prior to deciding whether specific treatment is indicated; furthermore, identification of its mechanism allows the physician to target antiarrhythmic therapy more precisely. Once an arrhythmia is identified, it is particularly useful to confirm its temporal association with clinical symptoms, especially in the case of benign or potentially lethal arrhythmias, since that relationship may influence the decision to treat. When antiarrhythmic treatment is warranted, baseline markers (i.e., positive tests) of that individual's susceptibility to the arrhythmia can be identified and used serially with subsequent therapies to assess efficacy. For example, the reproducible presence of nonsustained ventricular tachycardia (VT) on Holter monitoring can be used as a marker for infrequent sustained VT. In that example, repeat Holters are obtained once therapeutic antiarrhythmic drug levels are achieved and compared to the pretreatment Holter. Suppression of the marker on the drug can be used as an end point for therapy, predicting long-term benefit.

Identification of underlying structural heart disease and metabolic factors is also an important goal in patient evaluation. Congestive heart failure, electrolyte imbalances, and other potentially reversible causes for the arrhythmia should be addressed early. The presence of these factors also predicts suitability of many treatment options. Patients with severe ventricular dysfunction are not candidates for antiarrhythmic agents with pronounced negative inotropic effect and similarly may not be eligible for certain surgical procedures.

Noninvasive determination of the risk of sudden cardiac death helps the physician to select the appropriate level of aggressiveness in management. The worst clinical arrhythmia for that individual is identified. Then the anatomic substrate for the arrhythmia is defined to predict the likelihood of more serious arrhythmias in the future. Left ventricular dysfunction, potential areas of ventricular reentry, and autonomic nervous system imbalance each increases the risk of lethal arrhythmias [1].

Methods for achieving these three objectives are discussed in this chapter. Several of the procedures described serve more than one purpose.

I. **Twelve-lead electrocardiogram.** The 12-lead ECG is an essential tool in evaluating arrhythmias. Although unlikely to document fleeting arrhythmias in its 10-second duration, it can occasionally capture longer-lasting arrhythmias. The three-dimensional picture of cardiac electrical activity provides more information than either single- or two-channel recordings about the atrioventricular (AV) relationship, activation sequence of the atria, and QRS morphology, thus facilitating identification of the arrhythmia mechanism.

The ECG is also used to screen for organic heart disease, such as coronary disease, ventricular hypertrophy, or atrial enlargement. Their presence may suggest a substrate for arrhythmias, such as previous myocardial infarction (MI) or ventricular aneurysm, prolonged Q–T interval [2], or hypertrophic obstructive cardiomyopathy. A snapshot of conduction system abnormalities may suggest the potential for serious bradyarrhythmias. The therapeutic and toxic effects of cardioactive drugs and other treatments may be measured electrocardiographically when baseline tracings are available.

Computer-based ECG interpretation is now widely accepted and utilized. Compared to interpretation by cardiologists, computer algorithms are somewhat less reliable; however, individual programs vary widely in their accuracy. Thus, we recommend over-reading of computer-read tracings by trained cardiologists.

Table 10-1. Relationship between duration of monitoring and detection of premature ventricular complexes

Type of monitoring	Duration	% with premature ventricular complexes
12-lead ECG	1 min	10–14
Trendscription	30 min	40
Exercise stress test	15–20 min	56
Holter	24 h	85–88

Source: Adapted from B Lown, Cardiovascular collapse and sudden cardiac death. In E Braunwald (ed), *Heart Disease: A Textbook of Cardiovascular Medicine* (2nd ed). Philadelphia: Saunders, 1984.

II. **Long-term electrocardiographic recordings.** Ambulatory ECG recording for documentation of arrhythmias has had widespread application as a noninvasive tool in cardiology. As shown in Table 10-1, longer monitoring periods (trendscription, stress testing, and Holter monitoring) increase the likelihood of arrhythmia detection.

Since its original description by Holter in the 1950s, Holter monitoring has been the most widely used for this purpose. Lightweight (less than 1 kg), battery-powered ECG recorders are worn continuously for 24 or more hours during routine activity. They may be either cassette or reel-to-reel devices attached to a belt or shoulder strap. An internal clock, a patient diary of activity and symptoms, and a manual symptom-indicator button are used to establish the temporal relationship between ECG events and symptoms. Negative correlations between the two are as useful as positive correlations in managing patients [3].

Two-lead systems are more sensitive than single-lead systems in documenting aberrancy and ST-segment abnormalities and more accurate in screening out artifactual abnormalities (Fig. 10-1). The second channel can also be used to record simultaneous atrial activity in patients with arrhythmias that are difficult to interpret. This can be performed by having the patient swallow an esophageal pill electrode to record atrial activity on the second channel. The AV relationship during the arrhythmia, especially at the onset and termination, and during any changes in rate, frequently establishes the correct diagnosis.

Placement of the electrodes for Holter monitoring must be done properly in order to prevent inadvertent disconnection of leads. The skin is prepared by shaving and cleansing in order to minimize artifact. Impedance is measured with a 10-Hz signal and should be less than 5000 ohms. Modifications of leads V_1 and V_5 are most commonly used [4]. The modified V_1 lead reliably yields recognizable P waves and is helpful in differentiating right from left bundle branch block (Fig. 10-2). When ST-segment analysis is conducted, the leads are selected on the basis of the coronary artery suspected to be affected.

Recorded data are electronically scanned and automatically analyzed on a computer-based system with minimal quantitative error. The different types of beats are classified and counted. A technician reviews the scan and edits the classifications. The system then reanalyzes and quantitates heart rate, premature atrial and ventricular complexes, and runs of tachycardia. Pacemaker activity, ST-segment trends, and heart rate variability may also be analyzed. Most scanners print out data in a trend or graph

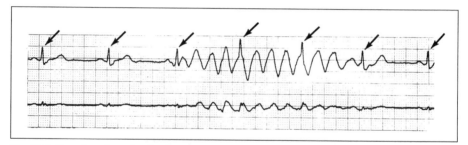

Fig. 10-1. Pseudotachyarrhythmia caused by electrode motion artifact. Note the true QRS complexes (*arrows*) marching through the apparent tachycardia.

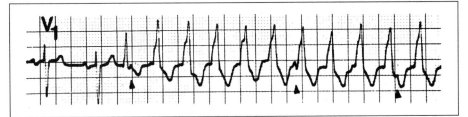

Fig. 10-2. Run of ventricular tachycardia with a right bundle branch block morphology documented in modified Holter lead V_1. Note intermittent P waves (*arrows*).

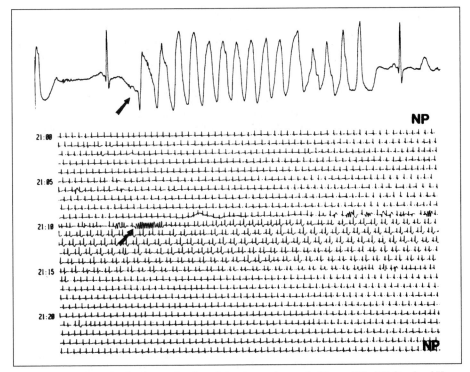

Fig. 10-3. *Top*: An episode of torsades de pointes (*arrow*) recorded in modified Holter lead V_5. Note the prolonged Q–T interval, pause dependency, and polymorphic appearance. *Bottom*: Simultaneous full disclosure recording in the same lead. The same run of ventricular tachycardia is marked in the 25-minute recording (*arrow*).

format for the interpreting physician to review, along with representative ECG strips and samples (either normal or abnormal) during reported symptoms. The technician can interact with the system to print out additional strips that are felt to be informative. Figure 10-3 shows a strip of nonsustained VT recorded by Holter monitor during symptoms.

The interpreting physician correlates the data from these reports with the total clinical picture. It is common for 24-hour monitoring to show some abnormalities, even in asymptomatic patients with normal hearts. Marked sinus bradycardia (less than 40 beats/minute), sinus pauses, premature atrial and ventricular complexes, AV Wenckebach (especially during sleep), and short runs of atrial and ventricular tachycardia have each been recorded in normal populations [5]. Pronounced resting sinus bradycardia and sinus arrhythmia are particularly common in trained athletes. These normal variants should be kept in mind so that normal individuals who demonstrate them are not treated unnecessarily. Conversely, the recording of normal sinus rhythm during the most severe of a patient's symptoms should prompt a search for a nonarrhythmic etiology.

Electrocardiographics artifacts, due to patient motion or electrical and mechanical malfunction, may mimic real arrhythmias. Pseudobradyarrhythmia, pseudotachyarrhythmia, and false AV block have been reported (Fig. 10-1) [4]. Poor electrode placement, broken lead wires and patient cables, tape jamming, erratic revolution of the tape, and defective batteries can cause these artifacts. The use of two simultaneous leads is helpful in identifying spurious results, since the abnormality may be isolated to a single lead.

Indications for Holter monitoring are listed in Table 10-2. The primary use of ambulatory monitoring is for the evaluation of known or suspected cardiac rhythm disturbances. Since arrhythmias are usually intermittent, the sensitivity varies, depending on the duration of the recording and the frequency of the arrhythmia. A 24-hour Holter monitoring permits the recording of cardiac rhythm during both sleeping and awake states. The diurnal variation of arrhythmia and the effects of physical and emotional stress can be demonstrated. Sleep is usually associated with sinus bradycardia and reduction in premature ventricular complex frequency.

A. Ventricular arrhythmias. Holter recordings are used in a serial fashion to judge the efficacy of antiarrhythmic drug treatment for ventricular arrhythmias. A baseline recording of 24–48 hours is obtained prior to initiation of therapy and/or after complete washout of previous drugs. The dosage is then titrated to achieve therapeutic blood levels, desired ECG effect, or maximum tolerated dosage. Then the Holter recording is repeated. Significant interval reduction or elimination of spontaneous arrhythmia is taken as an indication of beneficial effect. This noninvasive approach may be complemented by attempts to provoke the arrhythmia with exercise testing or invasive electrophysiologic testing.

The Holter approach is limited by spontaneous day-to-day variability in arrhythmia frequency. Figure 10-4 shows the hourly and daily variation in premature ventricular complex frequency on three consecutive days of Holter monitoring in a patient taking no antiarrhythmic medication. Although the patient had frequent ventricular ectopy during the first 48 hours, a spontaneous marked decrease occurred on the third day. This frustrating fluctuation can mimic drug effect as well as proarrhythmia, leading to inappropriate confidence in the therapeutic result (Fig. 10-5). Similarly, patients with lethal ventricular arrhythmias may have very low rates of ambient ventricular ectopy for long periods of time, punctuated by episodes of sustained ventricular tachyarrhythmias. In this group of patients, serial Holter recordings inadequately portray the continuing risk of serious arrhythmia. In the recent Electrophysiologic Study versus Electrocardiographic Monitoring (ESVEM) trial, 83% of patients with a history of sustained ventricular tachyarrhythmias had sufficiently frequent baseline ventricular ectopy to qualify for statistically valid noninvasive evaluation of drug efficacy with serial Holter monitoring [6].

Drug effect is defined as a statistically significant change in the number of arrhythmic events associated with a drug. Drug effect is not synonymous with clinical drug effectiveness, an end point reached when drug therapy has been shown to eliminate the symptomatic or high-risk arrhythmia. In pooled data, an 83% reduction in ventricular premature complexes over a 24-hour recording is a statistically valid end point; however, the clinical end point in an individual patient is variable and depends on the density of the baseline arrhythmia. Guidelines for defining drug effect are shown in Table 10-3. The end point can be corrected downward with longer monitoring periods (control and treated) [7, 8]. Criteria for clinical drug effectiveness are not well defined. Graboys et al. found that a 100% reduction in spontaneously occurring runs of VT, a 90% reduction in ventricular couplets, and at least a 50% reduction in the number of ventricular premature complexes over 24 hours predicted a favorable therapeutic response in high-risk patients with baseline high-

Table 10-2. Indications for Holter monitoring

Detection and quantitation of known or suspected arrhythmia

Assessment of the effect of antiarrhythmic treatment

Risk stratification

Evaluation of pacemaker function

Evaluation of chest pain

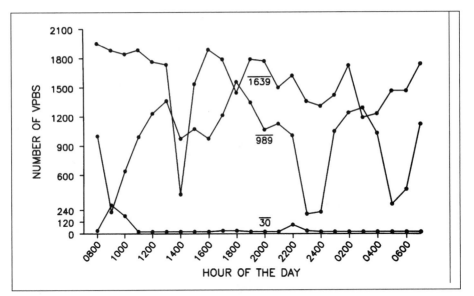

Fig. 10-4. Frequency of ventricular premature beats (VPBs) in a single patient undergoing Holter monitoring on 3 consecutive days without antiarrhythmic medication. Note the marked variability in VPB frequency, decreasing from a mean of 1639/hour during the first 24 hours to 989/hour and 30/hour during the second and third days, respectively. The low VPB frequency on the third day mimics drug effect.

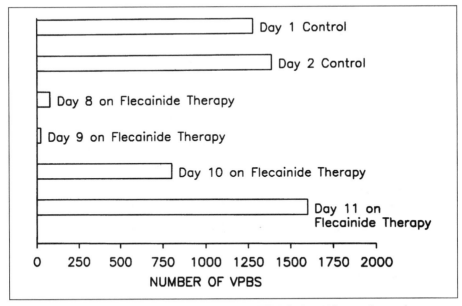

Fig. 10-5. Number of ventricular premature beats (VPBs) during 48 hours of control monitoring and 4 consecutive days of monitoring after therapeutic flecainide levels had been achieved. On days 8 and 9 of flecainide therapy, a 95% reduction of VPBs was observed, mimicking drug effect. On days 10 and 11, however, VPB frequency returned to baseline levels despite continuation of the drug.

density arrhythmia [9]. Criteria for drug effectiveness used in the Cardiac Arrhythmia Suppression Trial (CAST) were 80% reduction or more in ventricular premature complexes and 90% reduction or more in runs of VT in patients who had had at least six ventricular premature complexes/hour in the baseline study, but no runs of VT longer than 15 beats in duration [10].

The noninvasive approach to evaluation of drug effectiveness is less sensitive in predicting drug failure than is serial electrophysiologic testing. Many patients with adequate suppression of ventricular ectopy by Holter criteria may still demonstrate inducible sustained VT on drug therapy with invasive testing [11]. Thus, there is a lack of concordance between Holter monitoring and electrophysiologic testing for this end point. In patients whose clinical arrhythmias cannot be reproduced in the electrophysiology laboratory with programmed stimulation, Holter guidance may provide the only useful marker of electrical instability to follow with therapy. The ESVEM trial suggested that Holter-guided evaluation of drug therapy in patients with lethal ventricular arrhythmias is as predictive of clinical response as is invasive testing [6]. This study, however, has been criticized for employing electrophysiologic criteria for drug effectiveness less stringent than the current standard. Furthermore, only 83% of patients screened had a sufficient density of ventricular ectopy on baseline Holter recording to qualify for statistically valid noninvasive follow-up. Most agree that invasive electrophysiologic study should be used in conjunction with ambulatory monitoring in high-risk patients with infrequent ectopy.

Holter monitors are frequently used to determine whether a new cardioactive agent has deleterious proarrhythmic effects. Because of the spontaneous variability, such judgments should be made with caution. As in the case of predicting efficacy, longer monitoring periods are more accurate than a single 24-hour follow-up tracing. The criteria for detecting proarrhythmia by noninvasive techniques are controversial and may not predict adverse clinical events [12]. Table 10-4 lists the noninvasive criteria for diagnosing proarrhythmia employed in the Cardiac Arrhythmia Pilot Study (CAPS) trial [13]. Note that the threshold for increase in frequency of arrhythmia depends on the frequency observed on the control Holter study. As a general rule, we consider the following to be **clinically significant proarrhythmic responses:** development of a new ventricular tachycardia (including torsades de pointes), tachycardia that becomes incessant or noncardiovertible, or conversion of a nonsustained arrhythmia to a sustained one. Increases in spontaneous ventricular premature complex frequency are not life threatening; therefore, we do not consider these to be a clinically important proarrhythmia, unless they result in exacerbation of the patient's symptoms.

B. **Supraventricular arrhythmias.** Little attention has been directed toward the use of Holter monitoring in patients with supraventricular arrhythmias, partly due to technical problems in automatic discrimination of sinus rhythm and supraventricular arrhythmias. Accurate quantitation of premature atrial complexes and runs of supraventricular tachycardia is difficult to achieve. In addition, the typical patient with paroxysmal supraventricular tachycardia has very little daily atrial ectopy despite having relatively infrequent paroxysms of debilitating tachycardia. Therefore, 24-hour recordings are not very predictive of susceptibility to recurrence of the clinical arrhythmia. Transient symptomatic event recorders are more useful in this setting, unless the patient has incessant supraventricular tachycardia. In the incessant subset, serial Holter recordings can be used in assessment of drug effect; com-

Table 10-3. Holter monitoring: Guidelines for defining drug effect

Number of days monitoring before and after treatment	Reduction required to indicate drug effect (%)		
	PVCs	Couplets	Runs of VT
1	83	75	65
2	75	65	55
3	65	55	45

PVCs = premature ventricular complexes; VT = ventricular tachycardia.
Source: Data from EL Michelson, J Morganroth. Spontaneous variability of complex ventricular arrhythmias detected by long-term electrocardiographic recording. *Circulation* 61:690, 1980. J Morganroth et al. Limitations of routine long-term electrocardiographic monitoring to assess ventricular ectopic frequency. *Circulation* 58:408, 1978.

Table 10-4. Definitions of proarrhythmia by Holter criteria

PVCs

Baseline frequency (PVCs/h)	Increase defining proarrhythmia
10	10×
30	7×
100	4×
300	3×
1000	2×

Nonsustained VT

Baseline frequency (runs/day)	Frequency defining proarrhythmia
<5	≥50 runs/day
≥5	10× increase

New sustained VT

New torsades de pointes

PVC = premature ventricular complex; VT = ventricular tachycardia.
Source: CAPS Investigators. The cardiac arrhythmia pilot study. *Am J Cardiol* 57:91, 1986.

plete therapeutic efficacy requires 100% abolition of the arrhythmia on treated Holter. A 50% or greater reduction in frequency of the arrhythmia, slowing of the tachycardia rate, or shortening of the duration may qualify as partial efficacy [14]. In atrial fibrillation, Holter monitoring can help to establish whether the arrhythmia is paroxysmal or chronic, and whether the ventricular response is controlled during waking, sleeping, and exercising states. Sick sinus syndrome may be identified by the coexistence of sinus bradyarrhythmias with primary atrial tachyarrhythmias (Fig. 10-6).

Holter recording plays a more constant role in the evaluation of patients with Wolff-Parkinson-White syndrome than in those with other supraventricular arrhythmias. Intermittency of preexcitation, an observation useful in risk stratification, can be identified. When seen, intermittent preexcitation marks an accessory pathway with a longer refractory period and, thus, a lower risk of sudden cardiac death [15]. The presence of subclinical atrial arrhythmias may also warrant specific treatment in the Wolff-Parkinson-White patient.

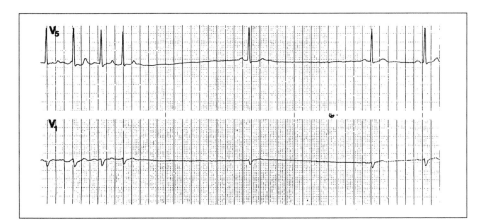

Fig. 10-6. Tachycardia-bradycardia syndrome. Modified Holter leads V_5 and V_1 demonstrate the termination of paroxysmal atrial flutter with a 2.9-second pause and a secondary pause.

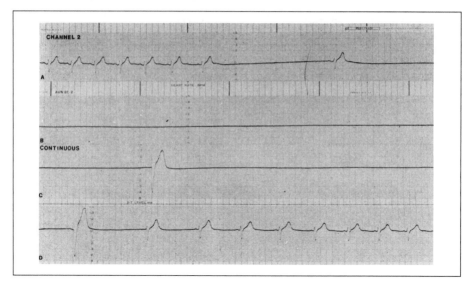

Fig. 10-7. Symptomatic bradycardia. Continuous strips in Holter lead II document sinus arrest with an 18-second pause, followed by a ventricular escape beat *(C)*, followed by a 12-second pause. The patient reported syncope at this time in the diary.

C. **Risk stratification.** Ambulatory monitors may be used for risk stratification in high-risk patients in whom the presence of an arrhythmia increases the likelihood of sudden death. Such clinical conditions include the post-MI period [16], congestive heart failure, dilated cardiomyopathy [17], hypertrophic obstructive cardiomyopathy [18], and prolonged Q–T syndromes (see Fig. 10-3) [2]. Holter monitoring is superior to treadmill testing in screening patients with coronary artery disease and hypertrophic obstructive cardiomyopathy for arrhythmias. It may also be useful in screening patients with the mitral valve prolapse and Wolff-Parkinson-White syndromes [15]. In contrast, Holter monitoring is not very sensitive in identifying patients with bifascicular block likely to develop higher degrees of block in the future [19].

Heart rate variability, the fluctuation of R–R intervals, can be quantitated with most modern Holter equipment, as well as with recordings of shorter duration. This parameter is an indirect measure of autonomic balance. Decreased heart rate variability indicates either reduced parasympathetic nervous system activity or resting sympathetic hyperactivity and is a poor prognostic sign in post-MI patients. Together with signal-averaged electrocardiography, left ventricular ejection fraction, and ventricular ectopy, it is useful in identifying ischemic heart disease patients with a high risk of sudden cardiac death [20].

D. **Bradyarrhythmias.** Holter monitors may also be used for screening patients with symptoms suggestive of impulse generation or conduction problems (Fig. 10-6). As in Fig. 10-7, in which the temporal correlation between symptoms and the occurrence of a bradyarrhythmia is established, the Holter recording can also be helpful in a negative sense (i.e., occurrence of symptoms during normal sinus rhythm). Zeldis et al. reported clinical syncope or presyncope during the Holter recording in 46% of patients presenting with these symptoms. Only 14% of the total group experienced an electrocardiographic abnormality at the time of the reported symptoms, whereas 32% had none that correlated with their symptoms [3]. In the latter group a workup of nonarrhythmic causes of syncope should be considered. Despite these limitations, Holter recordings do appear to have a higher diagnostic yield than exercise stress testing in syncope evaluations. Pacemaker patients with suspected device malfunction may require 24-hour monitoring to document an intermittent episode of failure to capture or sense, particularly if the malfunction is positional or due to intermittent environmental noise.

E. **Ischemic heart disease.** Many Holter systems are capable of quantitative ST-segment analysis. This feature can be useful in correlating episodes of chest pain with

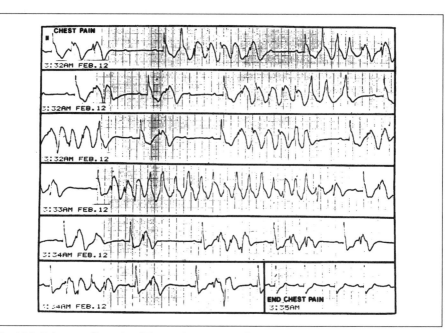

Fig. 10-8. Prinzmetal's angina. Noncontinuous recordings in Holter lead II documenting ST-segment elevation and runs of ventricular tachycardia during symptoms (3:32 AM). Note return of ST segments toward normal at end of chest pain (3:35 AM).

electrocardiographic abnormalities. For example, Prinzmetal's angina is associated with diagnostic ST-segment elevation in leads affected by the artery with spasm (Fig. 10-8). This variant angina is usually not provocable with exertion and typically occurs in the early morning hours or with emotional stress. Ambulatory monitoring can identify this special group of patients. Asymptomatic ST-segment depression in patients with known coronary disease indicates silent myocardial ischemia; however, the clinical significance of that finding is debated [21, 22]. Holter monitoring is much less sensitive and specific than exercise stress testing is for identifying new patients with obstructive coronary artery disease.

Reel-to-reel recorders have a better frequency response for analyzing ST-segment shifts. A two-lead system is highly recommended; the most useful combination for this purpose is a modified V_5 plus an inferior lead (II or III), although different lead combinations may be used in individuals, depending on the anatomy. Since ST segments may vary with position and hyperventilation, these conditions should be recorded at the beginning and end of each study and a 1-mV calibration signal should be recorded at regular intervals to correct for drift in the signal due to drying of the electrode gel. Playback of the recording at very rapid speeds (e.g., 60 times real time) can be helpful in distinguishing real from artifactual changes.

III. **Noncontinuous forms of electrocardiographic recording.** In patients with rare symptoms, even several consecutive days of Holter monitoring may be insufficient to document the corresponding clinical arrhythmia. A noncontinuous form of ambulatory recording will have a higher yield in this group and can be used for long-term surveillance of outpatients in their usual activities. Electrocardiographic recording is triggered either automatically (by detected arrhythmias or sampling at regular intervals) or, more commonly, manually by the patient when experiencing symptoms. Like devices used for transtelephonic monitoring of pacemaker function, transient symptomatic event recorders convert the electrocardiographic signal for transmission over the telephone. Audiophone signals are then converted back to an electrocardiographic signal at a central monitoring station. Typically, a nurse or trained technician receives the signal, interprets the tracing, and interacts with the patient. Busy monitoring centers triage the response to the call with a protocol designed to rate the urgency of the situation. Provisions for patient instruction or reassurance, urgent physician notification,

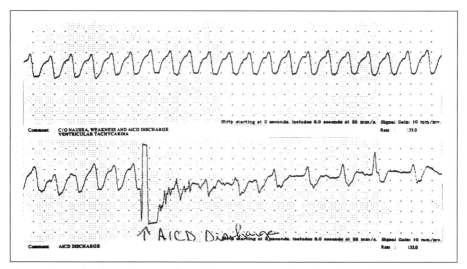

Fig. 10-9. Sustained ventricular tachycardia preceding implantable defibrillator discharge. The clinical arrhythmia was documented with a loop recorder automatically triggered by defibrillator activity.

initiation of emergency treatment in the field (e.g., self-injectable lidocaine), and summoning of local paramedical personnel, depending on the triage scale, may all be included in the response algorithm. Many centers have used this system with cardiac rehabilitation or other high-risk patients, combining routine calls with symptomatic ones. Follow-up of drug therapy can also be facilitated in this manner.

Several types of recorders have been used for transient symptomatic event detection. Most are highly portable (beeper or wristwatch configurations) and activated with minimal patient effort or delay. Simple lead systems may be engaged with either finger rings or bracelets or application to a bare patch of chest wall. Most modern devices have a memory capability and can record at least 30 seconds of information until the patient has access to a telephone to dump the recording; live recordings can also be transmitted. In order to extract the most benefit out of this device, the duration of the clinical arrhythmia must be sufficient to allow for recognition of symptoms and activation of the recorder. It is not suitable for evaluation of fleeting symptoms or those that rapidly incapacitate the patient. The patient must be aware of the symptom or rhythm of concern and alert enough to activate the device promptly. Less conscientious or intelligent patients may not be capable of effective usage.

More sophisticated devices, which require fixation of standard electrocardiographic cables, keep a loop of memory up to about 5 minutes in duration so that the rhythm preceding patients' symptoms is also recorded when manually activated. Thus, the more fleeting arrhythmias and those producing transient incapacitation can still be captured. Some loop recorders have been modified to make recordings triggered by the discharge of an automatic implantable cardioverter-defibrillator (Fig. 10-9). This feature can be invaluable in determining whether defibrillator discharges are appropriate, that is, triggered by VT. The main disadvantage of loop recorders is relatively poor patient acceptance; few patients can tolerate the inconvenience of the cables for more than a week or two at a time.

IV. **Exercise stress testing.** The exercise stress test is the most commonly used noninvasive technique for detecting latent coronary artery disease. Exertion induces myocardial ischemia in susceptible subjects by increasing myocardial oxygen demand in the presence of a limited supply. The purpose of the test is to provoke an electrocardiographic change suggestive of myocardial ischemia and to correlate these changes with symptoms suggestive of angina. Secondary motives include reproduction of clinical arrhythmias, evaluation of conduction abnormalities, and pacemaker prescription and follow-up.

A stress test is performed after obtaining baseline vital signs and 12-lead ECG. Additional baseline recordings during hyperventilation and standing are used to screen for

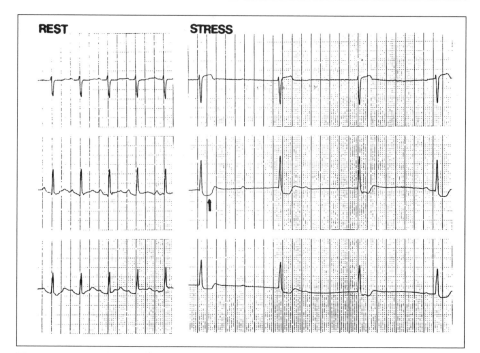

Fig. 10-10. Positive exercise stress in a patient with a history of chest pain. Leads V_1, II, and V_5 are shown at rest (*left*) and at peak exercise (*right*). During stress, 2- to 3-mm horizontal ST-segment depression is recorded in lead II (*arrow*) during symptoms. The patient also developed complete heart block with a junctional escape rhythm as a result of inferior ischemia.

labile ST–T wave segments unrelated to ischemia. The test is usually performed on a treadmill, although a bicycle ergometer can also be used. The Bruce protocol is frequently used [23], although many others are also standardized. Depending on the protocol, the rate and incline of the treadmill are increased at 2- to 3-minute intervals as the patient continues to exercise. Electrocardiographic and BP monitoring are continued throughout exercise and for several minutes into the recovery period. Exercise is continued until the patient develops incapacitating chest pain, fatigue, or dyspnea or achieves a target heart rate greater than 85% of the predicted maximum rate for an individual of that age and gender. Symptom-limited tests are preferred for maximizing sensitivity. Marked hypotension, long runs of VT, or marked ST-segment depression trigger premature termination of the test. In certain circumstances, patients are exercised only to an intermediate predetermined heart rate, for safety. For example, one rarely allows a patient to exceed 120 beats/minute after recent MI [24].

An exercise stress test is defined as positive for ischemia when 1 or more mm (0.1 mV) of horizontal, downsloping, or slow-upsloping ST-segment depression is recorded 80 msec after the J point, compared to the baseline tracing (Fig. 10-10). Raising the criteria for a positive result to 2 mm of ST-segment deviation increases the specificity of the test at the expense of its sensitivity. Additional criteria for a positive result that add to the sensitivity of the stress test include the development of hypotension, inversion of U waves, typical angina pectoris, or ventricular arrhythmias. The magnitude of ST-segment depression, the level of exercise at which ST-segment depression occurs, and the persistence of ST-segment abnormalities in the recovery period all provide an index of the severity of coronary artery disease. Interpretation of a positive stress test is limited in patients who have pretest ST-segment abnormalities, since they have a higher incidence of false-positive tests. Bundle branch block, left ventricular hypertrophy, mitral valve prolapse, overt Wolff-Parkinson-White syndrome, female gender, and the use of digitalis preparations each increase the likelihood of false-positives [25].

The predictive accuracy of a plain treadmill test is modest, with sensitivity averaging 68% and specificity of 77%, according to a meta analysis by Gianrossi et al. [26]. The predictive accuracy is considerably worse in women due to the very high rate of false-positive tests. According to Baye's theorem, the sensitivity and specificity of a test depend largely on the pretest likelihood of coronary artery disease as determined by history and physical examination [21, 27]. The optimal diagnostic yield is obtained in patients with an intermediate (40–60%) pretest likelihood of coronary disease—generally those with positive risk factors and atypical chest pain. There is evidence that the predictive accuracy of the test has worsened over the past decade as subjects with more classical presentations have been selected for more aggressive evaluation, thus being eliminated from the population undergoing stress testing [28].

A. **Stress nuclear studies.** Concomitant myocardial scanning with thallium 201 and newer isotopes, such as Tc 99m sestaMIBI and teboroxime, enhance the predictive accuracy of stress testing, particularly in subjects at risk for false-positive ECG tests. In addition to screening for the presence of coronary artery disease, stress nuclear studies can be very helpful in screening for reversible areas of ischemia in patients with known coronary disease in whom further intervention is being considered. Late imaging 24 hours after thallium 201 injection may be required to distinguish between viable myocardium and scar. Stress echocardiography provides similar information on reversible ischemia. Those who cannot easily perform physical exercise may undergo perfusion scanning with pharmacologic stress; agents useful for this purpose include intravenous (IV) dipyridamole, dobutamine, and adenosine.

   Positron emission tomography (PET) is a newer, more quantitative method of assessing myocardial perfusion and viability, as well as metabolism. ^{13}N ammonia, ^{15}O water, and rubidium 82 have been used to document myocardial perfusion [29]. PET studies may be performed with pharmacologic stress to detect coronary stenoses less than 50% of artery diameter. ^{13}N and ^{15}O radiopharmaceuticals must be manufactured in on-site cyclotron facilities, but rubidium 82 can be produced with a tabletop generator, thus expanding the practical venue of the procedure. ^{18}F fluorodeoxyglucose imaging is a sensitive indicator of myocardial viability.

B. **Evaluation of disability.** Exercise stress testing is also used for evaluating an individual's physical condition and New York Heart Association functional status. This application is useful for the patient who has valvular heart disease, especially mitral stenosis, since functional status is often used in determining the timing of prosthetic valve replacement. In cardiac rehabilitation programs, the presence of angina, dyspnea, or exercise-aggravated arrhythmia at a certain reproducible workload can be useful in limiting physical activity to a prescribed level.

C. **Risk stratification.** Submaximum stress testing has been found to be useful for risk stratification of patients 1 to 2 weeks after MI [1]. The occurrence of exercise-induced angina, ventricular arrhythmia, or diagnostic ST-segment changes is predictive of future anginal events, MI, and sudden death. Patients in these high-risk categories should be strongly considered for prophylactic beta-blocker protection and/or early cardiac catheterization and aggressive intervention to avert these serious sequelae.

D. **Ventricular arrhythmias.** In patients being evaluated for ventricular arrhythmias, we routinely recommend stress testing for three reasons. First, underlying coronary disease should be ruled out if coronary catheterization is not otherwise being considered. Exercise may provoke VT or ventricular fibrillation (VF) in coronary patients, occasionally as a direct consequence of acute ischemia (Fig. 10-11). More frequently, the arrhythmia occurs without preceding ST or T wave changes. Exercise enhances automaticity (normal, abnormal, and triggered), increases conduction velocity, and shortens refractoriness. Dispersion of refractoriness, due to either regional ischemia and scar or heterogeneous sympathetic nerve distribution, may facilitate reentry. Thus, the provocation of ventricular tachyarrhythmias with exercise is not specific for any particular mechanism. In those who do have active ischemia, cardiac catheterization and definitive management of the obstructive coronary disease are advisable, along with comprehensive antiarrhythmic therapy.

   Second, exercise provocation of VT can be used as a marker of arrhythmia susceptibility with serial drug or device therapy testing. Computerized treadmill equipment provides a stored record of arrhythmias, which can be quantified after completion of the test. The end point of serial testing is the suppression of the exercise-induced arrhythmia with adequate therapy [30]. Since VT is not always reproducible with exercise testing, documentation of its consistency as a marker with a second baseline treadmill test is preferable prior to serial drug testing.

   Third, stress testing is useful in identifying patients with idiopathic exercise-induced VT [31] (Fig. 10-12). This relatively uncommon condition tends to occur in

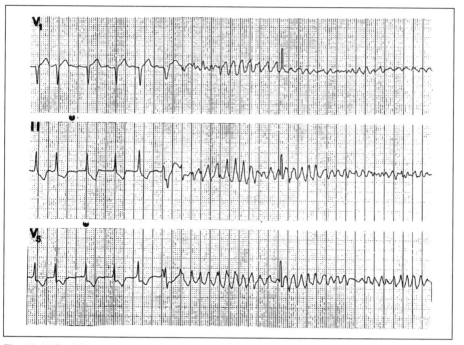

Fig. 10-11. Positive exercise stress test in a patient 1 month following anteroseptal myocardial infarction. In addition to ST-segment depression and T-wave inversion in leads II and V_5, ventricular fibrillation is induced with exertion. Coronary arteriography later documented occlusive left main and severe triple-vessel coronary artery disease.

younger patients without structural heart disease. The QRS during tachycardia typically has a left bundle branch block morphology. Mapping studies (usually requiring isoproterenol to facilitate tachycardia induction) demonstrate earliest activation in the area of the right ventricular outflow tract. A more uncommon variant of this syndrome has a right bundle branch block morphology with a superior axis and originates near the apex of the left ventricle. These arrhythmias are sensitive to catecholamines and can be blocked with beta-adrenergic blockers and calcium-channel antagonists, although circulating norepinephrine levels are no higher in these patients during VT than they are in control subjects, either at rest or with exercise. Cyclic adenosine monophosphate–mediated triggered automaticity, rather than reentry, is the presumed mechanism of the arrhythmia.

It is important to recognize this unusual form of VT because its management is atypical. The arrhythmia is potentially curable with radiofrequency catheter ablation at its origin. Beta-adrenergic blockers and calcium-channel antagonists are the treatments of choice when medical management is chosen; their efficacy can be monitored with serial stress testing.

Ventricular arrhythmias associated with exercise are not specific to disease states. Up to one-third of normal individuals may experience some ventricular arrhythmia with stress testing. Normal subjects may develop ventricular premature complexes or pairs with exercise but only rarely develop VT. In contrast to its occurrence in patients with coronary artery disease, more than 50% of whom will develop premature ventricular complexes during stress testing, ventricular ectopy is poorly reproducible in normal subjects and is not associated with an adverse prognosis [32]. Normal subjects tend to experience arrhythmia at higher heart rates with resolution in the recovery period.

E. **Supraventricular arrhythmias.** Exercise stress testing is of limited use in the screening of patients with supraventricular arrhythmias, since these abnormalities are rarely precipitated by exertion. The exception to this rule is the patient with Wolff-Parkinson-White syndrome, in whom much can be learned with an exercise evaluation. In those with overt or intermittent preexcitation, the degree of fusion

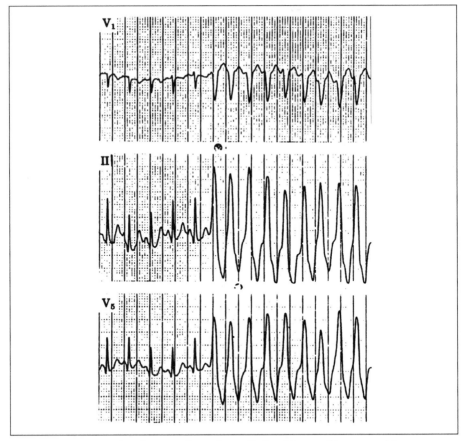

Fig. 10-12. Exercise-induced ventricular tachycardia in a 26-year-old woman with no structural heart disease. The arrhythmia had a left bundle branch block morphology with a normal axis. Propranolol treatment eliminated all recurrences.

represents the dynamic competition for antegrade conduction between the accessory pathway and the AV node at varying heart rates and autonomic states. Abrupt, but not gradual, loss of the delta wave at low levels of exercise correlates with a long refractory period of the accessory pathway in the antegrade direction [16] (Fig. 10-13). This finding implies a lower risk of sudden cardiac death and may obviate the need for invasive evaluation.

F. **Bradyarrhythmias and antiarrhythmic devices.** Stress testing is of limited use in the evaluation of known or suspected bradyarrhythmias. In patients with dizziness or syncope, it is inferior to Holter monitoring in detecting culprit arrhythmias but can be used adjunctively to increase diagnostic yield. On the other hand, exercise testing may be quite useful in the prescription and evaluation of antiarrhythmic devices. Sinus node competency can be evaluated by observing the appropriateness of sinus rates with graded exercise; this factor is useful in establishing whether dual chamber or rate-responsive pacing will be beneficial. In congenital heart block patients, the adequacy of the junctional escape rate with exertion is helpful in selecting the time for elective permanent pacemaker implantation. Sensor response to exercise provides feedback to the physician for optimizing the programming of rate-responsive pacemakers to settings comfortable for the individual patient after implantation. Stress testing also provides information about maximum supraventricular rates to be expected in patients with automatic implantable defibrillators. If overlap occurs in clinical VT rates and normal exercise rates, modifications of medical therapy or limitation of exercise may be indicated.

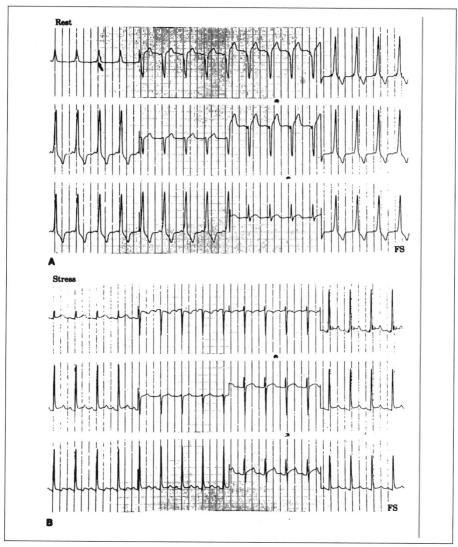

Fig. 10-13. Loss of preexcitation with exercise in a patient with Wolff-Parkinson-White syndrome associated with a paraseptal accessory pathway. **A.** 12-lead ECG at rest showing short P–R interval and delta wave (*arrow*). **B.** Electrocardiogram in the same patient during stress testing. Overt preexcitation disappeared abruptly as the heart rate increased to 100 beats/minute. This observation suggests a lower risk profile for the patient.

V. **Signal-averaged electrocardiography.** The anatomic substrate for sustained VT in most instances, especially in the setting of ischemic heart disease, is a heterogeneous area of viable, ischemic, and fibrotic tissue in the periphery of a myocardial scar. This mottled tissue, in which conduction may be slowed or tortuous, forms the nidus for reentrant VT. The high-resolution (signal-averaged) ECG is a special computerized analysis of the QRS complex designed to detect in normal sinus rhythm the late low-voltage electrical activity that is a marker of this condition (Fig. 10-14). It has been used to predict which patients are at high risk for sustained VT and sudden death. The technique and its interpretation will be discussed in detail in Chap. 11.

The presence of late potentials has been shown to predict inducibility of sustained VT in patients with syncope, those with asymptomatic ventricular ectopy, and in noncoronary disease patients with ventricular tachyarrhythmias [33]. Although the positive

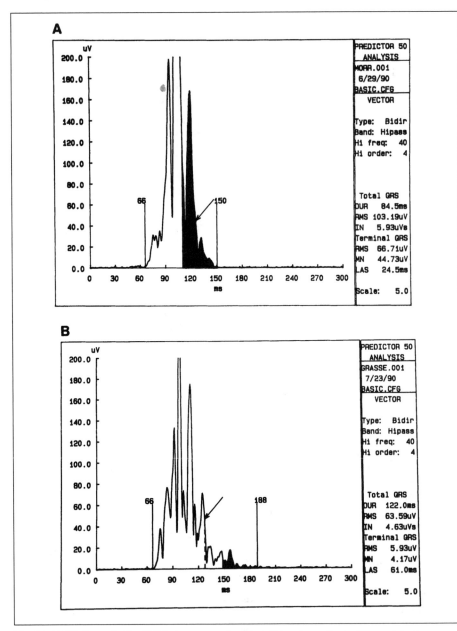

Fig. 10-14. High-resolution ECGs in a normal subject *(A)* and a patient with ventricular tachycardia *(B)*. The low-voltage late potential in *B* is identified by the three criteria of prolonged QRS duration (DUR), prolonged low-amplitude signal (LAS), and reduced root mean square (RMS) of the terminal portion of the QRS.

predictive accuracy is low in syncope patients, the negative predictive accuracy is quite high—in the range of 97–98%. Thus, a negative result can be very reassuring to both the patient and physician.

The signal-averaged ECG, a noninvasive low-cost screening procedure, has a significant role in risk stratification of patients following MI. Although 40–50% of those tested will have a positive test at some point, the highest predictive accuracy is seen at 2 weeks. The positive predictive value—that is, the likelihood that an individual with a positive test will subsequently have VT or sudden cardiac death—is fairly low (20%), but the negative predictive value is very high (97%) [34]. Thus, the procedure can be very useful in identifying a high-risk subset of post-MI patients and in reassuring the low-risk group, especially when the results are considered in conjunction with other risk factors (e.g., ejection fraction, ventricular ectopy, and heart rate variability).

This technique is limited by our inability with current commercial equipment to interpret the results in the presence of bundle branch block, preexcitation, or very high-density premature ventricular complexes. Late potentials do not typically disappear with effective antiarrhythmic therapy; thus, the procedure cannot be used in serial assessment of the efficacy of drug therapy.

VI. Echocardiography and Doppler. Structural heart disease may be either cause or consequence of cardiac arrhythmias. Thus, evaluation of one without the other is incomplete. Although many suggest that a cardiac catheterization be performed in all patients with sustained VT, there is general agreement that patients with complex ventricular arrhythmias should have at least some assessment of overall cardiac status. Both M-mode and two-dimensional echocardiography can be useful in identifying coronary artery disease, valvular stenosis and regurgitation, mitral valve prolapse, hypertrophic obstructive cardiomyopathy, pericardial disease, intracardiac tumors, arrhythmogenic right ventricular dysplasia, and congenital heart defects. Stress echocardiography is capable of detecting latent coronary artery disease by demonstrating the occurrence of new wall motion abnormalities with exercise. This technique is particularly useful in women. Doppler capability enhances the echocardiogram with more sensitive and quantitative measurements of myocardial function, valvular dysfunction, and intracardiac shunts. Table 10-5 lists potential abnormalities that may be documented with echo/Doppler techniques in arrhythmia patients.

Echocardiography is particularly useful in qualitative identification of ventricular dysfunction, either global or segmental, systolic or diastolic. Identification of a left ven-

Table 10-5. Echocardiographic and Doppler abnormalities potentially associated with arrhythmias

Left ventricular abnormalities
Dilated cardiomyopathy
Segmental wall motion abnormalities consistent with coronary artery disease
Concentric hypertrophy
Diastolic dysfunction
Hypertrophic cardiomyopathy

Right ventricular abnormalities
Dilated cardiomyopathy
Arrhythmogenic right ventricular dysplasia

Atrial abnormalities
Dilated atria
Atrial thrombi or hemostasis

Valvular abnormalities
Valvular stenosis
Valvular regurgitation
Mitral or tricuspid valve prolapse

Congenital abnormalities
Septal defects
Tetralogy of Fallot
Ebstein's anomaly

Intracardiac tumors

tricular aneurysm that is associated with lethal ventricular arrhythmias offers the affected patient a wider choice in treatment options, including those that may be curative. The presence of left ventricular dysfunction within any subclass of ventricular arrhythmia increases that individual's risk for sudden death and may render the decision for antiarrhythmic treatment more compelling. It also limits the choices for antiarrhythmic therapy, as many drugs have noticeable negative inotropic effects and may precipitate congestive heart failure in this group. The safety and applicability of surgical procedures are limited in patients with systolic dysfunction. As a quantitative tool for estimation of left ventricular ejection fraction, echo is limited by necessary assumptions about ventricular size and geometry and is less accurate in the presence of segmental wall motion abnormalities.

Echocardiography is a routine part of the evaluation of patients with paroxysmal or chronic atrial fibrillation. Left atrial dimension predicts the success of drug therapy; patients with markedly dilated atria are unlikely to experience conversion to sinus rhythm and to avoid recurrences with prophylactic antiarrhythmic therapy [35]. The likelihood of thromboembolic events is greatly increased in the presence of mitral valve stenosis but less so with mitral regurgitation [36]. Identification of intraatrial thrombi or stasis influences the aggressiveness of anticoagulant therapy. Although transthoracic echocardiography is relatively insensitive for this purpose, transesophageal echocardiography yields a clearer atrial image, allowing identification of blood stasis with a high sensitivity.

In the setting of Wolff-Parkinson-White syndrome, echocardiography can be very useful in screening for associated congenital and acquired defects, such as hypertrophic obstructive cardiomyopathy, atrial septal defect, mitral valve prolapse, and Ebstein's anomaly. The presence of Ebstein's anomaly increases the likelihood that the accessory pathway is right sided.

Echocardiography has a limited role in the evaluation of patients with syncope of undetermined etiology. The diagnostic yield is low in the absence of historical or physical findings suggestive of organic heart disease. In patients with a systolic murmur of left ventricular outflow tract obstruction, however, the echocardiogram can be diagnostic. Identifiable structural causes of syncope include aortic valve stenosis, hypertrophic obstructive cardiomyopathy, and left atrial myxoma.

VII. Radionuclide angiocardiography. The radionuclide angiocardiogram is an imaging tool for the quantitative assessment of global and regional left ventricular performance. Although ejection fraction can be measured using the first-pass technique, the gated equilibrium cardiac blood pool image is used more commonly. In this process, some of the patient's red blood cells are labeled with technetium 99m and imaged in transit through the heart with a gamma camera. Image acquisition is gated by the patient's ECG and the cardiac cycles divided into small intervals so that end diastole and end systole can be identified. Radioactive counts in the left ventricle during each fraction of the R–R interval, acquired over several hundred beats, are proportional to chamber blood volume and independent of geometry and segmental wall motion abnormalities. A representative cardiac cycle can be played back in a continuous loop format for visual analysis.

Left ventricular ejection fraction, a widely used index of systolic pump performance, is precisely quantitated, using the formula:

$$\frac{\text{Left ventricular end-diastolic counts} - \text{left ventricular end-systolic counts}}{\text{Left ventricular end-diastolic counts}}$$

A normal ejection fraction in most laboratories is 50% or more. This technique is accurate and reproducible ($\pm$ 6%) and correlates well with ejection fraction determinations from biplane angiography; it is more accurate than echocardiographic estimates of ejection fraction. The likelihood of measurement error is higher with rapid or irregular heart rates; the presence of atrial fibrillation with a rapid ventricular response or frequent premature ventricular complexes interferes with the gating process [37]. Like echocardiography, radionuclide angiocardiography can be repeated serially to measure the effects of clinical interventions.

Although it does not yield high-quality structural definition, cardiac blood pool imaging is an excellent method for evaluating regional wall motion. At least three views are analyzed (usually anterior, left anterior oblique, and left lateral) so that all coronary artery distributions are evaluated. Segmental hypokinesis, akinesis, or dyskinesis suggests an obstructive coronary process as the etiology of ventricular dysfunction, whereas global hypokinesis is more consistent with a dilated cardiomyopathy. The first-pass imaging technique is more appropriate for quantitative evaluation of right ventricular performance.

Like echocardiography, radionuclide angiocardiography can be used for risk stratification of patients with ventricular arrhythmias. A depressed ejection fraction is a marker of higher risk of both sudden and nonsudden death [1] and may stimulate more aggressive prophylactic antiarrhythmic therapy. Pharmacologic elimination of the arrhythmia, however, does not necessarily confer protection for sudden death, and in the Cardiac Arrhythmia Suppression Trial (CAST), it actually increased the risk [10]. In patients in whom antiarrhythmic therapy is contemplated, a depressed ejection fraction identifies those in whom drugs with negative inotropic activity should be avoided and those in whom aggressive surgical procedures may be inappropriate. In comparison to echocardiography, radionuclide angiocardiography has the advantage of being more quantitatively accurate in analyzing left ventricular function. In addition, qualitatively acceptable studies are easier to obtain in obese patients and in those with chronic obstructive pulmonary disease. On the other hand, radionuclide studies are not designed to identify structural abnormalities, such as valve lesions.

Because there is close electromechanical coupling in the heart, phase analysis of myocardial contraction sequence can be used as a mapping technique. Noninvasive identification of accessory pathway location and initiating areas of ventricular tachycardia has been reported.

VIII. **Head-up tilt-table testing.** The evaluation of the patient with syncope of undetermined etiology is typically unrewarding. Documentation of vital signs and arrhythmias during clinical events with unpredictable intermittency, the only certain way in which to exclude an arrhythmic cause, is tedious and may be impossible. Thus, provocative tests that attempt to reproduce clinical events under controlled circumstances are desirable.

The head-up tilt-table test is a maneuver designed to replicate neurocardiogenic syncope (especially vasovagal syncope, the common or "emotional" faint) [38]. In susceptible patients, the cardioinhibitory (bradycardic) and vasodepressor (hypotensive) components of neurocardiogenic syncope can be elicited. In addition, typical symptoms, including nausea, diaphoresis, pallor, and loss of consciousness, can be reproduced. The noninvasive test can be repeated serially with various interventions to evaluate their clinical effectiveness (see Chap. 5).

The test is performed on a tilt table capable of producing passive upright posture. Electrocardiogram and BP are continuously monitored for a 30-minute supine baseline period and throughout the procedure. The table is raised to an angle of 60–80 degrees for 20–45 minutes, with an end point of syncope, bradycardia, or hypotension. If symptoms do not occur, the procedure can be repeated with graded isoproterenol infusions for more aggressive provocation. If the test is positive, it can be repeated with IV infusion of esmolol to test the therapeutic effect of beta blockers in suppressing the vasovagal reaction. Alternatively, it can be repeated in serial fashion with oral trials of other agents, such as metoprolol, disopyramide, scopolamine, theophylline, or alpha agonists. The ability of these agents to suppress the response to tilt predicts their long-term success in suppressing symptoms.

Head-up tilt-table testing has a sensitivity and specificity in the range of 80–90%, depending on the population tested and the protocol used; however, the reproducibility is only in the range of 80%. Thus, the results should be interpreted in the light of the individual clinical picture. The role of tilt testing in the less common variants of neurocardiogenic syncope is not as well defined as it is in the case of the common faint. Although these figures are far from the ideal, they do have a diagnostic yield superior to that of any other diagnostic procedure in the evaluation of syncope.

References

1. Multicenter Postinfarction Research Group. Risk stratification and survival after myocardial infarction. *N Engl J Med* 309:331, 1983.
2. Schwartz PJ, et al. Diagnostic criteria for the long QT syndrome: An update. *Circulation* 88:782, 1993.
3. Zeldis SM, et al. Cardiovascular complaints: Correlation with cardiac arrhythmias on 24-hour electrocardiographic monitoring. *Chest* 78:456–462, 1980.
4. Kennedy HL. Long-term (Holter) electrocardiogram recordings. In DP Zipes, J Jalife (eds), *Cardiac Electrophysiology: From Cell to Bedside.* Philadelphia: Saunders, 1990. P 791.

5. Kennedy HL, et al. Long-term follow-up of asymptomatic healthy subjects with frequent and complex ventricular ectopy. *N Engl J Med* 312:193, 1985.
6. Mason JW. The Electrophysiologic Study versus Electrocardiographic Monitoring Investigators: A comparison of electrophysiologic testing with Holter monitoring to predict antiarrhythmic-drug efficacy for ventricular tachyarrhythmias. *N Engl J Med* 329:445, 1993.
7. Michelson EL, Morganroth J. Spontaneous variability of complex ventricular arrhythmias detected by long-term electrocardiographic recording. *Circulation* 61:690, 1980.
8. Morganroth J, et al. Limitations of routine long-term electrocardiographic monitoring to assess ventricular ectopic frequency. *Circulation* 58:408, 1978.
9. Graboys TB, et al. Long-term survival of patients with malignant ventricular arrhythmia treated with antiarrhythmic drugs. *Am J Cardiol* 50:437, 1982.
10. Investigators of the Cardiac Arrhythmia Suppression Trial: Preliminary report: Effect of encainide and flecainide on mortality in a randomized trial of arrhythmia suppression after myocardial infarction. *N Engl J Med* 321:406, 1989.
11. Kim SG, et al. Discordance between ambulatory monitoring and programmed stimulation in assessing efficacy of class IA antiarrhythmic agents in patients with ventricular tachycardia. *J Am Coll Cardiol* 6:539, 1985.
12. Task Force of the Working Group on Arrhythmias of the European Society of Cardiology et al. CAST and beyond: Implications of the Cardiac Arrhythmia Suppression Trial. *Circulation* 81:1123, 1990.
13. CAPS Investigators. The cardiac arrhythmia pilot study (CAPS). *Am J Cardiol* 57:91, 1986.
14. Naccarelli GV, et al. Assessment of antiarrhythmic drug efficacy in the treatment of supraventricular arrhythmias. *Am J Cardiol* 58:31C, 1986.
15. Klein GJ, Gulamhusein SS. Intermittent preexcitation in the Wolff-Parkinson-White syndrome. *Am J Cardiol* 52:292, 1983.
16. Bigger JT, Weld FM, Rolnitzky LM. The prevalence and significance of ventricular tachycardia detected by ambulatory ECG recording in the late hospital phase of acute myocardial infarction. *Am J Cardiol* 48:815, 1981.
17. Francis GS. Development of arrhythmias in the patient with congestive heart failure: Pathophysiology, prevalence and prognosis. *Am J Cardiol* 57:3B, 1986.
18. Maron BJ, et al. Prognostic significance of 24 hour ambulatory electrocardiographic monitoring in patients with hypertrophic cardiomyopathy: A prospective study. *Am J Cardiol* 48:252, 1981.
19. McAnulty SH, Rahimtoola SH, Murphy ES. A prospective study of sudden death in "high-risk" bundle branch block. *N Engl J Med* 299:209, 1978.
20. Malik M, Camm AJ. Heart rate variability: From facts to fancies. *J Am Coll Cardiol* 22:566, 1993.
21. Cohn PF. Silent myocardial ischemia: To treat or not to treat? *Hosp Pract* 18:125, 1983.
22. Crenshaw JH, et al. Interactive effects of ST–T wave abnormalities on survival of patients with coronary artery disease. *J Am Coll Cardiol* 18:413, 1991.
23. Bruce RA. Methods of exercise testing. *Am J Cardiol* 33:715, 1974.
24. Krone RJ, et al. Low-level exercise testing after myocardial infarction: Usefulness in enhancing clinical risk stratification. *Circulation* 71:80, 1985.
25. Kattus AA. Exercise electrocardiography: Recognition of the ischemic response, false positive and negative patterns. *Am J Cardiol* 33:721, 1974.
26. Gianrossi R, et al. Exercise-induced ST depression in the diagnosis of coronary artery disease. A meta analysis. *Circulation* 80:87, 1989.
27. Rifkin RD, Hood WB. Bayesian analysis of electrocardiographic exercise stress testing. *N Engl J Med* 297:681, 1977.
28. Patterson RE, Horowitz SF. Importance of epidemiology and biostatistics in deciding clinical strategies for using diagnostic tests: A simplified approach using examples from coronary artery disease. *J Am Coll Cardiol* 13:1653, 1989.
29. Soufer R, Zaret BL. Positron emission tomography and the quantitative assessment of regional myocardial blood flow. *J Am Coll Cardiol* 15:128, 1990.
30. Brugada P. Relative value of exercise electrocardiography, long-term electrocardiographic monitoring and programmed electrical stimulation of the heart in the treatment of cardiac arrhythmias. *Am Heart J* 8(Suppl D):305, 1987.
31. Sung RJ, et al. Clinical and electrophysiologic mechanisms of exercise-induced ventricular tachyarrhythmias. *PACE* 11:1347, 1988.
32. Busby MJ, Shefrin EA, Fleg JL. Prevalence and long-term significance of exercise-induced frequent or repetitive ventricular ectopic beats in apparently healthy volunteers. *J Am Coll Cardiol* 14:1659, 1989.

33. Kuchar DL, Thorburn CW, Sammel NL. Signal-averaged electrocardiogram for evaluation of recurrent syncope. *Am J Cardiol* 58:949, 1986.
34. Gomes JA, et al. The prognostic significance of quantitative signal-averaged variables relative to clinical variables, site of myocardial infarction, ejection fraction and ventricular premature beats: A prospective study. *J Am Coll Cardiol* 13:377, 1989.
35. Henry WL, et al. Relation between echocardiographically determined left atrial size and atrial fibrillation. *Circulation* 53:273, 1976.
36. Blackshear JL, et al. Mitral regurgitation decreases risk of thromboembolism in atrial fibrillation–associated left atrial enlargement. *J Am Coll Cardiol* 21:310A, 1993.
37. Pitt B, Strauss WH. Evaluation of ventricular function by radioisotope techniques. *N Engl J Med* 296:1097, 1977.
38. Almquist A, et al. Provocation of bradycardia and hypotension by isoproterenol and upright posture in patients with unexplained syncope. *N Engl J Med* 320:346, 1989.

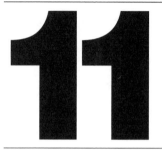

Signal-Averaged Electrocardiography

Stephen C. Vlay

Noninvasive methods of arrhythmia analysis are no longer limited to standard and ambulatory electrocardiography or exercise testing. The ability to record late potentials from carefully filtered ECGs has enhanced the ability to risk-stratify patients at risk for sudden cardiac death. Low-amplitude, high-frequency waveforms and abnormal components of the terminal QRS complex obtained through high-resolution electrocardiography are more likely to be found in patients with ventricular tachycardia (VT) and ventricular fibrillation (VF) than in individuals without risk of these arrhythmias. With current methods, signal averaging is able to distinguish low- and high-risk groups, although it is unable to specify the individual in the high-risk group who will experience the malignant ventricular arrhythmia.

Risk stratification is enhanced by the consideration of other variables, such as left ventricular function and the presence of arrhythmias on ambulatory ECG. The patient with late potentials on the signal-averaged ECG (SAECG), together with a left ventricular ejection fraction of 0.20, nonsustained VT on the Holter monitor, and prior myocardial infarction (MI) is at far greater risk of sudden death than the patient whose only abnormality is the abnormality on SAECG.

Heterogeneity of myocardium increases the distance the electrical impulse must travel, decreases the conduction velocity, and widens the interval between the times that individual islands of myocardium separated by fibrous tissue are activated. As a result, there may be fragmentation of local electrograms. The greater the heterogeneity of tissue is, the more possibilities there are for reentry, the more fragmented the electrogram, and the greater the risk for sustained ventricular arrhythmias. The SAECG represents another method for assessing an anatomic and electrical substrate. As noted in Chapter 1, sudden cardiac death occurs in the presence of an abnormal substrate and a trigger factor; the absence of the trigger factor explains why all patients with abnormal SAECG do not experience this fatal outcome.

Further research and developments are expected to improve the sensitivity and specificity of signal averaging.

I. **Technical aspects.** A task force of the European Society of Cardiology, the American Heart Association, and the American College of Cardiology published standards for analysis of ventricular late potentials using high-resolution or signal-averaged electrocardiography [1]. This scientific statement is a valuable addition to one's library and is the source for the following recommendations.

   A. **Leads and electrodes.** The electrodes of choice are silver–silver chloride since they have the lowest half-cell potential. Noise is one of the most common reasons preventing interpretation of the SAECG. Use alcohol or another solvent to cleanse thoroughly the area where the electrode will be applied, and lightly abrade the site to decrease impedance. It is recommended that impedance be less than 1000 ohms.

   The standard for time domain analysis is the bipolar X,Y,Z system:

   X lead: fourth intercostal space in both midaxillary lines
   Y lead: superior aspect manubrium and upper left leg or iliac crest
   Z lead: fourth intercostal space (V_2 position) and second electrode directly posterior on left side of vertebral column

   The positive leads are the left (X), inferior (Y), and anterior (Z).

   The leads used in the frequency domain analysis are the Frank leads and uncorrected orthogonal leads.

   B. **Amplification.** A low-noise amplifier is used to record ECG signals. Minimum band pass should be 0.5 Hz–250.0 Hz. Voltage calibration should be accurate to +/− 2%.

Range of linearity for input signals should be not less than +/− 2.5 mV. Sample data at not less than 1000 Hz and A/D convert with at least 12-bit precision. Record and convert all ECG leads concurrently.

C. **Signal averaging, noise reduction, and filters.** A template is formed, and newly acquired beats are aligned on the template before averaging. Averaging is calculated in real time. If alignment is not exact (termed *trigger jitter*), high-frequency signals are attenuated. Trigger jitter should be less than 1.0 msec and optimally 0.5 msec.

Noise is measured in the averaged signal over a 40-msec interval in the ST or TP segment with a four-pole Butterworth filter. It is recommended that noise be less than 1 μV with a 25-Hz high-pass cutoff or less than 0.7 μV with a 40-Hz high-pass cutoff as measured by the root mean squared (RMS) method from a vector magnitude of the X, Y, and Z leads.

For time domain analysis, a bidirectional filter with a high-pass corner frequency of 25 or 40 Hz is recommended to avoid artifact. For frequency analysis, the band pass should be 0.05–300.0 Hz. Notch filters (for power line interference) should not be incorporated into the systems hardware or software.

II. Data analysis

A. **Time domain analysis.** This method analyzes the vector magnitude of the filtered leads (square root of $x^2 + y^2 + z^2$), called the *filtered QRS complex*. The end of the filtered QRS complex is defined as the midpoint of a 5-msec segment in which the mean voltage exceeds the mean noise level plus three times the standard deviation of the noise sample. Measured values include:

1. *Filtered QRS duration.* The QRS duration on the SAECG is usually longer than on the standard ECG. Furthermore, it may be longer in patients with late potentials.
2. *Root mean square voltage of terminal 40 msec of filtered QRS.* This determination is made by adding the squares of the ECG signal amplitude at each measured time point and taking the square root of the sum. (RMS > 20 is generally considered normal.)
3. *Time-filtered QRS complex remains less than 40 μV.* The end of the QRS complex is determined and measured backward to the point at which the QRS signal amplitude first reaches 40 μV. (Low-amplitude signals [LAS] < 38 msec is generally considered normal.)

The committee has not yet standardized the definition of a late potential and scoring of the ECG as normal or abnormal and states that each laboratory must define its own normal values. Criteria for the existence of a late potential include:

1. Filtered QRS greater than 114 msec
2. Less than 20 μV of signal in last 40 msec of vector magnitude complex
3. Terminal vector magnitude complex less than 40 μV for more than 38 msec

B. **Frequency analysis.** An alternative method of analysis uses the fast Fourier transform, which provides a complete description of the ECG and information not seen in the output of a particular fixed-band filter. This method estimates scalar-lead spectra of the terminal QRS and ST segment of signal-averaged Frank X,Y,Z or uncorrected orthogonal leads, expressing the results as indexes of the relative contributions of specific frequencies comprising these ECG segments (Fig. 11-1).

Recently a new frequency analysis method, known as *spectral turbulence analysis*, has been described. Spectral analysis measures abnormalities anywhere in the entire QRS complex without dependence on any arbitrarily defined frequency, duration, or amplitude cutoffs. This technique may be used even in patients with bundle branch block [2].

C. **Reproducibility.** Engel found good short-term reproducibility in the measurement of duration in the absence of noise, although measurements of terminal voltage in the temporal domain were less consistent [3]. In the frequency domain, noise was critical to consistent voltage measurements but did not appreciably influence variation in duration [4]. Another study of immediate reproducibility (10 minutes apart) determined that the reproducibility of a normal or abnormal SAECG was high [5]. The highest reproducibility was noted with QRS duration. Terminal RMS voltage and low-amplitude signals varied by 13% and 7%, respectively. Moser et al. found that for individual parameters (QRS duration, terminal QRS RMS voltage, and terminal QRS low-amplitude signal duration), the incidence of false-positive tests ranged from 2% to 41% [6]. However, there were no false-positive tests for the combi-

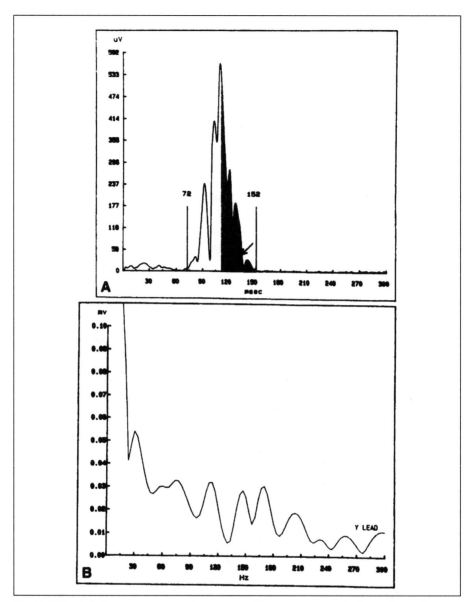

Fig. 11-1. Tracings from a representative patient with recurrent ventricular tachycardia whose signal-averaged ECG was normal when analyzed in the temporal domain *(A)*. A 25- to 250-Hz band-pass filter, high-frequency QRS was 80 ms, low-amplitude signals <40 µV was 16 ms (the *arrow* indicates where the QRS complex is last 40 µV), and root mean square voltage of the terminal 40 ms was 187 µV (filled-in portion of the QRS complex). However, when the tracing is analyzed in the frequency domain (as in *B*, which shows a representative lead), there is an excess of voltage >60 Hz. Mean high-frequency area was 0.8281 mV and 60 to 120 Hz/0–120 Hz was 0.0780 (7.8%), both indicating a risk for ventricular tachycardia. (From DL Pierce et al. Fast Fourier transformation of the entire low-amplitude late QRS potential to predict ventricular tachycardia. *J Am Coll Cardiol* 14:1731–1740, 1989. Reprinted with permission.)

nation of abnormal QRS duration plus either RMS voltage or low-amplitude signal duration. In this study, measurements were repeated after 6.4 months and were highly reproducible at all filter settings.

Recent data from Malik et al. indicate that reproducibility was higher for the time domain method than for spectral temporal mapping [7] (Fig. 11-2). In a series of reports from this same laboratory, time domain analysis identified patients with VT with significantly fewer false-positive results than either frequency analysis or spectral temporal mapping [8] (Fig. 11-3). These latter two techniques did not improve identification of postinfarction patients with VT and without bundle branch block. For the prediction of arrhythmic events after MI, time domain analysis was superior to spectral temporal analysis [9].

The latest report indicates that individual lead analysis can enhance the sensitivity of the SAECG by 10%. Lander et al. studied 73 patients without structural heart disease and 63 patients with VT [10]. The filtered QRS duration and amplitude of the terminal 40 msec of the QRS are related and were not considered independent measurements. The amplitude of the terminal 40 msec correlated with residual noise level. Noise reduction was unpredictable during averaging. They recommended a residual noise level of 0.2–0.3 µV RMS for maximizing sensitivity for VT. Furthermore, these investigators found that age and sex could be factored into criteria for VT risk assessment. Normal men had a longer QRS duration by an average of 8.7 msec, possibly because male hearts are larger and ventricular depolarization may take longer. In VT patients, women had a longer QRS duration by 8.0 msec, but the women they studied were significantly older. Also noted in the VT patients was the fact that the site of infarction influenced QRS duration.

III. Signal averaging in specific cardiac disorders

A. Coronary artery disease and myocardial infarction.
Solomon and Tracey reported that an abnormal SAECG in patients without known cardiac disease was predictive of underlying coronary artery disease [11]. The parameters suggestive of this condition included a filtered QRS greater than or equal to 100 msec, an RMS voltage below 50 µV, and low-amplitude signal duration over 28 msec. The sensitivity (62–76%), specificity (74–89%), and positive predictive value (75–87%) were able to distinguish this population from those without coronary disease. However, Turitto et al. found that transient myocardial ischemia did not generate a substrate for late potentials on the SAECG [12].

Winters et al. found that signal averaging was useful in the identification of patients with nonsustained VT or high-grade ventricular ectopy who will have inducible sustained VT during electrophysiology study [13]. Inducibility was unlikely in patients with a normal SAECG. Spontaneous sustained VT was unlikely in survivors of acute MI with a normal SAECG who were noninducible at EPS despite complex ventricular ectopy or nonsustained VT. Gomes et al. reported that the predictive value of the SAECG in patients with anterior wall MI was higher than that of ejection fraction [14] (Fig. 11-4). For inferior wall MI, the predictive value of both tests was equivalent. The most significant independent predictor of an arrhythmic event was the duration of the signal-averaged QRS complex followed by ventricular couplets and ejection fraction. Hammill et al. also concluded that SAECG was a better predictor than ejection fraction, but combining the two values increased the predictive accuracy [15]. In the study by Rodriguez et al., the strongest predictor of sustained VT or VF was the left ventricular ejection fraction, followed by the duration of the QRS complex on SAECG measured during the first 3 days of MI [16]. Sudden death was only predicted by left ventricular ejection fraction.

Thus, several studies provide conflicting data about which factor is the strongest predictor. Noteworthy, however, is that in each study, abnormalities on the SAECG were either the most important or second in importance (Fig. 11-5). Ho et al. attempted to increase sensitivity (to 70%) by using a 28-lead optimal array [17]. In this relatively young field, enhanced sensitivity should be expected to increase with improvements in methods of analysis and with combination of variables.

Farrell et al. found that impaired heart rate variability, late potentials, and repetitive ventricular forms were independent predictors of arrhythmic events in survivors of acute MI [18] (Fig. 11-6). These authors concluded that this combination of variables greatly improved the sensitivity over that of earlier studies. The combination of impaired heart rate variability and late potentials had a sensitivity of 58%, a positive predictive accuracy of 33%, and a relative risk of 18.5 for arrhythmic events. Further studies from this same laboratory evaluated the ability to predict sudden

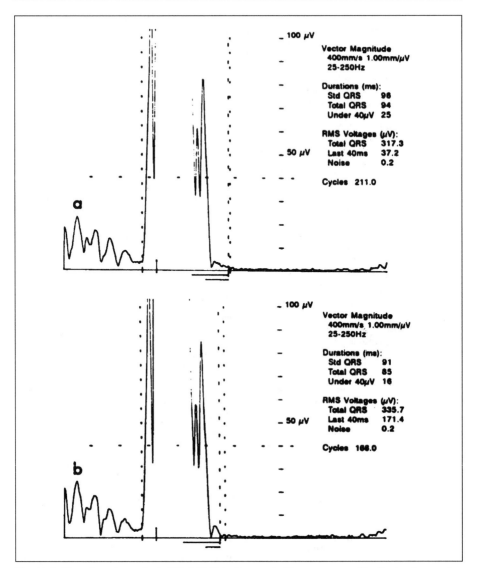

Fig. 11-2. Time domain analysis (25–250 Hz) of two recordings, separated by 5 minutes, made in a 28-year-old healthy male volunteer. The noise levels were equal in both recordings, and in both the duration of the standard (Std) QRS complex measured by the computerized algorithm was longer than the duration of the total QRS complex. The values for total QRS duration and terminal low-amplitude signal duration differed in both by 9 ms, whereas the terminal root-mean-square voltage (RMS) changed from 37.2 µV in recording *a* to 171.4 µV in recording *b*. (From M Malik et al, Frequency vs time domain analysis of signal-averaged electrocardiograms. I. Reproducibility of the results. *J Am Coll Cardiol* 20:127–134, 1992. Reprinted with permission.)

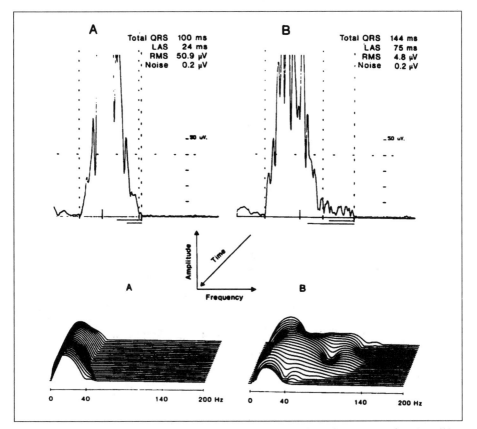

Fig. 11-3. Time domain and spectral temporal mapping recordings from a control patient *(A)* and from a patient with ventricular tachycardia *(B)*. The upper panel shows the time domain analysis. In the control patient *(A)* the recording is normal, whereas in the patient with ventricular tachycardia *(B)*, all time domain indexes are abnormal: late potentials are clearly visible at the end of the QRS complex and in the ST segment. The lower panel shows the spectral temporal maps obtained from the same patients. The frequency axis, ranging from 0 to 200 Hz, is horizontal, the amplitude axis is vertical, and the time axis is diagonal. The cutoff level is 0 dB. In the control patient *(A)* there was no frequency content between 40 and 140 Hz, and the factor of normality was 92%. In the patient with ventricular tachycardia, high-frequency components are present in the first 21 segments, whereas the last 4 segments show only low-frequency components characteristic for the ST segment. The normality factor is 9%. (LAS = low-amplitude signals; RMS = root-mean-square voltage of the last 40 ms of the QRS complex; total QRS = total QRS duration.) (From P Kulakowski et al, Frequency versus time domain analysis of signal-averaged electrocardiograms. II. Identification of patients with ventricular tachycardia after myocardial infarction. *J Am Coll Cardiol* 20:135–143, 1992. Reprinted with permission.)

death and VT [19]. For a sensitivity of 70%, the positive predictive accuracy was 31% for sudden death and 13% for VT. Recently in a stepwise logistic regression analysis, Nogami et al. found only low-amplitude signal duration under 30 µV (with a high pass filter setting, 80 Hz) and area ratio as independent predictors of sustained monomorphic VT [20]. They calculated 93% sensitivity, 81% specificity, and 72% positive and 95% negative predictive value, with an overall 85% predictive accuracy. Huikuri et al. also noted that spontaneous episodes of VT are preceded by changes in heart rate variability in the frequency domain [21].

Attempts to correlate abnormalities on the SAECG with success of reperfusion remain indecisive. Tranchesi et al. concluded that successful thrombolysis reduces the incidence of late potentials on SAECG but that the sensitivity and specificity

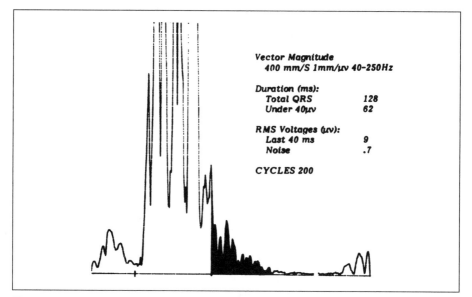

Fig. 11-4. Vector magnitude of a patient with an anterior wall infarction and an arrhythmic event. All quantitative signal-averaged ECG variables are abnormal. The total duration of the signal-averaged QRS complex is 128 ms, the duration of low-amplitude signals (*shaded area*) is 62 ms, and the root-mean-square (RMS) voltage of the terminal 40 ms is 9 µV. (From JA Gomes et al, The prognostic significance of quantitative signal-averaged variables relative to clinical variables, site of myocardial infarction, ejection fraction and ventricular premature beats: A prospective study. *J Am Coll Cardiol* 13:377–384, 1989. Reprinted with permission.)

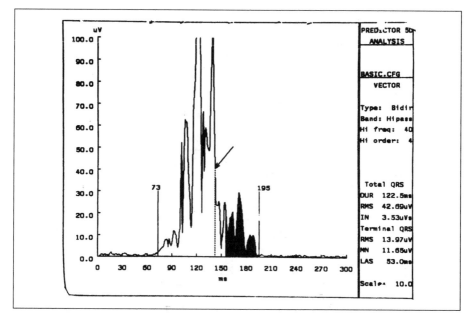

Fig. 11-5. Signal-averaged ECG from a 76-year-old male with coronary artery disease and recurrent episodes of symptomatic sustained ventricular tachycardia. He has an ischemic cardiomyopathy with a left ventricular ejection fraction of 0.46. The QRS is prolonged, the root mean square is low, and late potentials are present.

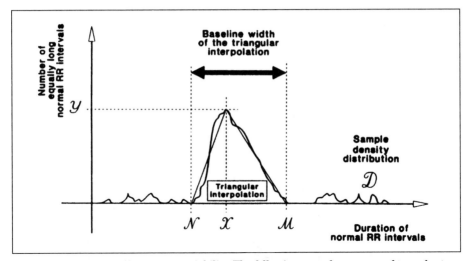

Fig. 11-6. Calculation of heart rate variability. The following procedure was used to evaluate heart rate variability from 24-hour ECG recordings: Two-channel 24-hour ECG recordings (modified leads III and CM_5) were made with use of a Tracker recorder (Reynolds Medical Ltd.). A commercially available system for long-term ECG analysis (Pathfinder III, Mk 2, Reynolds Medical Ltd.) was used to obtain the sequence of duration of intervals between adjacent QRS complexes of normal "supraventricular" morphology for each patient.

With this system, the duration of normal R–R intervals is measured on a discrete scale with the step of 1/128 second (~8 ms). This permitted the probability function D of the sample to be constructed by assigning the total number $D(w)$ of normal R–R intervals with the duration of w to each length w.

The maximal value $Y = D(X)$ of the function D was found:

$$Y = D(X) = {}_w^{\max} D(w).$$

Then the values N and M, $N < M$ are found, for which the sum

$$\sum_w [D(w) - T_{N,M}(w)]^2 dw$$

attained a minimum, where $T_{N,M}$ is the triangular linear function with values found by numeric approximation:

$$T_{N,M}(w) = 0, \qquad\qquad \text{for } w \leq N \text{ or } w \geq M$$

$$T_{N,M}(w) = y \left(\frac{w - N}{X - N} \right), \qquad \text{for } N < w \leq X$$

$$T_{N,M}(w) = y \left(\frac{M - w}{M - X} \right), \qquad \text{for } X < w \leq M$$

(From TG Farrell et al, Risk stratification for arrhythmic events in postinfarction patients based on heart rate variability, ambulatory electrocardiographic variables and the signal-averaged electrocardiogram. *J Am Coll Cardiol* 18:687–697, 1991. Reprinted with permission.)

were not high enough to allow reliable bedside monitoring of reperfusion [22]. Malik et al. noted that SAECG after acute MI was less informative in patients who had received thrombolytic therapy [23]. Chillou et al. noted that the incidence of abnormalities on the SAECG was not reduced by an early opening of the culprit vessel by percutaneous transluminal coronary angioplasty (PTCA) [24]. Ragosta et al. observed that among patients with successful reperfusion, those without late potentials at baseline had a greater extent of improved wall motion than those with late potentials [25]. They suggested that a normal SAECG in patients with a totally occluded coronary artery may signify the presence of viable myocardium. In reviewing these last four studies, it may be possible to explain some of the differences by

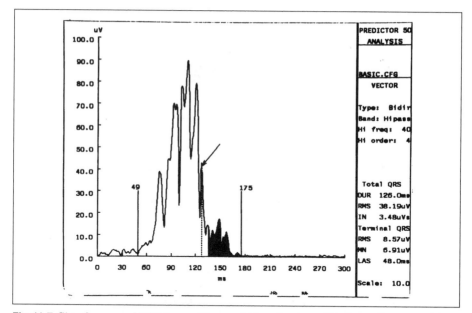

Fig. 11-7. Signal-averaged ECG from a 57-year-old female who suffered a cardiac arrest. Her coronary arteries are normal, but she has a nonischemic cardiomyopathy with a left ventricular ejection of 0.47. The QRS is prolonged, the root mean square is low, and late potentials are present.

the fact that abnormalities reflect viability of myocardium (which in turn affects activation) rather than the patency of a coronary artery.

B. **Signal-averaged electrocardiograms in cardiomyopathies.** In patients with **hypertrophic cardiomyopathy,** Cripps et al. found no association between an abnormal SAECG, a family history of premature sudden cardiac death, a history of syncope, symptomatic status, maximal left ventricular wall thickness, the presence of systolic anterior motion of the mitral valve, or the maximal rate of oxygen uptake on exercise [26]. However, in the four subjects in this study who had a cardiac arrest, three had an abnormal SAECG. The authors calculated a sensitivity of 50%, a specificity of 93%, and predictive accuracy of 77% for detecting patients with electrical instability.

Several studies have evaluated SAECG in patients with **nonischemic dilated cardiomyopathy.** Middelkauff et al. found that the incidence of arrhythmia substrate's producing late potentials depended on the etiology of the heart failure in the patient [27]. Keeling et al. observed that late potentials were seen more often in patients with as compared to without VT and in patients with sustained versus nonsustained VT, but the differences were not significant [28]. Time domain and spectral temporal mapping analysis were highly specific but had a low sensitivity. Mancini et al. reported that nonischemic cardiomyopathy patients with an abnormal SAECG had a statistically significant increase in sustained arrhythmias and/or sudden death over patients with a normal ECG or bundle branch block [29]. The prognosis of patients with a normal SAECG in this population suffered their adverse outcome from progressive heart failure (Fig. 11-7).

C. **Signal-averaged electrocardiogram in other conditions.** Jabi et al. performed SAECG in patients with **mitral valve prolapse** in the absence of other underlying heart disease [30]. Late potentials were a common and benign finding. As with other tests, the interpretation of the SAECG must be performed with the knowledge of the prevalence of disease in the population (Fig. 11-8).

Yotsukura et al. studied the SAECG in patients with **Duchenne's muscular dystrophy** [31]. Late potentials were associated with left ventricular dysfunction and may have represented the extent of myocardial derangement in this disease process. Sustained VT was not observed, but 3 of 66 patients had nonsustained VT.

Zimmerman et al. evaluated patients after surgical repair of **tetralogy of Fallot** [32]. The presence of both spontaneous ventricular ectopy and ventricular late

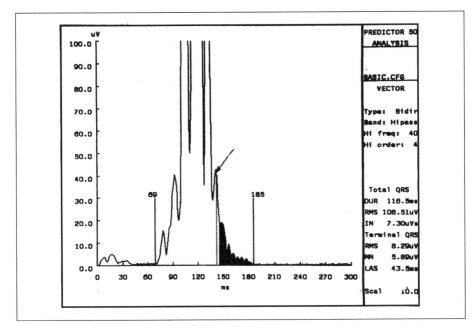

Fig. 11-8. Signal-averaged ECG from a 35-year-old female with mitral valve prolapse, mitral regurgitation, near-syncope, and inducible sustained ventricular tachycardia. The QRS is slightly prolonged, the root mean square is low, and late potentials are present.

potentials was associated with an increased incidence of inducible VT. If these factors were absent, the patient had a low risk of subsequent ventricular arrhythmias.

D. **Signal-averaged electrocardiograms in patients with bundle branch block.** Prolongation of the QRS by bundle branch block interferes with the detection of late potentials and makes the SAECG difficult to interpret. Lindsay et al. attempted to use frequency domain analysis (fast Fourier transform) to assist in the interpretation of the SAECG in patients with bundle branch block and were able to differentiate patients with and without VT [33]. Buckingham et al. used frequency domain analysis by the use of power law scaling [34]. This technique plots the power spectrum of the entire SAECG on a plot of log power versus log frequency and determines the slope by least-squares regression. Sensitivity, specificity, positive and negative predictive values, and predictive accuracy were superior to time domain analyses. Further improvements in the analysis of the SAECG in patients with bundle branch block will likely come from refinements of frequency domain rather than from time domain analysis.

E. **Effect of antiarrhythmic drugs on the signal-averaged electrocardiogram.** Signal averaging is a relatively new technique, so evaluation of drug effect on the SAECG has been limited. Freedman et al. reported that sotalol can alter QRS and late potential duration [35]. Prolongation of either the QRS or late potential duration may reflect slowing of conduction by sotalol.

Kulakowski et al. noted that procainamide prolonged the total and initial QRS complex and low-amplitude signal durations while the RMS voltage of the terminal QRS complex and the last 40 msec of the QRS was significantly reduced [36]. Procainamide prevented inducibility of sustained VT or prolonged the cycle length by over 100 msec. The fractional prolongation of the total QRS duration was greater in responders than in nonresponders and identified responders with a sensitivity of 94%, a specificity of 87%, and an overall predictive accuracy of 90% (Figs. 11-9, 11-10).

The studies with sotalol and procainamide should be considered preliminary, although promising, data. Further study is needed before we can completely understand the meaning of drug-induced changes on the SAECG and their implications for therapy.

IV. **Recommendations.** Signal averaging remains a promising new technique that will undergo further refinement to increase its sensitivity and specificity. It is useful in the risk stratification of patients with MI. A normal SAECG predicts a low risk of

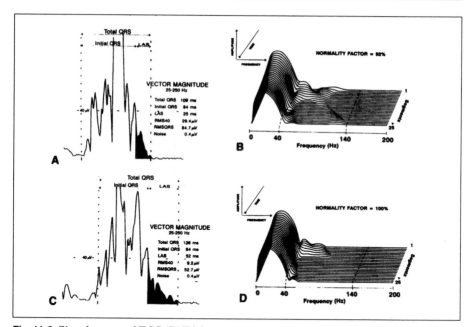

Fig. 11-9. Signal-averaged ECG (SAECG) recordings from a patient with an anterolateral infarction. The baseline time domain SAECG was normal *(A)*, and the results of the spectral temporal mapping were within normal limits (e.g., the normality factor in lead Z was 92%) *(B)*. Procainamide prevented inducibility of sustained ventricular tachycardia. After drug administration, all conventional time domain SAECG indexes became abnormal *(C)*. The prolongation of the total QRS duration (the fractional increase was 25%) was caused by prolongation of the low-amplitude signal duration, whereas the duration of the initial QRS complex remained unchanged. The results of the spectral temporal mapping were similar to those of the baseline recording (the normality factor in lead Z was 100%) *(D)*. (LAS = low-amplitude signal duration; RMS40 = the root-mean-square voltage of the last 40 ms of the QRS complex; RMSQRS = the root-mean-square voltage of the total QRS complex.) (From P Kulakowski et al, Effects of procainamide on the signal-averaged electrocardiogram in relation to the results of programmed ventricular stimulation in patients with sustained monomorphic ventricular tachycardia. *J Am Coll Cardiol* 21:1428–1439, 1993. Reprinted with permission.)

recurrent sustained ventricular arrhythmias. An abnormal SAECG indicates that the patient is in a higher-risk group but does not identify the individual who will suffer sudden death. Based on pooled data, 14–29% of patients recovering from MI with abnormal SAECG will experience sustained VT within 1 year, compared with only 0.8–4.5% of those whose SAECG is normal (standards for analysis of ventricular late potentials using high-resolution or signal-averaged electrocardiography) [1]. In this same population, another 3.6–4.0% of patients with late potentials will die suddenly, compared to 0–4.3% without late potentials. In terms of timing, there are data to suggest that obtaining the SAECG during the second week after MI may have the highest predictive accuracy.

The SAECG is useful in the risk stratification of patients with remote MI and those with nonsustained VT. In the evaluation of syncope, patients with abnormal SAECG are more likely to have inducible sustained VT during programmed electrical stimulation. However, the utility of the SAECG in syncope as well as other disorders such as cardiomyopathy has not yet been fully defined. Ongoing studies are evaluating the benefit in detecting rejection in patients with cardiac transplants.

Combining data from SAECG with other variables such as left ventricular ejection fraction increases sensitivity and specificity. Frequency domain methods of analysis improve the interpretation of the SAECG in specific problems, such as bundle branch block. Signal averaging should be viewed as another technique to evaluate and risk-stratify the patient with ventricular arrhythmias. In appropriate

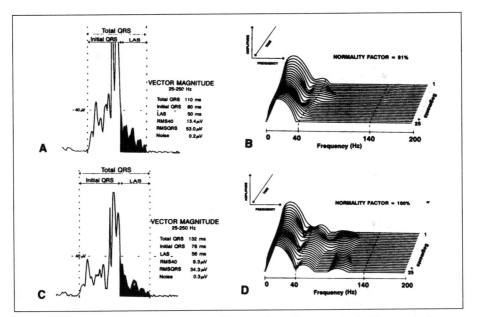

Fig. 11-10. The signal-averaged ECG (SAECG) recordings from a patient with an anterior infarction. The baseline time domain SAECG was abnormal *(A)*, whereas results of the spectral temporal mapping were within normal limits (for example, the normality factor in lead X was 91%) *(B)*. Procainamide prevented inducibility of sustained ventricular tachycardia. On the time domain SAECG *(C)*, the total QRS duration was prolonged by the drug by 22 ms (the fractional increase of 20%). The initial QRS prolongation was greater than the low-amplitude signal prolongation (17 vs. 6 ms, or 27% vs. 12%). The results of spectral temporal mapping were similar to those of the baseline recording (the normality factor in lead Z was 100%) *(D)*. Abbreviations as in Fig. 11-9. (From P Kulakowski et al, Effects of procainamide on the signal-averaged electrocardiogram in relation to the results of programmed ventricular stimulation in patients with sustained monomorphic ventricular tachycardia. *J Am Coll Cardiol* 21:1428–1439, 1993. Reprinted with permission.)

patients, it may identify who would benefit from further evaluation, such as electrophysiology study.

References

1. Breithardt G, et al. Standards for analysis of ventricular late potentials using high resolution or signal-averaged electrocardiography. *Circulation* 83:1481–1488, 1991.
2. Kelen GJ, et al. Spectral turbulence analysis of the signal-averaged electrocardiogram and its predictive accuracy for inducible sustained monomorphic ventricular tachycardia. *Am Heart J* 67:965–975, 1991.
3. Engel TR. High-frequency electrocardiography: Diagnosis of arrhythmia risk. *Am Heart J* 118:1302–1316, 1989.
4. Engel TR, Pierce DL, Patil KD. Reproducibility of the signal-averaged electrocardiogram. *Am Heart J* 122:1652–1660, 1991.
5. Sager PT, et al. A prospective evaluation of the immediate reproducibility of the signal-averaged ECG. *Am Heart J* 121:1671–1678, 1991.
6. Moser DK, Stevenson WG, Woo MA. Optimal late potential criteria for reducing false positive signal-averaged electrocardiograms. *Am Heart J* 123:412–416, 1992.
7. Malik M, et al. Frequency vs time domain analysis of signal-averaged electrocardiograms. I. Reproducibility of the results. *J Am Coll Cardiol* 20:127–134, 1992.
8. Kulakowski P, et al. Frequency versus time domain analysis of signal-averaged electrocardiograms. II. Identification of patients with ventricular tachycardia after myocardial infarction. *J Am Coll Cardiol* 20:135–143, 1992.

9. Odemuyiwa O, et al. Frequency versus time domain analysis of signal-averaged electro-cardiograms. III. Stratification of postinfarction patients for arrhythmic events. *J Am Coll Cardiol* 20:144–150, 1992.
10. Lander P, et al. Critical analysis of the signal-averaged electrocardiogram. *Circulation* 87:105–117, 1993.
11. Solomon AJ, Tracey CM. The signal-averaged electrocardiogram in predicting coronary artery disease. *Am Heart J* 122:1334–1339, 1991.
12. Turitto G, et al. Spontaneous myocardial ischemia and the signal-averaged electrocardiogram. *Am J Cardiol* 67:676–680, 1991.
13. Winters SL, et al. Role of signal averaging of the surface QRS complex in selecting patients with nonsustained ventricular tachycardia and high grade ventricular arrhythmias for programmed ventricular stimulation. *J Am Coll Cardiol* 12:1481–1487, 1988.
14. Gomes JA, et al. The prognostic significance of quantitative signal-average variables relative to clinical variables, site of myocardial infarction, ejection fraction and ventricular premature beats: A prospective study. *J Am Coll Cardiol* 13:377–384, 1989.
15. Hamill SC, et al. Establishment of signal-averaged electrocardiographic criteria with Frank XYZ leads and spectral filter used alone and in combination with ejection fraction to predict inducible ventricular tachycardia in coronary artery disease. *Am J Cardiol* 70:316–320, 1992.
16. Rodriguez LM, et al. Time course and prognostic significance of serial signal-averaged electrocardiograms after a first acute myocardial infarction. *Am J Cardiol* 66:1199–1202, 1990.
17. Ho DSW, et al. Signal-averaged electrocardiogram: Improved identification of patients with ventricular tachycardia using a 28-lead optimal array. *Circulation* 87:857–865, 1993.
18. Farrell TG, et al. Risk stratification for arrhythmic events in postinfarction patients based on heart rate variability, ambulatory electrocardiographic variables and the signal-averaged electrocardiogram. *J Am Coll Cardiol* 18:687–697, 1991.
19. Odemuyiwa O, et al. Differences between predictive characteristics of signal averaged ECG variables for postinfarction sudden death and ventricular tachycardia. *Am J Cardiol* 69:1186, 1992.
20. Nogami A, et al. Combined use of time and frequency domain variables in signal-averaged ECG as a predictor of inducible sustained monomorphic ventricular tachycardia in myocardial infarction. *Circulation* 86:780–789, 1992.
21. Huikuri HV, et al. Frequency domain measures of heart rate variability before the onset of nonsustained and sustained ventricular tachycardia in patients with coronary artery disease. *Circulation* 87:1220–1228, 1993.
22. Tranchesi B, et al. Usefulness of high-frequency analysis of signal-averaged surface electrocardiograms in acute myocardial infarction before and after coronary thrombolysis for assessing coronary reperfusion. *Am J Cardiol* 66:1196–1198, 1990.
23. Malik M, et al. Effect of thrombolytic therapy on the predictive value of signal-averaged electrocardiography after acute myocardial infarction. *Am J Cardiol* 70:21–25, 1992.
24. de Chillou C, et al. Effects on the signal-averaged electrocardiogram of the opening the coronary artery by thrombolytic therapy or percutaneous transluminal coronary angioplasty during acute myocardial infarction. *Am J Cardiol* 71:805–809, 1993.
25. Ragosta M, et al. Effects of late (1–30 days) reperfusion after acute myocardial infarction on the signal-averaged electrocardiogram. *Am J Cardiol* 71:19–23, 1993.
26. Cripps TR, et al. Signal-averaged electrocardiography in hypertrophic cardiomyopathy. *J Am Coll Cardiol* 15:956–961, 1990.
27. Middlekauff HR, et al. Comparison of frequency of late potentials in idiopathic dilated cardiomyopathy and ischemic cardiomyopathy with advanced congestive heart failure and their usefulness in predicting sudden death. *Am J Cardiol* 66:1113–1117, 1990.
28. Keeling PJ, et al. Usefulness of signal-averaged electrocardiogram in idiopathic dilated cardiomyopathy for identifying patients with ventricular arrhythmias. *Am J Cardiol* 72:78–84, 1993.
29. Mancini DM, Wong KL, Simson MB. Prognostic value of an abnormal signal-averaged electrocardiogram in patients with nonischemic congestive cardiomyopathy. *Circulation* 87:1083–1092, 1993.
30. Jabi H, et al. Late potentials in mitral valve prolapse. *Am Heart J* 122:1340–1345, 1991.
31. Yotsukura M, et al. Late potentials in progressive dystrophy of the Duchenne type. *Am Heart J* 121:1137–1142, 1991.
32. Zimmerman M, et al. Ventricular late potentials and induced ventricular arrhythmias after surgical repair of tetralogy of Fallot. *Am J Cardiol* 67:873–878, 1991.

33. Lindsay BD, et al. Identification of patients with sustained ventricular tachycardia by frequency analysis of signal-averaged electrocardiograms despite the presence of bundle branch block. *Circulation* 77:122–130, 1988.

34. Buckingham TA, et al. Power law analysis of the signal-averaged electrocardiogram for identification of patients with ventricular tachycardia: Effect of bundle branch block. *Am Heart J* 124:1220–1225, 1992.

35. Freedman RA, et al. Effects of sotalol on the signal averaged ECG in patients with sustained ventricular tachycardia: relation to suppression of inducibility and changes in tachycardia cycle length. *J Am Coll Cardiol* 20:1213, 1992.

36. Kulakowski P, et al. Effects of procainamide on the signal-averaged electrocardiogram in relation to the results of programmed ventricular stimulation in patients with sustained monomorphic ventricular tachycardia. *J Am Coll Cardiol* 21:1428–1439, 1993.

Bibliography

Deshmukh P, Winters SL, Gomes JA. Frequency and significance of occult late potentials on the signal-averaged elecrocardiogram in sustained ventricular tachycardia after healing of acute myocardial infarction. *Am J Cardiol* 67:806–811, 1991.

Jarrett JR, Flowers NC. Signal-averaged electrocardiography: History, techniques and clinical applications. *Clin Cardiology* 14:984–994, 1991.

Kennedy HL, Bavishi NS, Buckingham TA. Ambulatory (Holter) electrocardiography signal-averaging: A current perspective. *Am Heart J* 124:1339–1346, 1992.

Kremers MS, et al. Electrocardiographic signal-averaging during atrial pacing and effect of cycle length on the terminal QRS in patients with and without inducible ventricular tachycardia. *Am J Cardiol* 66:1095–1098, 1990.

McClements BM, Adgey AAJ. Value of signal-averaged electrocardiography, radionuclide ventriculography, Holter monitoring and clinical variables for prediction of arrhythmic events in survivors of acute myocardial infarction in the thrombolytic era. *J Am Coll Cardiol* 21:1419–1427, 1993.

Odemuyiwa O, et al. Differences between predictive characteristics of signal-averaged electrocardiographic variables for postinfarction sudden death and ventricular tachycardia. *Am J Cardiol* 1186–1192, 1992.

12

Electrophysiologic Testing

Stephen C. Vlay

Electrophysiologic testing is a complicated procedure that must be performed only by a clinician adequately trained and skilled in its performance. The treatment of rhythm disturbances was, to a large extent, empiric until the advent of invasive electrophysiologic testing. Initially, when measurement of only the His potential was routinely performed, the data obtained were used to assist in the decision to implant a permanent pacemaker. Certainly for most symptomatic patients who already had bradyarrhythmias, pauses, or heart block documented on the ECG, the His bundle study was not indicated. The value of recording intracardiac potentials in an individual whose arrhythmia could not be adequately diagnosed from the surface ECG soon became apparent. The best example is the situation of a wide-complex tachycardia in which P waves or atrioventricular (AV) dissociation cannot be demonstrated. Is the rhythm sinus with aberrant conduction or bundle branch block, an AV nodal reentrant tachycardia in a patient with bundle branch block, a reciprocating tachycardia with AV reentry, or ventricular tachycardia (VT)? Recording the His potential is helpful in making some of these distinctions but certainly not sufficient for evaluating all possibilities. With additional catheter electrodes in other locations and the observation that some arrhythmias could be induced and terminated by pacing, the era of programmed electrical stimulation (PES) began. Much of the methodology was made possible by basic electrophysiologic research.

I. **Indications for electrophysiologic studies (EPS).** Today there are four major conditions in which clinical electrophysiologic testing is commonly used [1–5]: (1) ventricular arrhythmias, (2) supraventricular arrhythmias, (3) conduction disturbances, and (4) syncope (when an exhaustive evaluation of other causes proves negative and there is a strong suspicion of one of the first three possibilities). New drugs are also evaluated by electrophysiologic testing. Assessment of patients who have survived VT or ventricular fibrillation (VF) and those with symptomatic supraventricular tachycardia (SVT) is the most frequent reason for referral to the clinical electrophysiologist [6]. Table 12-1 lists the indications for the procedure.

A. **General guidelines.** Guidelines for clinical intracardiac EPS were established in 1988 by a joint task force of the American College of Cardiology and the American Heart Association [7]:

Type I: Conditions for which there is general agreement that EPS provides information that is useful and important for patient management.

Type II: Conditions for which EPS is frequently performed but the usefulness of the information is less certain.

Type III: Conditions for which EPS does not provide useful information and is not warranted.

Every electrophysiology laboratory will determine which of the type II indications it will accept for study.

1. **Type I and type II**

a. **Patients with sinus node dysfunction.** The type I indication is for asymptomatic patients in whom sinus node dysfunction is suspected, but a causal relation between symptoms and sinus bradycardia, sinus pauses, or sinus node exit block cannot be documented by noninvasive means. Type II indications include the necessity for assessing antegrade and retrograde AV conduction when a pacemaker is indicated; to determine the severity or mechanism of sinus node dysfunction when it will affect therapy; and to exclude other mechanisms of arrhythmia when it is uncertain that the symptoms are due to sinus node dysfunction.

b. **Patients with acquired AV block.** The type I indication is for symptomatic patients (syncope or near-syncope) in whom His-Purkinje block is suspected but has not been documented by noninvasive means. In addition, patients with second- or third-degree AV block who remain symptomatic despite a pacemaker and in whom VT is suspected merit EPS. The type II indication involves EPS to determine the site or mechanism of AV block to guide therapy and to exclude pseudo AV block caused by concealed junctional extrasystoles.

c. **Patients with chronic intraventricular conduction delay (bundle branch block)** whose symptoms (syncope, near-syncope) are thought to be related to ventricular arrhythmia. EPS is a type I indication. The type II indication is when EPS may determine the site or severity of block and assist therapeutic decisions or assess prognosis.

d. **Patients with a narrow-complex tachycardia** (<120 msec) who have frequent, poorly tolerated, or poorly responsive to therapy. The type I indication is for EPS to document the origin, mechanism, and electrophysiological properties of the tachycardia. In addition, patients who prefer ablative therapy merit EPS. The type II indication applies when there is concern about the effects of antiarrhythmic drug therapy on the sinus node or AV conduction.

e. **Patients with symptomatic sustained wide-complex tachycardia.** EPS has a type I indication when the diagnosis is unclear and appropriate management is necessary. A type II indication is to evaluate the possibility of multiple bypass tracts in patients with suspected preexcitation and antidromic tachycardia.

f. **Patients with the long Q–T syndrome.** There is no type I indication. The type II indication involves identification of a proarrhythmic effect of antiarrhythmic drugs in the patient who has experienced the first episode of cardiac arrest or sustained VT while on the drug.

g. **Patients with Wolff-Parkinson-White (WPW) syndrome** with life-threatening or incapacitating arrhythmias or drug intolerance. EPS has a type I indication when nonpharmacologic treatment (e.g., ablation) is considered. Type II indications include obtaining information about the type of arrhythmia, localization, number and electrophysiologic properties of one or more accessory pathways, and determining the effect of antiarrhythmic drugs; evaluating asymptomatic patients with WPW syndrome involved in a high-risk profession or in whom there is a family history of premature sudden death; and when patients with WPW syndrome are undergoing cardiac surgery for other reasons.

h. **Patients with unexplained syncope.** EPS has a type I indication when the reason for syncope remains obscure despite noninvasive evaluation and the

Table 12-1. Indications for electrophysiologic study

1. Sudden cardiac arrest (ventricular fibrillation) not associated with acute myocardial infarction
2. Sustained ventricular tachycardia not associated with acute myocardial infarction
3. Severely symptomatic supraventricular tachycardia, particularly in Wolff-Parkinson-White syndrome (and with a very rapid ventricular rate) or in cases that have proved refractory to empiric drug therapy
4. Symptomatic cases in which ventricular tachycardia is strongly suspected but not documented
5. Syncope of unknown etiology after all other causes, including vascular, neurologic, and metabolic, have been completely excluded, and a comprehensive cardiac evaluation has been unrevealing
6. Diagnosis of an unknown tachyarrhythmia
7. Evaluation of a conduction disturbance in which the decision to implant a permanent pacemaker cannot easily be made on the basis of history and noninvasive testing
8. Evaluation of drug therapy for refractory arrhythmia
9. Evaluaton of mechanism and mapping prior to radiofrequency catheter ablation
10. Evaluation before and after implantation of an internal cardioverter-defibrillator device
11. Mapping prior to arrhythmia surgery

patient has known or suspected structural heart disease. The type II indication is the same except that structural heart disease is absent.

i. **Survivors of cardiac arrest.** EPS has a type I indication when there is no evidence of an acute Q wave myocardial infarction (MI) or if the arrest occurs more than 48 hours after acute MI. The type II indication is when the cardiac arrest is due to a bradyarrhythmia.

j. **Patients with unexplained palpitations.** The type I indication is documented inappropriate heart rate (usually >150 beats/minute) when the ECG fails to provide the diagnosis. The type II indication is when there is no documentation.

k. **EPS to guide drug therapy.** This use receives a type I indication for VT/VF not associated within 48 hours of acute MI or associated with the long Q–T syndrome, particularly if the patient has infrequent ectopy; WPW syndrome with atrial fibrillation associated with a rapid ventricular response, a short antegrade refractory period or cardiac arrest, or recurrent symptomatic reciprocating tachycardias unresponsive to empiric drug therapy; and finally for AV nodal reentrant tachycardia unresponsive to empiric drug therapy.

   Type II indications include recurrent symptomatic paroxysmal atrial fibrillation not prevented by empiric antiarrhythmic therapy; recurrent symptomatic inducible sinoatrial nodal reentrant tachycardia, intraatrial reentry, and ectopic atrial tachycardia unresponsive to empiric therapy; recurrent, nonsustained VT not associated with acute MI or the long Q–T syndrome; identification of proarrhythmia in patients experiencing the first episode of cardiac arrest or sustained VT on the drug; and risk stratification and consideration of therapy for the post-MI patient with reduced left ventricular function, frequent ventricular ectopy including nonsustained VT, especially if the signal-averaged ECG demonstrates late potentials.

l. **Patients who are candidates for or who have implantable electrical devices for arrhythmias.** The type I indication is prior to implantation and if necessary to reevaluate efficacy if changes in the therapy may affect the performance of the device. Type II indications involve testing to confirm acceptable device function. For patients with antibradycardia devices, testing AV and VA conduction as well as the most appropriate pacing site is a type II indication.

m. **Candidates for ablative therapy of arrhythmias.** These patients have a type I indication prior to the procedure and postprocedure to determine efficacy. Type II indications involve evaluation for symptoms compatible with arrhythmias that may be amenable to ablation in the presence of known anatomic substrates such as aneurysms, postoperative tetralogy of Fallot, and WPW syndrome.

2. **Type III.** There is general consensus that the type III indications are **inappropriate** for study:

   Symptomatic patients with sinus node dysfunction documented due to bradyarrhythmia
   Asymptomatic patients with sinus bradyarrhythmia or sinus pauses during sleep
   Symptomatic AV block documented on ECG
   Asymptomatic patients with transient AV block associated with sinus slowing (e.g., nocturnal type I second-degree block)
   Asymptomatic patients with intraventricular conduction delay
   Patients with intraventricular conduction defect whose symptoms are causally related to ECG events
   Patients with narrow-complex SVT in whom the ECG provides sufficient data to select appropriate treatment or those in whom vagal maneuvers or drug therapy can easily provide control without EPS
   Patients in whom the mechanism of wide-complex tachycardia can be clearly identified by ECG criteria
   Patients with congenital or acquired (due to identifiable cause) Q–T syndrome
   Asymptomatic WPW patients without high-risk occupations or without a family history of premature sudden death
   Asymptomatic patients with ventricular premature beats
   Patients with a known cause of syncope
   Survivors of cardiac arrest in the first 48 hours of MI or due to acute reversible ischemia or to another identifiable cause such as aortic stenosis or long Q–T syndrome

Patients in whom palpitations can be attributed to extracardiac causes
Assessment of pharmacologic therapy for isolated atrial premature beats,
multifocal atrial tachycardia, VT occurring in the acute phase of MI or associated with the long Q–T syndrome, asymptomatic nonrecurrent or drug-
responsive SVT or nonsustained VT

B. Ventricular arrhythmias. Much has been learned about the mechanism of tachycardia from EPS [8–12]. The most common mechanism for ventricular and supraventricular tachyarrhythmias is reentry. Characteristically, reentry is marked by the
ability to initiate and terminate an arrhythmia by programmed stimulation. Triggered activity is similar and difficult to distinguish but may be more likely to be
induced by rapid pacing. Automatic tachycardias do not terminate with programmed stimulation, although they may be temporarily suppressed by pacing at a
faster rate.

One of the most important goals in EPS is to reproduce the native arrhythmia, in
both rate and morphology, by programmed stimulation [13]. With aggressive stimulation techniques, a nonclinical tachycardia occasionally can be induced. To be accepted as a true positive result, the induced arrhythmia should be reproducible and
match features of the native arrhythmia, if recorded at the time of the clinical event.

Once it is ascertained that the arrhythmia can be reproduced, drug trials can be
initiated to determine whether inducibility can be suppressed. Usually this is performed at the time of initial EPS by the intravenous (IV) administration of drug and
repetition of stimulation. If the arrhythmia can no longer be induced, the drug is
expected to be protective against out-of-hospital recurrence as long as the same
blood level is maintained and the underlying cardiac substrate remains unchanged.
The risk of recurrent sudden cardiac arrest after successful suppressive therapy is
about 5–6%, compared with 25–30% if VT remains inducible. Some drugs, such as
amiodarone, may be effective in some patients in preventing clinical recurrence,
despite continued inducibility of the arrhythmias. In general, however, failure of
amiodarone predicts an increased chance of recurrence. These issues are addressed
in sec. **IV** on drug evaluation during EPS. It is important to note that drugs may
modify the tachycardia, particularly the rate—sometimes slowing, sometimes
accelerating it. Quite often these changes can be used to an advantage.

Some patients may not respond to drug therapy. It has been possible to refine the
EPS to the point that a relatively precise location of the irritable focus or tachycardia zone can be determined. This technique, called *mapping*, is performed in patients who are candidates for arrhythmia surgery and catheter ablation. At the time
of operation, the area is identified, from the mapping performed in the electrophysiology laboratory or during intraoperative mapping, and extirpated by subendocardial resection, cryoablation, or laser. Thus far, VT originating from the right ventricular outflow tract has the most favorable response from radiofrequency catheter
ablation. Further investigation will determine whether VT due to ischemic or nonischemic cardiomyopathy may benefit from this procedure.

C. Supraventricular arrhythmia. Electrophysiologic testing has become more frequent
for the management of supraventricular arrhythmias since the efficacy of catheter
ablation has been established. Two major groups of supraventricular arrhythmias
benefit from invasive electrophysiologic evaluation: paroxysmal supraventricular
tachycardias (PSVT) and arrhythmias related to accessory bypass tract conduction,
particularly the WPW syndrome. It is important to reiterate that PSVT is a comprehensive term for a group of arrhythmias, including AV nodal reentry, AV reentry
using a concealed bypass tract, sinus node reentry, intraatrial reentry, and automatic
atrial tachycardia. Accelerated junctional tachycardia owing to increased automaticity is another related arrhythmia. Electrophysiologic study assists in differentiating
the mechanism of these arrhythmias and excludes the possibility of a VT, particularly when the surface ECG is not diagnostic. Electrophysiologic evaluation of drug
therapy assesses efficacy without waiting for clinical recurrence. A section on electrophysiologic evaluation of supraventricular arrhythmias is included in Chap. 6.

Patients with accessory bypass tracts fall into four categories:

1. Those with atrio-Hisian (James) fibers with supraventricular arrhythmias: the
   Lown-Ganong-Levine syndrome.
2. Those with AV (Kent) bundles prone to reciprocating tachycardias: the WPW
   syndrome or those in whom the bypass tract conducts only in a retrograde (concealed bypass tract) manner.

3. Those with Mahaim, i.e., atriofascicular (and in some rare cases nodoventricular or fasciculoventricular) fibers.
4. Rare patients who may have both James and Mahaim fibers, simulating the clinical appearance of WPW. EPS may be necessary to sort these out.

Of this group, the WPW syndrome is the most common referral to the electrophysiologist. Clinical manifestations of this syndrome assume great importance when antegrade conduction down the accessory pathway occurs. Without the AV node to limit the number of impulses reaching the ventricle, the rapid 1:1 conduction with arrhythmias such as atrial fibrillation may result in a ventricular response of greater than 300 beats/minute—a de facto VT. If this rate accelerates, the rhythm may degenerate into VF. In patients with coronary artery disease (CAD), the rapid rate may induce VF on an ischemic basis. Since uncontrolled arrhythmias in this syndrome may be life threatening, the physician should consider electrophysiologic evaluation if the patient has experienced syncope or near-syncope. The patient who is mildly symptomatic with slight dizziness or palpitations may merit EPS if noninvasive testing indicates a very rapid ventricular rate during the nonsustained arrhythmia, suggesting a short, effective refractory period of the accessory pathway, a factor that may predispose to malignant arrhythmia and sudden cardiac death. Patients with persistent rather than intermittent preexcitation on the resting ECG during sinus rhythm may also represent a higher-risk group. Electrophysiologic testing in patients with accessory bypass tracts is performed to evaluate the type and location of the accessory bypass tract (often there is more than one) and then to perform catheter ablation.

Lifelong drug therapy is no longer the preferred treatment. For patients who require antiarrhythmic agents, it is important to induce atrial fibrillation to prove that the drug selected will block or slow conduction sufficiently to protect against a rapid ventricular response. Arrhythmia surgery has been replaced as a first-line treatment by catheter ablation, which can eliminate a lifelong need for antiarrhythmic drug therapy. The subject of the electrophysiology and management of accessory pathway syndromes is so important that it is considered separately in Chaps. 6, 7, and 13.

D. **Conduction disturbances.** Patients with documented symptomatic bradyarrhythmias or high-degree AV block do not require electrophysiologic testing to determine the need for permanent pacing. The clinical evidence is already sufficient. With respect to individuals with asymptomatic sinus bradycardia, data regarding the prognostic importance of normal or abnormal sinus node function are still limited. Consequently there is no reason to study these patients. In some patients suspected of having sick sinus syndrome but not having sufficient clinical evidence of symptomatic compromise or documented long pauses, assessment of sinus node function may offer some benefit.

Asymptomatic patients with chronic bifascicular block do not merit electrophysiologic measurement of the H–V interval since the rate of progression to complete heart block is difficult to predict. Prophylactic permanent pacing has not been demonstrated to make a major improvement in survival in this group of patients. If the cause of the bifascicular block is advanced CAD, and left ventricular dysfunction, mortality is commonly related to progression of disease, heart failure, and ventricular arrhythmias. Symptomatic patients with bifascicular block may benefit from EPS. If the H–V interval is severely prolonged (greater than 80–100 msec), the risk of progression to complete heart block is increased. Further evidence may be obtained by the demonstration of infrahisian block (i.e., block below the bundle of His) during atrial pacing. If these findings are present in the patient with dizziness or syncope, permanent pacing may be beneficial and is an indicated procedure.

Another common situation is the development of permanent high-degree AV block (Mobitz type II or greater) during anterior wall MI. These patients deserve permanent pacing and do not require EPS. Again, there is a high risk of death caused by ventricular arrhythmias. Patients who develop new bundle branch block during acute MI and are also noted to have first-degree AV block are considered by some to have an increased risk of progression to complete heart block (see Chap. 9). An extremely prolonged H–V interval at EPS may signal the potential need for permanent pacing.

Thus, the value of EPS in conduction system disease varies with the underlying cardiac problem and the presence of clinical symptoms that may already indicate a certain therapeutic intervention. In cases that are less clear, measurement of intracardiac intervals and the response to pacing may provide helpful prognostic information.

E. **Syncope.** Patients with syncope pose a common problem for the physician. (See Chap. 5.) The most life-threatening causes must be considered first: MI, arrhythmia, heart block, other cardiac disorders responsible for a decreased cardiac output, cerebrovascular accident or transient ischemic attack, hypoxia, hypoglycemia, and drug toxicity or overdose. Quite often, the diagnosis becomes readily apparent, and specific therapy, as indicated, is administered. When the cause is not readily apparent, a search for other factors, including electrolyte imbalance, abnormalities of the endocrine system, renal failure, and a variety of neurologic and vascular problems, must be carefully performed. If this search is unrevealing, further workup should begin with Holter monitoring, to document heart block or arrhythmia. The day-to-day variability of arrhythmias must be considered. If monitoring is unrevealing, an event recorder is recommended. This device consists of an endless-loop recorder that continuously records and erases the ECG. When the patient experiences a symptomatic episode, he or she pushes a trigger, which stores the electrogram. It is then transmitted via telephone to a central station that records hard copy and notifies the physician. The noninvasive evaluation of arrhythmias is discussed in Chap. 10. Conduction disorders similarly can be intermittent. If evidence of high-degree AV block on a Holter monitor tracing correlates with clinical symptoms, no further evaluation is necessary. Pacemaker therapy is indicated.

Should this comprehensive evaluation still prove unrevealing, it is not unreasonable to consider electrophysiologic testing with assessment of baseline conduction and testing of inducibility of atrial and ventricular arrhythmias. Previously unsuspected VT can account for a large number of syncopal episodes [14, 15]. If no arrhythmias or conduction disturbances can be documented at EPS, the patient must be referred back for more medical evaluation. Several studies have evaluated the efficacy of EPS for patients with syncope. They have noted that VT may be a major cause of syncope in patients with bifascicular block, as VT was induced at EPS in one-third of the patients [16, 17]. Similarly if the EPS results are negative, they point toward another cause of syncope.

Reiffel et al. pointed out that EPS was more frequently able to detect severe abnormalities responsible for recurrent syncope than was ambulatory monitoring [18]. A potential cause of syncope is least likely to be found in women without structural heart disease [19]. Teichman et al. suggested a protocol that includes the standard techniques already noted as well as evaluation for carotid sinus sensitivity by carotid sinus massage during intracardiac recording [20]. In their series of 150 patients, pathologic electrophysiologic findings that could explain syncope were found in 36%. If borderline abnormalities were considered, the yield increased to 75%. Thus, it is not unreasonable to consider EPS for this group of patients after the initial medical evaluation proves unrevealing. If specific electrophysiologic diagnoses can be made, patients can receive specific treatment that will prevent further episodes of syncope. In addition EPS can predict a population at low risk of cardiac syncope when PES results are negative [21].

II. **Electrophysiologic studies in the pediatric population.** Although most of the electrophysiology literature has dealt with arrhythmias and conduction disturbances in adults, there are indications for EPS in infants, children, and adolescents. The most frequent reasons for referral of this age group for EPS are primary conduction system disease; VT; SVT, particularly in WPW syndrome; and some cases of postoperative AV nodal dysfunction. Many of these patients have associated congenital heart disease and have undergone cardiac surgery.

A comprehensive evaluation of the use of EPS in the pediatric population at the University of Nebraska found that the technique was not only feasible but safe in these young patients [22]. It was effective in ascertaining the mechanism of the arrhythmia and predicting the efficacy (as well as immediate adverse reactions) of drug therapy.

The technique of EPS in children is similar to that used in adults, but vascular access must be obtained through smaller vessels. Drugs must be given at recommended pediatric doses.

III. **Technical aspects of electrophysiologic study**

A. **Instrumentation for electrophysiologic testing.** Instrumentation required for electrophysiologic testing includes a stimulator, amplifier, oscilloscope, and recording device [23] (Fig. 12-1). A variety of models are available. The stimulator must have the capability of pacing, delivering up to at least three extrastimuli, and rapid burst

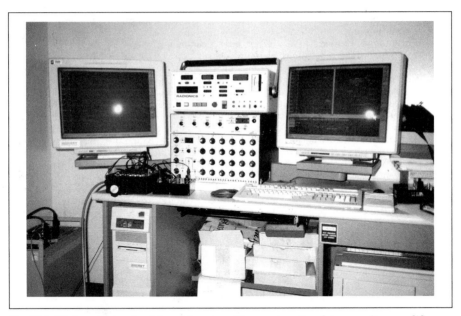

Fig. 12-1. Modern electrophysiology laboratory. Shown are a stimulator, monitor, amplifier, and recorder as well as instrumentation for radiofrequency ablation. The electrophysiology system includes an active screen for on-line monitoring and a second screen for data analysis. Data are stored on an optical disk. Not shown in this photo but common in this laboratory are the defibrillators (primary and back-up), crash cart, drug infusion pumps, and radiology equipment.

pacing, and must be relatively easy to manipulate. Currently the systems widely used are the Bloom stimulator and smaller hand-held stimulators with fewer options. Some of the new internal cardioverter-defibrillators (ICDs) have a noninvasive electrophysiology mode that allows stimulation.

The amplifier processes the intracardiac signals and delivers them to an oscilloscope and the recording device(s). The oscilloscope display permits constant monitoring of the surface and intracardiac signals in addition to the arterial pressure tracing. The electrograms are recorded on an optical disk on which the electrograms can be stored and retrieved for analysis.

Intracardiac signals are recorded using various electrode catheters. Most commonly, quadripolar pacing electrodes (No. 5 or 6 French) are employed. Recently special electrode catheters with multiple poles and deflectable curves have been developed to facilitate mapping and ablation, allowing more precise mapping of intracardiac electrograms (Fig. 12-2). Some electrode catheters have a movable core, which makes it easier to fashion a curve, as may be necessary when mapping an area in the ventricle whose position does not allow easy access. Electrode catheters can be custom-made to suit individual needs. The intraelectrode distance is usually 5–10 mm but may be customized. When the quadripolar pacing electrodes are used, one pair of electrodes is used to pace (usually the distal bipoles), and the other pair is used to record the electrogram.

Two cardioverter-defibrillator units should be available when performing electrophysiologic testing. In our experience, VT can be terminated by pacing techniques in greater than 65–85% of occurrences. Slower tachycardias generally respond better. However, in the remainder, cardioversion or defibrillation may be necessary. If the first defibrillator fails after VT or VF has been induced, a second must be readily available. Our laboratory utilizes adhesive defibrillator electrodes (one posteriorly in the area of the right scapula and the other near the apex) connected to the defibrillator, which avoids the problem of positioning the electrodes and contaminating a sterile field during an emergency situation. There seems to be less impedance with the adhesive electrodes as well as less of a burn.

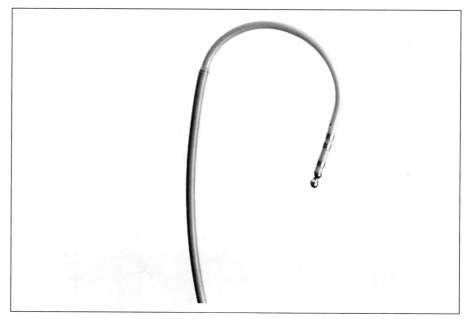

Fig. 12-2. Number 8 French-braided electrophysiology catheter. This electrode is deflectable, making it easier to position for mapping and catheter ablation. (Courtesy Cordis Webster, Inc, Baldwin Park, CA.)

Electrophysiologic study is ideally performed in a catheterization laboratory with c-arm fluoroscopy. The ability to move the fluoroscopy unit without moving the patient's position facilitates mapping (i.e., locating the position of the electrode). It is preferable to have a dedicated laboratory only for electrophysiology, as constant movement of the instruments always leads to mechanical problems.

B. Techniques of electrode insertion. The usual approach to insertion of the electrode catheters is via the femoral veins. Ordinarily, the number of entry sites is limited to two in each vein. For most conduction and VT studies, three electrode catheters will suffice and are inserted into the right and left femoral veins. In the evaluation of a patient with SVT, an additional electrode catheter is placed in the coronary sinus. Often this electrode is inserted through the internal jugular vein or rarely via the basilic vein, either percutaneously or by cutdown. Occasionally it can be manipulated into the coronary sinus via the femoral vein, but this method is more difficult. The other three electrode catheters are advanced to positions in the high right atrium (right atrial appendage), across the tricuspid valve adjacent to the bundle of His, and in the right ventricle (usually the apex or outflow tract) (Fig. 12-3). If ablation is performed, this fifth electrode will be positioned depending on the site of the pathway. Arterial pressure is monitored via a 16- or 18-gauge catheter percutaneously inserted into the femoral artery. Some centers utilize noninvasive BP monitoring, particularly for SVT studies.

C. Techniques of stimulation. The variety of techniques creates some difficulty in comparing the results of electrophysiologic studies from different institutions. This issue is considered in further detail in sec. **E.**

The pulse width of the impulse delivered is commonly 1 or 2 msec, but some laboratories have used 5 msec. Usually the stimulus strength for ventricular stimulation is set at twice diastolic threshold, but some laboratories use higher strengths. In our laboratory we utilize a pulse width of 1 msec and a stimulus strength of twice diastolic threshold. The stimulation site ideally has a threshold of 1 mA or less. It is important to recheck all the settings on the stimulator before starting each study.

A complete EPS includes measurement of the basic intervals (Table 12-2), atrial stimulation, and ventricular stimulation [24]. Measurement of the intervals is performed after obtaining the best catheter position near the bundle of His, so that a

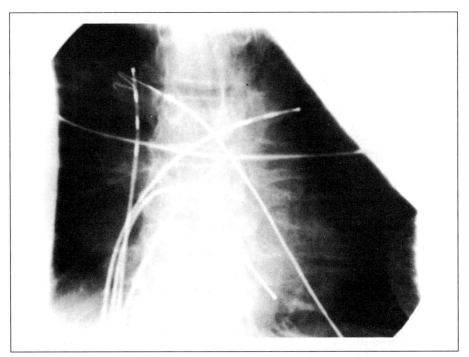

Fig. 12-3. Proper placement of catheters for electrophysiologic testing. Four quadripolar pacing electrodes are positioned in the high right atrium, His bundle position (across the tricuspid valve), right ventricle, and coronary sinus (in this case positioned via the femoral vein approach). Also seen is one of the adhesive pad electrodes (with the coil tip) connected to an external defibrillator, which would be used if pacing termination of a tachyarrhythmia was unsuccessful.

Table 12-2. Normal range of values for intracardiac intervals

Interval	Normal range (msec)
Surface	
P–R	120–200
QRS	60–100
Q–T	Depends on heart rate
Intracardiac	
HRA–LRA	10–40[a]
A–H	55–130
H–V	35–55
H (duration)	15–25
$Q-Tc = \left(\dfrac{\text{measured Q–T}}{\sqrt{\text{R–R interval [sec]}}} \right)$	Usually less than 420–440
Corrected sinus node recovery time (CSNRT)	<550
Sinoatrial conduction time (SACT)	50–125
Effective refractory period	
Atrium	180–320
Atrioventricular node	230–430
Ventricle	180–290

HRA = high right atrium; LRA = low right atrium.
[a]Intraatrial conduction time measurement depends on the location of the electrode in the right atrium.

large His deflection is seen (Fig. 12-4). Once these preliminary steps are completed, atrial stimulation can begin.

As expected, the stimulation threshold in the atrium is higher than in the ventricle, and it may be necessary to set the signal strength at 5–10 mA in some cases. Atrial stimulation is performed by pacing near the baseline cycle length to measure sinoatrial conduction time; decremental atrial pacing (premature extrastimuli) to assess AV nodal and distal conduction and induce arrhythmias; and rapid pacing to measure sinus node recovery times.

1. **Atrial stimulation.** Atrial pacing is accomplished via the pacing electrode in the high right atrium or right atrial appendage.

   a. **Decremental atrial pacing.** Programmed stimulation consists of a series of stimuli (usually eight beats) at a constant cycle length (A_1) followed by a premature stimulus (A_2). This is described as A_1A_2 (Fig. 12-5). After a dropout period of 4–5 seconds to assess the response, the cycle is repeated with A_2 more premature (i.e., closer to the previous A_1). This sequence of events is repeated until an arrhythmia is induced or the refractory period of first the AV node (demonstrated by failure to conduct to the bundle of His) and then the atrium (failure to produce an atrial electrogram) is reached. Occasionally the refractory period of the atrium occurs before the refractory period of the AV node.

   It is important to continue stimulation until the atrial effective refractory period (ERP) is reached, since a gap phenomenon may occasionally be seen with dual AV nodal pathways. The gap phenomenon is demonstrated by apparent achievement of the AV nodal refractory period and then capture again (i.e., conduction to the bundle of His) when the interval A_1–A_2 becomes even shorter. The gap phenomenon reflects functional differences in conduction or refractoriness in two or more regions of the conducting system. Stimulation is performed using at least two cycle lengths of the basic drive cycle (e.g., 600 msec, 500 msec). When testing a patient for supraventricular arrhythmias (particularly if an accessory pathway is present), up to five cycle lengths (400–800 msec) may be necessary to induce the arrhythmia.

   If an atrial arrhythmia is induced, it is evaluated in regard to type (i.e., atrial tachycardia, atrial flutter, atrial fibrillation), mechanism (AV nodal reentry, AV reentry, automatic), and method of initiation and termination. Sometimes it may be necessary to map the atrial activation sequence using the electrodes in the coronary sinus (to detect left atrial activity) and the right atrium to determine the mechanism. In certain cases, it may be extremely difficult to differentiate among the various possibilities, particularly when there is an accessory pathway. For example, one must distinguish between reentry restricted to the AV node with the accessory pathway inactive (i.e., bystander bundle of Kent) and reentry in a macrocircuit with the accessory pathway providing the retrograde limb of the loop.

   b. **Sinus node recovery time.** When atrial stimulation with the A_1A_2 technique is completed, the sinus node recovery time (SNRT) is measured [25, 26]. This may be accomplished by continuous pacing at a constant cycle length for 30–60 seconds and then abrupt termination of the pacing, so that the interval between the last atrial paced beat and the first atrial recovery beat can be measured (Fig. 12-6). Pacing for SNRT is also performed at several basic cycle lengths. As mentioned in Chap. 3, the SNRT is corrected for the resting sinus cycle length. One subtracts the baseline heart rate from the SNRT to obtain the corrected sinus node recovery time (CSNRT). A normal value is considered to be less than 550 msec. CSNRT is an index of intrinsic sinus node automaticity. Prolongation of the CSNRT reflects serious sinus node dysfunction. In the bradycardic patient whose symptoms are not absolutely diagnostic, abnormal CSNRT may be an additional factor to consider in the decision regarding permanent pacing.

   c. **Sinoatrial conduction time.** The other test of sinus node function is the sinoatrial conduction time (SACT), which measures impulse conduction through the peri-sinus-node tissue. Two methods may be used to calculate SACT. The method described by Strauss et al. uses a premature atrial stimulus to penetrate the sinus node and reset its pacemaker [27]. The return cycle length after the premature beat is measured, and the spontaneous cycle length is subtracted, leaving the time necessary to penetrate and again leave the sinus node tissue. SACT is half this interval—the time required by the impulse to conduct from the sinus node into the surrounding atrial tissue. However, if

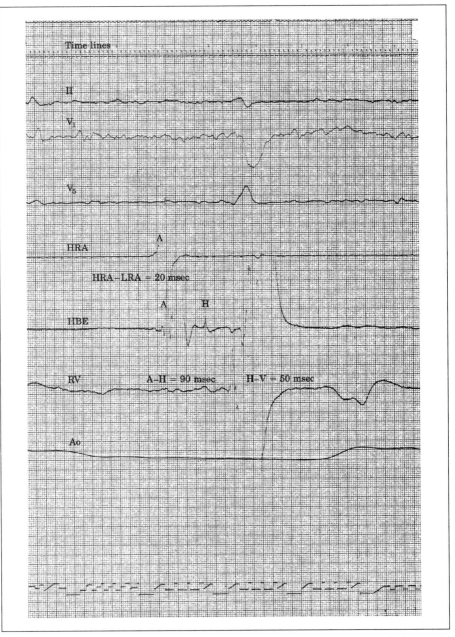

Fig. 12-4. Baseline electrophysiologic measurements. Time lines are seen on top; the interval between the small lines is 10 msec. The next three tracings are surface electrocardiographic leads II, V_1, and V_5. Then the endocardial electrodes record the high right atrium (HRA), the His bundle (HBE), and right ventricular (RV) electrogram. The aortic pressure (Ao) tracing is the last tracing.

Intraatrial conduction time	20 msec
A–H interval	90 msec
H duration	10 msec
H–V interval	50 msec

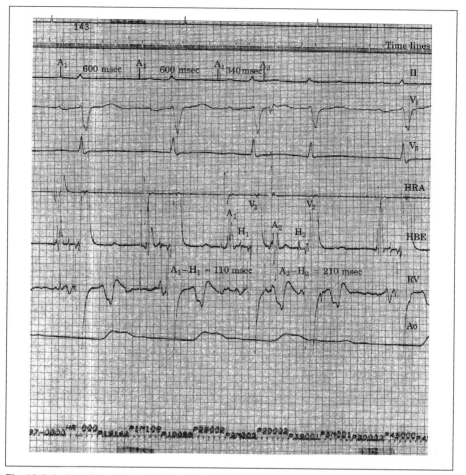

Fig. 12-5. A_1A_2 technique. This technique involves eight atrially paced beats at a constant cycle length (A_1), followed by a premature atrial extrastimulus (A_2), which is made more premature with each subsequent cycle. Note that A_2–H_2 (210 msec) is longer than A_1–H_1 (110 msec), but the H–V interval (55 msec) remains unchanged. (Format of tracings is explained in Fig. 12-4.)

conduction into and conduction out of the node are not equal, the calculation of SACT would be in error. Consequently, Narula et al. suggested brief overdrive pacing for eight beats before measuring the pause (with SACT then calculated as above) [28]. This method attempts to minimize changes in the basic sinus cycle.

d. **Value of SNRT and SACT.** SNRT is dependent on automaticity, SACT, and the presence of acetylcholine and norepinephrine, as well as the stimulation site of the exploring atrial electrode. Whereas CSNRT assesses automaticity of the sinus node, SACT assesses conduction through the tissue surrounding the sinus node. SACT may be abnormal (reflecting first-degree SA block) even if CSNRT is normal. The utility of these two indexes of sinus node dysfunction was assessed by Reiffel et al. [25]. With normal values for both CSNRT and SACT, symptoms were uncommon. Prolongation of CSNRT and SACT was common in patients who have or will develop symptoms associated with sinus bradycardia; however, it did not indicate which patients might become asymptomatic without pacemaker insertion. Finally, although it is possible to record the sinus node electrogram directly, in order to make direct measurements of sinus node function, doing so is hampered by technical difficulties. The sensitivities of CSNRT (54%) and SACT (51%) when combined are higher

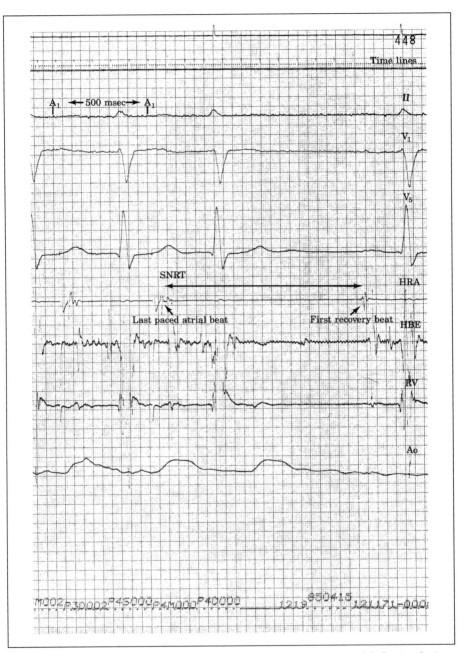

Fig. 12-6. Sinus node recovery time (SNRT) is measured from the last atrial deflection during pacing to the first sinus recovery beat and is corrected for rate by subtracting the resting sinus cycle length. In this tracing, SNRT = 1100 msec. (Format of tracings is explained in Fig. 12-4.)

The sensitivities of CSNRT (54%) and SACT (51%) when combined are higher (64%) and the specificity is 88% [29, 30].

2. Ventricular stimulation. Ventricular pacing is accomplished via the exploring electrode in the right ventricle. Formerly the premature extrastimuli were delivered while the patient was in sinus rhythm (in relation to a previous sinus beat) or after atrial pacing (the A_1V_2 technique) [31, 32]. The presence of repetitive responses or sustained arrhythmias was assessed. Owing to the low yield (see sec. E), these techniques are infrequently used. Current techniques use ventricular pacing with premature extrastimuli. Simultaneous atrial pacing at the same intervals is sometimes necessary to avoid competition from the intrinsic atrial pacemaker, which might interfere with the ventricular pacing (e.g., the sinus impulse might excite the ventricle before the ventricular-paced stimulus). Competition, however, is usually avoided by using a faster drive cycle length.

    a. Single extrastimuli. The first technique, V_1V_2, involves eight ventricular-paced beats at a constant drive cycle (usually 500, 400, and sometimes 350 msec) followed by a premature ventricular stimulus. V_2 is moved closer to V_1 (thus scanning diastole) with each repetition of the cycle until a sustained arrhythmia is induced or the refractory period of the ventricle is reached. Usually the decrement in the V_1–V_2 interval is 10–20 msec each time. Each cycle is followed by a 4- to 5-second dropout period to assess the response. Generally, more than one extrastimulus is required to induce VT.

    b. Double extrastimuli. The next technique, $V_1V_2V_3$, involves eight ventricular-paced beats at the constant drive cycle followed by premature double extrastimuli (Fig. 12-7). We arrive at the coupling intervals to start $V_1V_2V_3$ by adding 50 msec to the ventricular effective refractory period as determined by the V_1V_2 technique, to give us the new starting value for V_2. V_3 is entered at twice the value for V_2. Thus, if the ventricular ERP was 270 msec, V_2 is entered at 320 msec and V_3 at 640 msec. In this system, 320 msec is the time interval between V_1 and V_2, and 640 msec is the time interval between V_1 and V_3. Stimulation is started, and V_3 is brought closer to V_2 by 10-msec decrements until V_3 no longer conducts. Then V_2 is brought closer to V_1 by 10-msec decrements until V_3 conducts again. These cycles are repeated until V_2 reaches the refractory period of the ventricle. This technique and V burst (described below) uncover a relatively high yield of inducible ventricular tachyarrhythmias without causing nonclinical arrhythmias (Fig. 12-8).

    c. Triple extrastimuli. Since some patients still remain noninducible, triple extrastimuli were introduced. This technique increases sensitivity at the cost of lowering specificity. In other words, there is a higher risk of inducing a nonclinical arrhythmia. This technique is denoted as $V_1V_2V_3V_4$. Its starting values are derived as for $V_1V_2V_3$. To carry the same example further, the starting intervals would be V_2, 320 msec; V_3, 640 msec; and V_4, 960 msec. Stimulation is started with decrements in V_4 until V_3 no longer conducts; then V_3 is decremented until V_4 conducts again. Diastole is scanned by these premature triplets until the refractory period of the ventricle is reached by V_2 or a sustained tachyarrhythmia results. Stimulation with more than three extrastimuli is usually not performed, nor is it recommended because of a higher incidence of inducing nonclinical arrhythmias.

    d. Burst pacing. Another routine protocol is **V burst** (Fig. 12-9), which is a series of 10 paced ventricular beats at a constant cycle length, followed by evaluation of the response (Fig. 12-10). The paced cycle length is decremented on each repeat stimulation by 50–100 msec until reaching within 50 msec of the predicted ERP as determined by V_1V_2. Then the decrement proceeds by 10-msec intervals until ERP is achieved. Usually, the clinician does not pace below 200-msec cycle lengths even if ERP is not reached in uncommon patients.

    e. Induction of ventricular fibrillation. An additional electrophysiologic technique that uses **alternating current (AC)** is performed in certain situations [33] (Fig. 12-11). This technique is valuable when testing the ICD and in inducing tachyarrhythmias for intraoperative mapping when conventional techniques do not result in induction. One current source for AC is a standard line-operated battery charger, with its full wave-rectified output measured as 7 V over a 50-ohm load. Another source is a current limited fibrillator commonly used in cardiac surgery. The current is delivered through two

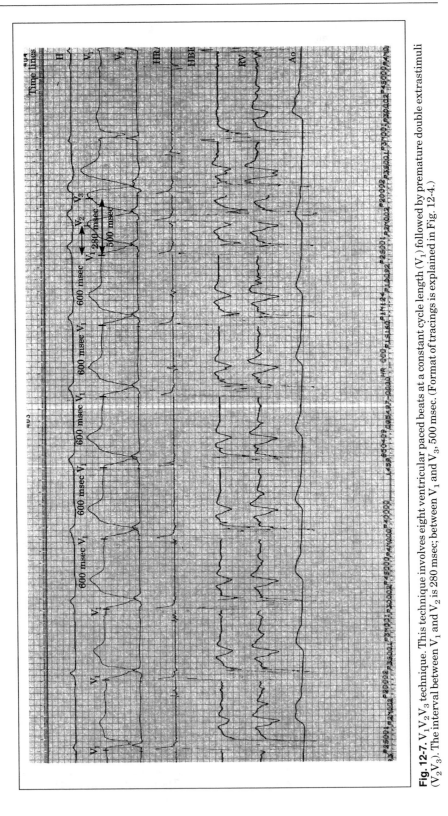

Fig. 12-7. $V_1V_2V_3$ technique. This technique involves eight ventricular paced beats at a constant cycle length (V_1) followed by premature double extrastimuli (V_2V_3). The interval between V_1 and V_2 is 280 msec; between V_1 and V_3, 500 msec. (Format of tracings is explained in Fig. 12-4.)

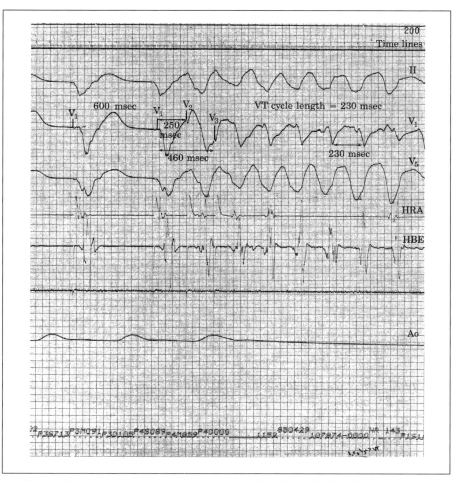

Fig. 12-8. Initiation of sustained ventricular tachycardia (VT) by the $V_1V_2V_3$ technique. Sustained monomorphic VT at a rate of 261 beats/minute is accompanied by symptomatic hypotension. (Format of tracings is explained in Fig. 12-4.)

bipoles of a catheter electrode or bipolar plunge electrodes in the ventricular myocardium. The arrhythmia is usually induced within the first second. No untoward outcomes have been noted in any of these patients. Today the newer ICDs induce VF via stimulation at cycle lengths of 30–50 msec or with a low energy shock delivered during the T wave.

f. **Isoproterenol.** Isoproterenol to facilitate induction of tachycardia has been used in the past when techniques, including $V_1V_2V_3$ and V burst, failed to induce clinical arrhythmias [34, 35]. The infusion rate is 1–2 µg/minute to increase the sinus rate 15–25 beats/minute. It is not absolutely certain how this catecholamine facilitates induction of VT. Possible mechanisms include shortening refractoriness, increasing conduction velocity, enhancing automaticity, causing afterdepolarizations, and causing ischemia.

Isoproterenol should be reserved for special situations, when routine testing does not induce a clinically documented arrhythmia or when a catecholamine-sensitive VT is suspected. It should be avoided if the patient is known to be ischemic.

Left ventricular stimulation is not used since the right ventricular stimulation techniques have sufficient sensitivity and specificity, avoiding the risk of left heart catheterization [36].

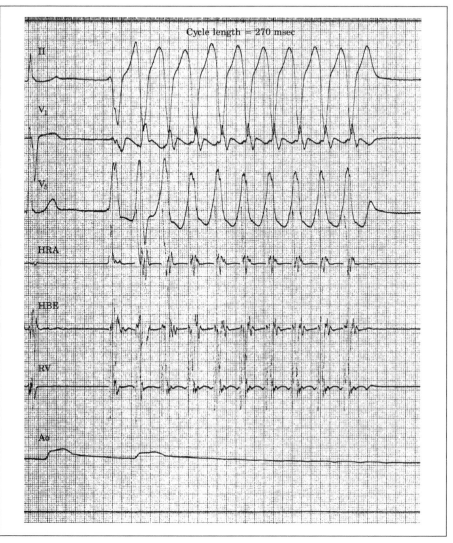

Fig. 12-9. V burst technique. Burst pacing involves 10 paced beats at a constant cycle length. Each time the technique is repeated, the cycle length is decreased until an arrhythmia is induced or the effective refractory period (ERP) of the ventricle is encountered (i.e., 2:1 conduction). Most electrophysiologists terminate V burst at a 200-msec cycle length even if the ERP is not reached. (Format of tracings is explained in Fig. 12-4.)

At this point, it is necessary to include a caveat: No physician should attempt to perform programmed electrical stimulation without rigorous training in a center performing a minimum number of studies. The inexperienced operator may create a hazard, in the improper performance of the study or in the incorrect interpretation of data. Recently standards have been recommended for the electrophysiology laboratory and for the stimulation protocols [23, 24].

Each electrophysiology laboratory will have to determine its own stimulation protocol using the techniques outlined in this section. It is useful to have a predetermined sequence, as is discussed in sec. **E**. Usually two sites are tested in the right ventricle (RV): the RV apex and the RV outflow tract (RVOT). EPS can be time-consuming, with different stimulation protocols necessary and

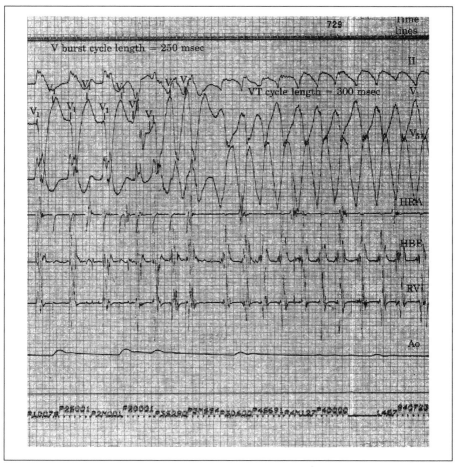

Fig. 12-10. Initiation of sustained monomorphic ventricular tachycardia (VT), rate 200 beats/minute, by the V burst technique. This VT corresponded to the patient's native arrhythmia in both morphology and rate. (Format of tracings is explained in Fig. 12-4.)

time required for drug infusion trials for suppression of inducible VT. The patient must be prepared for the study, and the entire electrophysiology staff must function as a team. In addition, the team must be prepared to deal with induced arrhythmias or any other emergency that may develop. Remember that the purpose of the study is to determine whether arrhythmias are inducible.

D. **Responses to programmed electrical stimulation.** Table 12-3 lists the possible responses to PES, as defined by a policy conference of the North American Society of Pacing and Electrophysiology on the evaluation of ventricular tachyarrhythmias [24]. With atrial stimulation, a variety of supraventricular arrhythmias may be induced, as discussed in Chaps. 6 and 7. Further elaboration of the mechanism of the tachycardia may be facilitated by the response to stimulation.

The major mechanisms for supraventricular and ventricular tachyarrhythmias are reentry and automaticity. Automaticity is a function of the spontaneous depolarization of cells. Automatic tachycardias result from enhanced spontaneous depolarization and usually cannot be initiated or terminated by PES. For reentry to occur, several conditions must be present, including dual pathways, unidirectional block, and slowed conduction. Reentrant tachycardias can be initiated or terminated by PES. Triggered activity may also demonstrate this property. Most VTs are due to reentry. If one examines the repetitive responses that occur after PES, some may be preceded by a His deflection. These are thought to represent macroreentry in the

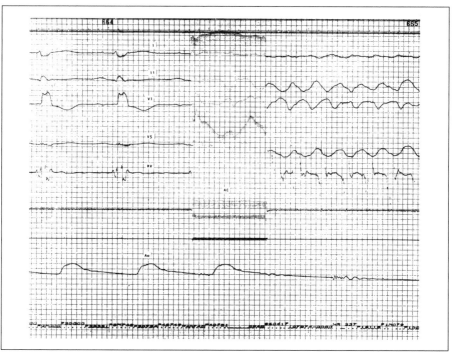

Fig. 12-11. Induction of monomorphic ventricular tachycardia (VT) by alternating current during a test of the automatic internal cardioverter-defibrillator. Note the immediate hemodynamic deterioration on the aortic pressure tracing. (Format of tracings is explained in Fig. 12-4.)

Table 12-3. Definitions of induced ventricular rhythms or beats

---

Sustained VT: VT >30 seconds or clinically requiring intervention to terminate the tachycardia

Nonsustained VT: VT >6 beats but <30 seconds, terminating spontaneously and not requiring intervention on a clinical basis

Monomorphic VT: VT with stable configuration of QRS complexes in at least three simultaneously recorded ECG leads, with a constant relation of inscription of the QRS complexes in the three recorded leads

Multiple monomorphic VT: ≥ 2 monomorphic VT in the same patient

Polymorphic VT: VT with an unstable (continuously varying) QRS complex configuration in any recorded ECG lead

VF: A ventricular tachyarrhythmia with absence of clearly defined QRS complexes in the body surface ECG. It may be indistinguishable from sustained polymorphic VT in some cases

Single ventricular response: One nonstimulated ventricular beat in response to a paced premature beat or beats

Repetitive ventricular responses: Two to five nonstimulated ventricular beats in response to a paced premature beat or beats

---

VT = ventricular tachycardia; VF = ventricular fibrillation.
Source: From AL Waldo et al., The minimally appropriate electrophysiologic study for the initial assessment of patients with documented sustained monomorphic ventricular tachycardia. Reprinted with permission from the American College of Cardiology. *(J Am Coll Cardiol* 6:1174, 1985.)

His-Purkinje system, usually a physiologic response. Also termed bundle branch reentry (BBR), it may be explained by retrograde conduction block in the right bundle and conduction through the myocardium to the left bundle, through which the impulse activates the His bundle in a retrograde fashion and is then propagated down the right bundle. Rarely, VT due to BBR is observed. In comparison, if no His potential is observed, it is likely that the repetitive response is due to intraventricular reentry (IVR), a pathologic state caused by microreentry in a circuit near the site of stimulation. Diagnostic and therapeutic decisions are based on induced sustained or nonsustained VT but not on the presence of 3–10 repetitive ventricular responses [37–40].

1. **Sustained and nonsustained ventricular tachycardia.** Sustained monomorphic VT is the most important response and has the highest predictive value, particularly if it reproduces the clinical arrhythmia in both rate and morphology. The laboratory of Josephson demonstrated that rapid and poorly tolerated ventricular arrhythmias could be initiated by PES in 61% of survivors of cardiac arrest [41]. Had they included nonsustained tachycardias, the yield would have been 70%. However, they did not consider the induction of brief and spontaneously terminating ventricular arrhythmias to be a bona-fide reproduction of the patient's clinical arrhythmia. This view is shared by Wellens et al., who consider the induction of nonsustained monomorphic VT to be of unknown importance [42].

   It is not clear whether the induction of nonsustained VT is truly an intermediate response between inducible VT (predictive of an unfavorable outcome) and noninducibility (predictive of a benign prognosis). Perhaps it would not be unreasonable to state that the induction of nonsustained VT may leave the physician with some concern. Swerdlow et al. addressed the issue of the number of induced responses predictive of therapeutic efficacy [43]. Continued induction of sustained VT was associated with a high risk of recurrence and sudden death. Outcome was favorable even if up to 15 beats of nonsustained VT were induced, but unfavorable if 16 or more beats resulted from PES. Platia and Reid found that five or more beats of nonsustained VT induced while the patient was receiving drug therapy for VT or VF had an increased risk of recurrent VT or sudden death [44]. Thus, this finding strengthened the predictive accuracy of the EPS and identified an inadequate drug regimen. In their review of the subject, Morady et al. concluded that the induction of sustained VT appeared to be specific to patients with clinical VT or VF, but nonsustained VT was not found to be predictive of later occurrence of clinical VT [19].

   Clearly, the individual with no underlying heart disease and no symptoms is expected to have negative results on EPS. In most cases, a negative EPS result indicates a favorable prognosis. However, occasional survivors of sustained VT or VF will be noninducible during EPS and are still prone to recurrence. In the past, the absence of $V_1V_2V_3V_4$ may have partially explained this response. For some patients, transient pathophysiologic abnormalities may trigger lethal arrhythmias. Usually these patients have underlying heart disease. If arrhythmias are noninducible, a drug regimen cannot be tested. If the patient is documented to be a survivor of VT or VF, then other measures, such as an ICD (see Chap. 18), may have to be considered. Thus, a negative result in EPS does not exclude the possibility of recurrent VT or VF.

2. **Polymorphic VT.** Polymorphic VT is frequently noted with very potent stimulation techniques. It is more likely with triple extrastimuli than with double or single extrastimuli. Quite often it does not reproduce the clinical arrhythmia, so most physicians see it as of limited prognostic value. Nevertheless, one group felt that polymorphic VT cannot be ignored [45]. When 88 patients (57%) with polymorphic VT were compared with 65 patients (43%) with monomorphic VT induced by PES, the total mortality and sudden death rate (12% and 7% for polymorphic, 10% and 5% for monomorphic) were similar. These researchers did use four extrastimuli in their protocol, which induced monomorphic VT in 36% and polymorphic VT in 64%. The similarity in outcome suggests that morphologic criteria cannot be used to discount completely a result from PES. Thus, when polymorphic VT is induced, the clinician must review the clinical history, the stimulation technique, and its reproducibility and then decide how likely it is to represent a clinical arrhythmia.

3. **Ventricular fibrillation.** Ventricular fibrillation is not usually induced during PES [46]. It is generally accepted that, in most cases, VT is the initiating mechanism in cardiac arrest [47, 48]. Ventricular tachycardia may degenerate to VF

(often quickly, even after only a few beats) because of related factors such as ischemia, hypoxia, or metabolic abnormalities or because of the rate of the VT.

If VF is induced during EPS, the clinician must consider the reason for referral. If the patient has never had clinical VT or VF and has no underlying heart disease, the induced VF is considered a nonspecific finding that does not mandate antiarrhythmic drug therapy. Obviously, this situation is different from that of the patient who has survived sudden cardiac arrest, in whom induced VF may be a more important finding. In general, however, the induction of VF is not felt to be a specific finding for identifying a definite course of chronic therapy.

4. **Repetitive ventricular responses.** One to five repetitive beats after programmed stimulation is felt to be a nonspecific finding. Initially it was hoped that a clinician would be able to uncover latent electrical instability without necessitating the induction of sustained VT. It soon became apparent that early techniques such as single ventricular extrastimuli during sinus rhythm were insensitive and that one to five induced beats was not predictive of outcome.

We note the presence of these responses during EPS and decide whether they represent IVR or BBR but do not use this information to guide therapy.

5. **Reproducibility.** The issue of reproducibility of EPS has been addressed in a number of recent studies. Cooper et al. found that the number of extrastimuli required for VT induction was significantly more reproducible during immediate repeat studies than from day to day [49]. Kudenchuk et al. found that induced ventricular arrhythmias were not reproducible in 45% of patients in whom the drug level was identical to the first study and not reproducible in 16% of patients with more variation in drug levels [50]. Bhandari et al., however, found that in survivors of acute MI, inducible sustained VT was a highly reproducible finding, but VF showed a significant day-to-day variability [51]. Volgman et al. noted that induction of sustained monomorphic VT was more reproducible than nonsustained VT or polymorphic VT and cautioned that the latter results not be used as end points to guide antiarrhythmic therapy [52]. Furthermore, sustained VT rate under 250 beats/minute was a more reproducible finding than sustained VT over 250 beats/minute.

6. **Recommendations.** The most predictive response is **sustained monomorphic VT.** It can be reliably used to guide therapy. In survivors of VT and VF, it is important to use even aggressive stimulation protocols to reproduce the initiating clinical arrhythmia in the laboratory. Nonsustained VT is considered to be a finding of unknown importance. However, it cannot be considered benign, and some physicians view it as valuable as a response in guiding drug therapy in patients with baseline inducible sustained VT. Polymorphic VT and VF are nonspecific findings that may have value in certain individuals. Repetitive ventricular responses provide little clinical information. A negative result usually indicates a favorable prognosis [53].

E. **Sensitivity and specificity of the various stimulation techniques.** Programmed electrical stimulation evolved from using single ventricular extrastimuli during sinus rhythm or atrial pacing (A_1V_2) to ventricular pacing with single (V_1V_2), double $(V_1V_2V_3)$, and triple $(V_1V_2V_3V_4)$ extrastimuli, as well as burst pacing and enhancement with faster drive cycle lengths or isoproterenol. To be accepted as a valid response, the induced arrhythmia should be reproducible. Nonclinical responses, which may occur with triple extrastimuli, must be excluded [54]. With varied responses in different patients, one must know the incidence of true-positive, false-positive, true-negative, and false-negative results. The majority of patients studied have underlying CAD. It is this group that is discussed in the majority of articles dealing with sensitivity and specificity of PES. Patients with cardiomyopathy and mitral valve prolapse are discussed separately.

1. **Nature of the response.** Enthusiasm for the A_1V_2 technique declined as it was felt to be relatively insensitive [37–40]. Better results were obtained with ventricular pacing with double extrastimuli $(V_1V_2V_3)$ and burst pacing, which were demonstrated to have the highest incidence of inducing sustained and nonsustained VT. The importance of the type of response was addressed. Although the repetitive ventricular response was sensitive, it had a low specificity in identifying patients with spontaneous VT. The induction of sustained VT had a moderate sensitivity but a very high specificity (98–100%). The experience of Josephson's laboratory confirmed that nonsustained repetitive responses caused by intra-

ventricular reentry were indeed a pathologic finding but of low sensitivity (65%) in identifying those with clinical ventricular tachyarrhythmias [3]. The specificity was somewhat higher (83%). In patients with a history of sustained VT, the arrhythmia was inducible during EPS in 95%, reproducing the rate and morphology of the native arrhythmia in most cases. In patients with only nonsustained VT clinically, the rate of inducibility during EPS was lower, 62%. Other studies indicated that sensitivity could be increased by exploring an additional right ventricular site, without sacrificing specificity [55]. In fact, by using a combination of RV sites, the sensitivity could be increased further: RV apex (65%), RVOT (76%), RV apex and RVOT together (89%); specificity remained at 100% for all [56]. Nevertheless, right ventricular stimulation alone was unable to identify all of the patients with spontaneous VT; left ventricular stimulation was necessary in 11%.

2. **More potent techniques.** To obtain the most precise data about patients at risk for VT or VF, more and more potent techniques were needed and utilized. With the addition of the third ventricular extrastimulus, the small increase in sensitivity came at the expense of specificity. $V_1V_2V_3V_4$ has a higher incidence of inducing a nonclinical arrhythmia, in particular, a polymorphic sustained or nonsustained VT with the potential for degeneration. In one series by Buxton et al., triple extrastimuli induced VT in 97% of those whose clinical presentation was sustained VT, in 81% with cardiac arrest, but also in 40% without documented spontaneous arrhythmias [57]. In the right ventricle, $V_1V_2V_3V_4$ induced VT in 22% of patients with sustained VT and in 46% with cardiac arrest. Stimulation of the left ventricle was required to induce VT in only 3% with stable tachycardia, compared to 19% with cardiac arrest. In 57% of patients without spontaneous arrhythmias, $V_1V_2V_3V_4$ induced polymorphic nonsustained VT. Morady et al. compared two protocols: (A) V burst, V_1V_2, $V_1V_2V_3$, and $V_1V_2V_3V_4$ at each of the following sites: (1) RV apex, (2) RVOT or septum, and (3) LV apex; (B) V burst, V_1V_2, and $V_1V_2V_3$ at the same sites, and if that failed to induce VT, $V_1V_2V_3V_4$, starting at site 1 [58]. Clinical VT was induced in 76% with protocol A and in 85% with protocol B, but the incidence of nonclinical VT (36–38%) was the same. The study indicated that with the use of $V_1V_2V_3V_4$ in the RV, it was often possible to avoid the need for LV stimulation. $V_1V_2V_3V_4$ seemed to be more effective in inducing clinical VT than LV stimulation. The initial use of V burst and $V_1V_2V_3$ made $V_1V_2V_3V_4$ or LV stimulation unnecessary in 53% of patients. Triple extrastimuli were necessary to induce clinical VT in 24%. In those without documented VT, $V_1V_2V_3V_4$ induced nonclinical VT in 45%. Double extrastimuli at two sites increased the chance of inducing clinical VT from 47% to 61%. No advantage was found with isoproterenol in patients without CAD, and there was increased risk of ischemia in those with CAD. In terms of deciding which stimulation techniques to use in the laboratory, protocol A was recommended for patients with well-documented VT and protocol B for those with suspected but undocumented VT.

In another study of drug efficacy, this same group of investigators concluded that a drug regimen that suppresses VT induction with both RV and LV stimulation results in a significantly better clinical response than suppression only in the RV [59].

Morady et al. assessed the value of EPS in patients without spontaneous VT using their stimulation protocol (RV and LV stimulation, up to three extrastimuli, 2-msec pulses, 5 mA) [60]. One to five repetitive beats was a nonspecific finding without predictive value. Nonsustained VT was induced in patients with structural heart disease but not in those without that finding. Thus, the induction of sustained VT appeared to be a response specific to patients with spontaneous VT or VF. Induction of VF was also noted infrequently in patients without spontaneous VT or VF.

3. **The European approach.** Brugada and Wellens reviewed the experience in their laboratory and recommended using three pacing rates at the RV apex, with $V_1V_2V_3V_4$ if necessary [61]. They were able to induce VT in 70–90% of those with recurrent, sustained VT with $V_1V_2V_3$. Adding $V_1V_2V_3V_4$ yielded induction in an additional 12–24%. With their protocol (including triple extrastimuli), they were able to induce clinically documented VT in 93%. No additional benefit was noted by increasing the stimulus strength to 20 mA. The nature of the underlying heart

disease was also important. The clinical arrhythmia was induced in 100% of those with CAD, 75–90% of those with idiopathic VT, but only 50–60% of those with cardiomyopathy or mitral valve prolapse. The induction of polymorphic VT was again noted to be a nonspecific response to an aggressive stimulation protocol. The induction of 3–10 beats of nonsustained VT was of unknown import. Sustained VT was initiated in 60% of all survivors of sudden cardiac death. A disquieting fact, however, is that sustained VT was induced in 45% of survivors of MI who had never manifested life-threatening arrhythmias. Thus, more than one-third of survivors of MI have an electrophysiologic substrate for VT but do not manifest clinical arrhythmias. The authors suggest that previous calculations of sensitivity and specificity did not look at the correct groups [62]. Instead of contrasting EPS-induced arrhythmic patients with normal individuals, the proper comparison would be EPS-induced arrhythmias in patients with clinical arrhythmias against EPS-induced arrhythmias in asymptomatic patients.

4. **Experience with additional provocative maneuvers.** To take the stimulation protocols another step, Mann et al. assessed the value of the third $(V_1V_2V_3V_4)$ and fourth $(V_1V_2V_3V_4V_5)$ extrastimulus [63]. Again an increase in the induction of clinical VT was accompanied by an increase in nonclinical VT. What was somewhat surprising was the 44% incidence of nonclinical VT with V burst (versus 72% incidence of clinical VT), somewhat higher than in other studies.

One final modification in the protocol was increasing the intensity of pacing to five times diastolic threshold, as reported by the group at Cedars-Sinai [64]. Their protocol includes (1) atrial pacing for 30 seconds from 600 to 300 msec in 50-msec decrements; (2) V burst at the RV apex; (3) V_1V_2, $V_1V_2V_3$, and $V_1V_2V_3V_4$ at 550- and 400-msec drive cycle lengths and twice diastolic threshold; (4) V_1V_2, $V_1V_2V_3$, and $V_1V_2V_3V_4$ at 400 msec and five times diastolic threshold; and (5) V_1V_2, $V_1V_2V_3$, and $V_1V_2V_3V_4$ at 400 msec and five times diastolic threshold at the second RV site, the outflow tract.

With this protocol, the researchers were able to induce VT in 92% of patients with clinical sustained VT and in 72% who survived sudden cardiac death. The protocol allowed induction of VT in 40% of patients with clinical VT using a maximum of two extrastimuli, in 77% with $V_1V_2V_3V_4$, and 92% using steps 4 and 5. The protocol had a low incidence of inducing nonclinical arrhythmias.

Several recent papers assess additional techniques. Belhassen et al. used a five-step approach: (1) A_1V_2, (2) V_1V_2 at three basic cycle drive lengths (600, 500, 400 msec), (3) $A_1V_2V_3$, (4) $V_1V_2V_3$ at three basic cycle drive lengths (600, 500, 400 msec), and (5) 3–5 seconds of V burst at 300, 265, and 240 msec [65]. The five-step protocol was done first at the RV apex and repeated at the RVOT if the patient was noninducible. The protocol had a sensitivity of 90% and specificity of 93%. Rapid right ventricular pacing increased the yield, particularly for patients with VF.

Summitt et al. found that a faster basic cycle drive length of 400 msec increased the yield of sustained monomorphic VT induced by one to three extrastimuli [66]. Simonson et al. used a short-long protocol with a short basic cycle drive length (400 msec) followed by a single stimulus at 600 msec, followed by up to two extrastimuli [67]. The yield was less than with standard protocols. However, when they used a second site protocol in which a standard basic drive cycle was delivered from site 1 and the extrastimuli were delivered from a second RV site, the yield increased.

Morady et al. used single, double, and triple extrastimuli at three basic cycle drive lengths (350, 400, 600 msec), first at the RV apex and then at a second RV site [68]. The yield with this accelerated protocol was 92% as compared to 89% for a standard protocol.

5. **Importance of the substrate CAD.** The majority of the studies I have cited considered patients with CAD. The findings in other disorders in the absence of CAD may differ. In patients in this category, Naccarelli et al. found that VT was induced less often than in those with CAD and less frequently in those with a history of nonsustained as compared to sustained VT [69]. In addition, although suppression of inducible VT appeared to predict drug efficacy, drug therapy guided by noninvasive testing appeared to be unreliable. This study considered patients with cardiomyopathy, mitral valve prolapse, and primary electrical disease.

6. **Nonischemic cardiomyopathy.** It is important to remember that ventricular arrhythmias, and nonsustained VT in particular, are common in dilated cardiomyopathy. The incidence of VT may not predict prognosis in these patients [70]. One study of patients with dilated cardiomyopathy failed to demonstrate a meaningful correlation between inducibility and clinical arrhythmias. However, this study limited stimulation to two sites in the right ventricle [71]. Poll et al. were able to induce sustained VT with PES and observed that the arrhythmia remained inducible despite drug therapy [72]. Brembilla-Perrot prospectively evaluated 103 patients with idiopathic dilated cardiomyopathy with up to triple extrastimuli and isoproterenol [73]. Sustained monomorphic VT was induced in 8 of 11 patients with spontaneous VT, in none of 35 without significant clinical arrhythmias, and in 9 of 56 with salvos of ventricular premature beats. In the follow-up period, there were eight sudden deaths in patients who initially had syncope, inducible sustained VT, or both, and three episodes of sustained VT in patients who initially had clinical nonsustained VT and inducible sustained VT. They found that the sensitivity of EPS in these patients increased from 73% to 91% with the use of isoproterenol.

   Patients with dilated nonischemic cardiomyopathy may die suddenly even before a problem with arrhythmias becomes apparent. EPS may be used to guide therapy if sustained EPS is induced. If suppressed by antiarrhythmic drugs, the prognosis is more favorable. If not, an ICD may be recommended. If the patient is noninducible, some patients will still die from VT/VF, but which individual will experience this outcome cannot be predicted. For asymptomatic patients with nonsustained VT, therapy presents a dilemma. Currently a study in Germany with ICD therapy is addressing this issue (Dilated Cardiomyopathy Trial) and may offer guidance as to the cost-benefit ratio of ICDs for these patients. Patients with end-stage hearts may not survive because of their poor LV function, even if an ICD can terminate episodes of VT/VF.

   In contrast, the presence of complex ventricular arrhythmias, particularly nonsustained VT, seems to indicate higher risk of sudden cardiovascular collapse for the individual with hypertrophic obstructive cardiomyopathy. Anderson et al. demonstrated unusually high vulnerability to induction of ventricular arrhythmias at EPS and warned of a higher risk to the patient (i.e., causing intractable VF) during programmed stimulation [74].

7. **Mitral valve prolapse.** Two studies addressed the issue of programmed stimulation in mitral valve prolapse. In the first, patients with asymptomatic ectopy and no inducible arrhythmias had a good outcome without therapy [75]. However, VT or VF was inducible in 65% of patients with transient symptoms and documented nonsustained VT or ventricular premature beats (VPBs). Most often the inducible arrhythmia was polymorphic VT, the importance of which, however, was unclear.

   The most recent report found that the majority of symptomatic patients had inducible ventricular tachyarrhythmias but could not demonstrate a correlation between this response and subsequent outcome [76].

8. **General comments and guidelines.** Previous studies have commented on the difficulty of inducing arrhythmias in patients with the prolonged Q–T syndrome in the electrophysiology laboratory [77]. **Thus, it is important to determine the underlying anatomic substrate so that one may assess the appropriateness of EPS in the individual patient. The sensitivity and specificity will be highest in patients with CAD; nevertheless, this does not mean that EPS is of no value in patients with other conditions. It does, however, indicate that the results may be somewhat more limited, and the clinician must be cautious in interpretation.**

   It would be ideal to have one universal protocol that all physicians could agree on. Certainly this is partially the intention of the authors of the most recent articles and my reason for presenting their protocols in such detail. Already some conclusions can be drawn. **The repetitive ventricular response as an end point is inadequate. Responses owing to BBR are usually physiologic, while those related to intraventricular reentry are pathologic. Induced polymorphic ventricular tachycardia is frequently a nonclinical arrhythmia and should not be used to guide therapy unless it is reasonably certain that it represents a clinical arrhythmia. Induced sustained monomorphic VT that is identical to the native arrhythmia has the highest sensitivity and specificity. Suppression of** this response with drugs constitutes an acceptable and desirable end point. The importance of nonsustained VT remains controversial. Certainly the longer the duration is of this induced response, the greater the possibility is that prognosis may be affected. Ventricular fibrillation induced at EPS is also a nonspecific finding [78].

9. **Noninducibility in cardiac arrest survivors.** Finally it is important to address the issue of the patient who has survived VT or VF and is noninducible at the time of EPS. Poole et al. assessed the long-term outcome of 241 survivors of out-of-hospital VF [79]. EPS induced VF (group 1 = 16%), sustained VT (group 2 = 27%), and nonsustained VT (group 3 = 14%); 42% were noninducible (group 4). The researchers administered antiarrhythmic drugs to 91% of group 1, 92% of group 2, and 47% of group 4. Ventricular fibrillation recurred in 28% of group 1, 21% of group 2, 12% of group 3, and 16% of group 4. Survival for patients with inducible VT/VF suppressed by antiarrhythmic drug therapy guided by EPS was not different from patients whose arrhythmia was not suppressed. The presence of congestive heart failure was an independent predictor of outcome in these patients. Inducibility at baseline EPS was dependent on left ventricular function and did not independently predict outcome.

Kim et al. evaluated 26 patients with sustained VT or VF with a variety of underlying disorders [80]. They found that noninducibility was associated with relatively preserved left ventricular function. Andresen et al. studied 60 noninducible survivors of VT/VF and found that the outcome was benign if the left ventricular ejection fraction was greater than 40% and worse when the fraction was poor [81].

The long-term benefit of EPS-guided antiarrhythmic therapy was addressed by Sousa et al. in 56 survivors of cardiac arrest [82]. They noted a 53% rate of sudden death over 3 years with antiarrhythmic drug therapy (either EPS guided or empiric) as compared to 9% with ICD devices.

Fogoros et al. analyzed 217 survivors of cardiac arrest [83]. The incidence of sudden death was similar for patients who were noninducible, drug responders, and drug nonresponders. Patients stratifed as high risk by EPS and treated with ICDs had mortality similar to those in low-risk groups. **Thus, survivors of VF may be more likely to be noninducible during EPS, and EPS-guided therapy may not provide as accurate a prediction as in patients whose arrhythmia is sustained monomorphic VT. Inducibility is related to left ventricular function. These patients deserve consideration for ICDs.**

10. **Recommendations for individual centers.** Until a consensus is reached, every laboratory will have to determine the limits of its stimulation protocol, and in part this will depend on the particular patient studied. Our protocol involves pacing at twice diastolic threshold, using a 1-msec pulse width and two basic cycle drive lengths (500 and 400 msec). Two sites in the right ventricle, the apex and outflow tract, are explored with four techniques in the following sequence: V_1V_2, $V_1V_2V_3$, V burst, and $V_1V_2V_3V_4$. V_1V_2 is performed first to determine the refractory period of the ventricle for calculation of further intervals with double extrastimulus techniques, as well as to assess the response of the ERP to drugs. We have obtained the best results with double or triple extrastimuli and pacing. $V_1V_2V_3V_4$ does increase the risk of inducing nonclinical VT. If the patient is a survivor of sudden cardiac death or sustained VT and right ventricular stimulation does not induce sustained VT, we will use a third basic cycle length (350 msec). If still noninducible, isoproterenol is used unless the patient is ischemic. Each patient is evaluated individually.

F. **Techniques for terminating ventricular tachycardia and ventricular fibrillation.** Just as pacing may initiate reentrant arrhythmias, it also may terminate them. Once a patient develops a sustained arrhythmia, the electrophysiologist must immediately assess whether there is hemodynamic compromise. This can be done immediately by viewing the arterial pressure tracing on the oscilloscope.

1. **Maintenance of blood pressure with coughing.** Our patients are instructed to cough on command (with practice sessions before PES). Coughing causes changes in the pressure difference between the intra- and extrathoracic veins, facilitating the circulation of blood. In fact, even patients with VT or VF can maintain their BP in this manner, without causing cerebral hypoperfusion. Therefore, if the induced arrhythmia causes severe hypotension, coughing main-

tains the circulation, allowing more time for pacing maneuvers to restore sinus rhythm. Certainly if the arrhythmia is VF, defibrillation is immediately performed without attempts at pacing.

2. **Defibrillation.** The patient is told to stop coughing while the defibrillator is charged. In this 10-second interval, the patient often loses consciousness and is amnesic for the event. Cardiopulmonary resuscitation, if necessary, is continued until the time of defibrillation. The patient is not compromised by these maneuvers. For the patient who must undergo repeated induction for evaluation of different drug regimens, every uncomfortable episode of arrhythmia and electrical countershock may cause reluctance to proceed with the study. These procedures are much less threatening when the shock is not remembered, as is discussed in Chap. 20.

   Use of the adhesive chest electrodes for cardioversion or defibrillation is recommended. They are in place when needed and one does not delay, positioning external paddles in an emergency. Adhesive electrodes make contamination of a sterile field less likely, and there is less chance of dislodging the pacemaker electrodes from their fixed positions. As well, there appears to be less of a burn with the adhesive chest electrodes. The energy used for cardioversion or defibrillation is standard. With VT, 50–100 joules may terminate the arrhythmia, whereas for defibrillation 200–300 joules should be used initially. Although some only recommend that a second defibrillator unit be available, I consider it mandatory to have a second in the laboratory. EPS is a relatively safe procedure. But if one induces the clinical arrhythmia and then pacing and the external defibrillator fail to terminate it, the situation could be catastrophic. Most electrophysiologists can probably recall at least one incident in which the backup defibrillator was lifesaving.

3. **Pacing.** Pacing terminates the tachycardia in 65–85% of occurrences. Quite often termination depends on the rate of the tachycardia, with faster rates more difficult to terminate. Other factors to consider include the site of stimulation in relation to the tachycardia zone, ventricular conduction, and refractoriness. Sometimes pacing accelerates the tachycardia, important information if antitachycardia pacing is being considered.

   Two methods are available for pacing termination if the patient tolerates the arrhythmia (Fig. 12-12). Mode 1 couples single or double ventricular extrastimuli to the tachycardia, scanning diastole until the refractory period of the ventricle is reached. Mode 2 uses burst pacing to overdrive the tachycardia, but there is a greater chance of acceleration than with the first mode. Roy et al. found that mode 1 was useful when the cycle length was longer than 300 msec, and mode 2 was required when the cycle length was less than 300 msec [84]. Gardner et al. suggested a combination of rapid pacing and extrastimuli to terminate tachycardias refractory to modes 1 and 2 [85]. Waxman et al. also pointed out that increasing the current strength from twice diastolic threshold to 5–10 mA further facilitated termination of the tachycardia [86].

4. **Trains.** Fisher et al. suggested ultrarapid single-capture train stimulation for termination [87]. Trains of 10 bipolar stimuli were delivered every eighth VT beat, beginning in the refractory period. Intervals between successive stimuli were 10, 20, and 40 msec with 100, 50, and 25 Hz, respectively. The researchers concluded that PES and trains were equally effective, but trains were more efficient because the VT was usually terminated with the first capture.

   Pacing termination is influenced by tachycardia rate. It is recognized that antiarrhythmic drugs may also influence the tachycardia rate. Slowing of the rate by drugs may facilitate pacing termination, as reported by Keren et al. [88] and as frequently observed in the electrophysiology lab. Of course in some patients, antiarrhythmic drugs may also make pacing termination more difficult.

5. **Entrainment.** Waldo et al. described the method of entrainment for both SVTs and VTs [89]. Transient entrainment is an increase in the rate of the tachycardia with rapid pacing. The intrinsic tachycardia rate resumes when the pacing rate is slowed or pacing is discontinued unless the arrhythmia is terminated. In some cases, rapid atrial pacing can result in transient entrainment of a sustained VT [90]. Entrainment also depends on the pacing site, as entrainment may be possible from one site but not another [91].

   Thus, a variety of methods of terminating VT or VF are available. Which will be used first depends on the hemodynamic state of the patient. The availability of

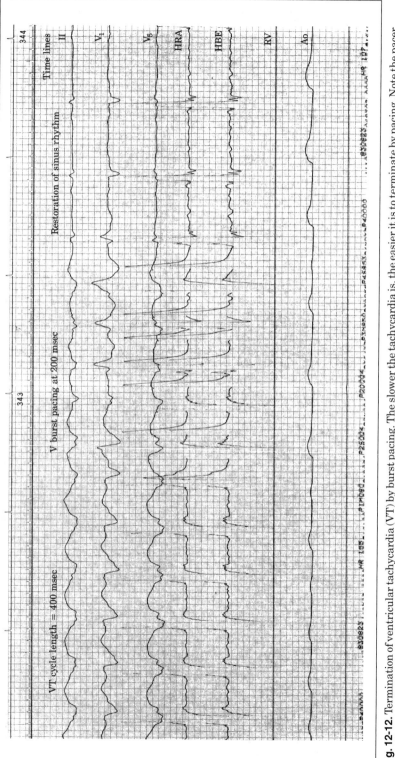

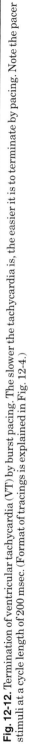

Fig. 12-12. Termination of ventricular tachycardia (VT) by burst pacing. The slower the tachycardia is, the easier it is to terminate by pacing. Note the pacer stimuli at a cycle length of 200 msec. (Format of tracings is explained in Fig. 12-4.)

burst pacing modes on the stimulator may make some modes easier than others. Burst pacing may increase the risk of acceleration [92]. It is important that the electrophysiologist be prepared to deal with the tachyarrhythmia when induced, sometimes with a planned sequence of maneuvers.

G. **Complications in electrophysiologic study.** The electrophysiologic study is a relatively safe procedure. Induced arrhythmias should not be considered a complication of the procedure.

Electrophysiologic study has a lower risk and complication rate than does cardiac catheterization for coronary disease or valvular problems. DiMarco et al. reported the experience at Massachusetts General Hospital [93]. Twenty complications were observed in 1062 EPS procedures (<2%): thromboembolism (9), infection (6), and pneumothorax (5). These were related to the catheterization procedure, not to the technique of PES. It is important to note that these investigators did not administer heparin (except when stimulating the left ventricle) and often used the subclavian vein approach.

Horowitz et al. reviewed the complication rates in 1000 patients in their experience: 1 death (0.1%); 12 vascular problems, consisting of 4 arterial injuries (0.4%), 6 cases of thrombophlebitis (0.6%), and 2 severe hematomas (0.2%); 1 systemic embolus (0.1%); 3 pulmonary emboli (0.3%); 2 cardiac perforations (0.2%); and 20 cases of hypotension (2.0%) [94]. Catheter-induced permanent complete heart block occurred in one patient. Nonclinical atrial fibrillation requiring therapy occurred in 10 patients. In 397 patients undergoing drug studies for VT, severe proarrhythmic events occurred in 12 (3.0%). In patients undergoing baseline studies, electrical cardioversion was required for termination of ventricular tachyarrhythmias in 179 patients (53% of patients with inducible arrhythmia). Cardioversion was necessary at least once in an additional 35 patients during follow-up studies.

These results are typical and applicable to most laboratories. The need for electrical cardioversion versus pacing termination of arrhythmias depends on the induced arrhythmia (monomorphic VT versus polymorphic VT or VF).

In our laboratory, heparin is routinely used in all cases, and the subclavian vein is not entered, which may explain why thromboembolism and pneumothorax have not been a problem. In addition there has been no incidence of infection. The only complication we have noted is an occasional groin hematoma or bruising, which is self-limited and requires no therapy. One must be extremely careful when performing retrograde entry into the left ventricle (for mapping or ablation) through an atherosclerotic or aneurysmal aorta.

IV. **Electrophysiologic evaluation of drug efficacy.** The ability of EPS to provoke a clinical arrhythmia provides a situation in which the effect of drugs on the tachycardia can be studied. Furthermore, clinical follow-up of chronic drug therapy with the regimen selected at EPS allows correlation with acute drug testing. Initial studies using conventional antiarrhythmic drugs available at the time revealed that a drug that suppressed reinduction of the tachyarrhythmia prevented recurrences of the clinical arrhythmia when administered chronically. Thus, EPS provided a rapid determination of the benefits of the drug, without having to wait a prolonged period for a clinical event, possibly with an unfortunate outcome if the arrhythmia occurred outside the hospital [6, 95]. These general principles hold true for supraventricular and ventricular tachyarrhythmias. Electrophysiologic management of SVT and WPW syndrome is further discussed in Chaps. 6, 7, and 13. The remainder of this section is concerned with ventricular tachyarrhythmias.

Wellens et al. reported the effect of procainamide on tachycardia, which is to reduce its rate and lengthen the effective refractory period of the ventricle [96]. Horowitz et al. reported suppression of VT, with chronic drug therapy preventing clinical recurrence if antiarrhythmic drug levels were maintained [97]. Similar results were reported by virtually all centers using PES to guide drug therapy [98, 99]. Attempts were then made to determine if the response to one drug would predict the response to another, in order to avoid repeated studies. To determine how electropharmacologic drug trials should be performed to select therapy for patients with VT, Kavanagh et al. evaluated patients using trials of 1A, 1B, combination of 1A and 1B agents, 1C, propranolol, and sotalol [100]. The probability of identifying predicted effective therapy was higher with the first trial and significantly lower with each succeeding trial. They concluded that the electropharmacologic approach should be abandoned after three unsuccessful trials. **Today with the availability of tiered-therapy ICDs, many physicians abandon drug trials after the second unsuccessful trial.**

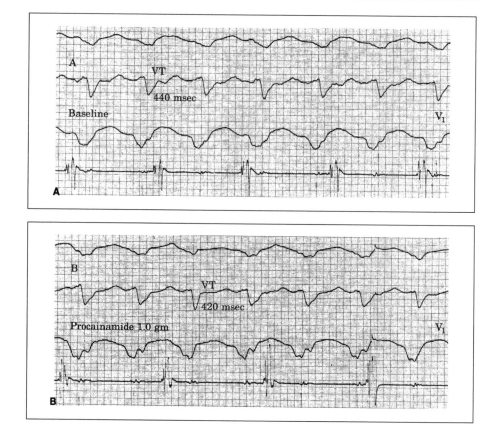

Fig. 12-13. Serial electrophysiologic testing. This figure is a compilation of lead V_1 tracings during serial drug tests in a patient with refractory ventricular tachycardia (VT). A variety of antiarrhythmic drugs (B–G) failed to suppress the VT, so the patient underwent subendocardial resection of the tachycardia zone. Note the different rates obtained with the various drugs.

Tracing	Rate of induced VT (beats / minute)	Cycle length (msec)
A. Baseline (and native)	136	440
B. Procainamide 1.0 g	142	420
C. Procainamide 1.75 g	136	440
D. Procainamide 2.00 g	127	460
E. Quinidine	150	400
F. Tocainide	150	400
G. Amiodarone	150	400
H. Two years after endocardial resection (left ventricular stimulation was required; no drug therapy)	333	180

Note how low-dose procainamide actually accelerated the tachycardia before a higher dose (2.0 g) slowed it. Therapeutic doses of quinidine, tocainide, and amiodarone failed to suppress inducibility. Since the induced tachyarrhythmia was just as fast with amiodarone as with other drugs that failed, it was felt unwise to rely on this drug for out-of-hospital protection, and the patient underwent subendocardial resection after endocardial mapping. Twelve years after surgery, the patient is alive and well and has had no clinical recurrence of VT.

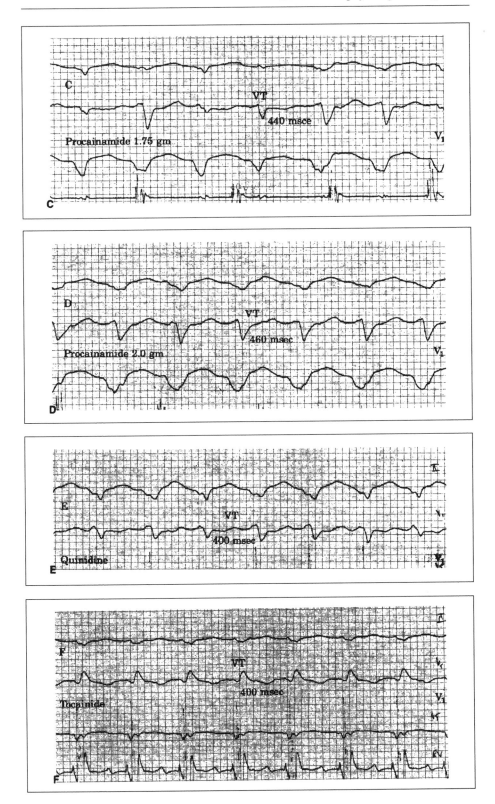

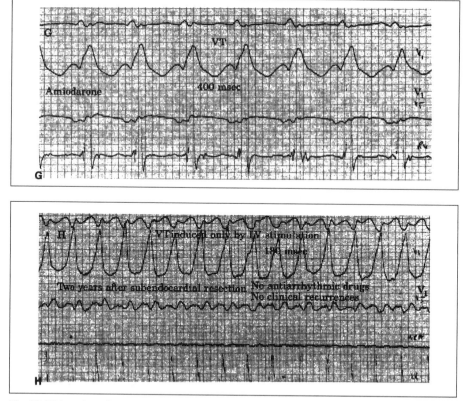

Fig. 12-13 (continued)

A. **Serial drug trials.** If an agent is found to be effective during acute drug testing, there is no guarantee that it will be tolerated chronically, even if it suppresses the tachyarrhythmia. Idiosyncratic or toxic reactions may occur and may mandate discontinuation. At that point, the patient may have to be hospitalized for further EPS.

Previously, some centers performed multiple drug trials at the time of initial study. (The cost of this approach today is prohibitive.) Thus, if an antiarrhythmic drug had to be stopped, another already proved at EPS was easily substituted. The problem with this approach was that it necessitated repeated studies that may not be necessary if the first drug to suppress sustained VT or VF was tolerated chronically. Today, after a successful drug regimen is found, the patient is discharged with return to the electrophysiology laboratory in the future if toxicity develops or is then considered for an ICD. At this point, the patient has already gone through multiple evaluations, including noninvasive studies and cardiac catheterization. The patient may remember the first termination of his or her clinical arrhythmia (possible CPR, defibrillation) and have had one or more electrophysiology studies. This person is psychologically drained. Furthermore, a repeat study at a later date may have a different result if the patient's heart disease progresses and the electrophysiologic substrate for VT or VF changes. Studies valid months ago may no longer be useful in the patient who has suffered another MI, or whose congestive heart failure has deteriorated. Every center must develop its own philosophy and recommendations to the patient after the first successful regimen is encountered.

Serial testing (Fig. 12-13) necessitates consideration of drug half-life, since one could not distinguish whether drug efficacy was related to one agent or a combination of drugs if given during the same test. It is necessary to allow five half-lives to pass after discontinuation of the preceding drug before considering another. Today it is not unreasonable to consider combination drug therapy, as discussed further in Chaps. 8 and 14. Consequently if the first drug causes a partial response, perhaps slowing the tachycardia but not completely suppressing it, and it is unwise to

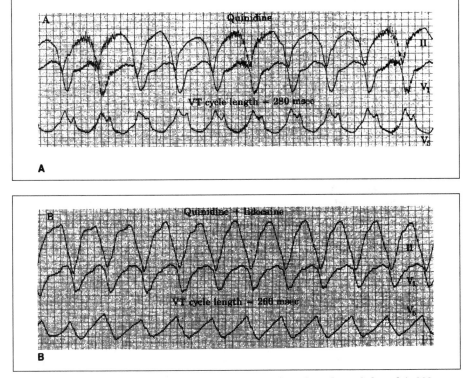

Fig. 12-14. Effect of drugs on cycle length. **A.** With quinidine alone the cycle length is 280 msec (214 beats/minute.) **B.** With quinidine and lidocaine together, the ventricular tachycardia (VT) cycle length is faster—260 msec (231 beats/minute). This graphically illustrates how drugs can modify the underlying rhythm disturbance.

administer a higher dose, the addition of another drug may be considered. Certainly the second drug would have to be compatible with the first and not increase toxicity. For example, the addition of IV quinidine to IV procainamide already administered in maximal dosage would be potentially dangerous and should not be considered. A drug such as lidocaine, with different electropharmacologic properties from the type 1A agents, might more safely be administered in addition to either procainamide or quinidine and the combination assessed by PES (Fig. 12-14).

Currently, a limited number of drug combinations can be administered IV during EPS. With the availability of ICDs, most electrophysiologists limit the number of drugs tested before recommending a device.

B. Predictors of survival. Before returning to the subject of individual drugs, it may be useful to review the multiplicity of factors that predict survival in patients undergoing EPS for life-threatening arrhythmias. Using a stepwise logistic regression analysis, Swerdlow et al. identified three variables independently predictive of drug response: fewer coronary arteries with a 70% or greater stenosis, female sex, and fewer episodes of arrhythmia [101]. In another analysis, this same center demonstrated that the two most important predictors of both sudden death and cardiac death were a high New York Heart Association functional class and the failure of any therapy to be identified as potentially effective on the basis of EPS [102]. The severity of heart failure was the strongest independent predictor of mortality.

Another independent predictor of survival was the response to therapy directed by EPS. The group from the University of Pennsylvania described four factors associated with successful medical therapy: age under 45 years, ejection fraction over 50%, hypokinesia as the only contraction abnormality, and the absence of organic heart disease [103]. Four factors were associated with failure of medical therapy:

induction of VT with V_1V_2 (a relatively mild stimulus), H–V interval over 60 msec, presence of left ventricular aneurysm, and Q waves on baseline ECG. A function incorporating eight variables in a discriminant analysis was able to classify 81% of the patient population correctly.

The group at the Massachusetts General Hospital correlated the presenting arrhythmia with the ability to induce and suppress the arrhythmia [104]. In patients with clinical sustained VT, 89% had inducible ventricular arrhythmias with PES, compared with only 61% with clinical nonsustained VT and 66% with clinical VF. Complete suppression was achieved only in 52% of patients with sustained VT but in 73% of those with nonsustained VT and 75% of those with VF. Clearly, sustained VT was the easiest arrhythmia to reproduce and the most difficult to suppress. The benign prognosis of patients whose life-threatening arrhythmias were suppressed by drug therapy and evaluation by PES was also demonstrated by the study of Benditt et al. [105].

Another concern in serial studies is progression of disease that causes a change in the electrophysiologic substrate for VT or VF. Schoenfeld et al. showed a striking concordance in 17 patients reexamined a mean of 18 months after the initial study [106]. None had had MI or cardiac surgery in the interim. Thus, if there is no change in the substrate, the EPS results are expected to be reproducible. Investigators at Yale questioned the reproducibility of VT provoked by three extrastimuli (56%), whereas the reproducibility of VT provoked by V_1V_2 or $V_1V_2V_3$ was 95% [54]. Part of this discrepancy may be related to the potency of $V_1V_2V_3V_4$ and the higher chance of a nonclinical arrhythmia.

C. **Individual drug trials to suppress ventricular tachycardia.** Quinidine was evaluated by DiMarco et al., who found it to prevent inducibility in 30% as a single agent and in an additional 10% when combined with another antiarrhythmic agent [107]. Procainamide was evaluated by Waxman et al., who noted that if it failed to suppress the inducible tachyarrhythmias, successful therapy was possible by only 7% of other drug regimens [108]. Earlier, Greenspan et al. pointed out that very high-dose procainamide occasionally was required to suppress the arrhythmia [109]. These conclusions represent generalizations; every electrophysiologist can remember exceptions. It was also shown that failure of IV procainamide to suppress inducibility might not predict efficacy of oral procainamide, because higher procainamide concentrations were achieved with the oral drug, which was then able to suppress inducibility. However, the procainamide concentration had to be at least 3 μg/ml higher [110]. The Hahnemann experience generally supports the conclusions of Waxman et al.; however, the Hahneman researchers point out that occasional patients may respond to either individual agents or combinations of agents [111]. The therapeutic implications are as follows. **One cannot exclude the drug efficacy of an agent not evaluated. All conventional agents without contraindications should be evaluated before considering investigational agents or agents with greater toxicity. A combination of agents may be more effective than individual agents alone.** This same group of investigators noted that the most successful combinations were procainamide or quinidine in combination with mexiletine [112]. Beta blockers are not often used as first-line antiarrhythmic agents, but LeClerq et al., using nadolol, found that it was suitable for EPS evaluation in patients with inducible sustained VT, although they urged caution if left ventricular function was impaired [113].

In contrast to the prediction of efficacy with procainamide or quinidine, amiodarone therapy proved unpredictable. Some patients may remain inducible but still have a good clinical response. On the other hand, suppression of induced VT by amiodarone still predicts a favorable outcome. Clinical recurrence of VT in a population of refractory VT patients whose sustained VT is suppressed by amiodarone is unlikely unless the underlying substrate changes. Wellens, among others, has suggested that if a patient's VT remains inducible during amiodarone therapy, other factors may indicate a favorable drug effect [42]. These include slowing of the tachycardia rate or induction only with a more potent stimulation technique. These indicators have not yet been entirely validated. Certainly inducibility only into nonsustained VT, but not into sustained VT, would seem to be a potentially favorable predictor of a successful outcome. Propafenone also has been compared to amiodarone in its ability to provide a favorable clinical outcome despite continued inducibility.

As a final note in regard to electropharmacologic testing, a recent study of MI patients with remote VT/VF observed that a patent infarct-related artery was associated with antiarrhythmic drug response more frequently than was an occluded artery [114]. Although only a small study, it would support the benefit of a patent artery post-MI. The effect may be related to a number of factors, including drug delivery to the zone as well as a different substrate (perhaps less scarring) than with an occluded artery.

V. Potential indications for electrophysiologic study

A. Nonsustained ventricular tachycardia. Although there is a clear indication to recommend EPS to patients who have survived sudden cardiac arrest or sustained VT and those with other symptomatic arrhythmias, the absolute indication for EPS in nonsustained VT in the absence of hemodynamic embarrassment is less well defined. In a study by Buxton et al., PES was shown to reproduce nonsustained VT in most patients with spontaneous arrhythmias [115]. In some, sustained VT was induced, most often in those with CAD and left ventricular aneurysm. The importance of this finding was not clear, although there was a suspicion that patients with clinical nonsustained VT and inducible sustained VT might be at higher risk. In the long-term follow-up of patients with nonsustained VT, sudden death occurred in 4 of 15 with inducible sustained VT, 2 of 37 with inducible nonsustained VT, and 4 of 31 with noninducible VT. However, the most powerful predictor of risk for sudden cardiac death was a left ventricular ejection fraction of 0.40 or less [116]. Nevertheless, the presence of inducible sustained VT was an independent risk factor for sudden death, although it did not identify the individual patient who would die. Another important finding in this study was that the underlying heart disease was important. Inducibility at EPS correlates with outcome in patients with CAD but not necessarily in those with cardiomyopathy.

Similar findings were reported by the Johns Hopkins group [117]. Asymptomatic patients with nonsustained VT were more likely to have inducible VT and future clinical arrhythmic events if underlying cardiac disease was present. Ejection fraction again predicted subsequent cardiac death and clinical arrhythmias, whereas inducibility did not. Spielman et al. found that patients with nonsustained VT and chronic left ventricular dysfunction had a high incidence of inducible sustained VT or VF [118]. Actually, inducibility correlated with the presence of akinesia or aneurysm but not with ejection fraction or the presence or absence of CAD.

Two other studies examined patients without symptomatic arrhythmias. Kowey et al. studied patients with CAD by EPS and found three or more repetitive responses in 14 of 32 patients with stable CAD [119]. Of the 14, 86% had an ejection fraction of less than 50% or regional wall motion abnormalities. In the 18 patients with fewer than three repetitive responses, only 22% had left ventricular dysfunction. Only 4 patients with three or more repetitive responses and 1 with fewer than three had complex ectopy on ambulatory monitoring. Long-term follow-up was not provided.

In a similar analysis, Gomes et al. assessed 73 asymptomatic patients with high-grade ectopy on Holter monitoring [120]. PES identified 27% with inducible VT or VF and 73% who were noninducible or had only two to four repetitive responses. Although there was no difference in the amount of ectopy on Holter monitoring between the groups, those with inducible VT or VF had more atherosclerotic heart disease, prior MI, and ejection fraction below 40%. Patients with inducible VT or VF were treated by antiarrhythmic drugs based on EPS efficacy results, whereas those with noninducible VT were randomly treated with prophylactic antiarrhythmic therapy. Patients with inducible VT or VF had a higher incidence of subsequent sustained VT or sudden death than the noninducible VT group (31% versus 2%). In those who were noninducible, no difference in survival was noted between the treated and untreated subjects. Patients without inducible tachyarrhythmias and ejection fraction over 40% had excellent survival and a low incidence of sudden death.

Kowey et al. evaluated EPS in 205 asymptomatic survivors of acute MI who continued to have nonsustained VT on ambulatory monitoring 1 month after the event [121]. Programmed stimulation was performed with up to three extrastimuli. In this population, 36% were noninducible, 29% had nonsustained VT, 33% had sustained VT, and 2% had polymorphic VT or VF. When outcome was considered, only left ventricular function discriminated those with sustained arrhythmia or death from those that did not. EPS did not have predictive value, but the conclusions were limited by the fact that patients received antiarrhythmic therapy based on the findings at EPS.

Kowey et al. further calculated sensitivity (54%), specificity (70%), and positive (18%) and negative (93%) predictive accuracy in a meta analysis of 926 patients with nonsustained VT and concluded that EPS was valuable if negative, but the low predictive accuracy of a positive result limited its clinical utility [122].

Finally Kadish et al. evaluated management of nonsustained VT in 280 patients with differing underlying substrates: coronary disease, idiopathic dilated cardiomyopathy, no structural heart disease, and miscellaneous (mostly valvular) heart disease. Ventricular tachycardia was most often inducible in patients with coronary disease and least when structural heart disease was absent [123]. Mortality was highest in idiopathic dilated cardiomyopathy, intermediate in coronary or miscellaneous heart disease, and lowest when structural heart disease was absent. Left ventricular ejection fraction and inducibility on the predischarge EPS were independent predictors of sudden death. Patients effectively treated with an antiarrhythmic drug that suppressed inducibility did not experience sudden death, whereas 4 of 27 patients not suppressed died. Dilated idiopathic cardiomyopathy patients with continued inducible sustained VT despite antiarrhythmic therapy were at substantial risk of sudden death.

1. **Lessons regarding nonsustained VT.** These studies indicate some common findings in patients with nonsustained VT. **The results of PES are more predictive for patients with CAD than for those with other types of heart disease. Even patients with a minimum of ectopy on ambulatory monitoring may have inducible sustained or nonsustained VT at EPS, particularly if there is underlying heart disease with left ventricular dysfunction. The worse the LV dysfunction is and the lower the ejection fraction, the poorer is the chance of survival. Inducibility into sustained VT is an independent risk factor but may not identify the individual patient who will die.** The combination of indexes of left ventricular function and results of EPS may permit risk stratification that will identify the patient who may obtain the greatest benefit from further evaluation and intervention. **Patients without inducible VT or VF and with good left ventricular function may not need prophylactic antiarrhythmic drug therapy even if the ambulatory ECG reveals complex ventricular ectopy.**

   The rationale for treating patients who have never demonstrated symptomatic ventricular tachyarrhythmias (sudden cardiac arrest, sustained hypotensive VT, syncope, near-syncope) but who have inducible sustained VT or VF and serious underlying heart disease deserves comment. Wellens and Brugada noted the problem of patients with an electrophysiologic substrate for VT but no clinical arrhythmia, when they discussed the sensitivity and specificity of the techniques of PES [61, 62]. While we may be able to classify a group of patients who are at very high risk of sudden cardiac death, it may be difficult to identify individual patients who will die. This problem recalls the considerations discussed in Chap. 1. Additional trigger factors that may be transiently present in the setting of an anatomic substrate will cause VT or VF. Since we do not fully understand the triggering mechanism but are fully cognizant of the end results (300,000–500,000 annual sudden deaths), should that risk not lead to a more aggressive approach? Perhaps all patients who go through the risk stratification process and fall into the very high-risk category should be treated with suppressive antiarrhythmic drugs or ICDs. Patients with inducible tachyarrhythmias in the absence of both clinical arrhythmias and structural heart disease fit into a different category, however, and it is not reasonable to consider aggressive treatment for them [124].

B. **Electrophysiologic study after myocardial infarction.** A number of studies have addressed the issue of electrophysiologic testing in patients after MI, some with and some without clinical arrhythmias in the acute or periinfarction period. No uniform conclusions have resulted, partially because of the differences in stimulation protocols and in the intervals after MI that the study was performed.

   Hamer et al. examined 70 patients 7–20 days after MI [125]. Twenty had repetitive ventricular responses to PES, 12 of them with sustained or nonsustained VT. Of these 12 patients, 5 died.

   A subsequent study by the same group analyzed 9 patients resuscitated from VT or VF within 3 months of acute MI [126]. Sustained VT was induced by PES in 5 and nonsustained VT in 1. In the clinical follow-up, 1 patient was treated successfully by coronary artery bypass graft and aneurysmectomy, 2 did well with empiric therapy, 1 responded to permanent overdrive pacing and drug therapy, and 2 died—1 because of failure to take medication and the other despite medication.

Richards et al. studied 165 patients 6–28 days after infarction [127]. Thirty-eight had electrical instability at EPS, 4 of whom later experienced symptomatic VT. In this study, the accuracy of inducibility in predicting outcome was 98% if negative (i.e., no induction, no subsequent VT) and 32% if positive (i.e., inducibility, subsequent spontaneous VT or sudden death). The sensitivity and specificity were 86% and 83%, respectively. This study provides some of the strongest arguments for the routine utilization of PES to screen for ventricular irritability in the postinfarction period.

Conversely, Marchlinski et al. concluded that EPS was not predictive in their study of 46 patients 8–60 days after MI [128]. Rather, left ventricular aneurysm and left ventricular ejection fraction were better prognostic indexes of the risk of sudden cardiac death. However, the patients in this study group had a high incidence of aneurysm, which may explain the difference.

Santarelli et al. studied 50 patients 17–40 days after MI, of whom 23 had repetitive ventricular responses (including 10 with sustained VT) at EPS [129]. Although there were no deaths in this population, the inducible group had a higher incidence of nonsustained VT on subsequent Holter monitoring. Brugada and Wellens studied a group of patients 21 days after infarction [62]. In the group without documented arrhythmia, 12 of 20 had inducible sustained VT and 2 of 20 had inducible VF. No deaths had occurred by 6 months. However, 3 weeks after MI may be too early to study these patients, and even 6 months is a short follow-up. Bhandari et al. studied 45 patients 2 weeks after MI and found that PES induced sustained VT or VF in 20 [130]. These patients with inducible VT or VF had a higher incidence of left ventricular wall motion abnormalities, but survival was not different from the noninducible groups. The same comments regarding timing and follow-up are applicable.

Waspe et al. tested 50 survivors of acute MI at a mean of 16 days after infarction [131]. Patients with sustained or nonsustained VT during EPS had a 41% incidence of subsequent VT or sudden death; patients in the noninducible group remained asymptomatic. PES was sensitive, albeit nonspecific, for identifying survivors of MI at high risk of a late malignant arrhythmia.

Recently Roy et al. again concluded that lower ejection fraction, left ventricular aneurysm, and exercise-induced ectopy were predictors of sudden death and spontaneous VT, but inducible arrhythmias were not [132]. However, this study was performed at 12 days after MI and used only double extrastimuli.

Denniss et al. studied 228 clinically well survivors of acute MI 1–4 weeks after infarction [133]. Patients with inducible VT or VF had a higher mortality (26% versus 6%, p <.001) than those without inducible arrhythmia. Although these investigators also used double extrastimuli, they performed EPS both at twice diastolic threshold and at 20 mA. Bourke et al. evaluated 1209 survivors of uncomplicated MI 6–28 days post-MI with either two or up to four or five extrastimuli [134]. In the first year of follow-up, 19% of patients with inducible VT experienced spontaneous VT/VF as compared to 2.9% without inducible VT. In the extended follow-up period (median, 28 months), 25% of those with inducible VT had a spontaneous electrical event, and 37% of these died. The authors concluded that patients with a negative result (94%) can be reassured that there is little risk; those at risk justify a trial of prophylactic antiarrhythmic therapy.

Bhandari et al. evaluated 86 survivors of MI complicated by congestive heart failure, angina, or nonsustained VT with EPS at a mean of 14 days (±7 days) post-MI using single, double, and triple extrastimuli [135]. Arrhythmic events occurred in 32% of patients with inducible VT compared to 7% of the remaining patients. Multivariate analysis indicated that the occurrence of arrhythmic events was independently predicted by both inducible sustained VT and Killip class III–IV heart failure. The risk of events related to arrhythmia was 38.4% when both variables were present and only 4.4% when neither was present. The total cardiac mortality was best predicted by low left ventricular ejection fraction (< 30%).

Many differences in the stimulation protocols hamper comparison of these reports. EPS in many cases was performed before discharge during the initial hospitalization for acute MI. In some cases, it may have been very early in the healing process since the scarring (substrate changes) associated with acute MI may not yet be complete, adversely affecting sensitivity and specificity.

1. **General guidelines for EPS post-MI. Electrophysiologic study after MI is not routinely recommended in the absence of late sustained VT unless the patient is stratified to be at high risk for sudden death (nonsustained VT, low left ventricular ejection fraction, abnormal signal-averaged ECG).** In review, though, a

negative result (i.e., noninducibility) seems to identify a low-risk group. In some cases, inducibility into sustained VT may identify a higher risk for subsequent VT or sudden death, but this opinion is not shared by all. It may be prudent to wait at least 14 days post-MI before performing EPS to evaluate the risk in patients who have not demonstrated symptomatic ventricular tachyarrhythmias.

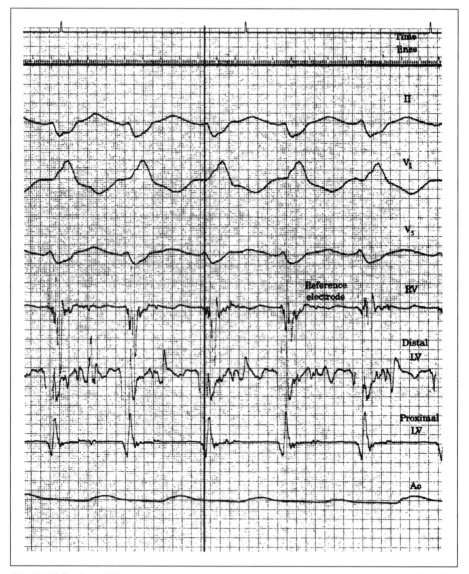

Fig. 12-15. Endocardial mapping. In this patient with refractory ventricular tachycardia (VT), endocardial mapping was done before surgery. At the time of surgery, monomorphic VT is quite often noninducible, and surgery must be directed by the preoperative map. This tracing is arranged as follows: surface ECG: II, V_1, and V_5; endocardial leads: right ventricle (RV), distal left ventricle (LV), and proximal LV exploring electrodes; aortic pressure tracing (Ao). Four sets of the 20 locations mapped are displayed. The earliest activation occurred in the posterobasal segment of the left ventricle. Continuous fractionated diastolic activity is noted in the electrogram closest to the irritable focus. The right ventricular electrogram is used as a reference point.

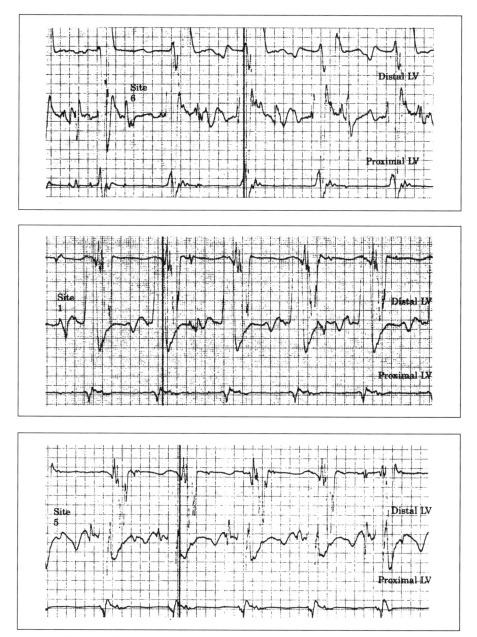

Fig. 12-15 (continued)

VI. **Mapping of the tachycardia zone.** Electrophysiologic testing allows evaluation of inducibility and prediction of the response to drug therapy. Further refinement in technique has permitted identification of the earliest site of activation during the tachycardia, which responds to its initiating site or focus (also described as the tachycardia zone). Endocardial mapping has aided in the evaluation of mechanisms of tachycardia and provides the basis for surgical therapy (and the potential for catheter ablation). Patients who fail to respond to medical therapy and are able to tolerate open heart surgery may have the tachycardia zone extirpated by a variety of methods.

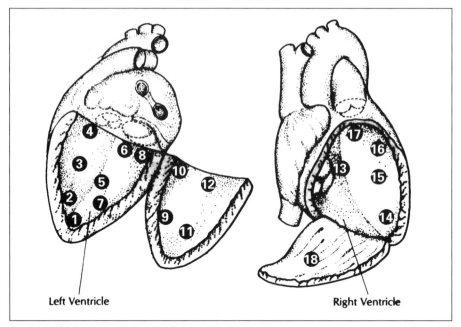

Left Ventricle   Right Ventricle

Fig. 12-16. Map diagram. Sites of catheter placement in mapping studies. (From ME Josephson, LN Horowitz, Recurrent ventricular tachycardia: An electrophysiologic approach. *Hosp Pract* 15(9):56, 1980. Artist: Nancy Lou Gahan Makris.)

Mapping is performed by a variety of methods. Again, this discussion focuses on VT, with SVT and WPW syndrome discussed in Chaps. 6 and 7. Mapping may be performed by recording the ventricular electrogram in various sites during VT, sinus rhythm, or pacing.

The exploring electrode is positioned in as many as 20 sites in the ventricle being mapped. In patients with ischemic heart disease, the site of origin is more often in the left ventricle, less commonly in the right ventricle (Fig. 12-15). Specific problems such as arrhythmogenic right ventricular dysplasia [136] would have the tachycardia zone in the right ventricle.

A. Catheter mapping. The electrograms from the 20 sites produced during VT are reviewed with relation to a fixed point on a surface or intracardiac electrogram. It is determined whether the onset of activation of the exploring electrogram precedes or follows the fixed point and what the time interval is. The earliest activation site corresponds to the electrode nearest the tachycardia zone. That location is determined. If performed correctly, mapping should be accurate to within 2–4 cm². At the time of surgery, the tachycardia zone is most often found to be 4–6 cm².

Sites of origin of the tachycardia in patients with ischemic heart disease are usually found in the periinfarction zone or in the border of a left ventricular aneurysm [137]. It is important to localize the position of the catheter when performing mapping. Mapping studies are facilitated by using a map diagram popularized by the University of Pennsylvania (Fig. 12-16) and by confirming the position of the catheter by fluoroscopy in two views. Josephson et al. emphasized the limitations of the surface ECG in localizing the site of origin [138]. In 10 VTs with a right bundle branch block (RBBB) morphology, the earliest site of activation was the LV or septum. In 11 VTs with a left bundle branch block (LBBB) morphology, the earliest site breaks down as follows: the RV (4), the LV (5), and the septum (2). Selected features of the surface ECG did provide some clues, however. Epicardial breakthrough points do not necessarily correspond to the endocardial activation site [139]. In fact, one endocardial site may have multiple epicardial breakthrough points, depending on timing, refractoriness, cycle length, and the effect of drugs. Therefore, one cannot correctly define ventricular ectopy as multifocal from the surface ECG alone [140]. The proper term is **multiform.** Certainly, more than one endocardial activation site is possible, particularly in the presence of diffuse myocardial disease. However, endocardial mapping is required to demonstrate multifocal ventricular ectopy [141, 142].

Mapping with one electrode is time-consuming, and a variety of different electrode systems have been proposed, including 30 endocardial electrodes attached to a balloon (which is inflated in the ventricle) and a set of 30–100 surface electrodes attached to a "sock" that is placed on the epicardial surface of the ventricle. Isochronic maps may be constructed to localize the origin of the tachycardia [143, 144].

B. Pace mapping. There are limitations to mapping, particularly if the induced arrhythmia is very rapid and associated with hemodynamic compromise. The ideal situation for mapping is a nonhypotensive VT in which the electrode can be moved to multiple sites without requiring abrupt termination of the arrhythmia. Quite often, certain antiarrhythmic drugs will facilitate this process. Other times ventricular tachyarrhythmias will be induced, one or two sites recorded, the arrhythmia terminated for hypotension, and another site selected. This process is most unacceptable if the VT cannot be terminated by pacing. Consequently, attempts have been made to reproduce the tachycardia by ventricular pacing in various sites. Studies revealed that pace mapping can help locate the area of the tachycardia zone but not precisely localize it. It was concluded that pace mapping was potentially useful in patients whose VT was noninducible or who could not tolerate routine catheter mapping, but was neither easier, nor more accurate, nor quicker than mapping during VT [145, 146].

C. Sinus mapping. An attempt was made to localize the tachycardia zone by exploring local electrograms during sinus rhythm. Various degrees of abnormality, fractionation, and late activation were noted, but none of these findings demonstrated a positive predictive value greater than 33%. These electrograms may be associated with, but are not specific for, tachycardia zones. Therefore, data from **sinus mapping** should not be used to guide endocardial extirpation during surgery and might lead to prolongation of the procedure with little gain [147–150].

D. Intraoperative mapping. At the time of surgery, it is desirable to confirm the location of the tachycardia zone with intraoperative mapping [151, 152]. Some limitations are involved, such as the time the surgeon will permit for the procedure (usually 20–40 minutes) and the ability to reproduce the arrhythmia when the heart is open and the patient under anesthesia. Some arrhythmias are no longer inducible. In fact, severe provocative maneuvers such as induction with AC are occasionally used. The surgeon utilizes a variety of electrodes for localization. Many of these are custom designed at individual centers; popular varieties are ring or probe electrodes. The arrhythmia is induced by the electrophysiologist, and the electrograms are recorded and immediately analyzed.

The group at Birmingham Medical Center has defined several terms used in intraoperative mapping [153]: **Delayed activation** occurs more than 100 msec after the onset of QRS. **Fractionation** of the bipolar electrogram was polyphasic, primarily low-amplitude deflection. **Double potentials** were two clearly separated deflections.

There is good correlation between the site identified at endocardial mapping and that identified during intraoperative mapping [151]. If intraoperative mapping is unsuccessful, the surgeon has to proceed on the basis of data obtained in the electrophysiology laboratory or perform a blind resection. Another report suggested that **cryothermal mapping** may provide some additional information [154]. Activation sites are cooled to determine whether induction can be prevented. The advantage is that it provides immediate information about efficacy. If the cooling does not terminate the VT, unnecessary excision may be avoided, since the process is reversible. If it abolishes inducibility, that site would be extirpated. In addition, the cryotermination site does not always correlate with the site of early activation. More data are necessary before the utility of this technique can be fully evaluated.

VII. Role of electrophysiologic study in surgical ablative procedures for ventricular tachyarrhythmias. Until the late 1970s, failure of medical therapy for refractory ventricular tachyarrhythmias left few viable alternatives. A new era of surgical procedures then began. This section concentrates on surgery for ventricular arrhythmias; surgery for accessory pathways is discussed in Chaps. 7 and 19.

It had become apparent that coronary artery bypass grafting alone or the incomplete resection of an aneurysm failed to provide effective therapy for refractory ventricular arrhythmias and was associated with high mortality [155–158]. Thus, newer approaches based on the concept of an identifiable tachycardia zone were developed [159].

Two recent reports addressed the issue of surgical coronary revascularization for survivors of out-of-hospital cardiac arrest. Kelly et al. retrospectively studied 50 patients who had experienced cardiac arrest in the absence of acute MI [160]. Preoperative EPS was performed in 41, and 80% had inducible ventricular arrhythmias. After aortocoronary bypass, 30 of these patients had a postoperative EPS off antiarrhythmic drugs, and induction was suppressed in 14. Multivariate analysis revealed that the only significant predictor of arrhythmia suppression by coronary surgery was inducible VF at the initial EPS. Inducible VT remained inducible in 80% of those whose preoperative EPS revealed this finding. After a 39-month follow-up period, there were four arrhythmia recurrences, one of them fatal. Poor LV function and advanced age were predictive of death. Thus, in a small subgroup, aortocoronary bypass was associated with noninducibility at postoperative EPS and a good outcome.

Every et al. evaluated 85 survivors of sudden cardiac arrest who underwent aortocoronary bypass after recovery and compared them to 180 similar patients treated medically [161]. In a multivariate analysis, coronary bypass had a significant effect in reducing the incidence of subsequent cardiac arrest in the subsequent follow-up period.

Several comments may apply to both reports. Both were retrospective, neither was randomized, and patients who undergo surgery are always carefully selected. In terms of EPS, it has been established that EPS may not always induce VT/VF in patients whose baseline arrhythmia is VF. Consequently, it is difficult to draw conclusions. With the knowledge that some patients remain at risk for recurrent cardiac arrest, many electrophysiologists will consider ICD therapy even if surgical coronary revascularization is successful. Finally, left ventricular function remains an important predictor of survival. Nevertheless, myocardial ischemia is a known trigger of arrhythmia, and successful revascularization certainly can alleviate this factor. Patients with normal left ventricular function who have been successfully revascularized may be different from those who have prior MI with heterogeneous tissue from scarring, providing the substrate for reentry. In patients with a discrete aneurysm, arrhythmia zone extirpation in addition to bypass may be necessary for a successful outcome.

A. **Subendocardial excision or resection.** On the basis of pre- and intraoperative mapping, Josephson et al. localized the tachycardia zone in 12 patients with refractory VT [162]. The surgeon excised the area (8–25 cm^2, 1–4 mm deep) with scissors in the 10 patients who survived, sustained ventricular arrhythmias were no longer inducible at repeat EPS, with a good clinical result at 9–28 months [163]. Many patients had associated coronary artery bypass grafts, if necessary. Further studies provided additional data on efficacy, the value of mapping, and tolerability in patients with LV dysfunction.

Ambulatory ECG monitoring failed to predict the long-term response in patients who underwent endocardial excision and in whom VT was noninducible at repeat EPS [164]. Thus, continued ventricular ectopy on Holter monitoring is not a cause for alarm. A review of the postoperative ECG revealed infrequent abnormalities such as changes in R wave amplitude, ST-segment shifts, or bundle branch block [165]. Left bundle branch block was a serious complication of inferoposterobasal resection. Further EPS also disclosed that some patients had a good outcome despite continued inducibility after subendocardial resection [166]. Thus, neither complex ectopy nor continued inducibility would seem to preclude a favorable outcome.

One important question that arose concerned the value of mapping. Since the surgeon could visually identify areas of subendocardial scar, was it necessary to perform a time-consuming electrophysiologic test? Mason et al. noted that arrhythmia recurrence was greater when the only procedure used was aneurysm resection in comparison to resection or incision guided by mapping procedures [167].

An important consideration when contemplating surgery is whether the patient can tolerate the procedure. Many of these patients have extensive CAD and left ventricular dysfunction. Those with the greatest potential gain (i.e., patients with refractory VT or VF and a poor ejection fraction) also have the highest risk. In a group of such patients with a preoperative mean ejection fraction of 28%, Martin et al. found that aneurysmectomy and endocardial resection were able to be performed with a low operative mortality [168]. Ventricular tachyarrhythmias were controlled, and left ventricular function quite often increased. However, a patient with an ejection fraction of 15–20% and a diffuse aneurysm presents a much higher risk, and the surgeon may be somewhat reluctant to consider arrhythmia surgery. Nevertheless, in patients with moderately but not severely compromised left ventricular function, activation-guided endocardial resection provides long-term effective therapy for malignant ventricular tachyarrhythmias refractory to medical therapy. An actuarial survival curve predicted 62% survival at 40 months in Josephson's series [169].

Wiener et al. suggested that the surgical approach could be enhanced by identifying and excising areas of fragmented electrical activity in the endocardial border zone of ventricular aneurysms [170]. The potential advantage is shortening the time required for intraoperative mapping.

In reviewing the first 100 patients at the University of Pennsylvania, several variables were found to correlate with failure of subendocardial resection [171]. These included multiple sites or tachycardia zones (>5 cm between mapped sites of origin) and the presence of multiple morphologically distinct spontaneous tachycardias. Other factors predictive of failure included inferior wall sites of origin and RBBB morphology of VT. One might consider adjunctive procedures (such as an ICD) in high-risk patients.

Although initially arrhythmia surgery was performed in patients long after MI, Garan et al. described the utility of guided endocardial excision in 10 patients with refractory ventricular tachyarrhythmias occurring 2–15 days after acute MI [172]. Two patients died immediately after surgery, and 1 died later of heart failure. The 7 patients who survived remained asymptomatic after surgery, 6 of them without antiarrhythmic drugs. Similar success in terms of operative mortality and control of VT was also reported by Miller et al. [173]. In addition, they noted that VT early after acute MI seemed to have faster rates and multiple morphologies. No clinical, angiographic, or hemodynamic variables were able to identify this group.

1. **General guidelines for the utilization of surgery for ventricular arrhythmias.** The first 15 years of experience with subendocardial resection indicate that it can be performed with a reasonable operative risk in patients with moderately severe left ventricular dysfunction and refractory ventricular tachyarrhythmias. Survival was improved, and patients had fewer recurrences of VT. Resection guided by mapping is superior to blind resection. Patients may have a good outcome despite continued complex ectopy or inducibility at EPS. However, the availability of ICD devices, the limited number of ideal candidates with discrete aneurysms, and the risk associated with surgery make its selection infrequent today.

B. **Encircling endocardial ventriculotomy.** The other major approach to refractory ventricular tachyarrhythmias was introduced by Guiraudon et al. in 1978 [174]. This technique identifies the tachycardia zone and involves a full-thickness section sparing the epicardium and coronary vessels. The encircling endocardial ventriculotomy completely surrounds the diseased zone at the edge of endocardial fibrosis, thus excluding the VT from the remainder of the ventricle. This technique has been used with considerable success (in preventing recurrent VT) and acceptable mortality, although it is a more extensive process than subendocardial resection and more likely to be associated with ventricular dysfunction.

It has been applied with particular success to selected patients with arrhythmogenic right ventricular dysplasia (ARVD) refractory to medical treatment. As described by Guiraudon et al., the right ventricular free wall was totally disconnected from the right ventricle and repaired [175]. The success of this procedure was attested to by the confinement of the ventricular flutter to the right ventricle while the rest of the heart remained in sinus rhythm (Fig. 12-17).

The encircling endocardial ventriculotomy has a higher incidence of a low-output syndrome postoperatively. Consequently, the subendocardial resection may be preferable in many cases. For limited aneurysms, especially in the posterior left ventricular wall or in cases of ARVD, encircling endocardial ventriculotomy may remain an option. As with subendocardial resection, one must determine the risk-benefit ratio as compared to an ICD alone.

C. **Cryosurgery and laser ablation.** There are limitations to the ability to resect tissue inside the ventricle. Areas in the ventricular septum or around the papillary muscle pose particular difficulty. Cryoablative procedures provide an alternative method to obtain similar extirpation of conductive tissue without creating major alteration in the basic collagen matrix. A cryoprobe freezes an area of tissue (usually 1.5–2.0 cm in diameter) to $-70°C$. With cryoablative techniques, the surgeon may complete the destruction of the tachycardia zone not permitted by subendocardial resection or encircling ventriculotomy alone [176–180]. Thus, the combination of techniques may be most effective.

Laser techniques have also been similarly applied.

VIII. **Surgical techniques for supraventricular arrhythmias (other than Wolff-Parkinson-White syndrome).** Surgery for supraventricular tachyarrhythmias [176, 181] is seldom

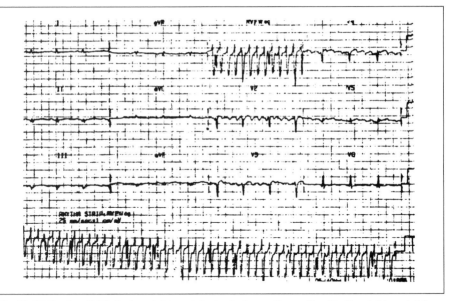

Fig. 12-17. Surface ECG during right ventricular tachycardia confined to the right ventricle after right ventricular disconnection in a patient with right ventricular dysplasia. (RVFW eg = unipolar right ventricular free-wall electrogram.) (From GM Guiraudon et al., Total disconnection of the right ventricular free wall: Surgical treatment of right ventricular tachycardia associated with right ventricular dysplasia. *Circulation* 67:468, 1983.)

necessary and has been replaced to a great extent by radiofrequency catheter ablation. It is discussed in Chaps. 7, 13, and 19.

IX. **Catheter ablation.** The success of surgical extirpative procedures and the ability to record intracardiac potentials (particularly the His bundle) and localize tachycardia zones by mapping led to the concept of catheter ablation. If energy could be delivered to a precise area within the heart via a percutaneous electrode, with resulting tissue injury and an effect on conduction, surgery might not be necessary. This section deals with the early aspects of catheter ablation using direct current. Chapter 13 describes the current experience and use of radiofrequency ablation.

Initial studies of ablation of the AV conduction system were performed in patients with refractory and disabling SVTs [182–184]. The catheter electrode was positioned in the usual His position and manipulated to obtain the largest His deflection. The electrode was then connected to a cardioverter, with a back paddle near the left scapula acting as the anode. After general anesthesia, a synchronized 150- to 400-joule discharge was delivered. A standby temporary pacemaker in the ventricle was then turned on, after observation of the initial escape rhythm.

In an initial registry report, Scheinman et al. described the initial experience in 127 patients [185]. A single shock was effective in 45 patients, but two or more shocks were necessary in another 45 patients. Immediate complications included VF (1), pericardial tamponade (2), and transient hypotension (1), all of which were immediately treated successfully without chronic sequelae. Late complications included VT (3), sepsis in the pacemaker pocket (2) or from the temporary pacemaker (1), thrombophlebitis or thrombosis (2), and hemothorax (2). All but 10% of the population derived complete or partial benefit from the procedure. There were late complications, including sudden cardiac death, when direct current cardioversion was used.

Reports also indicated the utility of this procedure in infants [186] and those with reentry through a nodoventricular tract [187]. Hartzler considered the technique for patients with VT [188]. Certainly this application requires precise localization by mapping for fear of potentially creating a tachycardia zone if the discharge was delivered to normal myocardium. Ruffy et al. reported the catheter ablation of a fascicular tachycardia by using three 300-joule shocks in the posterobasal region of the left ventricular septum [189].

Catheter ablation was then applied to accessory pathways [190] and automatic atrial tachycardias [191, 192]. Ablation of the AV conduction system [193] was the most successful. Examination of the catheter electrode itself after direct current ablation indicated the destructive potential of the technique. Delivery of the shock through the coronary sinus caused rupture with pericardial tamponade.

Scheinman and Davis summarized recommendations in 1986 [194]. Catheter ablation of the AV junction was as effective as surgery and was obtained at lower morbidity, mortality, and cost. In patients with accessory pathways, ablation through the coronary sinus was unacceptable. Free-wall accessory pathways were better treated surgically, but there was a role for ablation in patients with posteroseptal pathways. In regard to ventricular tachyarrhythmias, the results have been mixed and the procedure was not yet recommended, except for further investigation.

X. Other ablation techniques. Recently the utilization of intracoronary ethanol selectively injected into a segment of coronary artery supplying a critical area of myocardium has been reported. The initial studies, of a limited number of patients, have revealed a moderate degree of efficacy, but complications, including complete heart block and pericarditis, have been reported [195, 196]. The potential utility of this technique will hinge on the ability to deliver the alcohol subselectively to a very small coronary vessel supplying the critical tachycardia zone.

XI. Economic aspects of electrophysiologic study. Electrophysiologic testing is expensive in terms of time required for performance and analysis, personnel, instrumentation, and disposable equipment. These issues have been addressed by Ross et al. [197] and Ferguson et al. [198]. Although the studies are difficult, time-consuming, and expensive, therapy guided by EPS may shorten or prevent subsequent hospitalization, avoid recurrent malignant tachyarrhythmias, and possibly avert sudden cardiac death.

The time factor varies with the problem being investigated. The study in a patient with syncope who turns out to have no inducible arrhythmias may be relatively fast. The patient with VT in whom multiple drugs are tested or the patient with complicated accessory pathway conduction may have a study lasting 5 hours. The more complicated the arrhythmia is, the longer is the subsequent analysis of the recorded tracings. Fluoroscopy time is needed, but this is usually minimal for a routine diagnostic study when compared with cardiac catheterization. Ablation requires longer fluoroscopy times.

Currently the cost of an extensive initial EPS evaluation will include a professional fee of $2500–3500, and repeat limited studies for testing additional drugs may be an additional $1500–2000. In addition there will be charges for the electophysiology lab submitted by the hospital. The hourly cost should be calculated. For example, $2500 for an initial EPS lasting 2 hours, with 1 hour of further analysis and an additional 1 hour examining and counseling, is quite modest in today's economy. Considering the cost of hospitalization, if a patient were admitted with recurrent VT, a 10-day hospital stay would cost more than $10,000. Thus, the EPS becomes cost-effective even if it prevents one recurrent hospitalization.

Economic aspects, however, must not cloud the tremendous benefit in health care that EPS has provided to patients with life-threatening arrhythmias. Many patients are alive and active today because of the ability to guide therapy through EPS. It is a relatively safe study. There are definite indications, which continue to expand.

References

1. Kastor JA, et al. Clinical electrophysiology of ventricular tachycardia. *N Engl J Med* 304:1004–1020, 1981.
2. Josephson ME, Horowitz LN. Electrophysiologic approach to therapy of recurrent sustained ventricular tachycardia. *Am J Cardiol* 43:631–642, 1979.
3. Horowitz LN, et al. Role of programmed stimulation in assessing vulnerability to ventricular arrhythmias. *Am Heart J* 103:604–608, 1982.
4. Scheinman MM, Morady F. Invasive cardiac electrophysiologic testing: The current state of the art. *Circulation* 67:1169–1173, 1983.
5. Wiener I. Current applications of clinical electrophysiologic study in the diagnosis and treatment of cardiac arrhythmias. *Am J Cardiol* 49:1287–1292, 1982.
6. Ruskin JN, DiMarco JP, Garan H. Out of hospital cardiac arrest, electrophysiologic observations and selection of long term antiarrhythmic therapy. *N Engl J Med* 303: 607–613, 1980.

7. *J Am Coll Cardiol* 14:1827–1842, 1989.
8. Wellens HJ, Schuilenburg RM, Durrer D. Electrical stimulation of the heart in patients with ventricular tachycardia. *Circulation* 46:216–226, 1972.
9. Wellens HJ. Pathophysiology of ventricular tachycardia in man. *Arch Intern Med* 135: 473–479, 1975.
10. Wellens HJ, Duren DR, Lie KI. Observations on mechanisms of ventricular tachycardia in man. *Circulation* 54:237–244, 1976.
11. Wellens HJ. Value and limitations of programmed electrical stimulation of the heart in the study and treatment of tachycardias. *Circulation* 57:845–853, 1978.
12. Josephson ME, et al. Recurrent sustained ventricular tachycardia: 1. Mechanisms. *Circulation* 57:431–440, 1978.
13. Vandepol CJ, et al. Incidence and clinical significance of induced ventricular tachycardia. *Am J Cardiol* 45:725–731, 1978.
14. Hess DS, Morady F, Scheinman MM. Electrophysiologic testing in the evaluation of patients with syncope of undetermined origin. *Am J Cardiol* 50:1309–1315, 1982.
15. Olshansky B, Mazuz M, Martinus JB. Significance of inducible tachycardia in patients with syncope of unknown origin: A long-term follow-up. *J Am Coll Cardiol* 5:216–223, 1985.
16. Morady F, et al. Electrophysiologic testing in bundle branch block and unexplained syncope. *Am J Cardiol* 54:587–591, 1984.
17. Ezri M, et al. Electrophysiologic evaluation of syncope in patients with bifascicular block. *Am Heart J* 106:693–697, 1983.
18. Reiffel JA, et al. Electrophysiologic testing in patients with recurrent syncope: Are results predicted by prior ambulatory monitoring? *Am Heart J* 110:1146–1153, 1985.
19. Morady F, et al. Long term followup of patients with recurrent unexplained syncope evaluated by electrophysiologic testing. *J Am Coll Cardiol* 2:1053–1059, 1983.
20. Teichman SL, et al. The value of electrophysiologic studies in syncope of undetermined origin: Report of 150 cases. *Am Heart J* 110:469–479, 1985.
21. Doherty JV, et al. Electrophysiologic evaluation and followup characteristics of patients with recurrent unexplained syncope and presyncope. *Am J Cardiol* 55:703–708, 1985.
22. Kugler JD, et al. Drug-electrophysiology studies in infants, children, and adolescents. *Am Heart J* 110:144–154, 1985.
23. Gettes LS, et al. AHA committee report: Personnel and equipment required for electrophysiologic testing. *Circulation* 72:023–A, 1985.
24. Waldo AL, et al. The minimally appropriate electrophysiologic study for the initial assessment of patients with documented sustained monomorphic ventricular tachycardia. *J Am Coll Cardiol* 5:1174–1177, 1985.
25. Reiffel JA, et al. Electrophysiologic studies of the sinus node and atria. In Cardiac Arrhythmias: Electrophysiologic Techniques and Management. *Cardiovascular Clinics*. Philadelphia: Davis, 1985. Pp 37–59.
26. Greenspon AJ. Electrophysiologic studies for pacemaker selection. In Cardiac Arrhythmias: Electrophysiologic Techniques and Management. *Cardiovascular Clinics*. Philadelphia: Davis, 1985. Pp 119–137.
27. Strauss HC, et al. Premature atrial stimulation as a key to the understanding of sinoatrial conduction in man. *Circulation* 47:86, 1973.
28. Narula OS, et al. A new method for measurement of sinoatrial conduction time. *Circulation* 58:706, 1978.
29. Breithardt G, Speipel L, Loogen F. Sinus node recovery time and calculated sinoatrial conduction time in normal subjects and patients with sinus node dysfunction. *Circulation* 56:43–50, 1977.
30. Gann D, Tolentino A, Samet P. Electrophysiologic evaluation of elderly patients with sinus bradycardia. A long-term follow-up study. *Ann Intern Med* 90:24–29, 1979.
31. Greene HL, Reid PR, Schaeffer AH. The repetitive ventricular response in man: A predictor of sudden death. *N Engl J Med* 299:729–734, 1978.
32. Greene HL, Reid PR, Schaeffer AH. Mechanism of the repetitive ventricular response in man. *Am J Cardiol* 45:227–235, 1980.
33. Mower MM, et al. Use of alternating current during diagnostic electrophysiologic studies. *Circulation* 67:69–71, 1983.
34. Reddy CP, Gettes LS. Use of isoproterenol as an aid to elective induction of chronic recurrent ventricular tachycardia. *Am J Cardiol* 44:705–712, 1979.
35. Freedman RA, et al. Facilitation of ventricular tachyarrhythmia induction by isoproterenol. *Am J Cardiol* 54:765–770, 1984.
36. Robertson JF, et al. Anatomic and electrophysiologic correlates of ventricular tachycardia requiring left ventricular stimulation. *Am J Cardiol* 48:263–268, 1981.

37. Mason JW. Repetitive beating after single ventricular extrastimuli: Incidence and prognostic significance in patients with recurrent ventricular tachycardia. *Am J Cardiol* 45:1126–1131, 1980.
38. Ruskin JN, DiMarco JP, Garan H. Repetitive responses to single ventricular extrastimuli in patients with serious ventricular arrhythmias: Incidence and clinical significance. *Circulation* 63:767–772, 1981.
39. Platia EV, et al. Sensitivity of various extrastimulus techniques in patients with serious ventricular arrhythmias. *Am Heart J* 106:698–703, 1983.
40. Livelli FD, et al. Response to programmed ventricular stimulation: Sensitivity, specificity and relation to heart disease. *Am J Cardiol* 50:452–458, 1982.
41. Roy D, et al. Clinical characteristics and long term followup in 119 survivors of cardiac arrest: Relation to inducibility at electrophysiologic testing. *Am J Cardiol* 52:969–974, 1983.
42. Wellens HJ, Brugada P, Stevenson WG. Programmed electrical stimulation of the heart in patients with life-threatening ventricular arrhythmias: What is the significance of induced arrhythmias and what is the correct stimulation protocol? *Circulation* 72:1–7, 1985.
43. Swerdlow CD, Winkle RA, Mason JW. Prognostic significance of the number of induced ventricular complexes during assessment of therapy for ventricular tachyarrhythmias. *Circulation* 68:400–405, 1983.
44. Platia EV, Reid PR. Nonsustained ventricular tachycardia during programmed ventricular stimulation: Criteria for a positive test. *Am J Cardiol* 56:79–83, 1985.
45. Torres V, Flowers D, Somberg J. The clinical significance of polymorphic ventricular tachycardia provided at electrophysiologic testing. *Am Heart J* 110:17–23, 1985.
46. Spielman SR, et al. Ventricular fibrillation during programmed ventricular stimulation: Incidence and clinical implications. *Am J Cardiol* 42:913–918, 1978.
47. Josephson ME, et al. Electrophysiologic and hemodynamic studies in patients resuscitated from cardiac arrest. *Am J Cardiol* 46:948–955, 1980.
48. Josephson ME, et al. Mechanism of ventricular fibrillation in man. *Am J Cardiol* 44:623–631, 1979.
49. Cooper MJ, et al. Comparison of immediate versus day-to-day variability of ventricular tachycardia induction by programmed stimulation. *J Am Coll Cardiol* 13:1599–1607, 1989.
50. Kudenchuk PF, et al. Day-to-day reproducibility of antiarrhythmic drug trials using programmed extrastimulus techniques for ventricular tachyarrhythmias associated with coronary artery disease. *Am J Cardiol* 66:725–730, 1990.
51. Bhandari AK, et al. Day to day reproducibility of electrically inducible ventricular arrhythmias in survivors of acute myocardial infarction. *J Am Coll Cardiol* 15:1075–1081, 1990.
52. Volgman AS, et al. Reproducibility of programmed electrical stimulation responses in patients with ventricular tachycardia or fibrillation associated with coronary artery disease. *Am J Cardiol* 70:758–763, 1992.
53. Morady F, et al. Clinical features and prognosis of patients with out of hospital cardiac arrest and a normal electrophysiologic study. *J Am Coll Cardiol* 4:39–44, 1984.
54. McPherson CA, Rosenfeld LE, Batsford WP. Day to day reproducibility of responses to right ventricular programmed electrical stimulation: Implications for serial drug testing. *Am J Cardiol* 55:689–695, 1985.
55. Doherty JU, et al. Programmed ventricular stimulation at a second right ventricular site: An analysis of 100 patients, with special reference to sensitivity, specificity and characteristics of patients with induced ventricular tachycardia. *Am J Cardiol* 52:1184–1189, 1983.
56. Doherty JU, et al. Discordant results of programmed ventricular stimulation at different right ventricular sites in patients with and without spontaneous sustained ventricular tachycardia: A prospective study of 56 patients. *Am J Cardiol* 54:336–342, 1984.
57. Buxton HE, et al. Role of triple extrastimuli during electrophysiologic study of patients with documented sustained ventricular tachyarrhythmias. *Circulation* 69:532–540, 1984.
58. Morady F, et al. A prospective comparison of triple extrastimuli and left ventricular stimulation in studies of ventricular tachycardia induction. *Circulation* 70:52–57, 1984.
59. Morady F, Hess D, Scheinman MM. Electrophysiologic drug testing in patients with malignant ventricular arrhythmias: Importance of stimulation at more than one ventricular site. *Am J Cardiol* 50:1055–1060, 1982.
60. Morady F, et al. Programmed ventricular stimulation in patients without spontaneous ventricular tachycardia. *Am Heart J* 107:875–882, 1984.

61. Brugada P, Wellens HJ. Comparison in the same patient of two programmed ventricular stimulation protocols to induce ventricular tachycardia. *Am J Cardiol* 55:380–383, 1985.

62. Brugada P, Wellens HJ. Programmed electrical stimulation of the heart in ventricular arrhythmias. *Am J Cardiol* 56:187–190, 1985.

63. Mann DE, et al. Induction of clinical ventricular tachycardia using programmed stimulation: Value of third and fourth extrastimuli. *Am J Cardiol* 52:501–506, 1983.

64. Oseran DS, et al. Mode of stimulation versus response: Validation of a protocol for induction of ventricular tachycardia. *Am Heart J* 110:646–651, 1985.

65. Belhassen B, et al. Programmed ventricular stimulation using up to two extrastimuli and repetition of double extrastimulation for induction of ventricular tachycardia: A new highly sensitive and specific protocol. *Am J Cardiol* 65:615–622, 1990.

66. Summitt J, et al. Effect of basic drive cycle length on the yield of ventricular tachycardia during programmed ventricular stimulation. *Am J Cardiol* 65:49–52, 1990.

67. Simonson JS, et al. Increasing the yield of ventricular tachycardia induction: A prospective, randomized comparative study of the standard ventricular stimulation protocol to a short-to-long protocol and a new two-site protocol. *Am Heart J* 121:68–76, 1991.

68. Morady F, et al. Prospective comparison of a conventional and an accelerated protocol for programmed ventricular stimulation in patients with coronary artery disease. *Circulation* 83:764–773, 1991.

69. Naccarelli GV, et al. Role of electrophysiologic testing in managing patients who have ventricular tachycardia unrelated to coronary artery disease. *Am J Cardiol* 50:165–171, 1982.

70. Huang SK, Messer JV, Denes P. Significance of ventricular tachycardia in idiopathic dilated cardiomyopathy: Observations in 35 patients. *Am J Cardiol* 51:507–512, 1983.

71. Meinertz T, et al. Determinants of prognosis in idiopathic dilated cardiomyopathy as determined by programmed electrical stimulation. *Am J Cardiol* 56:337–341, 1985.

72. Poll DS, et al. Sustained ventricular tachycardia in patients with idiopathic dilated cardiomyopathy: Electrophysiologic testing and lack of response to antiarrhythmic drug therapy. *Circulation* 70:451–456, 1984.

73. Brembilla-Perrot B, et al. Diagnostic value of ventricular stimulation in patients with idiopathic dilated cardiomyopathy.

74. Anderson KP, et al. Vulnerability of patients with obstructive hypertrophic cardiomyopathy to ventricular arrhythmia induction in the operating room. *Am J Cardiol* 51:811–816, 1983.

75. Morady F, et al. Programmed ventricular stimulation in mitral valve prolapse: Analysis of 36 patients. *Am J Cardiol* 53:135–138, 1984.

76. Rosenthal ME, et al. The yield of programmed ventricular stimulation in mitral valve prolapse patients with ventricular arrhythmias. *Am Heart J* 110:970–976, 1985.

77. Denes P, et al. Electrophysiologic studies in patients with chronic recurrent ventricular tachycardia. *Circulation* 54:229–236, 1976.

78. DiCarlo LA, et al. Clinical significance of ventricular fibrillation—flutter induced by ventricular programmed stimulation. *Am Heart J* 109:959–963, 1985.

79. Poole JE, et al. Long-term outcome in patients who survive out of hospital ventricular fibrillation and undergo electrophysiologic studies: Evaluation by electrophysiologic subgroups. *J Am Coll Cardiol* 16:657–665, 1990.

80. Kim SG, et al. Prognosis of patients with ventricular tachycardia or fibrillation and a normal electrophysiologic study. *Am Heart J* 12:77–80, 1991.

81. Andresen D, et al. Prognosis of patients with sustained ventricular tachycardia and survivors of cardiac arrest not inducible by programmed stimulation. *Am J Cardiol* 70:1250–1254, 1992.

82. Sousa J, et al. Results of electrophysiologic testing and long-term prognosis in patients with coronary artery disease and aborted sudden death. *Am Heart J* 122:1001–1006, 1991.

83. Fogoros R, et al. Long-term outcome of survivors of cardiac arrest whose therapy is guided by electrophysiologic testing. *J Am Coll Cardiol* 19:780–788, 1992.

84. Roy D, et al. Termination of ventricular tachycardia: Role of tachycardia cycle length. *Am J Cardiol* 50:1346–1350, 1982.

85. Gardner MJ, et al. Termination of ventricular tachycardia: Evaluation of a new pacing method. *Am J Cardiol* 50:1338–1344, 1982.

86. Waxman HL, et al. Termination of ventricular tachycardia with ventricular stimulation: Salutary effect of increased current strength. *Circulation* 65:800–804, 1982.

87. Fisher JD, et al. Ultrarapid single-capture train stimulation for termination of ventricular tachycardia. *Am J Cardiol* 51:1334–1338, 1983.

88. Keren G, Mivra DS, Somberg JC. Pacing termination of ventricular tachycardia: Influence of antiarrhythmic-slowed ectopic rate. *Am Heart J* 107:638–643, 1984.
89. Waldo AL, et al. Demonstration of the mechanism of transient entrainment of ventricular tachycardia with rapid atrial pacing. *J Am Coll Cardiol* 2:422–430, 1984.
90. Almendual JM, et al. Entrainment of ventricular tachycardia by atrial depolarizations. *Am J Cardiol* 55:298–304, 1985.
91. Mann DE, et al. Importance of pacing site in entrainment of ventricular tachycardia. *J Am Coll Cardiol* 5:781–787, 1985.
92. Naccarelli GV, et al. Influence of tachycardia cycle length and antiarrhythmic drugs on pacing termination and acceleration of ventricular tachycardia. *Am Heart J* 105:1–5, 1983.
93. DiMarco JP, Garan H, Ruskin JN. Complications in patients undergoing cardiac electrophysiologic procedures. *Ann Intern Med* 97:490–493, 1982.
94. Horowitz LN, et al. Risks and complications of clinical cardiac electrophysiologic studies: A prospective analysis of 1,000 patients. *J Am Coll Cardiol* 9:1261–1268, 1987.
95. Mason JW, Winkle RA. Electrode catheter induction of ventricular tachycardia: Observations on the technique and its use in choosing and assessing the efficacy of antiarrhythmic drugs in patients with recurrent ventricular tachycardia. *Circulation* 58:971–985, 1978.
96. Wellens HJ, et al. Effect of procainamide, propranolol and verapamil on the mechanism of tachycardia in patients with chronic recurrent ventricular tachycardia. *Am J Cardiol* 40:579–585, 1977.
97. Horowitz LN, Josephson ME, Farshidi A. Recurrent sustained ventricular tachycardia. 3. Role of the electrophysiologic study in selection of antiarrhythmic regimens. *Circulation* 58:986–997, 1978.
98. Heger JJ, et al. Clinical efficacy and electrophysiology during long term therapy for recurrent ventricular tachycardia or ventricular fibrillation. *N Engl J Med* 305:539–545, 1981.
99. Swiryn S, et al. Prediction of response to class I antiarrhythmic drugs during electrophysiologic study of ventricular tachycardia. *Am Heart J* 104:43–50, 1982.
100. Kavanagh KM, et al. Drug therapy for ventricular tachyarrhythmias: How many electropharmacologic trials are appropriate? *J Am Coll Cardiol* 17:391–396, 1991.
101. Swerdlow CD, et al. Clinical factors predicting successful electrophysiologicpharmacologic study in patients with ventricular tachycardia. *J Am Coll Cardiol* 1:409–416, 1983.
102. Swerdlow CD, Winkle RA, Mason JW. Determinants of survival in patients with ventricular tachyarrythmias. *N Engl J Med* 308:1436–1442, 1983.
103. Spielman SR, et al. Predictors of the success or failure of medical therapy in patients with chronic recurrent sustained ventricular tachycardia: A discriminant analysis. *J Am Coll Cardiol* 1:401–408, 1983.
104. Schoenfeld MH, et al. Determinants of outcome of electrophysiologic study in patients with ventricular tachyarrhythmias. *J Am Coll Cardiol* 6:298–306, 1985.
105. Benditt DG, et al. Prevention of sudden cardiac arrest: Role of provocative electropharmacologic testing. *J Am Coll Cardiol* 3:418–425, 1983.
106. Schoenfeld MH, et al. Long-term reproducibility of responses to programmed cardiac stimulation in spontaneous ventricular tachyarrhythmias. *Am J Cardiol* 54:564–568, 1984.
107. DiMarco JP, Garan H, Ruskin JN. Quinidine for ventricular arrhythmias: Value of electrophysiologic testing. *Am J Cardiol* 51:909–915, 1983.
108. Waxman HL, et al. The response to procainamide during electrophysiologic study for sustained ventricular tachyarrhythmias predicts the response to other medications. *Circulation* 67:30–37, 1983.
109. Greenspan AM, et al. Large dose procainamide therapy for ventricular tachyarrhythmias. *Am J Cardiol* 46:453–462, 1980.
110. Marchlinski FE, et al. Comparative electrophysiologic effects of intravenous and oral procainamide in patients with sustained ventricular arrhythmias. *J Am Coll Cardiol* 6:1247–1254, 1984.
111. Rae AP, et al. Limitations of failure of procainamide during electrophysiologic testing to predict response to other medical therapy. *J Am Coll Cardiol* 6:410–416, 1985.
112. Rae AP, Greenspan AM, Spielman SR. Antiarrhythmic drug efficacy for ventricular tachyarrhythmias associated with coronary artery disease as assessed by electrophysiologic studies. *Am J Cardiol* 55:1494–1499, 1985.
113. LeClercq JF, et al. Predictive value of electrophysiologic studies during treatment of ventricular tachycardia with the beta-blocking agent nadolol. *J Am Coll Cardiol* 16:413–417, 1990.

114. Hii JTY, et al. Infarct artery patency predicts outcome of serial electropharmacologic studies in patients with malignant ventricular arrhythmias. *Circulation* 87:764–772, 1993.

115. Buxton AE, et al. Electrophysiologic studies in nonsustained ventricular tachycardia: Relation to underlying heart disease. *Am J Cardiol* 52:985–991, 1983.

116. Buxton AE, et al. Prognostic factors in nonsustained ventricular tachycardia. *Am J Cardiol* 53:1275–1279, 1984.

117. Veltri EP, et al. Programmed electrical stimulation and long-term followup in asymptomatic nonsustained ventricular tachycardias. *Am J Cardiol* 56:309–314, 1985.

118. Spielman SR, et al. Electrophysiologic testing in patients at high risk for sudden cardiac death: I. Nonsustained ventricular tachycardia and abnormal ventricular function. *J Am Coll Cardiol* 6:31–39, 1985.

119. Kowey PR, et al. Programmed electrical stimulation of the heart in coronary artery disease. *Am J Cardiol* 51:531–536, 1983.

120. Gomes JAC, et al. Programmed electrical stimulation in patients with high-grade ventricular ectopy: Electrophysiologic findings and prognosis for survival. *Circulation* 70: 43–51, 1984.

121. Kowey PR, et al. Value of electrophysiologic testing in patients with previous myocardial infarction and nonsustained ventricular tachycardia. *Am J Cardiol* 65:594–598, 1990.

122. Kowey PR, et al. Does programmed stimulation really help in the evaluation of patients with nonsustained ventricular tachycardia? Results of a meta-analysis. *Am Heart J* 123:481–485, 1992.

123. Kadish A, et al. Management of nonsustained ventricular tachycardia guided by electrophysiologic testing. *PACE* 16:1037–1050, 1993.

124. Brugada P, et al. Results of a ventricular stimulation protocol using a maximum of 4 premature stimuli in patients without documented or suspected ventricular arrhythmias. *Am J Cardiol* 52:1214–1218, 1983.

125. Hamer A, et al. Prediction of sudden death by electrophysiologic studies in high risk patients surviving myocardial infarction. *Am J Cardiol* 50:223–229, 1982.

126. Hamer A, et al. Electrophysiologic studies in survivors of late cardiac arrest after myocardial infarction. *Am Heart J* 105:921–927, 1983.

127. Richards DA, Cody DV, Denniss AR. Ventricular electrical instability: A predictor of death after myocardial infarction. *Am J Cardiol* 51:75–80, 1983.

128. Marchlinski FE, et al. Identifying patients at risk of sudden death after myocardial infarction: Value of the response to programmed stimulation, degree of ventricular ectopic activity and severity of left ventricular dysfunction. *Am J Cardiol* 52:1190–1196, 1983.

129. Santarelli P, et al. Ventricular arrhythmias induced by programmed ventricular stimulation after acute myocardial infarction. *Am J Cardiol* 55:391–394, 1985.

130. Bhandari AK, et al. Frequency and significance of induced sustained ventricular tachycardia or fibrillation two weeks after acute myocardial infarction. *Am J Cardiol* 56:737–742, 1985.

131. Waspe LE, et al. Prediction of sudden death and spontaneous ventricular tachycardia in survivors of complicated myocardial infarction: Value of the response to programmed stimulation using a maximum of three ventricular extrastimuli. *J Am Coll Cardiol* 5: 1292–1301, 1985.

132. Roy D, et al. Programmed ventricular stimulation in survivors of an acute myocardial infarction. *Circulation* 72:487–494, 1985.

133. Denniss AR, et al. Value of programmed stimulation and exercise testing in predicting one year mortality after acute myocardial infarction. *Am J Cardiol* 56:213–220, 1985.

134. Bourke JP, et al. Routine programmed electrical stimulation in survivors of acute myocardial infarction for prediction of spontaneous ventricular tachyarrhythmias during follow-up: Results, optimal stimulation protocol and cost-effective screening. *J Am Coll Cardiol* 18:780–788, 1991.

135. Bhandari AK, et al. Prognostic significance of programmed ventricular stimulation in patients surviving complicated acute myocardial infarction: A prospective study. *Am Heart J* 124:87–96, 1992.

136. Belhassen B, et al. Extensive endocardial mapping during sinus rhythm and ventricular tachycardia in a patient with arrhythmogenic right ventricular dysplasia. *J Am Coll Cardiol* 6:1302–1306, 1984.

137. McFarland TM, et al. Relation between site of origin of ventricular tachycardia and relative left ventricular myocardial perfusion and wall motion. *Am J Cardiol* 51:1329–1333, 1983.

138. Josephson ME, et al. Recurrent sustained ventricular tachycardia: 2. Endocardial mapping. *Circulation* 57:440–447, 1978.
139. Josephson ME, et al. Recurrent sustained ventricular tachycardia: 4. Pleomorphism. *Circulation* 59:459–468, 1979.
140. Josephson ME, et al. Sustained ventricular tachycardia: Role of the 12 lead electrocardiogram in localizing site of origin. *Circulation* 64:257–272, 1981.
141. Miller JM, et al. Morphologically distinct sustained ventricular tachycardia in coronary artery disease: Significance and surgical results. *J Am Coll Cardiol* 4:1073–1079, 1984.
142. Horowitz LN, Josephson ME, Harken AH. Epicardial and endocardial activation during sustained ventricular tachycardia in man. *Circulation* 61:1227–1238, 1980.
143. de Bakker JMT, et al. Endocardial mapping by simultaneous recording of endocardial electrograms during cardiac surgery for ventricular aneurysm. *J Am Coll Cardiol* 5:947–953, 1983.
144. Downar E, et al. On line epicardial mapping of intraoperative ventricular arrhythmias: Initial clinical experience. *J Am Coll Cardiol* 4:703–714, 1984.
145. Waxman HL, Josephson ME. Ventricular activation during ventricular endocardial pacing: 1. Electrocardiographic patterns related to the site of pacing. *Am J Cardiol* 50:1–10, 1982.
146. Josephson ME, et al. Ventricular activation during ventricular endocardial pacing: II. Role of pace mapping to localize origin of ventricular tachycardia. *Am J Cardiol* 50:11–22, 1982.
147. Cassidy DM, et al. The value of catheter mapping during sinus rhythm to localize site of origin of ventricular tachycardia. *Circulation* 69:1103–1110, 1984.
148. Cassidy DM, et al. Endocardial mapping in humans in sinus rhythm with normal left ventricles: Activation patterns and characteristics of electrograms. *Circulation* 70:37–42, 1984.
149. Kienzle MG, et al. Intraoperative endocardial mapping during sinus rhythm: Relationship to site of origin of ventricular tachycardia. *Circulation* 70:957–965, 1984.
150. Cassidy DM, et al. Catheter mapping during sinus rhythm: Relation of local electrogram duration of ventricular tachycardia cycle length. *Am J Cardiol* 55:713–716, 1985.
151. Josephson ME, Horowitz LN, Spielman SR. Comparison of endocardial catheter mapping with intraoperative mapping of ventricular tachycardia. *Circulation* 61:395–404, 1980.
152. Wiener I, Mindich B, Pitchon R. Determinants of ventricular tachycardia in patients with ventricular aneurysms: Results of intraoperative epicardial and endocardial mapping. *Circulation* 65:856–861, 1982.
153. Klein H, et al. Intraoperative electrophysiologic mapping of the ventricles during sinus rhythm in patients with a previous myocardial infarction: Identification of the electrophysiologic substrate of ventricular arrhythmias. *Circulation* 66:847–852, 1982.
154. Gallagher JD, et al. Cryothermal mapping of recurrent ventricular tachycardia in man. *Circulation* 71:733–739, 1985.
155. Gallagher JJ. Surgical treatment of arrhythmias: Current status and future direction. *Am J Cardiol* 41:1035–1044, 1978.
156. Lehrman KL, et al. Effect of coronary arterial bypass surgery on exercise induced ventricular arrhythmias. *Am J Cardiol* 44:1056–1060, 1979.
157. Ricks WB, et al. Surgical management of life-threatening ventricular arrhythmias with coronary artery disease. *Circulation* 56:38–42, 1977.
158. Buda AJ, Stinson EB, Harrison DC. Surgery of life-threatening ventricular tachyarrhythmias. *Am J Cardiol* 44:1171–1177, 1979.
159. Horowitz LN, et al. Surgical treatment of ventricular arrhythmias in coronary artery disease. *Ann Intern Med* 95:88–97, 1981.
160. Kelly P, et al. Surgical coronary revascularization in survivors of prehospital cardiac arrest: Its effect on inducible ventricular arrhythmias and long-term survival. *J Am Coll Cardiol* 15:267–273, 1990.
161. Every NR, et al. Influence of coronary bypass surgery on subsequent outcome of patients resuscitated from out of hospital cardiac arrest. *J Am Coll Cardiol* 19:1435–1439, 1992.
162. Josephson ME, Harken AH, Horowitz LN. Endocardial excision: A new surgical technique for the treatment of recurrent ventricular tachycardia. *Circulation* 60:1430–1439, 1979.
163. Horowitz LN, et al. Ventricular resection guided by epicardial and endocardial mapping for treatment of recurrent ventricular tachycardia. *N Engl J Med* 302:539–543, 1980.
164. Herling IM, Horowitz LN, Josephson ME. Ventricular ectopic activity after medical and

surgical treatment for recurrent sustained ventricular tachycardia. *Am J Cardiol* 45:633–639, 1980.

165. Kienzle MG, et al. Electrocardiographic changes following endocardial resection for ventricular tachycardia. *Am Heart J* 104:753–761, 1982.

166. Kienzle MG, et al. Subendocardial resection for refractory ventricular tachycardia: Effects on ambulatory electrocardiogram, programmed stimulation and ejection fraction, and relation to outcome. *J Am Coll Cardiol* 2:853–858, 1983.

167. Mason JW, et al. Surgery for ventricular tachycardia: Efficacy of left ventricular aneurysm resection compared with operation guided by electrical activation mapping. *Circulation* 65:1148–1154, 1982.

168. Martin JL, et al. Aneurysmectomy and endocardial resection for ventricular tachycardia: Favorable hemodynamic and antiarrhythmic results in patients with global left ventricular dysfunction. *Am Heart J* 103:960–965, 1982.

169. Josephson ME, Harken AH, Horowitz LN. Long-term results of endocardial resection for sustained ventricular tachycardia in coronary disease patients. *Am Heart J* 104: 51–56, 1982.

170. Wiener I, Mindich B, Pitchon R. Fragmented endocardial electrical activity in patients with ventricular tachycardia: A new guide to surgical therapy. *Am Heart J* 107:86–90, 1984.

171. Miller JM, et al. Subendocardial resection for ventricular tachycardia: Predictors of surgical success. *Circulation* 70:624–631, 1984.

172. Garan H, et al. Refractory ventricular tachycardia complicating recovery from acute myocardial infarction: Treatment with map guided infarctectomy. *Am Heart J* 107:571–577, 1984.

173. Miller JM, et al. Subendocardial resection for sustained ventricular tachycardia in the early period after acute myocardial infarction. *Am J Cardiol* 55:980–984, 1985.

174. Guiraudon G, et al. Encircling endocardial ventriculotomy: A new surgical treatment for life-threatening ventricular arrhythmias resistant to medical treatment following myocardial infarction. *Ann Thorac Surg* 26:438–444, 1978.

175. Guiraudon GM, et al. Total disconnection of the right ventricular free wall: Surgical treatment of right ventricular tachycardia associated with right ventricular dysplasia. *Circulation* 67:463–470, 1983.

176. Cox JL. The status of surgery for cardiac arrhythmias. *Circulation* 71:413–417, 1985.

177. Gallagher JJ, et al. Cryoablation of drug resistant ventricular tachycardia in a patient with a variant of scleroderma. *Circulation* 57:190–197, 1979.

178. Camm J, et al. The successful cryosurgical treatment of paroxysmal ventricular tachycardia. *Chest* 75:621–624, 1979.

179. Cox JL, Gallagher JJ, Ungerleider RM. Encircling endocardial ventriculotomy for refractory ischemic ventricular tachycardia: IV. Clinical indications, surgical technique, mechanism of action, and surgical results. *J Thorac Cardiovasc Surg* 83:865, 1982.

180. Cox JL. Anatomic-electrophysiologic basis for the surgical treatment of refractory ischemic ventricular tachycardia. *Ann Surg* 198:119, 1983.

181. Josephson ME, et al. Surgical excision of automatic atrial tachycardia: Anatomic and electrophysiologic correlates. *Am Heart J* 104:1076–1085, 1982.

182. Gallagher JJ, et al. Catheter technique for closed chest ablation of the atrioventricular conduction system. *N Engl J Med* 306:194–200, 1982.

183. Scheinman MM, et al. Catheter-induced ablation of the atrioventricular junction to control refractory supraventricular arrhythmias. *JAMA* 248:851–858, 1982.

184. Wood DL, et al. Catheter ablation of the atrioventricular conduction system in patients with supraventricular tachycardia. *Mayo Clin Proc* 58:791–796, 1983.

185. Scheinman MM, et al. Catheter ablation of the atrioventricular junction: A report of the percutaneous mapping and ablation registry. *Circulation* 70:1024–1029, 1984.

186. Gillette PC, et al. Junctional automatic ectopic tachycardia: New proposed treatment by transcatheter His bundle ablation. *Am Heart J* 106:619–623, 1983.

187. Bhandari A, et al. Catheter-induced His bundle ablation in a patient with reentrant tachycardia associated with a nodoventricular tract. *J Am Coll Cardiol* 4:611–616, 1984.

188. Hartzler GO. Electrode catheter ablation of refractory focal ventricular tachycardia. *J Am Coll Cardiol* 2:1107–1113, 1983.

189. Ruffy R, Kim SS, Lal R. Paroxysmal fascicular tachycardia: Electrophysiologic characteristics and treatment by catheter ablation. *J Am Coll Cardiol* 5:1008–1014, 1985.

190. Morady F, et al. Efficacy and safety of transcatheter ablation of posteroseptal accessory pathways. *Circulation* 72:170–177, 1985.

191. Gillette PC, et al. Treatment of atrial automatic tachycardia by ablation procedures. *J Am Coll Cardiol* 6:405–409, 1985.
192. Silka MJ, et al. Transvenous catheter ablation of a right atrial automatic ectopic tachycardia. *J Am Coll Cardiol* 5:999–1001, 1985.
193. Josephson ME. Catheter ablation of arrhythmias. *Ann Intern Med* 101:234–237, 1984.
194. Scheinman MM, Davis JC. Catheter ablation for treatment of tachyarrhythmias: Present role and potential promise. *Circulation* 73:10–13, 1986.
195. Brugada P, et al. Transcoronary chemical ablation of ventricular tachycardia. *Circulation* 79:475–482, 1989.
196. Kay GN, et al. Intracoronary ethanol ablation for the treatment of recurrent sustained ventricular tachycardia. *J Am Coll Cardiol* 19:159–168, 1992.
197. Ross DL, et al. Comprehensive clinical electrophysiologic studies in the investigation of documented or suspected tachycardias: Time, staff, problems and costs. *Circulation* 61:1010–1016, 1980.
198. Ferguson D, et al. Management of recurrent ventricular tachycardia: Economic impact of therapeutic alternatives. *Am J Cardiol* 53:531–536, 1984.

Bibliography

Dreifus LS. In AN Brest (ed-in-chief). *Cardiac Arrhythmias: Electrophysiologic Techniques and Management: Cardiovascular Clinics.* Philadelphia: Davis, 1985.

Fogoros R. *Electrophysiologic Testing.* 2nd ed. Boston: Blackwell Scientific Publications, 1994.

Josephson ME. *Clinical Cardiac Electrophysiology: Techniques and Interpretations* (2nd ed). Philadelphia: Lea & Febiger, 1993.

Josephson ME, Wellens HJJ (eds). *Tachycardias: Mechanisms, Diagnosis, Treatment.* Philadelphia: Lea & Febiger, 1984.

Surawicz B, Reddy CP, Prystowsky EN (eds). *Tachycardias.* Boston: Martinus Nijhoff, 1984.

Zipes DP, Jalife J (eds). *Cardiac Electrophysiology: From Cell to Bedside.* Philadelphia: Saunders, 1990.

Radiofrequency Catheter Ablation

Stephen C. Vlay

The ability to identify the location of reentrant pathways by mapping allowed surgical approaches to arrhythmia control. The next logical step was to attempt interruption of the reentrant circuit by a nonsurgical means. Initial efforts to extirpate specific locations in the heart were limited by difficulty in reaching the area by the catheters available at the time and by complications of direct current ablation. Both of these limitations have been largely overcome. The development of new mapping electrodes has resulted in improved localization of accessory pathway signals. Newly designed mapping electrodes have a larger distal tip for delivery of energy and are deflectable for better positioning.

Direct current catheter ablation was associated with barotrauma—literally, a tiny explosion at the site of current application and, in addition, a risk of ventricular fibrillation (VF). Perforation of the heart was occasionally noted. Furthermore, there was a 1.5% risk of sudden cardiac death, which occurred from 3 days to 6 months after the procedure. For these reasons, direct current catheter ablation is not routinely used in most electrophysiology laboratories, and the discussion in this chapter will center on radiofrequency ablation. (See Chap. 12 for historical data on direct current catheter ablation.)

Radiofrequency energy sources utilize signals of 300–1000 kHz delivered at amplitudes of 20–60 V root mean square (RMS) with a time duration of seconds to minutes. Radiofrequency output may be monitored by voltage, pulse duration, or catheter tip temperature. Tissue effect is minor compared with direct current and allows the delivery of a discrete, carefully defined lesion.

I. Overall considerations for radiofrequency catheter ablation

A. Efficacy and complications.
In a 1991 review of reported series, the NASPE Ad Hoc Committee on Catheter Ablation analyzed the efficacy of radiofrequency catheter ablation for various arrhythmias. For **accessory atrioventricular (AV) pathways,** success as defined by ablation of pathway function and tachycardia control without medications ranged from 88–99%. In 787 patients, complications included 3 cases of coronary arterial spasm with myocardial infarction (MI) in 1, 2 with aortic valve damage, 3 with pericardial tamponade requiring pericardiocentesis, and 3 with AV block after ablation of septal pathways. The risk of thrombosis seems low, with only 1 systemic and 1 pulmonary embolus. There were no procedure-related deaths and no postprocedure sudden deaths.

For **AV nodal modification,** selective block in the slow or fast pathway of the AV node, success, defined by cure of tachycardia without the creation of complete heart block, ranged from 85–99%. When complete heart block occurred, it resulted from attempts at ablation of the fast pathway. In 315 patients, there were 18 cases of complete heart block, 1 pulmonary embolus, 1 deep venous thrombosis of the lower extremity, and 1 asymptomatic pericardial effusion. It is acknowledged that the actual incidence of complications (e.g., heart block) as a result of ablation procedures may be higher than reported (Table 13-1).

The highest success rate is associated with persistence, meticulous mapping, and identification of pathway potentials at the site of ablation, but at the expense of lengthier studies and increased radiation exposure.

B. Radiation burden.
The radiation burden to the patient and to the physician is dependent on the fluoroscopy time. For the patient, Calkins et al. estimated that each hour of fluoroscopic imaging is associated with a lifetime risk of developing a fatal malignancy of 0.1% and a risk of developing genetic defect of 20 per 1 million births [1]. In the absence of radiation exposure, the expected incidence of fatal malignancies is 20%. For the catheter operator, the amount of radiation was small

and fell well below the occupational radiation exposure guidelines. With an average of 44 minutes of fluoroscopy time per case, they calculated that a single operator should be limited to 15 ablation procedures per month (based on radiation exposure at the maxilla) or to 42 procedures per month (based on radiation exposure to the left hand). The number of cases allowed would be reduced if fluoroscopy time per case is longer. Pulse fluoroscopy can reduce radiation exposure by 30%, and proper collimation of the field can further limit radiation burden.

C. **Cost considerations.** In addition to avoiding the risks, complications, and prolonged recovery time of open chest surgery, catheter ablation lowers the overall expenditure of the health care dollar. An assessment of a patient treated medically would have to include the cost, inconvenience, and long-term side effects of medications, as well as the cost of subsequent hospitalizations for uncontrolled arrhythmias. Consequently, both electrophysiology study and radiofrequency catheter ablation seem reasonable in cost and risk to the patient. In fact, when one considers the lifelong necessity for antiarrhythmic drug therapy with potentially proarrhythmic drugs, it seems difficult to justify drug therapy unless the patient has complete control and no adverse effects with either digoxin or an inexpensive beta blocker.

II. **Paroxysmal supraventricular tachycardias: AVNRT and AVRT**
A. **Atrioventricular nodal reentrant tachycardia (AVNRT).** Anatomic considerations are critical in the management of this arrhythmia. The AV node was initially considered to be a discrete structure that contained more than one internal pathway in some patients, providing a substrate for reentry. Recent advances in ablation of this structure have indicated that some of the pathways may not be internal and in fact are perinodal.

Perhaps a good analogy is to regard the AV node as a major train depot in which multiple tracks converge on a central station. While the majority of tracks travel in a single direction, some side tracks also lead to the same end point. Traditionally, fast and slow pathways have been described in the AV node, and recently some data have suggested the presence of multiple slow pathways. Since it is becoming more accepted that conduction in the region of the AV node involves not only a concentration of fibers in the node but also contributory fibers in the surrounding tissue, some electrophysiologists suspect that many, if not all, individuals have the potential to have AV nodal reentry. The clinical arrhythmia may occur in some due to the number of perinodal fibers as well as differences in autonomic tone, plus undefined variables.

The AV node is located at the apex of the triangle of Koch in the lower atrial septum. This location was described by Koch in 1909. The base of the triangle is delineated by the coronary sinus and the sides by the tricuspid annulus and the tendon of Todaro. It is within this area that the ablation electrode is positioned to locate and record potentials from the slow and fast pathways (Fig. 13-1).

Initial attempts to control AVNRT involved complete ablation of the AV node and the implantation of a permanent pacemaker. Today, selective ablation of one of the pathways allows abolition of the substrate for reentry but retention of AV conduction. Ablation of the fast pathway is likely to result in heart block, but ablation of the slow pathway results in abolition of AVNRT without the need for a pacemaker (Figs. 13-2 and 13-3).

Complete heart block is not desirable except for selected patients with refractory atrial arrhythmias and a rapid ventricular response. For example, extremely symptomatic patients with atrial fibrillation whose ventricular response is extremely dif-

Table 13-1. Potential complications of radiofrequency catheter ablation

1. The usual complications of electrophysiology study
2. Failure to ablate pathway
3. Complete heart block requiring a permanent pacemaker
4. Exposure to radiation

Fortunately the following are rare:
5. Perforation of a heart valve
6. Perforation of the heart causing pericardial tamponade
7. Myocardial infarction as a result of injury to a coronary artery
8. Injury to the coronary sinus
9. Pulmonary embolus
10. Cerebrovascular accident
11. Death

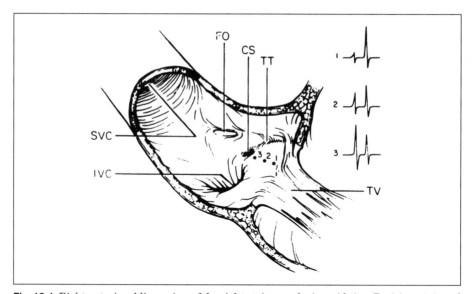

Fig. 13-1. Right anterior oblique view of the right atrium and tricuspid ring. Positions 1, 2, and 3 on the atrium represent three consecutive sites of ablation during a pullback. These would initially be placed along the 6 o'clock plane of the left anterior oblique view of the tricuspid ring. The corresponding electrograms of positions 1, 2, and 3 demonstrate the increasing size of the atrial electrogram relative to the ventricular electrogram. Following position 3, the catheter would be moved into the right ventricle and pulled back along the 5 o'clock plane of the tricuspid ring, once again applying sequential lesions. (CS = coronary sinus ostium; FO = foramen ovale; IVC = inferior vena cava; SVC = superior vena cava; TT = tendon of Todaro; TV = tricuspid valve.) (From M Wathen et al., An anatomically guided approach to atrio-ventricular node slow pathway ablation. *Am J Cardiol* 70:887, 1992. Reprinted with permission.)

ficult to control with drugs may obtain relief after catheter ablation of the AV node and implantation of a rate-responsive ventricular pacemaker.

1. **Diagnostic electrophysiologic considerations.** Before attempting ablation, the electrophysiologist must be certain about the mechanism of the tachycardia and have excluded AV reentry (accessory pathways as in the Wolff-Parkinson-White syndrome). After baseline measurements are performed, antegrade and retrograde AV nodal functional assessment is performed.

   Antegrade assessment is performed with the A_1A_2 technique (eight-beat drive train with single extrastimuli). A_2H_2 is plotted against A_1A_2, constructing an antegrade AV nodal function curve and looking for discontinuity. By definition, an increase in the A_2H_2 interval more than 50 msec after a decrement in the A_1A_2 coupling interval of 10 msec is defined as a discontinuous curve and evidence of dual antegrade AV pathways [2, 3].

   Retrograde assessment is performed with the V_1V_2 technique (eight-beat drive train with single extrastimuli). One looks for retrograde conduction from the ventricle to the His to the atrium. H_2A_2 is plotted against V_1V_2. As above, by definition, a discontinuous retrograde conduction curve is defined by an increase in the H_2A_2 interval more than 50 msec after a decrement in the V_1V_2 coupling interval of 10 msec. If the H_2A_2 interval does not increase by more than 10 msec from the longest to the shortest V_1V_2 intervals, the retrograde AV nodal function curve is considered nondecremental.

   The diagnosis of AVNRT is established by tachycardia initiation dependent on a critical A–H delay, earliest retrograde activation in the His bundle electrogram (shortest ventriculoatrial interval <70 msec), and inability to advance the subsequent atrial deflection with ventricular pacing at a time the His bundle is refractory to retrograde conduction (this latter finding would suggest an accessory AV pathway).

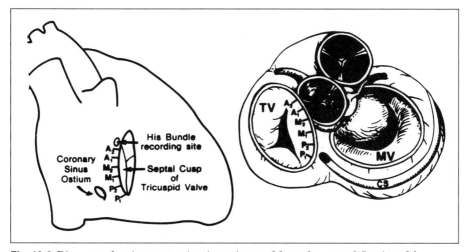

Fig. 13-2. Diagrams showing anatomic orientation used for catheter modification of the atrioventricular (AV) node. The schemata depict right anterior oblique (*left panel*) and left anterior oblique (*right panel*) projections for anatomic localization of fast and slow pathways. The fast pathway ablation is accomplished near the His bundle recording site. For the slow pathway, the ablation is started at the most posterior (P) location (P_1), and additional exploration is done only if lesion at P_1 fails. P_2 is a more anterior location than P_1, as are M_1 and M_2 (medial). The area labeled A_1, A_2 (anterior) should be avoided because a more anterior location could carry a higher chance of AV block as one begins to approach the more compact portion of the AV node. (TV = tricuspid valve; MV = mitral valve; CS = coronary sinus.) (From M Akhtar et al., Atrioventricular nodal reentry. *Circulation* 88:292, 1993. Reprinted with permission.)

The common form of AVNRT involves antegrade conduction down the slow pathway and retrograde conduction up the fast pathway. The timing of the subsequent atrial impulse in relation to the His potential distinguishes the common and atypical forms of AVNRT. When retrograde conduction is fast (H–A usually <50 msec), the subsequent atrial deflection is early, as is the p wave. In the atypical form of AVNRT, in which antegrade conduction occurs down the fast pathway and retrograde conduction up the slow pathway, retrograde conduction to the atria is longer and associated with a long R–P interval (hence the term *long R–P tachycardia*) (Fig. 13-4).

Unless there is a reason to attempt complete ablation of the AV node, most electrophysiologists would agree that selective ablation of the slow pathway is desirable. Identification of the slow pathway potential provides an optimal target for the ablation catheter. It may also be approached anatomically, in relationship to the triangle of Koch.

2. **Ablation.** The catheter approach to the slow pathway involves positioning the tip along the tricuspid annulus anterior to the ostium of the coronary sinus at the base of the triangle of Koch. Some position the electrode to record initially the largest His bundle electrogram and then curve the tip downward in the clockwise direction until the His deflection is no longer visible and the ratio of atrial to ventricular deflection is below 1. One report described the slow pathway potentials as uniphasic or biphasic.

In sinus rhythm, the largest, sharpest, and latest slow pathway potential is often recorded along the posteroseptal right atrium, close to the tricuspid annulus, where the atrial potential is small and the ventricular potential is large. It may also be recorded after atrial activation in the proximal coronary sinus. Not all series describe the ability to record slow pathway potentials. (Fig. 13-5).

After identification of the potentials, Jackman et al. note the response to late atrial extrasystoles, which advance atrial potentials on the His bundle electrogram but do not alter timing of the slow pathway potential [4]. The ablation electrode is positioned at the site of the largest, sharpest, and earliest slow pathway potential (from the distal pair of electrodes) during retrograde slow pathway con-

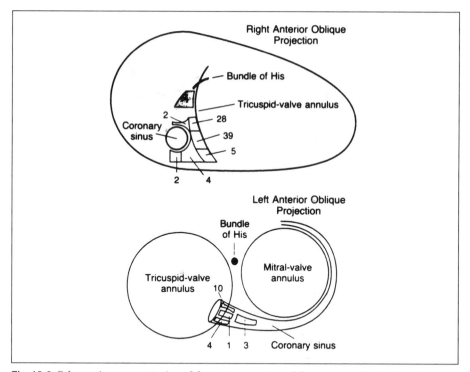

Fig. 13-3. Schematic representation of the septum as viewed fluoroscopically in the right and left anterior oblique projections, showing the 98 sites of successful slow pathway ablation in the 78 patients. Numbers indicate the number of sites of successful ablation in each region. During selective retrograde fast pathway conduction, the earliest atrial activation was recorded in the anterior septum, near the bundle of His (*shaded region*). During selective retrograde slow pathway conduction, the earliest atrial potential was recorded in the posterior septum or proximal coronary sinus (*unshaded regions*). (From WM Jackman et al., Treatment of supraventricular tachycardia due to atrioventricular nodal reentry by radiofrequency catheter ablation of slow pathway conduction. *N Engl J Med* 327:313–318, 1992. Reprinted with permission.)

duction or during sinus rhythm. Some electrophysiologists position the ablation electrode "anatomically," near the os of the coronary, which serves to identify the location of the slow pathway.

Radiofrequency current (550–750 kHz) is delivered at 45–70 V between the catheter tip electrode and an adhesive electrosurgical dispersive electrode pad applied to the posterior left chest. Current is applied for 45 seconds or longer but is terminated immediately if the impedance rises or catheter movement occurs (Fig. 13-6). Some electrophysiologists deliver a second or "insurance burn" even if the first application of radiofrequency energy has been successful. Electrophysiologic testing is repeated 30–45 minutes after the procedure to verify that AVNRT is no longer inducible.

If the goal is to ablate the fast pathway, the electrode is positioned to record the largest His deflection at the triangle of Koch. It is slowly withdrawn, maintaining clockwise torque, until the His deflection is no longer visible and the ratio of atrial to ventricular deflections is over 1. With this approach, there is a high chance of producing complete AV block.

Kay et al. described functional characteristics of the pathways after slow pathway ablation [5]. There was no change in the A–H interval during sinus rhythm. The AV Wenckebach rate was unchanged. The antegrade effective refractory period of the fast pathway shortened after slow pathway ablation. The retrograde effective refractory period of the VA conduction system demonstrated no significant change. The VA Wenckebach rate was unchanged. In four patients

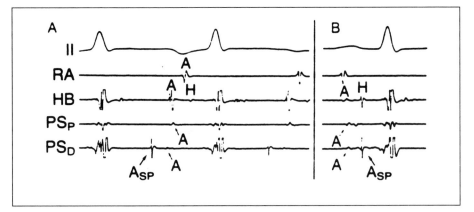

Fig. 13-4. Characteristic potentials recorded from the posterior septum at the site of successful slow pathway ablation in a patient with both common (slow–fast) and uncommon (fast–slow) forms of atrial ventricular nodal reentry tachycardia (AVNRT). From the top, the figure shows a tracing from lead II and electrograms recorded from the right atrial appendage (RA), the His bundle region (HB), and the proximal (PS$_P$) and distal (PS$_D$) pairs of electrodes of the mapping catheter, positioned against the posteroseptal right atrium between the coronary-sinus ostium and the tricuspid annulus. During fast–slow AVNRT (*panel A*), retrograde conduction occurred over the slow pathway, and the earliest retrograde atrial potential was recorded from the PS$_D$ electrodes, which showed a small atrial potential (A), nearly coincident with the atrial potentials in the PS$_P$ and HB electrograms. It was preceded by a large A$_{SP}$ potential (*large arrow*) recorded 60 msec before the onset of the P wave. During sinus rhythm (*panel B*), when the slow pathway was activated in the antegrade direction, the order of the two potentials in PS$_D$ was reversed, with the A potential still coincident with the other atrial potentials. The application of radiofrequency current at this site eliminated antegrade and retrograde slow pathway conduction and both forms of AVNRT. (H = His bundle potential.) (From WM Jackman et al., Treatment of supraventricular tachycardia due to atrioventricular nodal reentry by radiofrequency catheter ablation of slow pathway conduction. *N Engl J Med* 327:313–318, 1992. Reprinted with permission.)

with fast pathway ablation, the A–H interval was prolonged, but the antegrade effective refractory period of the slow pathway and the AV Wenckebach rate were unchanged. However, retrograde conduction remained intact, suggesting that only part of the AV node was affected rather than selective ablation of a distinct fast pathway.

Wu et al. described criteria for successful ablation: no evidence of or marked depression of retrograde fast pathway conduction with no induction of slow-fast form of AV node reentrant echoes or tachycardia [6]. No evidence of anterograde slow pathway conduction with no induction of slow-fast AV node reentrant echoes or tachycardia.

Jackman et al. note that it is not necessary to eliminate all slow pathway conduction to eliminate AVNRT [4]. Atrial stimulation at the end of the study is often able to induce AV nodal reentrant atrial echo beats, but tachycardia was noninducible and remained noninducible after more than 1 year of follow-up.

Catheter ablation of AVNRT is safe and relatively uncomplicated; it may be the treatment of choice for patients who are symptomatic and do not wish to take or cannot tolerate antiarrhythmic medications.

B. **Atrioventricular reentrant tachycardia (AVRT).** Catheter ablation has replaced surgery and antiarrhythmic drugs as the treatment of choice for AVRT. Chap. 7 on preexcitation discusses the options and choices in depth. In this section, the discussion centers on radiofrequency modification of the accessory pathway.

Today when a patient with preexcitation is referred for electrophysiology study, the location of the accessory pathway can be fairly well determined by morphologic characteristics of the delta wave, the resting ECG, and the ECG during tachycardia. Patients with concealed conduction (retrograde conduction through the accessory pathway) present somewhat more of a diagnostic challenge. For overt left-sided pathways, Kuck and Schluter have proposed a single catheter technique, provided

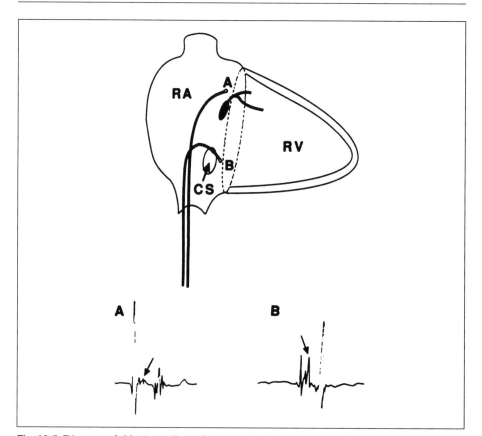

Fig. 13-5. Diagram of ablation catheter locations during the anterior (A) and posterior (B) approaches to radiofrequency atrioventricular nodal modification and representative target site electrograms. In this right anterior oblique projection, the tricuspid anulus is represented by a dashed line, and the atrioventricular node and specialized conduction system are represented by the shaded area. Note the presence of a diminutive His bundle potential (*left arrow*) at the effective site using the anterior approach (A). There is a fractionated atrial electrogram at the effective site using the posterior approach (B). Note the presence of a discrete late component of the signal (*arrow*), the slow pathway potential. (CS = ostium of the coronary sinus; RA = right atrium; RV = right ventricle.) (From JJ Langberg et al., A randomized prospective comparison of anterior and posterior approaches to radiofrequency catheter ablation of atrioventricular nodal reentry. *Circulation* 80:1527–1535, 1989. Reprinted with permission.)

that proper positioning and accessory pathway potentials can be obtained [7]. Although this approach may be applicable for specific locations and in experienced hands, the vast majority of ablations for accessory pathways involve classic mapping prior to ablation. However, it is reasonable to combine the diagnostic and therapeutic studies.

Many laboratories use four diagnostic electrodes and one ablation electrode. The electrodes are positioned in the high right atrium or right atrial appendage, in the coronary sinus (to record left atrial activity), across the His bundle, and in the right ventricle. Depending on the location of the accessory pathway, the ablation catheter is positioned in the right ventricle near the tricuspid annulus or in the left ventricle. Left-sided pathways may be approached retrograde through the aortic valve or via a transseptal sheath. Ablation catheters have a large tip and a deflectable curve to facilitate positioning.

The largest potentials are obtained by recording signals parallel to the impulse over a small area of myocardium. Jackman et al. reported the use of a catheter with

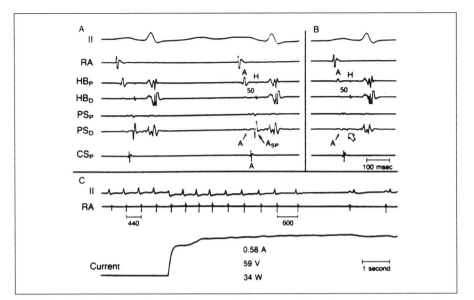

Fig. 13-6. Effects of slow pathway ablation on the A_{SP} potential and fast pathway conduction. The tracings shown were recorded from a patient with slow–fast atrioventricular nodal reentry tachycardia (AVNRT) and no retrograde slow pathway conduction. Before ablation (*panel A*), the largest, sharpest, and latest A_{SP} potential during sinus rhythm was recorded from the posteroseptal catheter (PS_D electrogram), positioned near the tricuspid annulus, posterior to the coronary sinus ostium. The A_{SP} potential was recorded after atrial activation in the proximal coronary sinus (the A potential in the CS_P electrogram). Radiofrequency current applied at this site (*panel C*) eliminated slow pathway conduction. Immediately after ablation (*panel B*), the A_{SP} potential (*open arrow*) was markedly attenuated. The antegrade fast atrioventricular nodal pathway conduction time, as measured by the atrial–His bundle (A–H) interval in the HB_P electrogram, was unchanged from the preablation value of 50 msec. During slow–fast AVNRT, 59 V of radiofrequency current (current, 0.58 A; power, 34 W) was applied to the large-tip electrode on the PS catheter, which recorded the large A_{SP} potential in panel A. The bottom tracing in panel C indicates the root-mean-square output of current from the radiofrequency generator. Beginning 2 seconds after the start of delivery of current, the cycle length of the tachycardia increased progressively from 440 to 600 msec, and tachycardia ended at 5 seconds. The increase in cycle length and the termination of tachycardia resulted from the prolongation of conduction time and then from conduction block in the slow pathway. After the termination of tachycardia, the P–R interval was not prolonged during sinus rhythm, indicating that ablation did not affect antegrade fast pathway conduction (RA = right atrium; HB = His bundle.) (From WM Jackman et al., Treatment of supraventricular tachycardia due to atrioventricular nodal reentry by radiofrequency catheter ablation of slow pathway conduction. *N Engl J Med* 327:313–318, 1992. Reprinted with permission.)

orthogonal electrodes that permitted selection of the best and largest signals regardless of the orientation of the electrode in the coronary sinus [8]. Three sets of four electrodes are spaced equally around the circumference of the electrode, each set spaced 10 mm from the next. The coronary sinus electrode is usually positioned from above via the internal jugular vein but may also be inserted via the subclavian or antecubital veins.

Mapping the tricuspid annulus is accomplished with a deflectable electrode catheter. This catheter may be inserted via a femoral vein or from above. The approach to an undiagnosed arrhythmia involves first assessing baseline conduction, finding clues for accessory pathway conduction, and then examining retrograde and antegrade conduction. One uses ventricular and atrial pacing to determine the path of conduction, which part of the conduction system is activated the earliest, and why conduction occurs when part of the system should be refractory (e.g., when retrograde conduction over the His bundle is blocked, conduction to the atria may occur over the accessory pathway). The diagnosis and localization of the

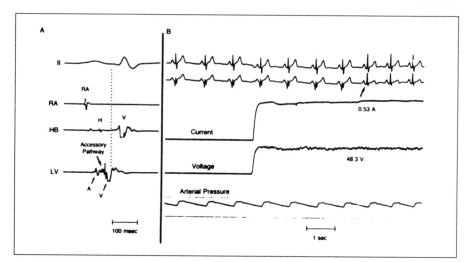

Fig. 13-7. Ablation of a posterior left free-wall accessory atrioventricular pathway.
A. Recordings from the ablation electrode during sinus rhythm. From the top, the tracings are lead II (and lead III in *panel B*) and electrograms recorded from the right atrial appendage (RA), the His bundle region (HB), and the ablation electrode (LV), which was positioned against the mitral annulus, beneath the mitral leaflet. The large potential resulting from atrial activation (A) indicates proximity to the atrium and therefore to the mitral annulus. Note the distinct potentials resulting from accessory pathway activation (*large arrow*). Left ventricular activation (V) began 20 msec before the onset of the delta wave (*dotted vertical line*). **B.** The tracings were recorded when radiofrequency current was applied to the large-tip electrode on the left ventricular catheter at 48.3 V and 0.53 A (calculated power, 25.6 W). Accessory pathway conduction ceased 3.9 seconds after the onset of the application of radiofrequency current (*arrow*), reflected by the lengthening of the P–R interval and normalization of the QRS complex. Arterial pressure was unaffected by the application of radiofrequency current. (From WM Jackman et al., Catheter ablation of accessory atrioventricular pathways (Wolff-Parkinson-White syndrome) by radiofrequency current. *N Engl J Med* 324:1605–1611, 1991. Reprinted with permission.)

accessory pathway require deductive reasoning. Tachycardia is induced and the relationship of conduction assessed during the tachycardia. Accessory pathway potentials are mapped and verified. The ablation catheter is positioned as close as possible to the accessory pathway and radiofrequency current applied. Current is terminated if the electrode position moves or if the impedance rises. With successful ablation of pathways that previously displayed overt preexcitation, the delta wave disappears, and only normal conduction remains on the ECG.

Catheter ablation of left-sided pathways has been the most successful and right-sided pathways the most difficult, mostly because of location and difficulty in positioning the ablation catheter. Accessory pathway locations include left free wall (60%), posteroseptal (24%), right free wall (9%), and anteroseptal (7%) [9].

C. **Various approaches to atrioventricular pathways**
  1. **Left free-wall pathways**
     a. Retrograde femoral artery approach across the aortic valve and positioning beneath the mitral leaflet high against the annulus at the site of the accessory pathway.
     b. As above but positioned above the mitral leaflet.
     c. Transseptal approach or through a patent foramen ovale with the ablation catheter above the leaflet along the mitral annulus.
     d. The ablation catheter inserted into the coronary sinus via the femoral vein (for left lateral AP) (Fig. 13-7).
  2. **Anteroseptal accessory pathways**
     a. The ablation catheter is inserted via the right subclavian vein and positioned under the septal or anterior leaflet of the tricuspid valve (ventricular aspect).

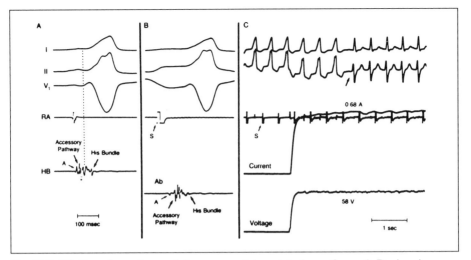

Fig. 13-8. Ablation of an anteroseptal accessory atrioventricular pathway. **A.** During sinus rhythm, the bipolar electrode in the His bundle region (HB) recorded activation potentials from both the accessory pathway and His bundle, indicating the close proximity of these two structures. **B.** During right atrial (RA) pacing at a cycle length of 450 msec (S denotes pacing-stimulus artifact), the ablation electrode (Ab) was positioned beneath the tricuspid leaflet, high against the tricuspid annulus and slightly anterior to the His bundle. At this site, the accessory pathway activation potential is still prominent, and the His bundle potential is much smaller than on the electrogram recorded at the true His bundle position. Note that the atrial potential (A) is smaller than on the His bundle electrogram in panel A, because the tip electrode approached the atrium from the ventricular side of the annulus. **C.** Radiofrequency current (power, 39.4 W) was applied to the large-tip electrode on the ablation catheter (Ab) during atrial pacing at cycle length 450 msec. Accessory pathway conduction ceased 1.7 seconds after the onset of the application of radiofrequency current (*arrow*). (From WM Jackman et al., Catheter ablation of accessory atrioventricular pathways (Wolff-Parkinson-White syndrome) by radiofrequency current. *N Engl J Med* 324:1605–1611, 1991. Reprinted with permission.)

  b. The ablation catheter is inserted via the right femoral vein and placed parallel to the His bundle catheter (Fig. 13-8).
3. **Posteroseptal accessory pathways**
  a. The ablation catheter is inserted via the right femoral vein with the tip against the tricuspid annulus or around the margin of the coronary sinus ostium.
  b. Retrograde femoral artery approach across the aortic valve with the tip positioned against the mitral annulus, close to the septum.
  c. The ablation catheter is inserted via the right subclavian vein with the tip in a venous branch (e.g., middle cardiac vein) of the coronary sinus.
  d. Bipolar tricuspid-mitral annulus electrode configuration with the tricuspid position at or anterosuperior to the os of the coronary sinus (but posterior to the AV node–His bundle position) and the mitral position posterior to the AV node in the region opposite the coronary sinus os. With this approach, the radiofrequency energy is delivered between two ablation electrodes, rather than between an ablation catheter and an indifferent electrode on the posterior or chest.
4. **Right free-wall pathways**
  a. The ablation catheter is inserted via the right subclavian vein and curved beneath the tricuspid valve.
  b. The ablation catheter is positioned above the tricuspid valve via the right subclavian or femoral vein (Fig. 13-9).
5. **Accessory pathway potentials.** Verification of the accessory pathway position facilitates successful ablation and avoids injury to critical adjacent structures (e.g., the AV node, particularly when attempting ablation of septal accessory

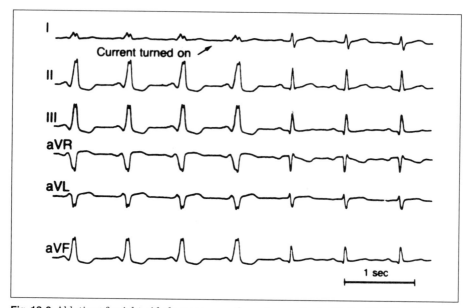

Fig. 13-9. Ablation of a right-sided accessory pathway in a patient with the Wolff-Parkinson-White syndrome. The tracings from the frontal plane leads are shown, in which a short P–R interval and prominent delta waves are evident. Radiofrequency current (36 W) was delivered for 20 seconds to the atrial side of the anterior portion of the tricuspid annulus during sinus rhythm at a rate of 74 beats/minute. Shortly after, the delta waves disappeared and the P–R interval normalized to 0.18 second. (From H Calkins et al., Diagnosis and cure of the Wolff-Parkinson-White syndrome of paroxysmal supraventricular tachycardias during a single electrophysiologic test. *N Engl J Med* 324:1612–1618, 1991. Reprinted with permission.)

pathways). At the annulus, both atrial and ventricular electrograms are recorded. Discrete accessory pathway potentials occur between atrial and ventricular activation.

Obtaining the optimal position and recording the accessory pathway potential may be the most time-consuming aspect of this procedure. In patients with left-sided pathways in whom the optimal position is not obtained with the retrograde aortic valve approach, transseptal catheterization allows supravalvular access to the mitral annulus. It may be easier to manipulate the electrode from the left atrial side, but the transseptal approach must be performed only by an experienced individual because of the risks of cardiac perforation and injury to the aorta.

The physician must be able to recognize accessory pathway potentials. They are sometimes hidden within other electrograms. Sometimes pacing will separate out these potentials. Adjustment of the gain also may improve the visualization of the potential (Fig. 13-10).

D. **Ablation.** For left-sided pathways, the patient should be heparinized. Once the ablation site has been confirmed, radiofrequency energy is delivered between the catheter tip and the standard adhesive electrosurgical adhesive electrode on the posterior chest. Most studies deliver 45–60 V for 45 seconds, or until a sudden rise in impedance occurs (indicative of coagulation). If the impedance rises but accessory pathway conduction persists, the catheter must be removed and cleaned before further attempts at ablation. Some electrophysiologists perform a second application of radiofrequency energy ("insurance burn") even if the first is successful. Electrophysiologic stimulation is repeated 30–45 minutes after the procedure to determine if accessory pathway conduction has returned.

E. **Recommendations.** For symptomatic patients with AVRT, catheter ablation offers a safe and effective alternative to surgical therapy. It is certainly preferable to life-long therapy with antiarrhythmic therapy, which is inconvenient, costly, and associated with potentially serious side effects. The number of patients with Wolff-Parkin-

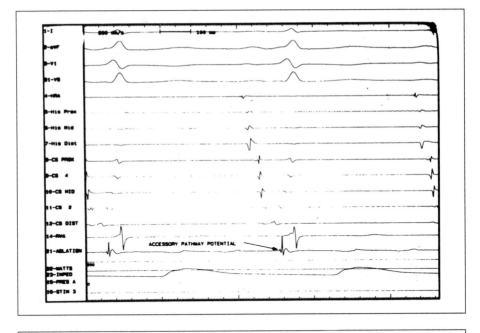

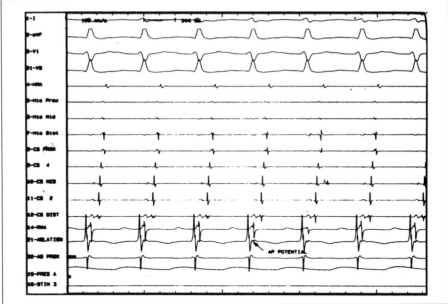

Fig. 13-10. *Top:* In a patient with Wolff-Parkinson-White syndrome and a left anterolateral free-wall pathway, the accessory pathway potential is seen on the ablation electrode recording and precedes the QRS complex during sinus rhythm. *Bottom:* During orthodromic reciprocating tachycardia, the accessory pathway potential is the earliest deflection following the QRS complex.

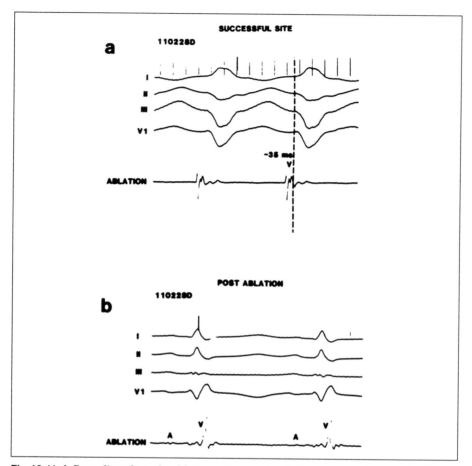

Fig. 13-11. A. Recordings from the ablation catheter when the tip was positioned under the tricuspid valve in a right posterolateral location in the right ventricle. Ventricular activation during tachycardia preceded the onset of the QRS complex by 35 msec. Atrial activation is not clearly identified on the recording. **B.** After elimination of the accessory pathway, an atrial electrogram is recorded, confirming that the ablation catheter tip was at the annulus on the ventricular side. Note that right ventricular activation now is recorded in the terminal portion of the QRS complex, the delay in part due to the right bundle branch block. Right bundle branch conduction subsequently recovered and was therefore thought to be due to catheter trauma. (From LS Klein et al., Radiofrequency catheter ablation of Mahaim fibers at the tricuspid annulus. *Circulation* 87:738–7 47, 1993. Reprinted with permission.)

son-White syndrome in the United States is estimated to be 375,000–750,000, with an annual increase of 6000–12,000 per year, considering the birth rate [10]. While not all of these are symptomatic, those that are should be given the option of catheter ablation. Perhaps one of the future questions will be to determine the optimal age for the symptomatic infant or child to undergo catheter ablation [11–13].

III. Mahaim fibers. Mahaim fibers are now thought to originate in the atrial free wall and insert at or adjacent to the distal right bundle branch (atriofascicular pathway). Usually conduction occurs only in the antegrade direction as part of an antidromic AVRT with a left bundle branch morphology [14] (Fig. 13-11). Decremental conduction may be present at the level of the tricuspid annulus.

The catheter ablation technique has now been applied to these tachyarrhythmias. It is possible to record potentials from Mahaim fibers, although there are few published reports. The ablation site is usually close to the tricuspid annulus at the insertion site of the pathway. Radiofrequency energy is delivered as noted in **II.D.**

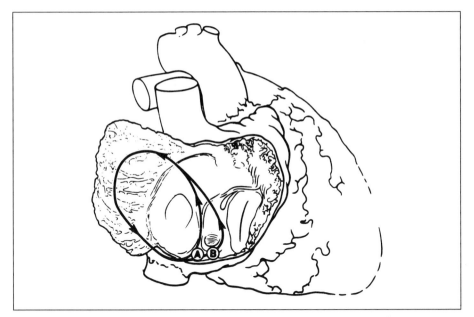

Fig. 13-12. Schematic cut-away view of the right atrium from a right anterior oblique projection. The typical direction of activation during atrial flutter is noted by the arrows. The usual locations where radiofrequency ablation terminated atrial flutter are indicated by the open circles posterior (A) or inferior (B) to the ostium of the coronary sinus. Ablation at site A was successful in seven patients and at site B in three patients. (From GK Feld et al., Radiofrequency catheter ablation for the treatment of human type 1 atrial flutter. *Circulation* 86:1233–1240, 1992. Reprinted with permission.)

IV. **Atrial flutter and other atrial tachycardias. Atrial flutter** is thought to be a macroreentrant arrhythmia involving the right atrium. Catheter ablation has been evaluated after endocardial mapping. Cosio et al. have described a large right atrial reentry circuit surrounding a central obstacle formed by the inferior vena cava and adjacent areas of functional conduction block [15]. Feld et al. identified the area of slow conduction by prolonged low-amplitude fragmented electrical activity and long stimulus-to-p-wave intervals [16]. It was located in the posteroseptal right atrium.

   After identification of the earliest potentials, radiofrequency energy is delivered in a similar fashion as described for AVNRT and AVRT. Multiple applications of energy in a linear fashion are sometimes necessary. Although the experience with atrial flutter is limited, selected patients with atrial flutter may benefit from this procedure (Fig. 13-12).

   Atrial fibrillation, a much more chaotic arrhythmia, presents a major challenge; it is one of the remaining frontiers for catheter ablation. The hope would be that the equivalent of a MAZE-type procedure could be performed noninvasively. At the 1995 NASPE meeting, Dr. John Schwartz of Tulsa, Oklahoma provided initial data on a limited number of patients that had successful ablation of chronic atrial fibrillation by a percutaneous MAZE procedure. However, at this time, for the majority of patients, radiofrequency catheter ablation can offer modification of the AV junction to patients whose lives are disabled by recurrent episodes of atrial fibrillation or those in whom the ventricular response is rapid and difficult to control. Patients with **multifocal atrial tachycardia** may present a similar challenge. After modification of the AV node to slow conduction or the creation of complete AV block, it is necessary to implant a permanent pacemaker, preferably with rate-responsive programmability to maintain an appropriate ventricular response.

   Ectopic atrial tachycardia and **sinoatrial reentrant tachycardia** are amenable to catheter ablation because it is possible to map the atrium and locate the earliest activation times. Kay et al. described successful ablation of both arrhythmias [17]. The diagnosis of ectopic atrial tachycardia is made if the p wave axis and configuration of the ECG documented tachycardia were different than observed during sinus rhythm. Atrial activation sequence during tachycardia was different than during sinus rhythm. AV block during the tachycardia were observed with a constant p wave configuration and

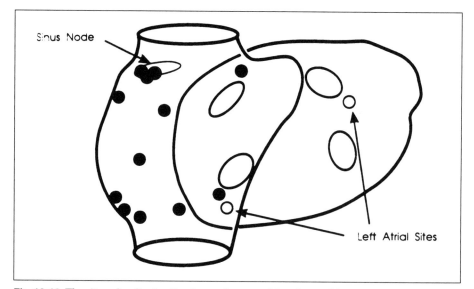

Fig. 13-13. The sites of earliest activation and successful catheter ablation are shown for ectopic atrial tachycardia or sinus node reentry arising in the right (*black circles*) and the left (*open circles*) atrium. One patient had two sites of origin within the left atrium. The successful ablation site for sinus node reentry was over an area 3 to 5 mm in length in the region of the sinus node. (From GN Kay et al., Radiofrequency catheter ablation for treatment of primary atrial tachycardias. *J Am Coll Cardiol* 21:901–909, 1993. Reprinted with permission.)

persistence of the tachycardia. Ventricular pacing during the tachycardia was associated with dissociation of the ventricles from the atria or with a change in the sequence of atrial activation in the presence of VA conduction (Fig. 13-13).

For sinoatrial reentrant tachycardia, the p wave axis, configuration, and sequence of atrial activation were the same as in sinus rhythm and tachycardia. The intraatrial conduction time were constant. Tachycardia was initiated and terminated by timed electrical extrastimuli within the critical zone of coupling intervals. Tachycardia onset and termination were associated with an abrupt change in atrial rate. Initiation and termination of the tachycardia were independent of AV conduction [18].

After identification of the earliest site of activation, the ablation catheter was positioned and radiofrequency energy applied in a similar manner to that described for AVNRT and AVRT. For ectopic atrial tachycardia, sites of origin have been located in both the right and left atria. Left atrial foci can be approached either retrograde across the aortic and mitral valves or by the transseptal approach. Several reports have noted the origin of the tachycardia in the atrium near the pulmonary veins. For sinoatrial nodal reentry, it was necessary to apply radiofrequency energy within an arc spanning 3–5 mm in the region of the sinus node in the right atrium, suggesting the involvement of perinodal atrial tissue (Fig. 13-14).

For ectopic atrial tachycardia, both Walsh et al. and Chen et al. note that positioning the ablation catheter at the area where local electrical activity precedes the onset of the surface p wave by 20–60 msec correlated with the highest rate of success [19, 20]. Thus, careful mapping facilitates success with this procedure too.

Automatic atrial tachycardia represents another mechanism that may be amenable to catheter ablation. With this mechanism, programmed stimulation is unable to initiate or terminate the tachycardia. The ability to map the atria and localize the earliest area of activation may allow successful catheter ablation.

A. **Recommendations.** For the patient with symptomatic drug-refractory atrial tachycardias, catheter ablation may represent an alternative. Nevertheless, the experience of catheter ablation with these arrhythmias is far less than with AVNRT or AVRT. The success rate may not be as high, and there are too few published reports to calculate statistics.

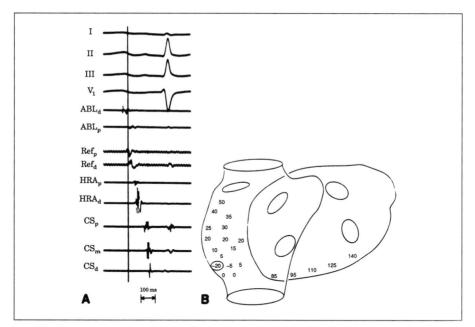

Fig. 13-14. A. Standard ECG leads I, II, III, and V_1 recorded simultaneously with bipolar intracardiac electrograms. The electrograms from the distal (ABL_d) and proximal (ABL_p) electrode pairs of a deflectable tip quadripolar ablation catheter positioned in the anterolateral right atrium are recorded simultaneously with electrograms from the proximal (Ref_p) and distal (Ref_d) pairs of electrodes of a nearby second deflectable tip quadripolar catheter used as a reference. Intracardiac electrograms from the proximal (HRA_p) and distal (HRA_d) electrode pairs of a quadripolar catheter positioned at the high right atrium, and from the proximal (CS_p), mid-(CS_m), and distal (CS_d) electrode pairs of a hexapolar catheter within the coronary sinus are also shown. Note that earliest atrial activation is recorded from the ABL_d electrode pair where the first rapid deflection in the electrogram crosses the baseline 20 ms before the onset of the p wave in the surface ECG (*vertical line*). Application of radiofrequency current at the ABL_d site resulted in successful ablation of ectopic atrial tachycardia (Patient 4). A 100-ms interval marker is demonstrated. **B.** Diagram illustrating the approximate intracardiac location of recording electrode pairs with their corresponding activation times relative to the onset of the p wave in the surface ECG during the same tachycardia. (From GN Kay et al., Radiofrequency ablation for treatment of primary atrial tachycardias. *J Am Coll Cardiol* 21:901–909, 1993. Reprinted with permission.)

V. **Permanent form of junctional reciprocating tachycardia.** The permanent form of junctional reciprocating tachycardia is thought to represent an AVRT involving retrograde conduction over an extra AV nodal pathway with decremental conduction properties localized to the posteroseptal area in the region of the coronary sinus os [21]. These investigators confirmed the diagnosis by demonstrating prolonged AV conduction time during tachycardia (280–350 msec) and the earliest site of atrial activation at the coronary sinus os. Critically timed ventricular premature depolarizations during the tachycardia when the His bundle was refractory advances atrial depolarization and demonstrates the presence of an accessory pathway.

The ablation catheter is positioned near the coronary sinus os and energy delivered in the standard manner. Chien et al. used direct current shocks, but today the preferred source of energy is radiofrequency current [21].

VI. **Ventricular tachycardia.** The success rate of catheter ablation for VT is significantly less than for AVNRT or AVRT. Among other reasons, the electrical substrate of the supraventricular arrhythmias is more compact and strictly delineated, and it provides a well-defined target for ablation. The majority of VTs are associated with extensive coronary artery disease, diffuse left ventricular dysfunction, and occasionally multiple foci of arrhythmias.

Only carefully defined VTs have been successfully treated with catheter ablation. These include VT related to bundle branch reentry and right ventricular ouflow tract tachycardia. Belhassen et al. described localization of right bundle branch-left axis deviation or left bundle branch-left axis deviation VT to discrete areas of myocardium in patients status post-MI [22]. In this early study, direct current ablation was successful. Limited or partial success with radiofrequency catheter ablation has been observed with other ventricular tachycardias associated with coronary artery disease.

A. **Mechanisms.** Mechanisms of VT include **classic reentry** provocable by programmed electrical stimulation and not suppressed by verapamil. Ventricular tachycardia due to **triggered activity** is inducible by atrial and ventricular pacing, and induction can be suppressed by verapamil. **Catecholamine-sensitive VT** due to **automaticity** cannot be induced or terminated by programmed stimulation but can be induced by the infusion of isoproterenol [23].

   In VT due to **bundle branch reentry** (BBR), AV dissociation occurs during tachycardia, a His or right bundle branch (RBB) deflection or both preceded each QRS complex, spontaneous His-to-His and RBB-to-RBB cycle length variations precede changes in VT cycle length, and the duration of the H–V interval was the same or longer during tachycardia. Ventricular extrastimuli delivered during inscription of the His bundle resulted in termination of the tachycardia. During tachycardia, His-to-RBB conduction time is the same as or shorter than at baseline [24].

B. **Mapping.** Morady et al. summarized the variety of mapping techniques that are used to localize the origin of the VT [25]. In **classic endocardial activation mapping,** the earliest endocardial activation relative to the onset of the QRS is noted (usually 70 msec earlier). Occasionally the clinician is able to detect an **isolated discrete potential** in diastole during VT. Pacing is unable to dissociate the potential from the VT [26]. The potential may represent activation of a segment of the slow conducting region of the ventricular reentrant circuit, which is critical to the continuation of the VT.

   Concealed entrainment of the VT at cycle lengths 30–100 msec shorter than the tachycardia with a stimulus to QRS morphology over 90 msec without change in the morphology of the VT provides further evidence for the origin of the tachycardia [27]. The pacing site is thought to be in an area of slow conduction of the reentry circuit. In **pace mapping,** ventricular pacing at the site of origin of the tachycardia results in a similar or identical morphology compared with the clinical VT.

C. **Ablation.** In patients with **bundle branch reentrant ventricular tachycardia,** the site of ablation is the RBB. Criteria for localization include a sharp deflection occurring more than 20 msec after the His deflection and no atrial electrogram on the RBB recording. Radiofrequency energy is applied to the RBB at 15–20 W for up to 60 seconds, or until an increase in impedance occurs.

   For patients with **right ventricular outflow tract (RVOT) tachycardia,** earliest activation is usually localized to the high RVOT (anteroseptal in the majority; other sites are anterolateral and anterior) and in some patients to the right ventricular inflow tract. The VT morphology is usually left bundle branch block with an inferior axis, but others have included left bundle branch block with a rightward axis or right bundle branch block with a superior axis [28]. These investigators did not find it necessary to identify areas of concealed entrainment or middiastolic potentials. Earliest activation or pace mapping provided the best localization. In patients without coronary disease, the earliest endocardial activation times were later than in patients with VT associated with coronary artery disease. Radiofrequency current is delivered at 40–60 V for 30–60 seconds, or until an impedance rise occurred. In related observations, there was no difference in signal-averaged ECGs.

   Calkins et al. found that radiofrequency ablation was successful in ablating 100% of VT originating from the RVOT but only in 50% originating at other sites in the right or left ventricle [29]. In this study, pace mapping was the primary mapping technique, with careful attention paid to both major (changes in a component that was >50% of total QRS amplitude) and minor (notching, Q,R, or S changes <25% of peak to peak QRS amplitude, changes in slope) differences in the paced tachycardia as compared to the clinical tachycardia (Figs. 13-15, 13-16).

   In patients with **VT due to coronary artery disease,** Morady et al. used all four mapping techniques to localize the site of origin of the tachycardia [25]. Radiofrequency energy is delivered during VT if possible using 30–35 W for 10 seconds (Fig. 13-17). If VT terminates, radiofrequency is continued for a total of 30 seconds. If VT does not terminate after 10 seconds, another site is selected. A second application is delivered at the successful site for insurance. The mean number of applications of

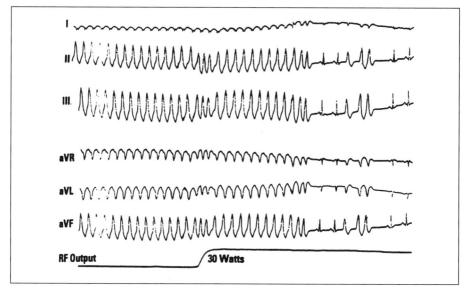

Fig. 13-15. Delivery of radiofrequency (RF) energy at successful ablation site during sustained ventricular tachycardia. Six limb leads and power (watts) of RF energy used for ablation are shown. Sustained ventricular tachycardia terminated 6 seconds after onset of RF energy delivery. (From H Calkins et al., Relation between efficacy of radiofrequency catheter ablation and site of origin of idiopathic ventricular tachycardia. *Am J Cardiol* 71:827–833. Reprinted with permission.)

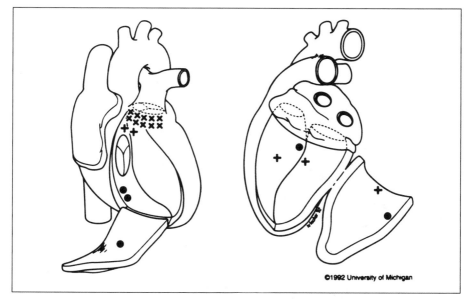

Fig. 13-16. Schematic drawing of heart showing site of origin of 20 ventricular tachycardias for which radiofrequency catheter ablation was attempted. Ten ventricular tachycardias were located in outflow tract of right ventricle, and 10 were located at other sites in left and right ventricles. (X = ventricular tachycardias that were successfully ablated; *closed circles* = ventricular tachycardias that were not successfully ablated.) (From H Calkins et al., Relation between efficacy of radiofrequency catheter ablation and site of origin of idiopathic ventricular tachycardia. *Am J Cardiol* 71:827–833. Reprinted with permission.)

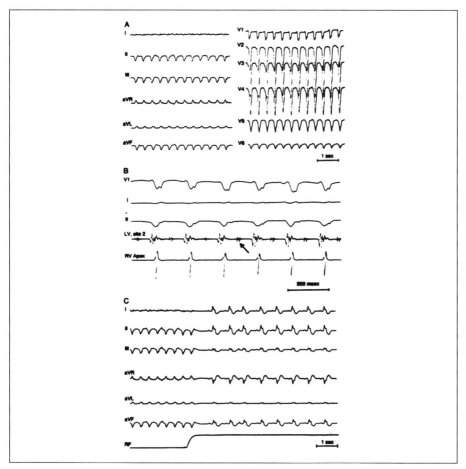

Fig. 13-17. Traces show target site for catheter ablation of ventricular tachycardia (VT) selected based on the presence of an isolated middiastolic potential. **A.** Twelve-lead ECG of the VT induced in the electrophysiology laboratory. The VT had a left bundle branch block configuration and a cycle length of 380 msec and was identical in configuration to the VT that had been occurring spontaneously. **B.** An isolated middiastolic potential (*arrow*) was recorded during VT in the left ventricle (LV) at site 2 (apical septum). (RV = right ventricular.) **C.** The VT, which had never previously terminated spontaneously, terminated less than 1 second after the onset of a 32-W application of radiofrequency (RF) energy at site 2. Afterward, the VT was no longer inducible by programmed stimulation. (From F Morady et al., Radiofrequency catheter ablation of ventricular tachycardia in patients with coronary artery disease. *Circulation* 87:363–372, 1993. Reprinted with permission.)

radiofrequency energy was 4.2 (range, 2–15). Although effective in 73% of patients selected, the authors emphasized that the population represented less than 10% of patients referred for management of VT who could not be managed by pharmacological therapy or an internal cardioverter-defibrillator. Also the majority of patients still required other therapies for VT, and radiofrequency ablation was considered more an adjunctive therapy to control frequent or incessant tachycardias.

D. **Complications and limitations.** With radiofrequency ablation, complications have been relatively few, at least in the short term. It is a safe procedure and does not result in proarrhythmia. Only minimal elevation of creatine kinase (MB fraction) has been reported. Any left-sided ablation is performed with heparin anticoagulation. One of the major concerns is the inability to eliminate VT, hence the caution to be certain that the VT is eliminated before sending the patient home without pharmacologic or other device therapy.

Limitations of this technique in the treatment of VT include the fact that only a small percentage of patients with VT may be suitable. Patients with hemodynamically embarrassing VT may not be able to tolerate mapping. Some other patients may have clinical but not inducible VTs. Finally, since catheter ablation for VT is still a new technique, it may be unwise to rely on it as the only therapy for malignant ventricular arrhythmias.

E. **Recommendations for radiofrequency catheter ablation in VT.** Catheter ablation for ventricular tachycardia is particularly useful for RVOT or BBR tachycardias; the success rate may be higher than 90%. It may occasionally be useful for selected patients who have coronary artery disease, in particular as an adjunctive therapy, but the success rate may be only 70%. Our ability to employ this technique for VT may improve in the future.

References

1. Calkins H, et al. Radiation exposure during radiofrequency catheter ablation of accessory atrioventricular connections. *Circulation* 84:2376–2382, 1991.
2. Denes P, et al. Demonstration of dual AV nodal pathways in patients with paroxysmal supraventricular tachycardia. *Circulation* 48:549–555, 1973.
3. Rosen K, et al. Demonstration of dual atrioventricular nodal pathways in man. *Am J Cardiol* 33:291–294, 1974.
4. Jackman WM, et al. Treatment of supraventricular tachycardia due to atrioventricular nodal reentry by radiofrequency catheter ablation of slow pathway conduction. *N Engl J Med* 327:313–318, 1992.
5. Kay GN, et al. Selective radiofrequency ablation of the slow pathway for the treatment of atrioventricular nodal reentrant tachycardia. *Circulation* 85:1675–1688, 1992.
6. Wu D, et al. Nature of dual atrioventricular node pathways and the tachycardia circuit as defined by radiofrequency ablation technique. *J Am Coll Cardiol* 20:884–895, 1992.
7. Kuck KH, Schluter M. Single-catheter approach to radiofrequency current ablation of left-sided accessory pathways in patients with Wolff-Parkinson-White syndrome. *Circulation* 84:2366–2375, 1991.
8. Jackman W, et al. New catheter technique for recording left free-wall accessory atrioventricular pathway activation. *Circulation* 78:598–611, 1988.
9. Jackman WM, et al. Catheter ablation of accessory atrioventricular pathways (Wolff-Parkinson-White syndrome) by radiofrequency current. *N Engl J Med* 324:1605–1611, 1991.
10. Zipes DP. Arrhythmias on the endangered list. *J Am Coll Cardiol* 21:918, 1993.
11. Case CL, et al. Radiofrequency catheter ablation of incessant, medically resistant supraventricular tachycardia in infants and small children. *J Am Coll Cardiol* 20:1405–1410, 1992.
12. Dick M, et al. Use of radiofrequency current to ablate accessory connections in children. *Circulation* 84:2318–2324, 1992.
13. Saul JP, et al. Catheter ablation of accessory atrioventricular pathways in young patients: Use of long vascular sheaths, the transseptal approach and a retrograde left posterior parallel approach. *J Am Coll Cardiol* 21:571–583, 1993.
14. Klein LS, et al. Radiofrequency catheter ablation of Mahaim fibers at the tricuspid annulus. *Circulation* 87:738–747, 1993.
15. Cosio FG, et al. Radiofrequency ablation of the inferior vena cava-tricuspid valve isthmus in common atrial flutter. *Am J Cardiol* 71:705–709, 1993.
16. Feld GK, et al. Radiofrequency catheter ablation for the treatment of human type 1 atrial flutter. *Circulation* 86:1233–1240, 1992.
17. Kay GN, et al. Radiofrequency ablation for treatment of primary atrial tachycardias. *J Am Coll Cardiol* 21:901–909, 1993.
18. Wu D, et al. Demonstration of sustained sinus and atrial reentry as a mechanism of paroxysmal supraventricular tachycardia. *Circulation* 51:234–243, 1975.
19. Walsh EP, et al. Transcatheter ablation of ectopic atrial tachycardia in young patients using radiofrequency current. *Circulation* 86:1138–1146, 1992.
20. Chen SA, et al. Radiofrequency catheter ablation of sustained intra-atrial reentrant tachycardia in adult patients. *Circulation* 88:578–587, 1993.
21. Chien WW, et al. Electrophysiologic findings and long-term follow-up of patients with the permanent form of junctional reciprocating tachycardia treated by catheter ablation. *Circulation* 85:1329–1336, 1992.

22. Belhassen B, et al. Transcatheter electrical shock ablation of ventricular tachycardia. *J Am Coll Cardiol* 7:1347–1355, 1986.
23. Morady F, et al. Long-term results of catheter ablation of idiopathic right ventricular tachycardia. *Circulation* 82:2093–2099, 1990.
24. Cohen TJ, et al. Radiofrequency catheter ablation for treatment for bundle branch reentrant ventricular tachycardia: Results and long-term follow-up. *J Am Coll Cardiol* 18: 1767–1773, 1991.
25. Morady F, et al. Radiofrequency catheter ablation of ventricular tachycardia in patients with coronary artery disease. *Circulation* 87:363–372, 1993.
26. Fitzgerald DM, et al. Electrogram patterns predicting successful catheter ablation of ventricular tachycardia. *Circulation* 77:806–814, 1988.
27. Morady F, et al. Identification and catheter ablation of a zone of slow conduction in the reentrant circuit of ventricular tachycardia in humans. *J Am Coll Cardiol* 11:775–782, 1988.
28. Klein LS, et al. Radiofrequency catheter ablation of ventricular tachycardia in patients without structural heart disease. *Circulation* 85:1666–1674, 1992.
29. Calkins H, et al. Relation between efficacy of radiofrequency catheter ablation and site of origin of idiopathic ventricular tachycardia. *Am J Cardiol* 71:827–833, 1993.

Bibliography

Akthar M, et al. Atrioventricular nodal reentry. *Circulation* 88:282–295, 1993.

Avitall B, et al. Physics and engineering of transcatheter cardiac tissue ablation. *J Am Coll Cardiol* 22:921–932, 1993.

Bardy GH, Sawyer MS. Biophysical and anatomic consideration for safe and efficacious catheter ablation of arrhythmias. *Clin Cardiol* 13:425–433, 1990.

Bashir Y, et al. Radiofrequency current delivery by way of a bipolar tricuspid annulus–mitral annulus electrode configuration for ablation of posteroseptal accessory pathways. *J Am Coll Cardiol* 22:550–556, 1993.

de Buitleir M, et al. Cost of catheter vs surgical ablation in the Wolff-Parkinson-White Syndrome. *Am J Cardiol* 66:189–192.

Calkins H, Kim YN, Schmaltz S. Electrogram criteria for identification of appropriate target sites for radiofrequency catheter ablation accessory atrioventricular connections. *Circulation* 85:565–573, 1992.

Calkins H, et al. Diagnosis and cure of the Wolff-Parkinson-White syndrome or paroxysmal supraventricular tachycardias during a single electrophysiologic test. *N Engl J Med* 324:1612–1618, 1991.

Calkins H, et al. Radiofrequency catheter ablation of accessory atrioventricular connections in 250 patients. *Circulation* 85:1337–1346, 1992.

Camm AJ, Sneddon JF. High energy His bundle ablation: A treatment of last resort. *Circulation* 84:2187–2189, 1991.

Chen SA, et al. Selective radiofrequency catheter ablation of slow and fast pathways in 100 patients with atrioventricular nodal reentrant tachycardia. *Am Heart J* 125:1–10, 1993.

Chen X, et al. Characteristics of local electrogram predicting successful transcatheter radiofrequency ablation of left-sided accessory pathways. *J Am Coll Cardiol* 20:656–665, 1992.

Epstein LM, et al. Percutaneous catheter modification of the atrioventricular node. *Circulation* 80:757–768, 1989.

Evans GT, et al. Predictors of in-hospital mortality after DC catheter ablation of atrioventricular junction. *Circulation* 84:1924–1937, 1991.

Haissaguerre M, et al. Catheter ablation of Mahaim fibers with preservation of atrioventricular nodal conduction. *Circulation* 82:418–427, 1990.

Haissaguerre M, et al. Electrogram patterns predictive of successful catheter ablation of accessory pathways. *Circulation* 84:188–202, 1991.

Haissaguerre M, et al. Radiofrequency catheter ablation of left lateral accessory pathways via the coronary sinus. *Circulation* 86:1464–1468, 1992.

Haissaguerre M, et al. Elimination of atrioventricular nodal reentrant tachycardia using discrete slow potentials to guide application of radiofrequency energy. *Circulation* 85:2162–2175, 1992.

Jackman WM, et al. Catheter ablation of atrioventricular junction using radiofrequency current in 17 patients: Comparison of standard and large tip catheter electrodes. *Circulation* 83:1562–1576, 1991.

Jazayeri MR, et al. Selective transcatheter ablation of the fast and slow pathways using radiofrequency energy in patients with atrioventricular nodal reentrant tachycardia. *Circulation* 85:1318–1328, 1992.

Kalbfleisch SJ, Calkins H, Langberg JJ. Comparison of the cost of radiofrequency catheter modification of the atrioventricular node and medical therapy for drug-refractory atrioventricular node reentrant tachycardia. *J Am Coll Cardiol* 19:1583–1587, 1992.

Kalbfleisch SJ, et al. Safety, feasibility and cost of outpatient radiofrequency catheter ablation of accessory atrioventricular connections. *J Am Coll Cardiol* 21:567–570, 1993.

Kalbfleisch SJ, et al. Repolarization abnormalities after catheter ablation of accessory atrioventricular connections with radiofrequency current. *J Am Coll Cardiol* 18:1761–1766, 1991.

Klein L. Radiofrequency catheter ablation. *Circulation* 84:2594–2597, 1991.

Kuck KH, Schluter M, Gursoy S. Preservation of atrioventricular nodal conduction during radiofrequency current catheter ablation of midseptal accessory pathways. *Circulation* 86:1743–1752, 1992.

Langberg JJ, et al. Catheter ablation of the atrioventricular junction with radiofrequency energy. *Circulation* 80:1527–1535, 1989.

Langberg JJ, et al. Recurrence of conduction in accessory atrioventricular connections after initially successful radiofrequency catheter ablation. *J Am Coll Cardiol* 19:1588–1592, 1992.

Langberg JJ, et al. A randomized prospective comparison of anterior and posterior approaches to radiofrequency catheter ablation of atrioventricular nodal reentry tachycardia. *Circulation* 87:1551–1556, 1993.

Leather RA, et al. Radiofrequency catheter ablation of accessory pathways: A learning experience. *Am J Cardiol* 68:1651–1655, 1991.

Lee MA, et al. Catheter modification of the atrioventricular junction with radiofrequency energy for control of atrioventricular nodal reentry tachycardia. *Circulation* 83:827–835, 1991.

Lesh MD, et al. Comparison of the retrograde and transseptal methods for ablation of left free wall accessory pathways. *J Am Coll Cardiol* 22:542–549, 1993.

Lesh MD, et al. Curative percutaneous catheter ablation using radiofrequency energy for accessory pathways in all locations: Results in 100 consecutive patients. *J Am Coll Cardiol* 19:1303–1309, 1992.

McGuire MA, et al. Dimensions of the triangle of Koch in humans. *Am J Cardiol* 70:829–830, 1992.

Mitrani RD, et al. Radiofrequency ablation for atrioventricular node reentrant tachycardia: Comparison between fast (anterior) and slow (posterior) pathway ablation. *J Am Coll Cardiol* 21:432–441, 1993.

Morady F, et al. Catheter ablation of ventricular tachycardia with intracardiac shocks: Results in 33 patients. *Circulation* 75:1037–1049, 1987.

Morady F, et al. Concealed entrainment as a guide for catheter ablation of ventricular tachycardia in patients with prior myocardial infarction. *J Am Coll Cardiol* 17:678–689, 1991.

Morady F, et al. A prospective randomized comparison of direct current and radiofrequency ablation of the atrioventricular junction. *J Am Coll Cardiol* 21:102–109, 1993.

NASPE Ad Hoc Committee on Catheter Ablation. Catheter ablation for cardiac arrhythmias: Personnel and facilities. *J Arrhythmia Management* 30–38, Spring 1992.

Olgin JE, Scheinman MM. Comparison of high energy direct current and radiofrequency catheter ablation of the atrioventricular junction. *J Am Coll Cardiol* 21:557–564, 1993.

Rabbani LE, et al. Time course of improvement in ventricular function after ablation of incessant automatic atrial tachycardia. *Am Heart J* 121:816–819, 1991.

Ruskin JN. Catheter ablation for supraventricular tachycardia. *N Engl J Med* 324: 1660–1662, 1991.

Saoudi NS, et al. Catheter ablation of the atrial myocardium in human type 1 atrial flutter. *Circulation* 81:762–771, 1990.

Scheinman MM, et al. Current role of catheter ablative procedures in patients with cardiac arrhythmias. *Circulation* 83:2146–2153, 1991.

Scheinman MM. Catheter ablation. *Circulation* 83:1489–1498, 1991.

Schluter M, et al. Catheter ablation using radiofrequency current to sure symptomatic patients with tachyarrhythmias related to an accessory atrioventricular pathway. *Circulation* 84:1664–1661, 1991.

Schluter M, Kuck KH. Catheter ablation from right atrium of anteroseptal accessory pathways using radiofrequency current. *J Am Coll Cardiol* 19:663–670, 1992.

Schwartz JF, Tracy CM, Fletcher RD. Radiofrequency endocardial catheter ablation of accessory atrioventricular pathway atrial insertion sites. *Circulation* 87:487–499, 1993.

Tchou P, et al. Transcatheter electrical ablation of the right bundle branch: A method of treating macroreentrant ventricular tachycardia attributed to bundle branch reentry. *Circulation* 78:246–257, 1988.

Tebbenjohanns J, et al. Radiofrequency catheter ablation of a right posterolateral atrioventricular accessory pathway with decremental conduction properties (Mahaim fiber). *Am Heart J* 125:898–901, 1993.

Tracy CM, et al. Radiofrequency catheter ablation of ectopic atrial tachycardia using paced activation sequence mapping. *J Am Coll Cardiol* 21:910–917, 1993.

Wathen M, et al. An anatomically guided approach to atrioventricular node slow pathway ablation. *Am J Cardiol* 70:886–889, 1992.

Yeh SJ, et al. Radiofrequency ablation in multiple accessory pathways and the physiologic implications. *Am J Cardiol* 71:1174–1180, 1993.

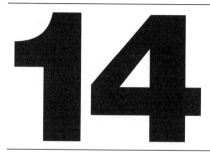

Pharmacology of the Antiarrhythmic Drugs

Stephen C. Vlay

I. **Antiarrhythmic drugs.** This chapter emphasizes the key aspects of drug therapy rather than presenting a comprehensive review of pharmacology.

   A. **Classification.** Antiarrhythmic drugs have been classified by their electrophysiologic properties, which offers some utility in selecting or combining them (Table 14-1). Vaughan Williams [1, 2] classified drugs that act on the fast sodium channels as type 1, beta-receptor antagonists as type 2, drugs that prolong the action potential and repolarization as type 3, and inhibitors of the slow calcium current as type 4. Further division of the type 1 drugs into types 1A, 1B, and 1C has allowed differentiation according to effects on the specialized conduction system tissue, ventricular refractoriness, and repolarization. In particular, this classification was designed to facilitate utilization of drugs while avoiding toxicity. A clinician would avoid prescribing a drug that prolonged repolarization (and the Q–T interval) to a patient with a widened Q–T at baseline. Should a combination of agents be advisable, selection of one that shortens with one that prolongs repolarization (and the Q–T interval) may result in greater efficacy with less toxicity. Combination of drugs is discussed in Chap. 8.

   The traditional Vaughan Williams classification is limited by the fact that many drugs fit into more than one category, only block is considered, and many basic electrophysiologic properties such as channels, pumps, and receptors are only partially considered. Consequently, to include these aspects, a new classification was devised by a group of eminent physicians who met in Palermo, Sicily, and published their consensus of opinion [3]. This article, entitled "The Sicilian Gambit," should be part of every electrophysiologist's library. Many of the features are summarized in Table 3-2 on basic electrophysiology. The new classifications are included for each drug.

   B. **Indications.** The goal of antiarrhythmic drug therapy is to prevent symptomatic arrhythmias and sudden cardiac death. Treating asymptomatic ectopy may not be necessary, and the antiarrhythmic agent may have the potential to exacerbate the arrhythmia and cause sudden cardiac death. The indications for antiarrhythmic drug therapy are discussed in Chaps. 6 through 8. The FDA has approved certain indications for each drug. New data frequently indicate utility of a drug for other-than-approved indications. As an example, amiodarone has been approved for ventricular tachyarrhythmias but may also be valuable for supraventricular tachyarrhythmias. It is not a first-line drug for the latter but may be considered if all else fails and one is willing to accept the potential toxicities. This decision rests on a clinical judgment that the risks are warranted, that conventional therapy has failed, that results of previous trials are documented, and that the clinical interests of the patient are well served. Obviously, this type of situation is ideally handled with informed consent and an approved protocol.

   Drug therapy involves responsibility for both the physician and the patient. The physician must be aware of the immediate and long-term toxicities of the drug. He or she must obtain the appropriate follow-up laboratory tests (e.g., CBC, chemistries, liver function tests) as well as other tests (such as pulmonary function tests with diffusion capacity in the case of amiodarone). It is the responsibility of the patient to report any serious problem to the physician in a timely fashion.

   The method of administration of each drug, either intravenous (IV) or oral, depends on the availability of the preparation, as well as the urgency of achieving a therapeutic effect. Intravenous administration quite often is limited by potential toxic electrophysiologic effects or by accompanying hypotension. The route chosen is dictated by the clinical situation, as is discussed in Chaps. 6 through 8.

Often drug therapy presents a lifelong commitment. Attention to certain pharmacotherapeutic principles (Table 14-2) may facilitate successful treatment. The physician should know the half-life of the drug. The elimination half-life is the time it takes to eliminate half the drug from the body or decrease its concentration by 50% and is determined by the drug's volume of distribution and its clearance. The time to steady state is determined by the elimination half-life. The physician must also realize that certain situations mandate adjustment of drug dosage. Among the most critical are drug management in (1) the **elderly,** (2) patients with **renal insufficiency or failure,** (3) patients with **hepatic insufficiency or failure,** (4) **pregnancy,** and (5) patients taking **multiple drugs that interact.**

The elderly have a reduced creatinine clearance, may be more sensitive to certain drugs, may have other systemic illnesses that complicate therapy, and may have slower rates of hepatic metabolism. However, with antiarrhythmic drug therapy, usually only minor adjustments need to be made. A reduced dosage of digoxin may be required in the elderly when renal function declines as a function of a reduced creatinine clearance. Similarly, lidocaine is more likely to result in CNS toxicity, partly owing to a reduction in hepatic blood flow and metabolism of the drug. The elderly may be more sensitive to beta-blocker therapy because of decreased clearance of the drug in the liver. Also some beta blockers may cause CNS depression, an undesirable consequence.

In the patient with renal or hepatic insufficiency or failure, drug toxicity is related to the metabolism of the drug. The physician must first reevaluate if continued drug therapy is necessary and then reduce the dosage appropriately. The subject of antiarrhythmic drugs in pregnancy is discussed in detail in Chap. 8. Combinations of drugs are discussed in individual sections as well as in Chap. 8.

C. **Proarrhythmic effects.** Perhaps the most important realization concerning antiarrhythmic drugs in the past 10 years has been growing appreciation of their ability to cause or exacerbate arrhythmias—a **proarrhythmic** effect. **Every antiarrhythmic drug has this potential.** The incidence ranges from 5–20% in most series, with an average incidence of **10%.** The effects vary from an increase in baseline ectopy, to precipitation of ventricular tachycardia (VT), to causing intractable VT or ventricular fibrillation (VF) refractory to all measures and resulting in death. Both ambulatory ECG recording and electrophysiology study can be used to quantitate proar-

Table 14-1. Antiarrhythmic drugs

Digitalis preparations
Digoxin
Digitoxin

Type 1: Sodium channel blockers
1A: Quinidine, procainamide, disopyramide, (imipramine)[a]
1B: Lidocaine, mexiletine, tocainide
1C: Flecainide, propafenone
Other: moricizine, (ajmaline)[b]

Type 2: Beta-adrenergic receptor blockers
Cardioselective: Acebutolol, atenolol, betaxolol, bisoprolol, esmolol, metoprolol
Noncardioselective: Carteolol, labetalol, nadolol, penbutolol, pindolol, propranolol, sotalol, timolol

Type 3: Potassium channel blockers
Bretylium, amiodarone, sotalol

Type 4: Calcium channel blockers
Verapamil, diltiazem, bepridil

Purinergic receptor blockers
Adenosine

Muscarinic receptor blockers
Atropine

[a]Imipramine is a tricyclic antidepressant that has 1A properties. It is not approved, however, for cardiac arrhythmias.
[b]Ajmaline is not available in the United States.

rhythmia. With ambulatory ECG, varying criteria have been used. A tenfold increase in the amount of ectopy is a general guideline. Smaller amounts may reflect day-to-day variability. Changes in the morphology of VT with drug suggest proarrhythmia. Drugs that prolong the Q–T interval (such as type 1A agents) frequently cause torsades de pointes, a type of polymorphic VT. Drugs that enhance conduction (type 1B agents) may result in a faster VT. With electophysiology study, induction with a less potent technique represents proarrhythmia (e.g., postdrug induction with double extrastimuli of an arrhythmia inducible only with triple extrastimuli at baseline). Another proarrhythmic effect is the development of sustained VT after drug in a patient with only nonsustained VT at baseline. In patients with baseline inducible VT, if the postdrug-induced arrhythmia is more hemodynamically unstable or difficult to terminate (by either pacing or defibrillation), the criteria for proarrhythmia are satisfied.

Arrhythmogenicity may be related to alteration of the dispersion of refractoriness, changes in the rate of impulse formation, prolongation of the effective refractory period (ERP), prolongation of repolarization, and nonuniformity of drug distribution in the myocardium. All of these factors may alter the reentrant pathways. In addition, depression of contractility, hypotension causing decreased coronary perfusion, and reflex sympathetic activity are hemodynamic variables that may exacerbate arrhythmias. Anticholinergic effects of some drugs may be contributory. Finally, electrolyte fluxes, acidosis, ischemia, and neural activity are influential. Thus, with more than a dozen variables, all of which may interact, is it any wonder that antiarrhythmic drugs have the potential to exacerbate arrhythmias? Therefore, the decision to treat a patient who has no or only borderline indications for antiarrhythmic drug therapy is attended by considerable hazard. With more serious and symptomatic arrhythmias, the risk of therapy becomes more acceptable, but the drug selected must be used properly and its efficacy evaluated correctly. Evaluation of efficacy can be performed at the time of electrophysiologic study (EPS) or by Holter monitoring, as described in prior chapters.

D. Drug levels. Assays to determine the plasma or serum level of an antiarrhythmic drug have a definite role in the management of an arrhythmia. Several important considerations must be remembered.

First, **therapeutic ranges for individual drugs are empirically derived, and individual patients may have therapeutic results outside these ranges.** The most common example of this situation is encountered in the patient with atrial fibrillation, who may require higher dosages of digoxin to control the ventricular response than someone in sinus rhythm would. Although the level may be high, the patient may not be digitalis toxic. Another such situation may be observed in the patient with refractory VT treated with high-dosage procainamide. Although the levels of procainamide and N-acetylprocainamide (NAPA) may be much higher than the upper limit of the therapeutic range, these levels may be required to suppress VT.

Table 14-2. Pharmacotherapeutic principles

Minimize the number of medications.
Choose convenient times of administration, if possible.
Avoid or minimize immediate and long-term toxicity.
Insist that the patient know the name of the medication as well as the indication for its
  use and its potential toxicities.
Select the least expensive preparation.
Document blood levels.
Document response to medication.
Use conventional drugs prior to investigational agents.
Electrophysiologic testing should be available (ideally).
Establish a firm physician-patient relationship for successful management.
Choose the investigational drug that electrophysiologically would be most likely to
  succeed, based on prior experience with conventional agents.
If this fails, choose the agent with the highest probability of success, even though
  conventional drugs with similar electrophysiologic characteristics were
  unsuccessful.

Source: From SC Vlay, PR Reid. Ventricular ectopy: Etiology, evaluation, therapy. *Am J Med* 73:905, 1982.

Thus, the blood level is useful in that it provides a guide to monitoring the patient. If the level is in the therapeutic range, the arrhythmia will be controlled in most patients. When the level is high, there is a greater possibility of a toxic effect, although the drug will still be therapeutic for some. When the level is low, there is a chance that the dosage is subtherapeutic, although some patients will have a good result.

Second, **a drug level in the therapeutic range does not guarantee clinical suppression of the arrhythmia or prevention of sudden cardiac death.** Nevertheless, several studies have suggested that patients with serious arrhythmias who maintain their drug levels in the therapeutic range may have a better outcome than those who do not. Studies in patients with malignant ventricular tachyarrhythmias will be discussed shortly.

Third, **the time of sampling is important.** I recommend measuring the blood level before the next dose is due. This timing provides the benefit of consistency when comparing samples obtained on different days. The predose level is close to the nadir (the level will continue to fall as the next dose is being absorbed if given orally, before increasing again).

Fourth, **if the patient has a recurrence of the arrhythmia, obtain a drug level assay at that time.** Similarly, if the patient is examined for symptoms that may be attributable to an arrhythmia although it is not manifest at the time, saving a blood specimen that can be analyzed later is prudent. If the blood level is within the therapeutic range for that patient (e.g., equivalent to that obtained during EPS in which induction was suppressed), it suggests that the drug is no longer effective. Possibly this may be attributed to progression of the underlying heart disease, but acute exacerbating factors such as myocardial infarction (MI) or ischemia and hypokalemia or other electrolyte disturbances must also be considered. If the level is high, one would have to consider a proarrhythmic effect. If the level is low, the possibilities include malabsorption of the drug and noncompliance.

Drug levels in VT and VF patients have been assessed for their ability to correlate with clinical outcome. Few studies have ever conclusively demonstrated improved survival if the level was in the therapeutic range. An early study with phenytoin after MI found similar outcomes in treated and control patients. A European study using aprindine in a similar subject population was unable to demonstrate survival differences. Three studies from the United States in patients with VT showed improved survival if the levels of antiarrhythmic drugs remained in the therapeutic range. The drugs were quinidine, procainamide, and aprindine.

In treating patients with potentially malignant arrhythmias, one must always attempt to optimize all factors: the underlying heart disease, the electrophysiologic substrate, and antiarrhythmic drug therapy. In regard to the last, the patient must be taking the medication correctly, the subsequent drug levels must match those obtained during successful acute drug trials, and no serious adverse effects should be present. **For some drugs, levels may have minimal value.** This statement may be particularly relevant for amiodarone. Obtaining levels is rarely helpful, and patient management is guided by an attempt to achieve efficacy with the lowest dose to avoid adverse effects.

E. **Format for specific drug listings.** The remainder of this chapter deals with specific drugs by class. The format used will provide the physician with the key facts but is **not** intended to represent a comprehensive list and does not substitute for reviewing the package insert or the listing in *Physicians' Desk Reference* or *The Pharmacological Basis of Therapeutics* [4] before prescribing the drug. **A physician who is uncomfortable about the treatment of an arrhythmia should obtain a consultation rather than treat with potentially dangerous drugs. The availability of tiered therapy cardioverter-defibrillator devices and techniques such as radiofrequency catheter ablation have made drug therapy a second choice for some arrhythmias.**

Each drug is summarized in outline form to present the salient points related to arrhythmia management. Not all of the adverse reactions of each drug are listed— only those most frequently seen in practice. All drugs have the potential for an unknown reaction. Similarly the proarrhythmic potential of each drug is not specifically mentioned again in detail unless it is a major concern. **Nevertheless, every drug may exacerbate the arrhythmia.**

Key references are listed at the end of the chapter and are limited to the most important recent additions to the literature. Further sources can be found in the reference sections of the review articles. Finally, drug dosages specified are for **adults.**

For specific recommendations in children and infants, consult the PDR or a textbook of pediatrics.

The format for drug listings in the remainder of this chapter is as follows:

Pharmacology: Class of agent.
New classification: according to "The Sicilian Gambit" [3].
Preparations: Chemical name, trade name, dosages.
Approved indications: Arrhythmia indications approved by the FDA.
Potential indications: Potential uses for the drug suggested by the medical literature and clinical practice.
Metabolism: Route.
Active metabolites: If any.
Half-life: Elimination half-life.
Therapeutic level: If known.
Common adverse reactions: Only the most common reactions.
Potentially life-threatening reactions: The potential reactions (in addition to possible proarrhythmic effect) that the physician must be aware of, even if they are rare.
Comments: General comments about the use of the drug in arrhythmias.

II. **Digitalis.** Digitalis, one of the most widely used cardiac drugs, is useful not only for cardiac arrhythmias but also for heart failure. It is extremely important for the physician to understand its pharmacology because of the considerable potential for toxicity. The subject of digitalis and its various preparations has been extensively studied and reviewed. The discussion here focuses on digoxin and highlights the key points of its effects on the cardiac rhythm. Digitalis inhibits the sodium-potassium ATPase pump. Other effects are indirect and are mediated through the autonomic nervous system, particularly by augmenting vagal activity.

Effects on the electrical activity of the heart are dose dependent and vary from a pharmacotherapeutic to a toxic effect. After a minimal increase in the action potential duration (APD) with an initial dose, the APD shortens—vagal stimulation activates the I K (ACh) channel in atrial tissue and nodal cells—as the dose is increased. The resting potential becomes less negative. Both the maximal rate of phase 0 depolarization and the amplitude of the action potential decrease. Digitalis has an effect on phase 4 that is related to the serum potassium. With low levels, the slope of phase 4 increases, resulting in increased automaticity. At high levels (greater than 4 mM), delayed afterdepolarizations may appear. These last two effects provide two different mechanisms for ectopic impulse formation [5].

Direct vagal effects on the sinoatrial (SA) and atrioventricular (AV) nodes include an increase in the effective refractory period and a decrease in the conduction velocity. Cyclic AMP–mediated sympathetic activity is antagonized by vagal effects by inhibition of adenyl cyclase and block of the L-type calcium channel. These reasons explain the effect of digitalis on AV nodal reentrant tachycardia (for both termination of the acute arrhythmia and prevention of its recurrence). Toxic doses may suppress sinus discharge and cause high-degree AV block. Specialized atrial fibers may demonstrate enhanced automaticity, as well as delayed afterdepolarizations. In atrial or ventricular muscle fibers, digitalis may cause delayed afterdepolarizations but not phase 4 depolarization. Both the refractory period and action potential amplitude of these fibers decrease.

Indirect effects of digitalis reflect cardiac responses to altered sympathetic and vagal tone. An increase in vagal tone and a decrease in sympathetic tone may slow the sinus rate. The interactions among these opposing autonomic neural factors may be different in patients with heart failure. Furthermore, some of the indirect effects of digitalis oppose the direct effects. In the AV node, however, both the direct effects (increase in ERP, decrease in conduction velocity) and the indirect effects (increased vagal tone) produce additive effects to slow conduction of supraventricular activity to the ventricles. In atrial fibrillation and atrial flutter, even those impulses that are not conducted to the ventricle provide additional local slowing of transmission, since subsequent impulses must await repolarization before they can be conducted. The indirect effects of digitalis predominate in the His-Purkinje system, although they usually do not play a major role. Finally, it is important to remember that the positive inotropic effects of digitalis on a patient with heart failure may modify the overall physiologic state, which indicates the complexity of actions on the heart.

A. **Use of digitalis in arrhythmias**
   1. **Atrial flutter.** Digitalis is the drug of choice for atrial flutter since it may terminate it as well as control the ventricular response. Digitalis increases the AV nodal ERP.

2. **Atrial fibrillation.** Unlike the situation in atrial flutter, digitalis alone usually does not terminate atrial fibrillation but does slow the ventricular response. If digitalis alone fails to slow the ventricular response sufficiently, a beta blocker or verapamil may add some benefit, but both have a negative inotropic effect that may be detrimental in patients with poor left ventricular function. Whether digitalis is effective in maintaining sinus rhythm after conversion remains controversial. The ability of digitalis to enhance automaticity and afterdepolarizations may even predispose to atrial fibrillation. The potential benefit of digitalis in preventing recurrent atrial fibrillation may result from decreasing atrial premature beats, which can cause the arrhythmia. Whether chronic digitalis therapy is even useful in limiting the ventricular response if atrial fibrillation recurs has also been questioned.

3. **Atrial tachycardia.** Atrial tachycardias may be terminated by drugs that enhance vagal tone at the AV node. For AV nodal reentrant tachycardia, adenosine is probably the drug of choice, although digitalis may have an effect. If the patient has Wolff-Parkinson-White (WPW) syndrome, digitalis is almost always contraindicated since it may increase the ERP of the AV node, shorten the ERP of the accessory pathway, and promote rapid conduction to the ventricle.

4. **Ventricular tachycardia.** Digitalis is more often a cause of VT than a treatment for it. If a patient has ventricular ectopy that was caused by heart failure, treating the failure may decrease the ectopy.

B. **Preparations of digitalis.** Although a variety of digitalis preparations are known (digoxin, digitoxin, ouabain, deslanoside, powdered digitalis, digitalis leaf), the one most frequently used is **digoxin.** Consequently this discussion is limited to its description. Because of the variation in absorption of different preparations, many physicians prefer to use a particular brand (such as Lanoxin) exclusively and not write a generic prescription. However, variation in biologic activity has not been a major problem lately. Absorption from the GI tract is usually about 75% unless an alcoholic elixir preparation (90% absorption) is used. Peak levels are achieved in 2–3 hours, with the greatest effect at 4–6 hours. The half-life of digoxin averages 36 hours.

When instituting therapy with digoxin, the physician must determine how soon it is necessary to achieve steady-state plasma levels. Without loading—that is, starting out with maintenance digoxin (0.25 mg PO daily)—steady state is achieved in 7–10 days. Loading involves administering 1.25 mg over the first 24-hour period. Quite often this loading dose is administered as 0.50 mg IV over a period of 10 minutes, with the remaining 0.75 mg given orally in three divided doses, one every 4–6 hours. This is a conservative recommendation, with specific situations requiring individualized therapy.

Digoxin is only minimally metabolized by the liver (12–15%). It is excreted, almost completely unchanged, by the kidney. Consequently patients in renal failure must receive a reduced maintenance dosage (usually ≦0.125 mg daily or every other day rather than 0.25 mg daily, but again this dosage depends on the individual case). The therapeutic plasma concentration is 0.5–2.0 ng/ml.

Although digitoxin is metabolized by the liver, knowledge of the pharmacokinetics of digoxin permits the latter to be used even in renal failure, at lower dosage. Most physicians prefer to use one preparation in all situations because of the ease of use.

It is important to recognize the interactions with other drugs. **Quinidine** may displace digoxin from its binding sites and increase the digoxin level. Quinidine may also reduce the renal and total body clearance of digoxin. The dosage of digoxin may require reduction, often by 50%. Other antiarrhythmic drugs that increase the digoxin level are verapamil, propafenone, and amiodarone.

C. **Digitalis toxicity.** Digitalis is effective and versatile but may result in **serious and potentially fatal adverse reactions.** Patients may complain of anorexia, nausea, or vomiting as GI manifestations of toxicity. Visual disturbances may be described as blurred vision or yellow-green (chromatopsia) tinting or haloes. Rarely, gynecomastia may be seen.

The most life-threatening adverse reactions are rhythm disturbances. Often an increase in ventricular ectopy may be one of the first manifestations. Ventricular tachycardia (particularly bidirectional) and VF may occur. Commonly, patients develop high-degree AV block or accelerated junctional rhythms. If a patient with chronic atrial fibrillation treated with digoxin suddenly develops a regular rhythm, one should suspect digitalis toxicity and a junctional rhythm. Atrial tachycardia with block is another rhythm frequently seen in digitalis toxicity. Sinus bradycardia or sinoatrial block may occur (see Chap. 8, **VII.I.1**).

Electrolyte disturbances, particularly hypokalemia, may exacerbate digitalis toxicity. Hypercalcemia may also contribute to toxicity. The combination of digitalis toxicity, hypokalemia, and quinidine (especially with a prolonged Q–T) can result in a catastrophic outcome. Hypomagnesemia, hypoxia, acid-base imbalance, and other drug toxicity may also be contributory. In the presence of hyperkalemia, high-degree AV block and cardiac arrest are possibilities. Electrolyte disturbances may be particularly prevalent in renal failure. Patients taking antimicrobials that eliminate bowel flora may have increased absorption of digoxin, which may further contribute to untoward effects. Finally, the effect of thyroid function must be mentioned. Both the toxic and therapeutic effects of digitalis preparations are inversely related to thyroxine levels. Hyperthyroid patients may be less responsive to usual doses, and hypothyroid patients may be susceptible to toxicity even with low doses.

D. **Management of digitalis toxicity.** The treatment of digitalis toxicity begins with recognition. Then digitalis is discontinued, cardiac monitoring ensues, and treatment of specific arrhythmias takes place. Ventricular ectopy that is asymptomatic may be observed. Ventricular tachycardia should be treated with lidocaine or phenytoin. The serum potassium should be corrected to the range of 4.0–4.5 mEq/liter. Symptomatic bradyarrhythmias may require atropine or temporary pacing. Patients who have ingested massive doses of digitalis and do not respond to conventional therapy are candidates for therapy with digoxin-specific antibody (Fab) fragments.

E. **Digitalis after myocardial infarction.** A controversial subject is the use of digitalis after MI. A number of studies suggest that the use of digitalis increases posthospital mortality in patients with left ventricular dysfunction and arrhythmias. Others seem to indicate that it was not the use of digitalis but rather the more extensive underlying heart disease that was the major determinant of mortality. This subject is still not totally resolved, which underscores the necessity of reviewing the indication for each drug administered, particularly in high-risk individuals. If there is a definite need for digitalis—in a patient with heart failure, to control the ventricular response in atrial fibrillation, or to prevent recurrent supraventricular tachycardia—then it should not be withheld.

F. **Digoxin**

Pharmacology: Digitalis glycoside.

New classification: High-potency blocker of Na/K ATPase. Stimulator of muscarinic subtype 2 receptors.

Preparations: Digoxin (Lanoxin) 0.125-mg (125 µg), 0.250-mg (250 µg), and 0.500-mg (500 µg) tablets; 0.05 mg/ml (50 µg/ml) pediatric elixir; 0.50 mg/2 ml (500 µg/2 ml), 0.100 mg/ml (100 µg/ml) injection; digoxin solution in 0.05-mg (50 µg), 0.10-mg (100 µg), 0.20-mg (200 µg) capsules (Lanoxicaps); digoxin (generic).

Approved indications: Atrial fibrillation, atrial flutter, paroxysmal atrial tachycardia, heart failure.

Metabolism: Excreted unchanged in urine.

Half-life: 36 hours.

Therapeutic levels: 0.5–2.0 ng/ml.

Adverse reactions: See text.

Comments: See text. Reduce dose in renal failure.

G. **Digitoxin**

Pharmacology: Digitalis glycoside.

Preparations: Digitoxin (Crystodigin) 0.05-mg, 0.1-mg, 0.15-mg, 0.2-mg tablets.

Approved indications: Atrial fibrillation, atrial flutter, supraventricular tachycardia, heart failure.

Metabolism: Hepatic.

Active metabolite: Digoxin (small fraction).

Half-life: 7–9 days.

Therapeutic levels: 10–35 ng/ml.

Comments: See text. Oral maintenance dosage is 0.1–0.15 mg daily.

III. **Beta blockers.** The application of beta blockers in the treatment of arrhythmias must be discussed in terms of the pharmacologic effects on supraventricular arrhythmias, suppression of ventricular premature beats (VPBs) and VT, elevation of the VF threshold, and prevention of sudden cardiac death.

A. **Pharmacologic properties of beta blockers.** Stimulation of the beta receptors increases the L-type calcium current, shifts pacemaker current to more positive potentials, and enhances the delayed rectifier currents (I K). Beta blockers antagonize these effects, resulting in decreased AV nodal conduction, suppressing ectopic pacemakers and some calcium-mediated triggered arrhythmias.

It may be useful to review the pharmacologic properties of beta blockers as they relate to arrhythmias (Table 14-3). **Cardioselectivity** is a property of several agents that have a selective effect on cardiac beta-1 receptors with relative sparing of the beta-2 receptors in the bronchial tree and vascular system, if used in low doses. Cardioselectivity is lost at high doses. The potential advantage is increased safety in patients who may have a bronchospastic component to their lung disease and theoretical benefit in patients with impairment of the peripheral circulation. Recently the issue of an increased risk of transient hypokalemia with cardioselective beta blockers has been raised. Catecholamines facilitate inward movement of potassium from the extracellular environment into the cell. The critical site for initiating transmembrane potassium migration is a beta-2 receptor site. Thus, a beta-1 selective blocker theoretically may not be as effective as a nonselective blocker in preventing transient hypokalemia. However, cardioselectivity is lost at the higher doses often necessary in the treatment of angina, hypertension, or arrhythmias. In addition, the transient hypokalemia associated with catecholamine release may be important only in the presence of clinical hypokalemia (e.g., that caused by diuretic therapy). An increased risk of malignant ventricular tachyarrhythmias with cardioselective beta blockers has never been demonstrated.

Membrane-stabilizing activity is the ability of certain agents to have a local anesthetic (quinidinelike) effect on the cardiac action potential. This activity usually occurs at high concentration of the drug. Despite the implication that this might have an effect on abnormal heart rhythms, there is no evidence that membrane-stabilizing activity is related to any important antiarrhythmic effect.

Intrinsic sympathomimetic activity (ISA) is the ability of some drugs to demonstrate partial agonist activity. These drugs still block the exercise-induced increases in heart rate and BP but provide less baseline depression of heart rate and contractility. These properties make them useful in patients with bradyarrhythmias or left ventricular dysfunction who require beta blockade. One theoretical disadvantage of beta blockers with ISA is that the elevation of the VF threshold may be less than with beta blockers without ISA.

Other pharmacologic properties such as **half-life** and **lipid solubility** determine ease of administration and tolerance. If there is a question whether the patient can tolerate beta blockade, a short-acting drug may be administered initially. If it is tolerated, a longer-acting preparation can be recommended. Beta blockers penetrate across the blood-brain barrier as a function of their lipid solubility (the more lipid soluble, the greater the CNS effect). Occasionally these effects may be manifest as fatigue, depression, nightmares, or hallucination. Switching to a hydrophilic (low-lipid-solubility) beta blocker may avoid these adverse reactions.

According to the new classification, propranolol is a low-potency blocker of the sodium channel with fast kinetics and a highly potent beta blocker. Nadolol also has highly potent beta receptor blocking activity but does not affect the sodium channel. Sotalol has highly potent beta receptor blocking activity and is a strong blocker of the potassium channel.

B. **Treatment of arrhythmias.** The major mechanism by which this class of drugs exerts antiarrhythmic activity is through beta blockade, particularly by blocking the action of circulating catecholamines. In addition, beta blockers slow the rate of discharge of pacemaker cells in the sinus node (as well as ectopic pacemakers). The functional refractory period of the AV node is increased. Beta blockers with ISA will have less of an effect in this regard.

1. **Supraventricular ectopy and tachycardia.** Atrial premature beats may respond minimally to beta blockers. Some physicians believe that supraventricular ectopy exacerbated by digitalis toxicity is more likely to respond than random ectopy. In both atrial flutter and atrial fibrillation, beta blockade will slow the ventricular response, occasionally facilitating diagnosis. Rare cases of atrial flutter may respond to beta blockade, but the drug of choice for this arrhythmia is digitalis. Some cases of paroxysmal supraventricular tachycardia (PSVT) (caused by AV nodal or AV reentry) respond to beta blockade (by creating block in the antegrade slow pathway), but the drug of choice for this arrhythmia is adenosine (unless the patient has WPW with antidromic conduction). If beta blockade

does not terminate the arrhythmia, it may assist in diagnosis by slowing the ventricular response. Beta blockers may be useful in preventing recurrent episodes of PSVT.

2. **Ventricular ectopy and tachyarrhythmias.** Beta blockers may have a variable effect on VPBs. These agents may suppress them partially or completely, or have no effect whatsoever. If the VPBs are ischemic, there is a better chance they will respond. Similarly, VPBs exacerbated by catecholamine excess may benefit from beta blockade. The negative inotropic effect of beta blockers may be partially responsible for VPB suppression in patients with mitral valve prolapse or hypertrophic cardiomyopathy. As a single agent for sustained VT, beta blockers usually are ineffective. Recently, combination of a beta blocker and a type 1 antiarrhythmic drug has been shown to improve the efficacy of VT suppression when either drug alone was unsuccessful. Beta blockers' ability to raise the VF threshold may partially explain the reduction in sudden cardiac death found in a number of studies.

C. **The beta blocker trials.** A number of studies have assessed the effect of beta blockers in the acute and convalescent phases of MI. The majority have demonstrated both short-term and long-term benefit. Patients receiving beta blockers have a reduced incidence of sudden cardiac death. The major explanations have included reducing ischemia, injury, and recurrent infarction; decreasing the incidence of arrhythmias—a direct antiarrhythmic effect; and increasing the VF threshold. The beta blockers studied in the convalescent phase are practolol, alprenolol, timolol, propranolol, and sotalol. In the acute phase, metoprolol, alprenolol, timolol, propranolol, and atenolol have been given IV. In addition to benefits in terms of mortality and chest pain, metoprolol seemed to decrease the incidence of supraventricular arrhythmias and VF.

D. **Choice of beta blocker.** Table 14-3 describes the beta blockers by their pharmacologic properties. Oxprenolol is not available in the United States. Practolol and alprenolol have been excluded because of potentially toxic adverse reactions. The FDA-approved indications are listed, although it is common knowledge that current clinical practice does not limit the use of the drug to these restrictions. In other words, a physician may use a drug for an indication not approved by the FDA since the drug seems to have clinical efficacy. This is a decision based on clinical judgment.

The clinical situation often determines the beta blocker chosen. A physician seeking to reproduce the results of the published clinical trials would have to prescribe the drug in the same dosage as in the study. For the acute phase of MI, metoprolol and atenolol are available in IV form. Intravenous propranolol, although also available, was not beneficial in acute MI. However, this study was limited by the administration late after the onset of the infarction. Esmolol, an ultra-short-acting beta blocker, is approved by the FDA for use in supraventricular tachycardia.

Currently, propranolol and acebutolol are also approved for arrhythmias. Propranolol is approved for supraventricular tachycardias, ventricular tachyarrhythmias caused by digitalis toxicity, and resistant tachyarrhythmia caused by catecholamine action during anesthesia. Sotalol is approved for ventricular arrhythmias and, as a result of the ESVEM trial, is one of the first antiarrhythmic drugs considered for the treatment of life-threatening VT/VF. Consult Chaps. 6 through 9 for further recommendations. Acebutolol is approved for ventricular arrhythmias.

E. **Metabolism.** The lipid-soluble drugs are absorbed almost completely from the small intestine and metabolized by the liver. The water-soluble drugs are excreted unchanged by the kidney since absorption through the GI tract is limited. In renal failure, reduced doses of drugs excreted by the kidney may be necessary. Similarly, some patients with severe hepatic dysfunction may require lower doses of the lipid-soluble beta blockers.

F. **Adverse effects.** This class of drug is generally well tolerated and perhaps one of the safest in terms of all antiarrhythmic agents. Adverse effects vary by beta blocker, depending on the individual pharmacologic properties. In general, adverse effects are related to the negative inotropic effect, negative chronotropic effect, and lipid solubility. Patients may develop congestive heart failure if there is serious left ventricular dysfunction and a limited cardiovascular reserve. Slowing of the heart rate is dose related and easily reversible on withdrawal. If the patient has underlying conduction system disease, it may be exacerbated by the beta blocker. Adverse cardiovascular effects may necessitate temporary support with vasopressors, atropine, or pacemakers.

Table 14-3. Beta blockers

Drug	Membrane-stabilizing activity	Intrinsic sympatho-mimetic activity	Lipid solubility	Elimination half-life	Preparations available in United States	Initial dose	Angina	Hypertension	Arrhythmia	MI	Migraine	Hypertrophic cardiomyopathy	Pheochromocytoma	Essential tremor
Cardioselective														
Acebutolol hydrochloride	+	+	Low	3–4 hr	Sectral 200-, 400-mg caps	200 mg bid or 400 mg qd		X	X					
Atenolol	0	0	Low	6–9 hr	Tenormin 50-, 100-mg tabs	50 mg qd		X						
Betaxolol	+	0	Low	14–22 hr	Kerlone 10-, 20-mg tabs	10 mg od		X						
Bisoprolol	0	0	Low	9–12 hr	Zebeta 5-, 10-mg tabs	5 mg od		X						
Esmolol	0	0	Low	10 min	Brevibloc 250 mg/ml in 10-ml ampules	Loading 500 µg/kg/min IV and then 50 µg/kg/min × 4 min			X					
Metoprolol tartrate	0	0	Intermediate	3–4 hr	Lopressor 50-, 100-mg tabs; 5-mg/5-ml vials for IV use; Toprol XL 50-, 100-, 200-mg tabs	50 mg bid; 15 mg IV*		X		X				

FDA-approved Indications

Noncardioselective

Drug					Preparations	Dose							
Carteolol	0	+	Low	6 hr	Cartol 2.5-, 5-mg tabs	2.5 mg od		X					
Labetalol hydrochloride	0	?	Intermediate	5–8 hr	Normodyne 200-, 300-mg tabs; 100-mg/20-ml vials for IV use; Trandate 200-, 300-mg tabs	100 mg bid; IV: 0.25/kg* (usually 20 mg)		X					
Nadolol	0	0	Low	14–24 hr	Corgard 40-, 80-, 120-, 160-mg tabs	40 mg qd	X	X					
Penbutolol	0	+	High	5 hr	Levatol 20-mg tabs	20 mg od		X					
Pindolol	+	2+3+	Intermediate	3–4 hr	Visken 5-, 10-mg tabs	5 mg bid		X					
Propranolol hydrochloride	2+	0	High	3–4 hr	Inderal 10-, 20-, 40-, 60-, 80-, 90-mg tabs; Inderal LA 80-, 120-, 160-mg caps; generic	Varies with each indication; usually 10–40 mg q6h	X	X	X		X	X	X
Sotalol hydrochloride	0	0	Low	8–12 hr		80 mg q12h				X			
Timolol maleate	0	0	Low	4–5 hr	Blocadren 5-, 10-mg tabs	10 mg bid		X	X			X	

FDA = Food and Drug Administration; MI = myocardial infarction.
*See precautions in *Physicians' Desk Reference* or package insert before IV administration.

Perhaps the most common and troublesome adverse reactions of beta blockers are related to the drug's crossing the blood-brain barrier. Patients complain of fatigue, depression, insomnia, and occasionally nightmares or hallucinations. The hydrophilic beta blockers (nadolol, atenolol) may be associated with a lower incidence of this problem. Beta blockers may cause a loss of sexual potency, a major reason patients may discontinue the drug.

Bronchospasm and a history of asthma are contraindications to beta blockers. Beta-1 selective blockers may be useful in a small minority of patients with asthma, but beta-1 selectivity is lost in doses usually required. It is important to distinguish patients with bronchospasm from those with chronic lung disease without bronchospasm.

Some physicians consider diabetes mellitus and peripheral vascular disease relative contraindications to beta blockers. If a diabetic patient taking insulin becomes hypoglycemic, the warning signs of sympathetic discharge may not be noticed. A decision to prescribe a beta blocker for a diabetic patient is dependent on the need for the drug. If it is the only drug that can prevent life-threatening arrhythmias or myocardial ischemia, the risk may be acceptable. The same sort of rationale may be used in patients with peripheral vascular disease, although this may be less of a problem. Unopposed alpha vasoconstriction with blockade of beta vasodilative ability, along with a decreased cardiac output, however, may be extremely detrimental in patients with very severe vascular compromise.

Most adverse effects are reversible on drug withdrawal. Abrupt withdrawal, however, may result in an exacerbation of underlying ischemic heart disease.

G. d,l Sotalol

Pharmacology: Beta blocker with type 3 activity.

New classification: Highly potent beta receptor blocker and strong blocker of the potassium channel (delayed rectifier I K).

Preparations: Sotalol (Betapace) 80-mg, 160-mg, 320-mg tablets.

Approved indication: Life-threatening ventricular arrhythmias.

Potential indications: Atrial arrhythmias including PSVT and prevention of paroxysmal atrial fibrillation.

Metabolism: Excretion by the kidney in unchanged form.

Active metabolites: None.

Half-life: 12 hours.

Therapeutic level: Not determined.

Common adverse reactions: Beta blocker effects.

Potentially life-threatening reactions: Proarrhythmia, including torsades de pointes, heart failure, and conduction disturbances.

Comments: Start with a low dosage, and allow several days before further increases, to allow for achievement of steady state. Due to the potential for proarrhythmia, this drug should be avoided in patients with a prolonged Q–T. It should be started in the hospital on a monitored unit. The l-isomer accounts for most of the beta-blocking activity. Both isomers have type 3 activity, but these are seen only at dosages above 160 mg. It is not cardioselective and does not have either intrinsic sympathomimetic or membrane stabilizing activity.

IV. Calcium antagonists. Calcium antagonists, a unique class of drugs, interfere with the transmembrane flux of calcium during the plateau phase of the cardiac action potential. Slow inward currents carried by both calcium and sodium use the same membrane slow channel, which is different from the fast sodium channel, mediated by another gating mechanism. The calcium antagonists block the L-type calcium channel in a **use-dependent** and **voltage-dependent** way. The references list several comprehensive reviews of the action of these drugs to uncouple excitation-contraction at the cellular level. The discussion here focuses on their clinical utility in the management of arrhythmias.

The effects of these agents in isolated muscle preparations may differ from the effect in vivo, since the latter is dependent on a complex interaction among hemodynamic variables, including preload, afterload, contractility, heart rate, and coronary blood flow. In turn, these factors may depend on the extent and severity of coronary artery disease and left ventricular dysfunction. Table 14-4 describes the pharmacologic properties in the patient.

In the treatment of arrhythmias, nifedipine, amlodipine, and felodipine have little utility since they have no negative dromotropic or negative chronotropic properties. They may be useful only if the event precipitating the arryhythmia was coronary spasm. In those rare patients with pure vasospastic (Prinzmetal's) angina, myocardial ischemia and injury precede sustained VT. Prevention of vasospasm and ischemia may prevent ventricular tachyarrhythmia.

Verapamil, with its potent negative dromotropic effect, remains an option for paroxysmal supraventricular tachycardia caused by AV nodal reentry. Diltiazem has less potent effects but has been shown to have clinical efficacy in an IV preparation and may be particularly useful for controlling the ventricular response to atrial fibrillation. Verapamil terminates AV nodal reentrant arrhythmias by slowing or blocking the antegrade conduction of the circulating wave front in one of the dual AV nodal pathways. In a patient with an accessory pathway (WPW syndrome), verapamil may be effective if antegrade conduction occurs through the AV node. Prolongation of the effective refractory period of the AV node may allow interruption of the reentry loop. Since the accessory pathway is not calcium channel dependent, verapamil will have little effect if antegrade conduction occurs via the accessory pathway (wide-complex tachycardia). In fact, if the patient has atrial fibrillation, increasing the effective refractory period of the AV node will facilitate conduction down the accessory pathway, sometimes with deleterious hemodynamic consequences.

Rarely, verapamil has been found effective for VT, particularly those in whom the mechanism is related to afterdepolarizations. Some of these tachycardias originate in the right ventricular outflow tract and have a left bundle branch block morphology. In the vast majority of cases, it is ineffective, which is probably related to different mechanisms involved. For VT related to vasospastic angina, verapamil and diltiazem may be useful, like the dihydropyridine calcium blockers. Verapamil slows the ventricular response to atrial flutter and atrial fibrillation. Effective conversion to sinus rhythm occurs only in a few cases, usually when the atrial arrhythmia is of short duration and the left atrium is not enlarged.

Bepridil blocks not only the slow calcium channel but also the fast sodium channel. It impairs AV conduction and slows the sinus rate. In the atrium, the amplitude and upstroke velocity of the atrial action potential are decreased. The atrial effective refractory period is prolonged. Bepridil has been approved for the treatment of angina pectoris, but its potential to prolong the Q–T interval and cause torsades de pointes has limited its utilization. In the new classification, bepridil is considered a highly potent blocker of the calcium channel, a low-potency blocker of the sodium channel with fast kinetics, and a moderate-potency blocker of the potassium channel.

A. Nifedipine, amlodipine, felodipine

Pharmacology: Dihydropyridine calcium antagonists.

Preparations: Nifedipine (Procardia) 10- and 20-mg capsules; Procardia XL 30-, 60-, and 90-mg tablets; Adalat 10-mg capsules; amlodipine (Norvasc) 2.5-, 5.0-, and 10.0-mg tablets; felodipine (Plendil) 5-, 10-mg tablets.

Potential indications: Arrhythmias triggered by vasospastic angina.

Metabolism: Rapidly absorbed, converted to inactive metabolites and eliminated by the kidneys (nifedipine 80%, amlodipine 60%, felodipine 70%).

Half-life: Nifedipine, 2–5 hours; amlodipine, 30–50 hours; felodipine, 11–16 hours.

Table 14-4. Clinical pharmacology of the calcium antagonists in patients

Drug	Negative dromotropic activity[a,b]	Vasodilatation[b]	Negative inotropic activity[b,c]
Dihydropyridines Amlodipine Felodipine Isradipine Nicardipine Nifedipine	0	4+	0
Verapamil	4+	3+	4+
Diltiazem	2+	2+	2+
Bepridil[d]	1+	2+	2+

[a]Slows conduction.
[b]Strength of effect on a scale of 0–4.
[c]Depresses contractility.
[d]Also blocks sodium current.

Common adverse reactions: Flushing, headache, dizziness, nausea, peripheral edema (related to vasodilatory effect and fluid retention).

Potentially life-threatening reactions: Hypotension.

Comments: These drugs are primarily useful as therapy for the underlying problem rather than as a specific antiarrhythmic agent. Because of their vasodilatory properties, some may cause a sinus tachycardia. Therapy is individualized with each agent.

B. Verapamil

Pharmacology: Calcium antagonist.

New classification: Highly potent blocker of the calcium channel, low-potency blocker of the sodium channel with fast kinetics, and moderate alpha-receptor blocking activity.

Preparations: Verapamil hydrochloride (Isoptin): 80-, 120-mg tablets; 5 mg/2 ml, 10 mg/4 ml for IV use; (Calan) 80-mg, 120-mg tablets; (Verelan) 120-, 180-, 240-mg capsules.

Approved indications: IV: paroxysmal supraventricular tachycardias, control of ventricular response in atrial fibrillation or atrial flutter unassociated with accessory pathway syndromes.

Potential indications: Chronic suppression of above arrhythmias with oral preparations.

Metabolism: Hepatic with metabolites excreted in urine (70%) and in feces (16%) 12 N- and O-dealkylated metabolites.

Active metabolite: Norverapamil.

Half-life: IV 4 minutes, oral 4.5–12.0 hours.

Therapeutic level: 0.10–0.15 µg/ml.

Common adverse reactions: Usually minimal. Some patients will have hypotensive symptoms, headache, and constipation.

Potentially life-threatening reactions

1. Cardiovascular: bradycardia, high-degree AV block, asystole, hypotension, congestive heart failure.
2. In patients with Duchenne's muscular dystrophy, verapamil may cause respiratory failure.
3. The interaction between verapamil and disopyramide is poorly defined; concomitant administration should be avoided.
4. In patients with hypertrophic cardiomyopathy, verapamil should be avoided if there is severe obstruction to outflow and an elevated pulmonary capillary wedge pressure or a history of nocturnal dyspnea. The combination of quinidine and verapamil should be avoided in these patients.

Comments: Verapamil is a generally well-tolerated drug. The major potentially serious reactions relate to its negative inotropic and negative dromotropic effects. Patients with serious left ventricular dysfunction and a limited cardiovascular reserve may develop overt heart failure, necessitating withdrawal of the drug and temporary supportive treatment.

Because of the possibility of symptomatic bradycardia, high-degree AV block, or asystole, verapamil should be given via the IV route only in a setting where these consequences can be rapidly dealt with. Atropine, levarterenol, and cardiac pacing may occasionally be necessary. These severe cardiovascular effects are less common when verapamil is given orally.

Caution must be exercised when administering verapamil in combination with a beta blocker because of the combined effects on heart rate and contractility. Verapamil also raises the digoxin level by 50–70%, and this factor must be carefully monitored.

Oral therapy is usually initiated with 80 mg orally q8h. The usual daily dosage is 320–480 mg in divided doses. For IV use, the dose is 5–10 mg (0.075–0.150 mg/kg body weight) over a period of at least 2 minutes. An additional 10 mg may be given 30 minutes later, if necessary.

C. Diltiazem

Pharmacology: Calcium antagonist.

New classification: Moderate-potency blocker of the calcium channel.

Preparations: Diltiazem hydrochloride (Cardizem) 30-, 60-mg tablets. Cardizem CD: 120-, 180-, 240-, and 300-mg capsules. Cardizem SR: 60-, 90-, 120-mg sustained-release capsules. Cardizem injectable: 25 mg/5 ml and 50 mg/10 ml.

Indications: IV diltiazem is indicated for paroxysmal supraventricular tachycardias and temporary control of the ventricular response in atrial fibrillation or flutter. Cardizem has an indication for angina due to coronary artery spasm or chronic-stable angina. Cardizem SR has an indication for hypertension. Cardizem CD has an indication for both hypertension and angina.

Metabolism: Hepatic with excretion by the kidney and in bile.

Active metabolite: Desacetyl diltiazem.

Half-life: 3.5 hours.

Therapeutic level: 50–200 ng/ml.

Common adverse reactions: Minimal.

Potentially life-threatening reactions: Cardiovascular: bradycardia, high-degree AV block, hypotension.

Comments: Since diltiazem has less potent pharmacologic effects than the other calcium antagonists, the related adverse reactions are similarly less severe. Nevertheless, rare patients may be exquisitely sensitive to even small dosages, which may cause bradycardia or heart block and necessitate withdrawal.

Therapy is usually initiated with 30 mg q6h and titrated upward as necessary and as tolerated. The usual daily dosage is 180–240 mg in divided doses. The initial dose of diltiazem is 0.25 mg/kg as a bolus over 2 minutes. If the response is inadequate, a second bolus 0.35 mg/kg over 2 minutes may be given 15 minutes after the first dose. The initial IV maintenance dose is 10 mg/hour.

V. **Type 1A antiarrhythmic drugs.** The type 1A drugs are quinidine, procainamide, and disopyramide (and imipramine; see **VIII**). Electrophysiologically, they block the sodium channel and slow the upstroke velocity of the action potential, slowing conduction velocity. After binding to the sodium channel, the drugs dissociate at different rates specific to each agent (fast for type 1B, intermediate for type 1A, slowly for type 1C). When the rate of stimulation increases, sodium channel blockade may become incremental (use dependence). These drugs also block the delayed rectifier channel (I K). The APD increases, as does the refractory period. The ERP/APD ratio increases. A slight decrease in spontaneous automaticity is noted.

Quinidine, procainamide, and disopyramide have been available for many years and have demonstrated efficacy for both ventricular and supraventricular arrhythmias, but only quinidine has an FDA indication for supraventricular arrhythmias. In addition, the effects of these drugs on the ERP of accessory pathways make them effective in the WPW syndrome.

If specific arrhythmias need treatment, quinidine and procainamide are among the choices but may not be the agents of first choice. Procainamide can be administered IV, although this mode is usually reserved for emergencies or for drug infusions in the electrophysiology laboratory. The main concern is hypotension. Both quinidine and procainamide (and disopyramide) are available in a variety of preparations, some in slow-release forms that minimize the frequency of dosing. Both quinidine and procainamide may cause mild myocardial depression but usually do not precipitate heart failure. Disopyramide has a number of adverse reactions that make it unsuitable for the patient most frequently treated for arrhythmias: the middle-aged or older male with left ventricular dysfunction. Its negative inotropic activity may cause heart failure, and its anticholinergic effects may cause xerostomia, constipation, and urinary retention. The drug is best tolerated by the younger individual with a normal left ventricle and without prostate enlargement. In patients with hypertropic cardiomyopathy, however, the negative inotropy may be used to advantage.

All three drugs have been implicated in proarrhythmias, especially torsades de pointes, the particularly malignant form of VT in patients with Q–T prolongation. **Never** administer this group of drugs to a patient with a congenital prolonged Q–T syndrome. **Always** measure the Q–T interval before starting the drug. If the Q–T is normal at baseline but becomes more than 50% prolonged, reduce the dosage or discontinue the drug.

With quinidine, monitor the patient for the development of an idiosyncratic or immunologic reaction such as fever, thrombocytopenia, or hemolytic anemia. Since the most common adverse reaction is gastrointestinal, it may be wise to avoid quinidine in a patient with diarrhea, abdominal cramps, or ulcer disease. With procainamide, it is wise to obtain an antinuclear antibody (ANA) assay before starting the drug, since patients are at risk of developing a procainamide-induced lupuslike syndrome. A considerable number will later have a positive ANA result, but not all will develop the syndrome. It seems that patients who rapidly metabolize (acetylate) the drug have a low incidence of the syndrome, which is prevalent in slow acetylators. The metabolite NAPA has antiarrhythmic activity but is much less potent than the parent drug. It is also important to note the interactions with other drugs.

If these drugs do not completely suppress a VT, often a slowing of the rate may be observed. In other cases, no effect may be seen. Some individuals with distal conduction system disease may develop heart block. Quinidine in particular has vagolytic activity. Therefore, in patients with atrial fibrillation, digoxin is a necessary addition in order to control the ventricular response. Since these drugs may slow the rate of atrial flutter, conduction down the AV node may be facilitated—another reason for the prior administration of digoxin.

A. Quinidine

Pharmacology: Type 1A antiarrhythmic drug.

New classification: High-potency blocker of the activated state of the sodium channel with intermediate kinetics, moderately potent blocker of the potassium channel, low-potency blocker of the alpha and muscarinic subtype 2 receptors.

Preparations
1. Quinidine gluconate: (Quinaglute) 324 mg (202 mg quinidine base).
   Quinidine gluconate: (Duraquin) (206 mg quinidine base) (equivalent to 248 mg quinidine sulfate).
   Quinidine gluconate: (generic).
2. Quinidine sulfate: (Quinidex) 300 mg.
   Quinidine sulfate: (Quinora) 200 mg, 300 mg.
   Quinidine sulfate: (generic).
3. Quinidine polygalacturonate (Cardioquin) 275 mg (equivalent in quinidine content to 200 mg quinidine sulfate).

Approved indications
Ventricular arrhythmias: Life-threatening ventricular arrhythmias, including VT.
Junctional arrhythmias: Junctional ectopy and paroxsymal junctional tachycardia.
Supraventricular arrhythmias: Atrial ectopy, paroxysmal atrial tachycardia, atrial fibrillation, atrial flutter.
Metabolism: Hepatic (60–80%), renal excretion of unchanged drug (20–40%).
Active metabolite: 2-hydroxyquinidine.
Half-life: 4–10 hours in healthy individuals, prolonged in the elderly.
Therapeutic level: 2–5 µg/ml. Levels of 2–3 µg/ml usually are considered too low to be therapeutic.

Common adverse reactions
Gastrointestinal: Nausea, vomiting, abdominal pain, diarrhea.
Cinchonism: Tinnitus, headache, nausea, disturbed vision.

Rare but potentially life-threatening reactions
Cardiovascular: Widening of the QRS, cardiac asystole, ventricular ectopy, VT, VF, arterial embolism, hypotension.
Hematologic: Acute hemolytic anemia, thrombocytopenia, agranulocytosis, hypoprothrombinemia.
Hypersensitivity: Angioedema, acute asthma, vascular collapse, respiratory arrest, hepatotoxicity including granulomatous hepatitis.

Comments: Some physicians consider the gluconate preparation to cause less GI toxicity than the sulfate. Both are available in preparations that can be administered q8–12h, making dosage more convenient. When converting from the sulfate to the gluconate, determine the total amount of quinidine alkaloid the patient is taking (62% quinidine in the gluconate, 82% quinidine in the sulfate) to ensure an equivalent dosage.

Dosage is usually initiated with 324 mg PO q8h for quinidine gluconate or 200–300 mg PO q6h for quinidine sulfate. To administer an oral loading dose, 600–1000 mg quinidine may be given. Usual maintenance dosages are 300–600 mg PO q8h–q6h.

B. Procainamide

Pharmacology: Type 1A antiarrhythmic drug.

New classification: High-potency blocker of the activated state of the sodium channel with intermediate kinetics and moderate-potency blocker of the potassium channel.

Preparations
Procainamide hydrochloride (Procan SR) 250-mg, 500-mg, 750-mg, 1000-mg tablets. (Pronestyl) 250-mg, 375-mg, 500-mg capsules; 250-mg, 375-mg, 500-mg tablets. (Pronestyl) injection 1000 mg/10 ml, 1000 mg/2 ml. (Generic)

Approved indications: Life-threatening ventricular arrhythmias, including VT.
Potential indications: Atrial arrhythmias.
Metabolism: Hepatic, excreted in urine by active tubular secretion and glomerular filtration.
Active metabolite: *N*-acetylprocainamide (NAPA).
Half-life: Depends on preparation (usually 2–5 hours for procainamide), prolonged in renal failure.
Therapeutic levels: Procainamide 4–8 µg/ml, NAPA 10–20 µg/ml.

Common adverse reactions
Gastrointestinal: Nausea, vomiting, anorexia, bitter taste, diarrhea.
Cardiovascular: Hypotension after IV administration.
Multisystem: Lupuslike syndrome (incidence from 1 in 500 to 30% receiving chronic therapy—most often in slow acetylators).

Rare but potentially life-threatening reactions
Cardiovascular: Asystole, ventricular fibrillation after IV administration.
Hematologic: neutropenia, thrombocytopenia, hemolytic anemia, agranulocytosis.

Comments: Procainamide is most often initiated with a slow-release preparation at a dosage of 500 mg PO q6h. If oral loading is desired, up to 1000 mg may be given. Maintenance dosages are 500–1000 mg q6h. Rarely, very high doses (6–12 g) of procainamide have been used to treat refractory VT. The IV administration is 100 mg IV q5min until 1000 mg is given. If there is continued need for IV procainamide, a 1- to 4-mg/minute infusion is used. In the electrophysiology laboratory, 1000 mg is usually administered intravenously over a period of 20 minutes with careful attention to heart rate, blood pressure, and Q–T interval.

C. **Disopyramide phosphate**

Pharmacology: Type 1A antiarrhythmic drug.
New classification: High-potency blocker of the activated state of the sodium channel with intermediate kinetics, moderate-potency blocker of the potassium channel, and moderate blocker of muscarinic subtype 2 receptors.
Preparations: Disopyramide phosphate (Norpace) 100-mg, 150-mg capsules; (Norpace CR) 100-mg, 150-mg capsules.
Approved indications: Life-threatening ventricular arrhythmias.
Potential indications: Atrial arrhythmias.
Metabolism: Hepatic, 50% excreted unchanged in the urine.
Active metabolite: *N*-monodealkylated disopyramide.
Half-life: 4–10 (mean 6.7) hours in healthy individuals, 8–18 hours in renal dysfunction.
Therapeutic level: 2–4 µg/ml.

Common adverse reactions
Anticholinergic: Xerostomia, urinary retention.
Cardiovascular: Hypotension, congestive heart failure, QRS and Q–T prolongation.

Potentially life-threatening reactions: Torsades de pointes, hypoglycemia, heart block.

Comments: The common adverse reactions to disopyramide phosphate limit its utilization. Younger individuals without heart failure, patients without prostate problems, and those with hypertrophic cardiomyopathy are the best candidates. The starting dosage is 100–150 mg PO q6h. If oral loading is desired, 300–400 mg may be given. Maintenance dosages usually do not exceed 300 mg PO q6h. The slow-release equivalent dosage for 150 mg PO q6h Norpace is 300 mg PO q12h Norpace CR. Intravenous disopyramide is not available.
   One must be cautious about the use of disopyramide with any other drug that also depresses cardiac contractility. Severe anticholinergic toxicity may be treated with neostigmine if absolutely necessary.

VI. **Type 1B antiarrhythmic drugs.** The type 1B drugs are lidocaine, mexiletine, and tocainide. The affinity of these drugs for the inactive state is high. They dissociate rapidly from sodium channels after depolarization. Thus, sodium current blockade occurs only during rapid rates (as may occur in ischemia). Electrophysiologically, they cause only minimal change in the upstroke velocity of the action potential and decrease its duration. The ratio of the effective refractory period to the APD increases. Spontaneous automaticity decreases. Lidocaine may have more of an effect on abnormal than normal cells. Since lidocaine may enhance AV nodal conduction, caution must be exercised when administering it to patients with atrial tachyarrhythmias and an uncontrolled ventricular response.

Lidocaine is the drug of first choice for emergency treatment of ventricular ectopy and VT. Because of its extensive first-pass hepatic metabolism, it is not useful except in IV form. In general, the efficacy of type 1B drugs for supraventricular tachyarrhythmias is too poor to make them even a consideration.

The search for an oral lidocaine-like drug resulted in the development of tocainide and mexiletine. Although there may be electrophysiologic similarities, tocainide and mexiletine are dissimilar. Thus, failure to respond to one does not imply lack of success with the other.

The major concern with lidocaine is CNS activity. This side effect is dose related and is seen with tocainide and mexiletine as well. Both tocainide and mexiletine may have proarrhythmic effects, sometimes with a faster VT than at baseline (owing to the effects on conduction). However, these drugs may be less arrhythmogenic than other options. Thus, both tocainide and mexiletine may be considered for ventricular arrhythmias, particularly applicable if the patient has a prolonged Q–T interval. Due to the concern about agranulocytosis with tocainide, it is rarely used today.

Combination therapy of a 1B drug with a 1A drug has appeal in reducing the potential toxicity from prolonged repolarization, as well as increasing efficacy. Mexiletine and quinidine have been used together. Combination therapy may be worth examining in individual patients before considering drug therapy with far more toxic drugs such as amiodarone.

Phenytoin does not have a specific FDA-approved antiarrhythmic indication. In the past, before the availability of Fab antibodies for digitalis toxicity, phenytoin was used for digitalis toxic tachyarrhythmias. It is useful only rarely as a single drug for VT not related to digitalis toxicity, although it is occasionally effective in combination with a type 1A agent. If it is necessary to administer phenytoin, the PDR should be consulted for prescribing recommendations.

A. Lidocaine

Pharmacology: Type 1B antiarrhythmic drug.
New classification: Low-potency blocker of the sodium channel with fast kinetics.
Preparations: Lidocaine hydrochloride (Xylocaine and generic) 100-mg/5-ml ampules or prefilled syringes.
Approved indications: Ventricular arrhythmias.
Metabolism: Hepatic; less than 10% excreted unchanged in urine.
Active metabolites: Monoethylglycinexylidide, glycinexylidide.
Plasma half-life: 1.5–2.0 hours.
Therapeutic level: 1.5–5.0 µg/ml.
Common adverse reactions: Central nervous system: lightheadedness; nervousness; apprehension; euphoria; confusion; dizziness; drowsiness; tinnitus; blurred or double vision; vomiting; sensation of heat, cold, or numbness; twitching.

Rare but potentially life-threatening reactions
Cardiovascular: Bradycardia, hypotension, cardiovascular collapse.
Central nervous system: Tremors, convulsions, unconsciousness, respiratory depression and arrest.

Comments: Decisions about prophylactic treatment of patients with acute MI must weigh the benefits and risks of therapy. One must be particularly cautious if the patient is elderly or has congestive heart failure or hepatic dysfunction. Lidocaine dose must be decreased in the presence of cimetidine. Constant ECG monitoring is recommended.

The usual initial bolus is 50–100 mg IV (0.7–1.4 mg/kg) at a rate of 25–50 mg/minute. A second bolus may be administered 5 minutes later if the patient remains in VT, or 15 minutes later if the patient has responded but it is desirable to increase the drug level. An infusion of 1–4 mg/minute (0.014–0.057 mg/kg/minute) is started and titrated to control the arrhythmia but minimize side effects. Studies in which intramuscular injections were used en route to the hospital have usually recommended 300 mg (4.3 mg/kg), preferably in the deltoid muscle for its better absorption.

When discontinuing lidocaine, it is unnecessary to taper the drug. Simply stopping the drug will result in an automatic tapering due to the washout from tissue stores.

B. Mexiletine

Pharmacology: Type 1B antiarrhythmic drug.
New classification: Low-potency blocker of the sodium channel with fast kinetics.
Preparations: Mexiletine hydrochloride (Mexitil) 150-mg, 200-mg, 250-mg tablets.
Approved indications: Ventricular arrhythmias, VT.
Metabolism: Hepatic, 10% excreted unchanged in urine.
Active metabolites: None significant.
Plasma half-life: 10–12 hours; may be prolonged in patients with acute MI.
Therapeutic level: 0.5–2.0 µg/ml.

Common adverse reactions
Gastrointestinal: Nausea, vomiting.
Central nervous system: Dizziness, lightheadedness, tremor, nervousness.

Rare but potentially life-threatening reactions: Isolated case reports of severe hepatic injury.

Comments: Mexiletine is an antiarrhythmic drug without major negative inotropic effect. It shortens repolarization and the Q–T interval. The incidence of proarrhythmic events is relatively low. There are no serious interactions with other drugs. Cimetidine may raise mexiletine levels. Hepatic enzyme inducers may lower them. Mexiletine is as effective as other drugs for suppressing ventricular ectopy and may be effective in a minority of patients with truly refractory VT. Combination therapy with mexiletine and quinidine provides effective therapy in some cases.

There are no data to suggest a relationship between the response to lidocaine and the response to mexiletine. Failure of tocainide therapy does not necessarily imply future failure with mexiletine. The most common side effects of mexiletine are GI, followed by neurologic. Some physicians have noted a higher incidence of CNS reactions. Patients with high-degree AV block may require a pacemaker if mexiletine therapy is needed.

The usual oral dosage is 200–300 mg q8h. If a loading dose is desired, 400 mg may be given. The dose is titrated upward as necessary (by 50- to 100-mg increments), but few patients tolerate a total daily dosage of 1200 mg, which should not be exceeded. The dosage is titrated downward to minimize adverse drug reactions.

C. Tocainide

Pharmacology: Type 1B antiarrhythmic drug.
New classification: Low-potency blocker of the sodium channel with fast kinetics.
Preparations: Tocainide hydrochloride (Tonocard) 400-mg, 600-mg tablets.
Approved indications: Ventricular arrhythmias, VT.
Metabolism: 25% hepatic biotransformation to a glucuronide, 45% excreted unchanged in the urine.
Active metabolites: None.
Plasma half-life: 15 hours.
Therapeutic level: 4–10 µg/ml.

Common adverse reactions
Gastrointestinal: Nausea, vomiting.
Central nervous system (less common): Lightheadedness, dizziness, vertigo, nervousness.

Rare but potentially life-threatening reactions: Isolated reports of agranulocytosis and pulmonary fibrosis.

Comments: Tocainide is an antiarrhythmic drug without major negative inotropic effect. It shortens repolarization and the Q–T interval. The incidence of proarrhythmic events is relatively low. There are no serious interactions with other drugs.

Tocainide is as effective as other drugs for suppressing ventricular ectopy and may be effective in a minority of patients with truly refractory VT. Combination therapy of quinidine and tocainide was once reported as effective in a preliminary report.

Because of its effects on conduction, breakthrough ventricular tachyarrhythmias may be faster than the original arrhythmia.

The most common side effects encountered are GI, followed by neurologic. Taking the dose with food decreases GI toxicity. Uncommonly, some patients have developed a rash, which usually necessitates discontinuation.

The usual starting dosage is 400 mg PO q8h, which may be increased to 600 mg PO q8h. Few patients tolerate higher than a total daily dosage of 1800 mg. If GI or CNS side effects are observed, the dosage is titrated downward to determine if drug efficacy can be maintained while avoiding adverse reactions.

VII. Type 1C antiarrhythmic drugs. The currently available type 1C drugs are flecainide and propafenone. They are activation blockers of the sodium channel with very long recovery time constants (dissociation from the channel). Electrophysiologically, they slow the upstroke velocity of the action potential but cause only a minimal change in the APD. Consequently there is little change in the ratio of the effective refractory period to the APD. There seems to be no effect on spontaneous automaticity.

Flecainide and propafenone have an effect on both ventricular and supraventricular arrhythmias (although only flecainide has an FDA indication for SVT). They are effective in terminating up to 70% of recent-onset atrial fibrillation and may maintain sinus rhythm in up to 40% of patients who fail initial therapy. In addition, these drugs are effective in the treatment of ectopic atrial tachycardias and AV nodal and AV reentrant tachycardias. Although both of these drugs are indicated for the treatment of life-threatening ventricular arrhythmias, their efficacy is probably less than 20% in preventing induction during electrophysiology study.

This group of drugs is characterized by the ability to suppress or eradicate ventricular ectopy. Nevertheless, the ultimate goal of therapy is the prevention of sudden cardiac death. Eradication of ventricular ectopy does not necessarily prevent VF.

The initial trials of flecainide were halted when a serious proarrhythmic effect was observed in patients with refractory VT and heart failure who were receiving high doses of flecainide. The VT or VF that developed was incessant and refractory to all measures and caused death. This outcome is less likely to occur with lower doses and when patients with serious left ventricular dysfunction are excluded. Nevertheless, flecainide acetate must be used with extreme caution because of the potential severity of the proarrhythmic effect. The potential for proarrhythmia was again seen in the Cardiac Arrhythmia Suppression Trial (CAST) study. Encainide, another type 1C drug also used in CAST, was then withdrawn from the market. Thus, flecainide should not be considered a drug of first choice for VTs. Other problems with flecainide include the occasional need for a pacemaker.

A. Flecainide

Pharmacology: Type 1C antiarrhythmic drug.

New classification: High-potency blocker in the activated state of the sodium channel with slow kinetics and low-potency blocker of the potassium channel.

Preparations: Flecainide acetate (Tambocor) 100-mg tablets.

Approved indications: Life-threatening ventricular arrhythmias, including sustained VT. Disabling supraventricular arrhythmias in the **absence** of structural heart disease: AV nodal and AV tachycardia, other supraventricular tachycardias, and paroxysmal atrial fibrillation.

Metabolism: Hepatic; 10–50% excreted unchanged in urine.

Active metabolite: O-dealkylated flecainide (potency 20% of parent drug).

Half-life: 20 hours (range 12–27 hours).

Therapeutic levels: 0.2–1.0 µg/ml. (Cardiovascular toxicity more likely above 0.7–1.0 µg/ml.)

Common adverse effects

Cardiovascular: P–R interval prolongation (25%), first-degree AV block (33%). QRS prolongation, bundle branch block, sinus node dysfunction.

Central nervous system: Dizziness, visual disturbance.

Uncommon but potentially life-threatening reactions

1. Death caused by proarrhythmic events (most common in patients with heart failure, low ejection fraction, or prior MI and with high doses of flecainide acetate).
2. Congestive heart failure caused by the negative inotropic effect of flecainide.
3. High-degree AV block.
4. Increase in endocardial pacing thresholds and suppression of escape rhythms.

Comments: Flecainide should be started at a dosage of 100 mg PO q12h. It should not be increased by more than 50 mg/dose every 4 days. The ECG must be carefully monitored. The maximal dosage should not exceed 200 mg PO q12h. Intravenous flecainide remains investigational, but loading doses of 1–2 mg/kg have been used.

The ideal candidate for flecainide therapy has no left ventricular dysfunction and needs antiarrhythmic therapy.

B. Propafenone

Pharmacology: Type 1C antiarrhythmic drug.

New classification: High-potency blocker of the activated state of the sodium channel with intermediate kinetics and moderate blocker of the beta receptor.

Preparations: Propafenone hydrochloride (Rythmol) 150-mg, 225-mg, 300-mg tablets.

Indications: Life-threatening ventricular arrhythmias, including VT.

Potential indications: Atrial arrhythmias, including prevention of paroxysmal atrial fibrillation and other SVTs. Potential use in arrhythmias associated with WPW syndrome.

Metabolism: Hepatic, excreted via feces (53%) and urine (18.5–38.0%).

Active metabolite: 5-hydroxypropafenone (possibly active).

Half-life: 6–7 hours with chronic administration.

Therapeutic level: 0.5–2.0 µg/ml.

Common adverse reactions

Gastrointestinal: Nausea, vomiting, metallic taste in the mouth.

Central nervous system: Dizziness, lightheadedness.

Rare but potentially life-threatening reactions

Cardiovascular: Ventricular tachycardia or VF (1.6–6%), bundle branch block, first- or second-degree AV block, congestive heart failure.

Hematologic: Granulocytopenia, agranulocytosis.

Immunologic: Positive ANA titer with lupuslike symptoms.

Comments: The usual starting dosage is 150 mg PO q8h, with an increase to 300 mg PO q8h if necessary. Therapy beyond a total of 900 mg daily is not recommended. Loading has been accomplished with 600–900 mg orally if desired. Propafenone hydrochloride has been reported to be effective in restoring 30–50% of paroxysmal atrial fibrillation to sinus rhythm. In addition, it has been effective in accessory pathway and other supraventricular arrhythmias. It has some beta-blocking activity as well. Propaferone increases the levels of digoxin, propranolol, and warfarin. Cimetidine increases the propafenone level.

VIII. New and unclassified type 1 agents. The agents considered in this section (moricizine, ajmaline, and imipramine) have not been used as extensively as the other type 1 drugs, at least not in the United States. Imipramine is a tricyclic antidepressant drug that may be useful for arrhythmias but has not received this indication from the FDA.

Moricizine is a phenothiazinelike drug with type 1 antiarrhythmic activity, blocking the inward sodium current with fast kinetics. It does not fall in any specific Vaughan Williams category of type 1 drugs. In terms of dissociation from the sodium channel, its rate is slower than the 1B agents but faster than the 1A agents. It does not block potassium channels. It shortens action potential duration (similar to 1B and 1C drugs). There is no significant dopamine-agonist activity or neuroleptic phenothiazine activity. It slows AV nodal and intraventricular conduction and increases P–R, QRS, and corrected Q–T intervals. No benefit was seen with moricizine in the CAST trials. Moricizine has been evaluated in both supraventricular and ventricular arrhythmias, but its value in symptomatic sustained VT or VF seems limited.

Ajmaline is a reserpine derivative with type 1 antiarrhythmic effects. It reduces the rate of phase 0 depolarization and prolongs the action potential. Its major use has been in the WPW syndrome. Ajmaline prolongs the effective refractory period of the accessory pathway.

Ajmaline has been used to determine whether a patient has a short effective refractory period of the accessory pathway. Abolition of preexcitation on the resting ECG after IV ajmaline is an indication of a long ERP of the accessory pathway, which places the patient at lower risk of sudden cardiac death.

Intravenous ajmaline has also been used to test for early signs of chagasic myocarditis, as it transiently may cause right bundle branch block with or without left anterior fascicular block, ventricular arrhythmias, or ischemic ST–T wave changes. Ajmaline is not available in the United States.

In addition to its activity as a tricyclic antidepressant, **imipramine** is similar in antiarrhythmic properties to quinidine, a type 1A agent. Imipramine prolongs intraventricular conduction and repolarization and may have a direct effect on the heart.

Imipramine prolongs the P–R, QRS, and Q–T intervals. It has the ability to suppress ventricular ectopy in certain individuals. Adding imipramine therapy for depression to a patient receiving a type 1 antiarrhythmic drug for arrhythmias is potentially hazardous. It is possible that a depressed patient needing therapy for both depression and ventricular ectopic control might benefit from imipramine alone. This should be attempted under monitored conditions. Imipramine has also been shown to have antiarrhythmic effects in patients without depression.

In addition to suppressing ventricular ectopy, imipramine has the ability to suppress VT in some patients, but its efficacy is as limited as that of the other 1A agents.

A. Moricizine

Pharmacology: Sodium channel blocker, decreases APD and ERP, decreases automaticity and triggered activity.

New classification: High-potency blocker of the inactivated state of sodium channel with fast kinetics.

Preparations: Moricizine (Ethmozine) 200-, 250-, 300-mg tablets.

Approved indications: Life-threatening ventricular arrhythmias.

Potential indications: Supraventricular arrhythmias.

Metabolism: Hepatic.

Half-life: 3–4 hours, prolonged to 6–13 hours in patients with arrhythmias and up to 47 hours in renal insufficiency.

Therapeutic level: 0.1–0.3 µg/ml.

Common adverse effects

Gastrointestinal: Nausea, vomiting.

Central nervous system: Dizziness.

Other: Urinary retention.

Potentially life-threatening adverse effects: 15% chance of proarrhythmia. Rare cases of thrombocytopenia.

Comments: Usual total dosage is 200–300 mg q8h, increasing the dosage every 3 days in 50-mg increments. Concomitant administration of cimetidine decreases clearance of moricizine and increases moricizine's half-life and plasma concentration. Moricizine increases plasma concentrations of theophylline.

B. Ajmaline

Pharmacology: Reserpine derivative.

Preparations: Ajmaline.

Potential indications: Supraventricular arrhythmias in the WPW syndrome.

Half-life: 1–3 minutes.

Therapeutic level: 1–3 µg/ml.

Potentially life-threatening reactions: Proarrhythmia, neutropenia.

Comments: Ajmaline may be useful only for diagnostic purposes because of its short half-life and side effect profile.

C. Imipramine

Pharmacology: Tricyclic antidepressant with type 1 antiarrhythmic properties.

Preparations: Imipramine pamoate (Tofranil-PM) 75-, 100-, 125-, and 150-mg capsules, and Tofranil 10-, 25-, and 50-mg.

Approved indication: Depression.

Potential indications: Ventricular arrhythmias.

Metabolism: Hepatic.

Active metabolites: Desmethylimipramine, 2-hydroxyimipramine, 2-hydroxydesmethylimipramine.

Half-life: Approximately 35 hours.

Therapeutic level: 100–300 ng/ml.

Potentially life-threatening reactions

Cardiac: Myocardial infarction, arrhythmias, stroke, heart block, precipitation of congestive heart failure.

Hematologic: Bone marrow depression, including agranulocytosis and thrombocytopenia.

Anticholinergic: Avoid use of imipramine in intraocular hypertension (glaucoma).

Do not use imipramine if the patient is receiving guanethidine or clonidine since their effects may be blocked.

Methylphenidate may inhibit metabolism of imipramine.

Comments: Cardiac toxicity increases with levels greater than 500 ng. Levels higher than 1000 ng/ml may be lethal.

IX. **Type 3 antiarrhythmic drugs.** The type 3 drugs include bretylium, amiodarone, and sotalol. Electrophysiologically, they cause a minimal change in the upstroke velocity of the action potential. They increase the effective refractory period and the ERP/APD ratio. Only a minimal effect is observed on automatic cells.

Bretylium, available only in IV form, is taken up by adrenergic nerve terminals, which is accompanied by the release of norepinephrine. Subsequently, it prevents the release of norepinephrine and may cause hypotension (particularly orthostatic). Some patients receiving bretylium tosylate may require a vasopressor such as phenylephrine if it is necessary to continue the former. Bretylium has been reputed to cause chemical defibrillation in patients refractory to other drug therapy. Bretylium may also be helpful in some refractory VTs, but it is not a first-line drug.

Oral bretylium as well as several analogues were evaluated but were not found to be effective with minimal side effects. The other drugs studied were bethanidine, clofilium, and meobentine.

Amiodarone, originally developed as a vasodilator, has type 1B, 2, 3, and 4 antiarrhythmic properties. It blocks sodium channels in the inactivated state and dissociates rapidly (like lidocaine). In addition, it causes noncompetitive beta-adrenergic blockade. It blocks the I K channel and the L-type calcium channel. It is approved by the FDA for refractory ventricular tachyarrhythmias. Amiodarone is perhaps the most effective antiarrhythmic agent available for supraventricular and ventricular arrhythmias but is also one of the most toxic. The most feared adverse reaction is an interstitial pulmonary process clinically manifest as progressive dyspnea and cough. Pulmonary toxicity usually occurs after 1 year of therapy in 2–15% of patients. In this group, there may be a 10% mortality. Some have found the use of steroids helpful in reversing pulmonary toxicity, but this use remains controversial. It is extremely important to follow these patients with pulmonary function studies, particularly the diffusion capacity. Evidence of a major change indicates the necessity of dosage reduction or withdrawal.

Many patients demonstrate abnormalities of hepatic enzymes but only rarely are symptomatic. Rare patients have experienced hepatic failure. One should become concerned if the baseline value triples. Amiodarone contains iodine and interferes with thyroid hormone by inhibiting the peripheral conversion of thyroxine (T4) to triiodothyronine (T3). The result is higher T4, lower T3, and higher inactive reverse T3. Amiodarone may cause hyper- or hypothyroidism. Mild elevation of T4 is usually not a cause for concern as long as the patient remains asymptomatic. Hypothyroidism may be treated with supplementation with thyroxine. Clinical hyperthyroidism may necessitate drug discontinuation.

Other effects are less serious. Corneal microdeposits occur in almost all patients receiving amiodarone but rarely cause impaired vision. Occasionally patients may notice halos or blurred vision. Corneal microdeposits are reversible on withdrawal. Usually patients do not require drug discontinuation. Dermatologic problems include photosensitization (usually necessitating sun barrier creams) in 10% and a blue-gray skin discoloration after long-term therapy.

Before starting a patient with amiodarone, the physician must be certain that the patient is truly refractory to all other antiarrhythmic drugs, alone or in combination. The physician must weigh the severity of the arrhythmia and the underlying heart disease. Is the patient a candidate for arrhythmia surgery, a tiered therapy internal cardioverter defibrillator? A particular concern is starting a young patient on amiodarone therapy because of the long-term toxicity. If the patient is elderly and too ill to undergo invasive procedures, amiodarone is more justifiable.

Amiodarone is very effective for refractory VT in a large number of patients. If amiodarone suppresses inducible VT, it implies a good clinical outcome. Failure to suppress inducible VT is a somewhat more controversial subject. Most consider it a poor outcome, yet others have commented that some patients continue to do well despite inducibility. Some of the discrepancies may be related to performing different times of EPS after the initiation of amiodarone therapy. If a patient continued to be inducible into the same monomorphic VT (in both rate and morphology), one might wish to consider other options, including combination therapy (amiodarone plus a type 1 drug), arrhythmia surgery, or an electronic device. If the rate of the induced VT is slower on amiodarone, it suggests some effect on the arrhythmia, possibly beneficial.

Amiodarone may be effective in up to 80–85% of refractory paroxysmal atrial tachyarrhythmias in patients who have a chance of remaining in sinus rhythm. Patients with severely enlarged left atria or who are in chronic atrial fibrillation do not fall into this category. Again the risk-benefit ratio must be evaluated.

Data are now available on sotalol, a beta blocker that lengthens repolarization and the effective refractory period. Sotalol (see **III.G**) decreases sinus rate; prolongs the Q–T and A–H intervals; and increases the ERP of the AV node, the relative refractory period of the His-Purkinje system (no change in the H–V interval), and the ERP of the atrium and ventricle. There seems to be promise for the treatment of ventricular tachyarrhythmias, but there is also the potential to cause torsades de pointes.

A. Bretylium

Pharmacology: Type 3 antiarrhythmic agent.

New classification: High-potency blocker of the potassium channel and biphasic activity initially to stimulate alpha and beta receptors by release of norepinephrine, followed by subsequent block of norepinephrine release and indirect antagonism of these receptors.

Preparations: Bretylium tosylate (Bretylol) 500 mg/10 ml.

Approved indications: Ventricular fibrillation and VT.

Metabolism: Eliminated intact by the kidneys.

Active metabolites: None.

Half-life: 8 hours; longer in renal failure.

Therapeutic level: 0.5–1.5 µg/ml.

Common adverse reactions

Hypotension.

Transient hypertension and increased arrhythmias owing to release of norepinephrine.

Possible aggravation of digitalis toxicity related to norepinephrine release.

Potentially life-threatening reactions: Because of renal excretion, the dosage must be reduced and administration intervals increased when the patient has impaired renal function.

Comments: Bretylium is a second-line agent when the patient has failed to respond to therapy with lidocaine or procainamide. Bretylium tosylate may be given at 5 mg/kg by rapid IV infusion. If VF persists, the dosage may be increased to 10 mg/kg. If continuous bretylium infusion is necessary, 500 mg of bretylium is diluted in a minimum of 50 ml D5W or saline and infused at a rate of 1–2 mg/minute.

B. Amiodarone

Pharmacology: Type 3 antiarrhythmic drug.

New classification: Low-potency blocker of the sodium channel with fast kinetics, low-potency blocker of the calcium channel, moderate-potency blocker of both the alpha- and beta-adrenergic receptors, and a high-potency blocker of the potassium channel.

Preparations: Amiodarone hydrochloride (Cordarone) 200-mg tablets; investigational use: amiodarone injection 150-mg/ml ampules.

Approved indications: Recurrent VT and VF.

Potential indications: Supraventricular tachyarrhythmias.

Metabolism: Hepatic.

Active metabolite: Desethylamiodarone (activity not completely established).

Half-life: 26–107 days (mean 53 days) for amiodarone, mean 61 days for desethylamiodarone.

Therapeutic level: 1.0–2.5 µg/ml.

Common adverse reactions

Corneal microdeposits.

Thyroid abnormalities.

Dermatologic problems.

Potentially life-threatening reactions

Pulmonary toxicity.

Hepatotoxicity (very rare).

Sinus bradyarrhythmias or AV block (may require pacemaker).

Torsades de pointes.

Comments: Many of the major considerations regarding amiodarone are discussed in the introduction to the type 3 antiarrhythmic drugs. In addition it is important to note several drug interactions. An interaction between amiodarone and warfarin (Coumadin) may increase the prothrombin time by 100%. Consequently the dosage of warfarin should be decreased by 30–50%. Amiodarone will increase the digoxin level, necessitating a 50% reduction in digoxin. If amiodarone is administered with quinidine, the quinidine should be discontinued or decreased 30–50%. Similarly if procainamide is the second drug, its dosage should be lowered 30%.

When amiodarone therapy is started, a loading dose of 800–1600 mg daily is necessary for 1–3 weeks, before reducing it to a maintenance level. My own experience has been successful with a conservative regimen of 1000 mg daily (600 mg AM, 400 mg PM) for days 1–7, 600 mg daily for days 8–14, and thereafter 400 mg daily for VT and 200 mg daily for SVT. Other drugs may remain necessary to control VT or VF until amiodarone takes effect. Prior investigational regimens for IV amiodarone have called for 5 mg/kg over a period of 15–20 minutes, followed by 10–20 mg/kg over the next 24-hour period. However, severe hypotension may accompany rapid administration. Perhaps the only indication for IV amiodarone may be intractable refractory life-threatening arrhythmias. A new preparation of IV amiodarone has just received FDA approval.

X. Other pharmacologic agents used in the management of arrhythmias. Adenosine and adenosine triphosphate (ATP) have recently been used in paroxysmal and supraventricular tachycardia with great success. These compounds provide a physiologic alternative to drugs with potentially greater toxicity. For completeness, the key facts for adenosine, atropine, edrophonium, and isoproterenol are mentioned. Atropine and isoproterenol are used for emergency treatment of bradyarrhythmias and are discussed in Chaps. 2 and 6. Edrophonium is included because of the rare possibility that a physician might wish to use it in SVT; however, its inclusion is more for historical perspective.

Adenosine and adenosine triphosphate have negative dromotropic and negative chronotropic effects on both the SA and AV nodes. Adenosine acts on the adenosine A1 receptor system and activates GTP binding proteins. Inhibitory G-proteins both inhibit adenyl cyclase and directly activate the I K (ACh,Ado) channel. Since adenosine and adenosine triphosphate (ATP) are physiologic substances and have a very short half-life, the electrophysiologic effects suggest a utility in paroxysmal supraventricular tachycardia that is particularly appealing.

The potent depressant effects on the AV node result in a high efficacy in terminating paroxysmal supraventricular tachycardia (PSVT) caused by AV nodal reentry. Data suggest that the block occurs in the slow antegrade AV nodal pathway or within the AV node in patients with concealed retrograde accessory pathway. The effects on the SA node cause sinus bradycardia.

The duration of action of these drugs is less than 1 minute, and the side effects are similarly brief. The side effects, which are more profound with ATP than with adenosine, include malaise, flushing, headaches, retching, and cough. Cardiac effects include sinus bradycardia, sinus arrest, AV block, and sinus tachycardia (owing to vasodilatation). Rarely ventricular ectopy including nonsustained VT may be seen.

Interestingly, potency of effects is related to the rate of administration and rapid degradation. If it is given rapidly, the negative dromotropic effects are seen. If it is given slowly, only the reflex tachycardia owing to vasodilatation is observed. Aminophylline, a competitive antagonist of adenosine, prevents the effect of adenosine and ATP, but atropine has no such effect. Adenosine and adenosine triphosphate may be potentially safer than verapamil in attempts to terminate PSVT because of the short duration of action.

A. Adenosine

Pharmacology: Adenine nucleoside.
New classification: Stimulator of purinergic receptor.
Preparations: Adenosine (Adenocard) 6-mg/2-cc vials.
Indication: Paroxysmal supraventricular tachycardia.
Metabolism: Adenosine is metabolized to inosine and adenosine monophosphate.
Half-life: Less than 10 seconds.

Common adverse reactions
Cardiac: Sinus bradycardia, sinus arrest, AV block.
Noncardiac: Malaise, flushing, headache, retching.

Comments: Very high success rate in terminating PSVT. Antagonized by methylxanthines (caffeine, theophylline) and potentiated by dipyridamole. Carbamazepine may increase the degree of heart block. May rarely cause bronchospasm.

B. Atropine

Pharmacology: Antimuscarinic agent.
New classification: Potent antagonist of muscarinic subtype 2 receptor.
Preparations: Atropine sulfate 1 mg/10 ml.
Approved indications: Abolition of reflex vagal cardiac slowing or asystole.
Metabolism: Most excreted in urine within 12 hours, in part unchanged.
Half-life: 2.5 hours.
Common adverse effects: Xerostomia, urinary retention, blurred vision.

Potentially life-threatening effects
Cardiac: Tachycardia (and its consequences in patients with ischemic heart disease).
Central nervous system: Hallucinations, delirium, coma.

Comments: Atropine is most often used in emergencies to treat bradyarrhythmias. Temporary pacing is quite often a preferable alternative to continued atropine administration. With initial low atropine doses, there is occasionally a decrease in rate due to central vagal stimulation or low doses that fail to achieve peripheral antimuscarinic effects.

C. Edrophonium

Pharmacology: Short-acting, rapidly acting cholinergic drug (anticholinesterase).
Preparations: Edrophonium chloride (Tensilon) 10-mg/1-ml ampule.
Approved indications: Diagnosis of myasthenia gravis; counteracting the neuromuscular block produced by curarelike drugs.
Potential indication: Termination of supraventricular tachycardias.
Metabolism: Not completely elucidated.
Half-life: 10 minutes.
Common adverse reactions: Nausea, vomiting.

Potentially life-threatening adverse reactions
Cardiac: Bradycardia, asystole.
Central nervous system: Seizures.
Respiratory: Increased tracheobronchial secretions, laryngospasm, paralysis of muscles of respiration, central respiratory paralysis.

Comments: Edrophonium was formerly used to terminate supraventricular tachycardia, but its use was limited by the accompanying nausea and vomiting. Now that verapamil is available, there is little reason to use edrophonium unless the patient cannot tolerate other available drugs.

D. Isoproterenol

Pharmacology: Potent beta-receptor agonist (almost no alpha activity).
Preparations: Isoproterenol hydrochloride 0.2 mg/1 ml.
Approved indications: Positive inotropic and chronotropic activity.
Metabolism: Hepatic.
Common adverse reactions: Lowering of peripheral vascular resistance, fall in diastolic pressure.
Potentially life-threatening reactions: Cardiac arrhythmias, including VT.

Comments: Isoproterenol is used for emergency treatment of bradyarrhythmias, particularly when a positive inotropic effect is also desirable. It is not desirable for prolonged use, and a pacemaker may have to be inserted after the patient is stabilized. Isoproterenol may be useful in torsades de pointes.

References

1. Vaughan Williams EM. Classification of antidysrhythmic drugs. *Pharm Ther* 1:115, 1975.
2. Vaughan Williams EM. A classification of antiarrhythmic actions reassessed after a decade of new drugs. *J Clin Pharm* 24:129, 1984.
3. Task Force. The Sicilian Gambit: A new approach to the classification of antiarrhythmic drugs based on their actions on arrhythmogenic mechanisms. *Circulation* 84:1831–1851, 1991.
4. Goodman AG. *Goodman & Gilman's The Pharmacologic Basis of Therapeutics* (8th ed). New York: McGraw-Hill, 1990.

5. Hoffman BF, Bigger JT. Digitalis and allied cardiac glycosides. In AG Gilman, et al. (eds), *Goodman and Gilman's The Pharmacological Basis of Therapeutics* (7th ed). New York: Macmillan, 1985. Pp 716–747.

Bibliography

Antiarrhythmic Drugs
Antonaccio MJ. *Cardiovascular Pharmacology* (3rd ed). New York: Raven Press, 1990.

Coromilas J. *The Pharmacotherapy of Sustained Arrhythmias.* New York: Creative Medical Communications, 1994.

Opie LH. *Drugs for the Heart* (3rd ed). Philadelphia: Saunders, 1991.

Perspectives on Proarrhythmia [symposium]. *Am J Cardiol* 59:no 11 (Suppl), 1987.

Vaughan Williams EM. Significance of classifying antiarrhythmic actions since the Cardiac Arrhythmia Suppression Trial. *J Clin Pharm* 31:123–135, 1991.

Digitalis Preparations
Antman EM, et al. Treatment of 150 cases of life-threatening digitalis intoxication with digoxin-specific Fab antibody fragments. *Circulation* 81:1744–1752, 1990.

Bigger JT. The quinidine-digoxin interaction. *N Engl J Med* 301:779–781, 1979.

Bigger JT, et al. Effect of digitalis treatment on survival after acute myocardial infarction. *Am J Cardiol* 55:623–630, 1985.

Bresnahan JF, Vlietstra RE. Digitalis glycosides. *Mayo Clin Proc* 54:675–684, 1979.

Byington R, Goldstein S, BHAT Research Group. Association of digitalis therapy with mortality in survivors of acute myocardial infarction: Observations in the beta blocker heart attack trial. *J Am Coll Cardiol* 6:976–982, 1985.

David D, et al. Inefficacy of digitalis in the control of heart rate in patients with chronic atrial fibrillation: Beneficial effect of an added beta adrenergic blocking agent. *Am J Cardiol* 44:1378–1382, 1979.

Doering W. Quinidine-digoxin interaction. *N Engl J Med* 301:400–404, 1979.

Falk RH, et al. Digoxin for converting recent-onset atrial fibrillation to sinus rhythm. *Ann Intern Med* 106:503–506, 1987.

Fisch C (guest ed). William Withering: An account of the foxglove, 1785–1985. *J Am Coll Cardiol* 5:1A–122A, 1985.

Hager WD, et al. Digoxin-quinidine interaction. *N Engl J Med* 300:1238–1241, 1979.

Leahey EB, et al. The effect of quinidine and other oral antiarrhythmic drugs on serum digoxin. *Ann Intern Med* 92:605–608, 1980.

Marcus FI. Use of digitalis in acute myocardial infarction. *Circulation* 62:17–19, 1980.

Marcus FI. Digitalis: Key references. *Circulation* 59:837–840, 1979.

Moss AJ, et al. Digitalis-associated cardiac mortality after myocardial infarction. *Circulation* 64:1150–1155, 1981.

Reid PR. Digoxin and the radioimmunoassay. *Md State Med J* 1975.

Smith TW. Digitalis glycosides. *N Engl J Med* 288:719–722, 942–946, 1973.

Smith TW, et al. Digitalis glycosides: Mechanisms and manifestations of toxicity. *Prog Cardiovasc Dis* 26:413–458, 495–540, 27:21–56, 1984.

Smith TW, et al. Treatment of life-threatening digitalis intoxication with digoxin-specific Fab antibody fragments. *N Engl J Med* 307:1357–1362, 1982.

Smith TW, Haber E. Digitalis. *N Engl J Med* 289:945–952, 1010–1015, 1063–1072, 1125–1129, 1973.

Beta Blockers

General
Anderson JL, Rodier HE, Green LS. Comparative effects of beta-adrenergic blocking drugs on experimental ventricular fibrillation threshold. *Am J Cardiol* 51:1196–1202, 1983.

Bigger JT, Coromilas J. How do beta blockers protect after myocardial infarction? *Ann Intern Med* 101:256–258, 1984.

Frishman WH. *Clinical Pharmacology of the Beta Adrenoceptor Blocking Drugs* (2nd ed). Norwalk CT: Appleton-Century Croft, 1984.

Frishman WH, Furberg CD, Friedewald WT. Beta adrenergic blockade for survivors of acute myocardial infarction. *N Engl J Med* 310:830–837, 1984.

Lefkowitz RJ. Beta adrenergic receptors: Recognition and regulation. *N Engl J Med* 295:323–328, 1976.

Lichstein E. Why do beta receptor blockers decrease mortality after myocardial infarction? *J Am Coll Cardiol* 6:973–975, 1985.

Singh BN, Venkatesh N. Prevention of myocardial reinfarction and of sudden death in survivors of acute myocardial infarction: Role of prophylactic beta adrenoceptor blockade. *Am Heart J* 107:189–199, 1984.

Staessen J, et al. Secondary prevention with beta adrenoceptor blockers in post myocardial infarction patients. *Am Heart J* 104:1395–1399, 1982.

Acebutolol

Aronow WS, et al. Treatment of premature ventricular complexes with acebutolol. *Am J Cardiol* 43:106–108, 1979.

deSoyza N, et al. Acebutolol therapy for ventricular arrhythmia. *Circulation* 65:1129–1133, 1982.

O'Reilly M. Chronic use of acebutolol in the treatment of cardiac arrhythmias. *Am Heart J* 121:1185–1194, 1991.

Williams DO, Tatelbaum R, Most AS. Effective treatment of supraventricular arrhythmias with acebutolol. *Am J Cardiol* 44:521–525, 1979.

Atenolol

Frishman WH. Atenolol and timolol, two new systemic beta adrenoceptor antagonists. *N Engl J Med* 306:1456–1462, 1982.

Heng MK, Zimmer I. Reduction of ventricular arrhythmias by atenolol. *Am Heart J* 109:1273–1280, 1985.

Bucindolol

Anderson JL, Gilbert EM, O'Connell JB. Long-term (2 year) beneficial effects of beta-adrenergic blockade with bucindolol in patients with idiopathic dilated cardiomyopathy. *J Am Coll Cardiol* 17:1373–1381, 1991.

Esmolol

Barth C, et al. Ultra short-acting intravenous beta-adrenergic blockade as add-on therapy in acute unstable angina. *Am Heart J* 121:782–788, 1991.

Byrd RC, et al. Safety and efficacy of esmolol (ASL-8052: an ultrashort-acting beta-adrenergic blocking agent) for control of ventricular rate in supraventricular tachycardias. *J Am Coll Cardiol* 3:394–399, 1984.

Esmolol Multicenter Study Research Group. Efficacy and safety of esmolol vs propranolol in the treatment of supraventricular tachyarrhythmias: A multicenter double blind clinical trial. *Am Heart J* 110:913–922, 1985.

Gray RJ, et al. Esmolol: A new ultrashort acting beta adrenergic blocking agent for rapid control of heart rate in postoperative supraventricular tachyarrhythmias. *J Am Coll Cardiol* 5:1451–1456, 1985.

Metoprolol

Brodsky MA, et al. Adjuvant metoprolol improves efficacy of class I antiarrhythmic drugs in patients with inducible sustained monomorphic ventricular tachycardia. *Am Heart J* 124:629–635, 1992.

Capucci A, et al. Tocainide and metoprolol: An efficacious therapeutic combination in the treatment of premature ventricular beats. *Clin Cardiol* 12:322–331, 1989.

Hjalmarson A, et al. Effect on mortality of metoprolol in acute myocardial infarction. *Lancet* 2:823–827, 1981.

Koch Weser J. Metoprolol. *N Engl J Med* 301:698–702, 1979.

Marchlinski FE, et al. Electrophysiologic effects of intravenous metoprolol. *Am Heart J* 107:1125–1130, 1984.

Miami Trial Research Group. Metoprolol in acute myocardial infarction (MIAMI). A randomized placebo controlled international trial. *Eur Heart J* 6:199–226, 1985.

Olsson G, Rehnquist N. Ventricular arrhythmias during the first year after acute myocardial infarction: Influence of long term treatment with metoprolol. *Circulation* 69:1129–1134, 1984.

Ravid S, Lampert S, Graboys TB. Effect of the combination of low-dose mexiletine and metoprolol on ventricular arrhythmia. *Clin Cardiol* 14:951–955, 1991.

Ryden L, et al. A double blind trial of metoprolol in acute myocardial infarction: Effects on ventricular tachyarrhythmias. *N Engl J Med* 308:614–618, 1983.

Nadolol
Frishman WH. Nadolol: A new beta adrenoceptor antagonist. *N Engl J Med* 305:678–682, 1981.

Oxprenolol
Bethge KP, et al. Effect of oxprenolol on ventricular arrhythmias: The European infarction study experience. *J Am Coll Cardiol* 6:963–972, 1985.

Pindolol
Frishman WH. Pindolol. A new beta adrenoceptor antagonist with partial agonist activity. *N Engl J Med* 308:940–944, 1983.

Propranolol
Beta Blocker Heart Attack Trial Research Group. A randomized trial of propranolol in patients with acute myocardial infarction: I. Mortality results. *JAMA* 247:1707–1714, 1982; II. Morbidity results. *JAMA* 250:2814–2819, 1983.

Roberts R, et al. Effect of propranolol on myocardial infarct size in a randomized blinded multicenter trial. *N Engl J Med* 311:218–225, 1984.

Shand DG. Propranolol. *N Engl J Med* 293:280–285, 1975.

Woosley RL, et al. Suppression of chronic ventricular arrhythmias with propranolol. *Circulation* 60:819–827, 1979.

Sotalol
Anastasiou-Nana MI, Gilbert EM, Miller RH. Usefulness of d,l sotalol for suppression of chronic ventricular arrhythmias. *Am J Cardiol* 67:511–516, 1991.

Dorian P, et al. Sotalol and type 1A drugs in combination prevent recurrence of sustained ventricular tachycardia. *J Am Coll Cardiol* 22:106–113, 1992.

Funck-Brentano C, et al. Rate dependence of sotalol-induced prolongation of ventricular repolarization during exercise in humans. *Circulation* 83:536–545, 1991.

Hohnloser SH, et al. Short- and long-term antiarrhythmic and hemodynamic effects of d,l sotalol in patients with symptomatic ventricular arrhythmias. *Am Heart J* 123:1220–1224, 1992.

Huikuri HV, Koistinen J, Takkunen JT. Efficacy of intravenous sotalol for suppressing inducibility of supraventricular tachycardias at rest and during isometric exercise. *Am J Cardiol* 69:498–502, 1992.

Jordaens L, et al. Efficacy and safety of intravenous sotalol for termination of paroxysmal supraventricular tachycardia. *Am J Cardiol* 68:35–40, 1991.

Juul-Moller S, Edvardsson N, Rehnqvist-Ahlberg N. Sotalol versus quinidine for the maintenance of sinus rhythm after direct current conversion of atrial fibrillation. *Circulation* 82:1932–1939, 1990.

Kus T, et al. Efficacy and electrophysiologic effects of oral sotalol in patients with sustained ventricular tachycardia caused by coronary artery disease. *Am Heart J* 123:82–89, 1992.

Rizos I, et al. Differential effects of sotalol and metoprolol on induction of paroxysmal supraventricular tachycardia. *Am J Cardiol* 53:1022–1027, 1984.

Sahar DI, et al. Efficacy, safety, and tolerance of d-sotalol in patients with refractory supraventricular tachyarrhythmias. *Am Heart J* 117:562–568, 1989.

Schwartz J, et al. The antiarrhythmic effects of d-sotalol. *Am Heart J* 114:539–544, 1987.

Senges J, et al. Electrophysiologic testing in assessment of therapy with sotalol for sustained ventricular tachycardia. *Circulation* 69:577–584, 1984.

Singh BN, Nademanee K. Sotalol: A beta blocker with unique antiarrhythmic properties. *Am Heart J* 114:121–138, 1987.

Timolol

Gundersen T, et al. Timolol related reduction in mortality in patients ages 65–75 years surviving acute myocardial infarction. *Circulation* 66:1179–1184, 1982.

International Collaborative Study Group. Reduction in infarct size with the early use of timolol in acute myocardial infarction. *N Engl J Med* 310:9–15, 1984.

Norwegian Multicenter Study Group. Timolol-induced reduction in mortality and reinfarction in patients surviving acute myocardial infarction. *N Engl J Med* 304:801–808, 1981.

Pedersen TR. Six year followup of the Norwegian multicenter study on timolol after acute myocardial infarction. *N Engl J Med* 313:1055–1058, 1985.

Calcium Antagonists

General

Antman EM, et al. Calcium channel blocking agents in the treatment of cardiovascular disorders: Basic and clinical electrophysiologic effects. *Ann Intern Med* 93:875–885, 1980.

Braunwald E. Mechanism of action of calcium channel blocking agents. *N Engl J Med* 307:1618–1627, 1982.

Braunwald E (ed). Seminar on calcium channel blockers. *Am J Cardiol* 46:1045–1067, 1980.

Kawai C, et al. Comparative effects of three calcium antagonists, diltiazem, verapamil and nifedipine on the sinoatrial and atrioventricular nodes. *Circulation* 63:1035–1042, 1981.

Stone PH, et al. Calcium channel blocking agents in the treatment of cardiovascular disorders: II. Hemodynamic effects and clinical applications. *Ann Intern Med* 93:886–904, 1980.

Verapamil

Belhassen B, Horowitz LN. Use of intravenous verapamil for ventricular tachycardia. *Am J Cardiol* 54:1131–1133, 1984.

Klein GJ, et al. Comparison of the electrophysiologic effects of intravenous and oral verapamil in patients with paroxysmal supraventricular tachycardia. *Am J Cardiol* 49:117–124, 1982.

Mangrardi LM, et al. Electrophysiologic and hemodynamic effects of verapamil. *Circulation* 57:366–372, 1978.

Mauritson DR, et al. Oral verapamil for paroxysmal supraventricular tachycardia. *Ann Intern Med* 96:409–412, 1982.

Rinkenberger RL, et al. Effects of intravenous and chronic oral verapamil administration in patients with supraventricular tachyarrhythmias. *Circulation* 62:996–1010, 1980.

Rosen MR, Wit AL, Hoffman BF. Electrophysiology and pharmacology of cardiac arrhythmias: VI. Cardiac effects of verapamil. *Am Heart J* 89:665–673, 1975.

Sung RJ, Elser B, McAllister RG. Intravenous verapamil for termination of reentrant supraventricular tachycardias. *Ann Intern Med* 93:682–689, 1980.

Waxman HL, et al. Verapamil for control of ventricular rate in paroxysmal supraventricular tachycardia and atrial fibrillation or flutter. *Ann Intern Med* 94:1–6, 1981.

Diltiazem

Beltriv A, et al. Beneficial effect of intravenous diltiazem in the acute management of paroxysmal supraventricular tachyarrhythmias. *Circulation* 67:88–93, 1983.

Bigger JT, et al. Effect of diltiazem on cardiac rate and rhythm after myocardial infarction. *Am J Cardiol* 65:539–546, 1990.

Ellenbogen KA, et al. A placebo-controlled trial of continuous intravenous diltiazem infusion for 24-hour heart rate control during atrial fibrillation and atrial flutter: A multicenter study. *J Am Coll Cardiol* 18:891–897, 1991.

Sternbach GL, et al. Intravenous diltiazem for the treatment of supraventricular tachycardia. *Clin Cardiol* 9:145–149, 1986.

Newer Agents

Eichler HG, et al. Tiapamil, a new calcium antagonist: Hemodynamic effects in patients with acute myocardial infarction. *Circulation* 71:779–786, 1985.

Levy S, et al. Bepridil for recurrent sustained ventricular tachycardias: Assessment using electrophysiologic testing. *Am J Cardiol* 54:579–581, 1984.

Rowland E, McKenna WJ, Kuekler DM. Electrophysiologic and antiarrhythmic actions of bepridil. *Am J Cardiol* 55:1513–1519, 1985.

Somberg J, et al. Prolongation of QT interval and antiarrhythmic action of bepridil. *Am Heart J* 109:19–26, 1985.

Upward JW, et al. Electrophysiologic, hemodynamic and metabolic effects of intravenous bepridil hydrochloride. *Am J Cardiol* 55:1589–1595, 1985.

Type 1A Antiarrhythmics

Quinidine

Bauman JL, et al. Torsade de pointes due to quinidine: Observations in 31 patients. *Am Heart J* 107:425–430, 1984.

Cohen IS, Jick H, Cohen SI. Adverse reactions to quinidine in hospitalized patients: Findings based on data from the Boston Collaborative drug surveillance program. *Prog Cardiovasc Dis* 20:151–163, 1977.

Coplen SE, et al. Efficacy and safety of quinidine therapy for maintenance of sinus rhythm after cardioversion. *Circulation* 82:1106–1116, 1990.

Drayer D. Basic clinical pharmacology of the antiarrhythmic drugs procainamide and quinidine. *Cardiovasc Rev Rep* 2:475–482, 1981.

Duff HJ, et al. Intravenous quinidine: Relations among concentration, tachyarrhythmia suppression and electrophysiologic actions with inducible sustained ventricular tachycardia. *Am J Cardiol* 55:92–97, 1985.

Kim SG, et al. Combination of procainamide and quinidine for better tolerance and additive effects for ventricular arrhythmias. *Am J Cardiol* 56:84–88, 1985.

Morganroth J, Goin JE. Quinidine-related mortality in the short-to-medium-term treatment of ventricular arrhythmias. *Circulation* 84:1977–1983, 1991.

Morganroth J, Horowitz LN. Incidence of proarrhythmic effects from quinidine in the outpatient treatment of benign or potentially lethal ventricular arrhythmias. *Am J Cardiol* 56:585–587, 1985.

Morganroth J, Hunter H. Comparative efficacy and safety of short-acting and sustained release quinidine in the treatment of patients with ventricular arrhythmias. *Am Heart J* 100:1176–1180, 1985.

Oseran DS, et al. Electropharmacologic testing in sustained ventricular tachycardia associated with coronary heart disease: Value of the response to intravenous procainamide in predicting the response to oral procainamide and oral quinidine treatment. *Am J Cardiol* 56:883–886, 1985.

Procainamide

Buxton AE, et al. Polymorphic ventricular tachycardia induced by programmed stimulation: Response to procainamide. *J Am Coll Cardiol* 21:90–98, 1993.

Engel TR, Meister SG, Luck JC. Modification of ventricular tachycardia by procainamide in patients with coronary artery disease. *Am J Cardiol* 46:1033–1038, 1980.

Giardina EGV, et al. Efficacy, plasma concentrations and adverse effects of a new sustained release procainamide preparation. *Am J Cardiol* 46:855–862, 1980.

Greenspan AM, et al. Large dose procainamide therapy for ventricular tachyarrhythmia. *Am J Cardiol* 46:453–462, 1980.

Interian A, et al. Paired comparisons of efficacy of intravenous and oral procainamide in patients with inducible sustained ventricular tachyarrhythmias. *J Am Coll Cardiol* 17:1581–1586, 1991.

Myerburg RJ, et al. Relationship between plasma levels of procainamide, suppression of premature ventricular complexes and prevention of recurrent ventricular tachycardia. *Circulation* 64:280–290, 1981.

Strasberg B, et al. Procainamide-induced polymorphous ventricular tachycardia. *Am J Cardiol* 47:1309–1314, 1981.

N-*acetylprocainamide*

Jaillon P, et al. Electrophysiologic effects of N-acetylprocainamide in human beings. *Am J Cardiol* 47:1134–1140, 1981.

Kluger J, et al. Acetylprocainamide therapy in patients with previous procainamide-induced lupus syndrome. *Ann Intern Med* 95:18–23, 1981.

Kluger J, et al. Long-term antiarrhythmic therapy with acetylprocainamide. *Am J Cardiol* 48:1124–1132, 1981.

Roden DM, et al. Antiarrhythmic efficacy, pharmacokinetics and safety of N-acetylprocainamide in human subjects: Comparison with procainamide. *Am J Cardiol* 46:463–468, 1980.

Sung RJ, Juma Z, Saksena S. Electrophysiologic properties and antiarrhythmic mechanisms of intravenous N-acetylprocainamide in patients with ventricular dysrrhythmias. *Am Heart J* 105:811–819, 1983.

Winkle RA, et al. Clinical pharmacology and antiarrhythmic efficacy of N-acetylprocainamide. *Am J Cardiol* 47:123–130, 1981.

Wynn J, et al. Electrophysiologic evaluation of the antiarrhythmic effects of N-acetylprocainamide for ventricular tachycardia secondary to coronary heart disease. *Am J Cardiol* 56:877–881, 1985.

Disopyramide

Danilo P, Rosen MR. Cardiac effects of disopyramide. *Am Heart J* 92:532–536, 1976.

Desai JM, et al. Electrophysiologic effects of disopyramide in patients with bundle branch block. *Circulation* 59:215–225, 1979.

Koch-Weser J. Disopyramide. *N Engl J Med* 300:957–962, 1979.

LaBarre A, et al. Electrophysiologic effects of disopyramide phosphate on sinus node function in patients with sinus dysfunction. *Circulation* 59:226–235, 1979.

Lerman BB, et al. Disopyramide: Evaluation of electrophysiologic effects and clinical efficacy in patients with sustained ventricular tachycardia or ventricular fibrillation. *Am J Cardiol* 51:759–764, 1983.

Morady F, Scheinman MM, Desai J. Disopyramide. *Ann Intern Med* 96:337–343, 1982.

Nicholson WJ, et al. Disopyramide-induced ventricular fibrillation. *Am J Cardiol* 43:1053–1055, 1979.

Podrid PJ, Schoenberger A, Lown B. Congestive heart failure caused by oral disopyramide. *N Engl J Med* 302:614–617, 1980.

Prystowshky E, Waldo AL, Fisher JD. Use of disopyramide by arrhythmia specialists after Cardiac Arrhythmia Suppression Trial: Patient selection and initial outcome. *Am Heart J* 121:1571–1582, 1991.

Swiryn S, et al. Effects of oral disopyramide phosphate on induction of paroxysmal supraventricular tachycardia. *Circulation* 64:169–175, 1981.

Type 1B Antiarrhythmics

Lidocaine

Antman EM, Berlin JA. Declining incidence of ventricular fibrillation in myocardial infarction: Implications for the prophylactic use of lidocaine. *Circulation* 86:764–773, 1992.

Davison R, Parker M, Atkinson AJ. Excessive serum lidocaine levels during maintenance infusions: Mechanisms and prevention. *Am Heart J* 104:203–208, 1982.

Knapp AB, et al. The cimetidine-lidocaine interaction. *Ann Intern Med* 98:174–177, 1983.

Kuo CS, Reddy CP. Effect of lidocaine on escape rate in patients with complete atrioventricular block: B. Proximal His bundle block. *Am J Cardiol* 47:1315–1320, 1981.

Reid PR. Lidocaine: To taper or not to taper. *J Clin Pharmacol* 16:162–164, 1976.

Ribner HS, Frishman WH. Prophylactic lidocaine therapy in acute myocardial infarction. *Cardiovasc Rev Rep* 2:395–401, 1981.

Wyman MG, et al. Multiple bolus technique for lidocaine administration during the first hours of an acute myocardial infarction. *Am J Cardiol* 41:313–317, 1978.

Wyman MG, et al. Multiple bolus technique for lidocaine administration in acute ischemic heart disease: II. Treatment of refractory ventricular arrhythmias and the pharmacokinetic significance of severe left ventricular failure. *J Am Coll Cardiol* 2:764–769, 1983.

Zito RA, Reid PR. Lidocaine kinetics predicted by indocyanine green clearance. *N Engl J Med* 298:1160–1163, 1978.

Tocainide

Anderson JL, et al. Clinical electrophysiologic effects of tocainide. *Circulation* 57:685–691, 1978.

Engler R, et al. Assessment of long-term antiarrhythmic therapy: Studies on the long-term efficacy and toxicity of tocainide. *Am J Cardiol* 43:612–618, 1979.

Hohnloser SH, et al. Short- and long-term therapy with tocainide for malignant ventricular tachyarrhythmias. *Circulation* 73:143–149, 1986.

Horowitz LN, Josephson ME, Farshidi A. Human pharmacology of tocainide, a lidocaine congener. *Am J Cardiol* 42:276–280, 1978.

Keefe DL, Somberg JC. New therapy focus: Tocainide. *Cardiovasc Rev Rep* 10:1014–1030, 1984.

Kutalek SP, Morganroth J, Horowitz LN. Tocainide: A new oral antiarrhythmic agent. *Ann Intern Med* 105:387–391, 1985.

Morganroth J, Nestico PF, Horowitz LN. A review of the uses and limitations of tocainide—a class 1B antiarrhythmic agent. *Am Heart J* 110:856–862, 1985.

Morganroth J, Oshrain C, Steele PP. Comparative efficacy and safety of oral tocainide and quinidine for benign and potentially lethal ventricular arrhythmias. *Am J Cardiol* 56:581–585, 1985.

Winkle RA, Meffin PJ, Harrison DC. Long-term tocainide therapy for ventricular arrhythmias. *Circulation* 57:1008–1016, 1978.

Mexiletine

DiMarco JP, Garan H, Ruskin JN. Mexiletine for ventricular arrhythmias: Results using serial electrophysiologic testing. *Am J Cardiol* 47:131–138, 1981.

Duff HJ, et al. Mexiletine in the treatment of resistant ventricular arrhythmias: Enhancement of efficacy and reduction of dose related side effects by combination with quinidine. *Circulation* 67:1124–1128, 1983.

Flaker GC, et al. Mexiletine for recurring ventricular arrhythmias: Assessment by long term electrocardiographic recordings and sequential electrophysiologic studies. *Am Heart J* 108:490–495, 1984.

Giardina EG, Wechsler ME. Low dose quinidine-mexiletine combination therapy versus quinidine monotherapy for treatment of ventricular arrhythmias. *J Am Coll Cardiol* 15:1138–1145, 1990.

Greenspan AM, et al. Efficacy of combination therapy with mexiletine and a type 1A agent for inducible ventricular tachyarrhythmias secondary to coronary artery disease. *Am J Cardiol* 56:277–284, 1985.

Heger JJ, et al. Mexiletine therapy in 15 patients with drug resistant ventricular tachycardia. *Am J Cardiol* 45:627–632, 1980.

Impact Research Group. International mexiletine and placebo antiarrhythmic coronary trial: I. Report on arrhythmia and other findings. *J Am Coll Cardiol* 6:1148–1163, 1984.

Manolis AS, et al. Mexiletine: Pharmacology and therapeutic use. *Clin Cardiol* 13:349–359, 1990.

Palileo EV, et al. Lack of effectiveness of oral mexiletine in patients with drug refractory paroxysmal sustained ventricular tachycardia. *Am J Cardiol* 50:1075–1081, 1982.

Podrid PJ, Lown B. Mexiletine for ventricular arrhythmias. *Am J Cardiol* 47:895–902, 1981.

Rutledge JC, et al. Clinical evaluation of oral mexiletine therapy in the treatment of ventricular arrhythmias. *J Am Coll Cardiol* 6:780–784, 1985.

Tepper D. Somberg JC. Mexiletine. An investigational antiarrhythmic agent. *Cardiovasc Rev Rep* 5:1138–1141, 1984.

Waspe LE, et al. Mexiletine for control of drug-resistant ventricular tachycardia: Clinical and electrophysiologic results in 44 patients. *Am J Cardiol* 51:1175–1181, 1983.

Type 1C Antiarrhythmics

Flecainide

Abitol H, et al. Use of flecainide acetate in the treatment of premature ventricular complexes. *Am Heart J* 105:227–230, 1983.

Anderson JL, Gilbert EM, Alpert BL. Prevention of symptomatic recurrences of paroxysmal atrial fibrillation in patients initially tolerating antiarrhythmic therapy. *Circulation* 80:1557–1570, 1989.

Anderson JL, Lutz JR, Allison SB. Electrophysiologic and antiarrhythmic effects of oral flecainide in patients with inducible ventricular tachycardia. *J Am Coll Cardiol* 2:105–114, 1983.

Anderson JL, Stewart JR, Parry BA. Oral flecainide acetate for the treatment of ventricular arrhythmias. *N Engl J Med* 305:473–477, 1981.

Cohen AA, et al. Hemodynamic effects of intravenous flecainide in acute noncomplicated myocardial infarction. *Am Heart J* 110:1193–1196, 1985.

Creamer JE, Nathan AW, Camm AJ. Successful treatment of atrial tachycardias with flecainide acetate. *Br Heart J* 53:164–166, 1985.

Falk RH. Flecainide-induced ventricular tachycardia and fibrillation in patients treated for atrial fibrillation. *Ann Intern Med* 111:107–111, 1989.

Fish FA, Gillette PC, Benson DW. Proarrhythmia, cardiac arrest and death in young patients receiving encainide and flecainide. *J Am Coll Cardiol* 18:356–365, 1991.

Flowers D, et al. Flecainide: Long-term treatment using a reduced dosing schedule. *Am J Cardiol* 55:79–83, 1985.

Helmy I, et al. Electrophysiologic effects of isoproterenol in patients with atrioventricular reentrant tachycardia treated with flecainide. *J Am Coll Cardiol* 16:1649–1655, 1990.

Henthorn RW, et al. Flecainide acetate prevents recurrence of symptomatic paroxsymal supraventricular tachycardia. *Circulation* 83:119–125, 1991.

Josephson MA, et al. Hemodynamic effects of intravenous flecainide relative to the level of ventricular function in patients with coronary artery disease. *Am Heart J* 109:41–45, 1985.

Lal R, et al. Short- and long-term experience with flecainide acetate in the management of refractory life-threatening ventricular arrhythmias. *J Am Coll Cardiol* 6:772–779, 1985.

Legrand V, et al. Hemodynamic effects of a new antiarrhythmic agent, flecainide (R818), in coronary artery disease. *Am J Cardiol* 51:422–426, 1983.

Marcus F. The hazards of using type 1C antiarrhythmic drugs for the treatment of paroxsymal atrial fibrillation. *Am J Cardiol* 66:366–367, 1990.

Meinertz T, et al. Long-term antiarrhythmic therapy with flecainide. *Am J Cardiol* 54:91–96, 1984.

Nathan AW, et al. Proarrhythmic effects of the new antiarrhythmic agent flecainide acetate. *Am Heart J* 107:222–228, 1984.

Oetgen WJ, et al. Clinical and electrophysiologic assessment of oral flecainide acetate for recurrent ventricular tachycardia: Evidence for exacerbation of electrical instability. *Am J Cardiol* 52:746–750, 1983.

Pieterson AH, Helleman H. Usefulness of flecainide for prevention of paroxysmal atrial fibrillation and flutter. *Am J Cardiol* 67:713–717, 1991.

Platia EV, et al. Flecainide: Electrophysiologic and antiarrhythmic properties in refractory ventricular tachycardia. *Am J Cardiol* 55:956–962, 1985.

Pritchett ELC, et al. Flecainide acetate treatment of paroxysmal supraventricular tachycardia and paroxysmal atrial fibrillation: Dose-response studies. *J Am Coll Cardiol* 17:297–303, 1991.

Pritchett ELC, Wilkinson WE. Mortality in patients treated with flecainide and encainide for supraventricular arrhythmia. *Am J Cardiol* 67:976–980, 1991.

Suttorp MJ, et al. The value of class 1C antiarrhythmic drugs for acute conversion of paroxysmal atrial fibrillation or flutter to sinus rhythm. *J Am Coll Cardiol* 16:1722–1727, 1990.

Symposium on flecainide acetate. *Am J Cardiol* 53:1B–122B, 1984.

Vik-Mo H, Ohm O, Lund-Johansen P. Electrophysiologic effects of flecainide acetate in patients with sinus nodal dysfunction. *Am J Cardiol* 50:1090–1094, 1982.

Propafenone

Brodsky MA, et al. Propafenone therapy for ventricular tachycardia in the setting of congestive heart failure. *Am Heart J* 110:794–799, 1985.

Chilson DA, et al. Electrophysiologic effects and clinical efficacy of oral propafenone therapy in patients with ventricular tachycardia. *J Am Coll Cardiol* 5:1407–1413, 1985.

Connolly SJ, et al. Clinical efficacy and electrophysiology of oral propafenone for ventricular tachycardia. *Am J Cardiol* 52:1208–1213, 1983.

Connolly SJ, et al. Clinical pharmacology of propafenone. *Circulation* 68:589–596, 1983.

de Soyza N, et al. Effect of propafenone in patients with stable ventricular arrhythmias. *Am Heart J* 108:285–289, 1984.

Dinh H, et al. Efficacy of propafenone compared with quinidine in chronic ventricular arrhythmias. *Am J Cardiol* 55:1520–1524, 1985.

Doherty JU, et al. Limited role of intravenous propafenone hydrochloride in the treatment of sustained ventricular tachycardia: Electrophysiologic effects and results of programmed ventricular stimulation. *J Am Coll Cardiol* 4:378–381, 1984.

Funck-Brentano C, et al. Propafenone. *N Engl J Med* 322:518–525, 1990.

Hernandez M, Reder RF, Marinchak RA. Propafenone for malignant ventricular arrhythmia: An analysis of the literature. *Am Heart J* 121:1178–1184, 1991.

Manz M, Steinbeck G, Luderitz B. Usefulness of programmed stimulation in predicting efficacy of propafenone in long term antiarrhythmic therapy or paroxysmal supraventricular tachycardia. *Am J Cardiol* 56:593–597, 1985.

Naccarella F, et al. Comparison of propafenone and disopyramide for treatment of chronic ventricular arrhythmias. Placebo-controlled, double blind, randomized cross-over study. *Am Heart J* 109:833–839, 1985.

Naccarella F, et al. Propafenone for refractory ventricular arrhythmias: Correlation with drug plasma levels during long-term treatment. *Am J Cardiol* 54:1008–1014, 1984.

Podrid P, Lown B. Propafenone: A new agent for ventricular arrhythmia. *J Am Coll Cardiol* 4:117–125, 1984.

Pritchett ELC, McCarthy EA, Wilkinson WE. Propafenone treatment of symptomatic paroxysmal supraventricular arrhythmias. *Ann Intern Med* 114:539–544, 1991.

Recent advances in antiarrhythmic therapy: Symposium on propafenone. *Am J Cardiol* 54:10D–71D, 1984.

Salerno DM, et al. A controlled trial of propafenone for treatment of frequent and repetitive ventricular premature complexes. *Am J Cardiol* 53:77–83, 1984.

Salerno DM, Hodges M. New therapy focus: Propafenone. *Cardiovasc Rev Rep* 6:924–931, 1985.

Shen EN, et al. Electrophysiologic and hemodynamic effects of intravenous propafenone in patients with recurrent ventricular tachycardia. *J Am Coll Cardiol* 3:1291–1297, 1984.

Yeung-lai-wah JA, et al. Propafenone-mexiletine combination for the treatment of sustained ventricular tachycardia. *J Am Coll Cardiol* 20:547–551, 1992.

Type 3 Antiarrhythmics

Bretylium

Duff HJ, et al. Bretylium: Relations between plasma concentrations and pharmacologic actions in high frequency ventricular arrhythmias. *Am J Cardiol* 55:395–401, 1985.

Greene HL, et al. Failure of bretylium to suppress inducible ventricular tachycardia. *Am Heart J* 105:717–721, 1983.

Haynes RE, et al. Comparison of bretylium tosylate and lidocaine in management of out of hospital ventricular fibrillation: A randomized clinical trial. *Am J Cardiol* 48:353–356, 1981.

Heissenbuttel RH, Bigger JT, Bretylium tosylate: A newly available antiarrhythmic drug for ventricular arrhythmias. *Ann Intern Med* 91:229–238, 1979.

Koch-Weser J. Bretylium. *N Engl J Med* 300:473–477, 1979.

Patterson E, Lucchesi BR. Bretylium: A prototype for future development of antidysrhythmic agents. *Am Heart J* 106:426–431, 1983.

Amiodarone

Coumel P, Fidelle J. Amiodarone in the treatment of cardiac arrhythmias in children: One hundred thirty-five cases. *Am Heart J* 100:1063–1069, 1980.

Dusman RE, et al. Clinical features of amiodarone-induced pulmonary toxicity. *Circulation* 82:51–59, 1990.

Evans SJL, et al. Highdose amiodarone loading: Electrophysiologic effects and clinical tolerance. *J Am Coll Cardiol* 19:169–173, 1992.

Fogoros RN, et al. Amiodarone: Clinical efficacy and toxicity in 96 patients with recurrent drug refractory arrhythmias. *Circulation* 68:88–94, 1983.

Gomes JAC, et al. Electrophysiologic effects and mechanisms of termination of supraventricular tachycardia by intravenous amiodarone. *Am Heart J* 107:214–221, 1984.

Greene HL, et al. Toxic and therapeutic effects of amiodarone in the treatment of cardiac arrhythmias. *J Am Coll Cardiol* 2:1114–1128, 1983.

Haffajee CI, et al. Clinical pharmacokinetics and efficacy of amiodarone for refractory tachyarrhythmias. *Circulation* 67:1347–1355, 1983.

Hamer A, et al. The potentiation of warfarin anticoagulation by amiodarone. *Circulation* 65:1025–1029, 1982.

Harris L, et al. Side effects of long-term amiodarone therapy. *Circulation* 67:45–51, 1983.

Heger JJ, et al. Amiodarone. Clinical efficacy and electrophysiology during long-term therapy for recurrent ventricular tachycardia or ventricular fibrillation. *N Engl J Med* 305:539–545, 1981.

Herre JM, et al. Long-term results of amiodarone therapy in patients with recurrent sustained ventricular tachycardia or ventricular fibrillation. *J Am Coll Cardiol* 13:442–449, 1989.

Horowitz LN, et al. Usefulness of electrophysiologic testing in evaluation of amiodarone therapy for sustained ventricular tachyarrhythmias associated with coronary heart disease. *Am J Cardiol* 55:367–371, 1985.

Kaski JC, et al. Long-term management of sustained, recurrent symptomatic ventricular tachycardia with amiodarone. *Circulation* 64:273–279, 1981.

Kim SG, et al. Rapid suppression of spontaneous ventricular arrhythmias during oral amiodarone loading. *Ann Intern Med* 117:197–201, 1992.

Marchlinski FE, et al. Amiodarone pulmonary toxicity. *Ann Intern Med* 97:839–845, 1982.

Marcus FI, et al. Clinical pharmacology and therapeutic applications of the antiarrhythmic agent, amiodarone. *Am Heart J* 101:480–493, 1981.

McGovern B, et al. Long-term clinical outcome of ventricular tachycardia or fibrillation treated with amiodarone. *Am J Cardiol* 53:1558–1563, 1984.

McGovern B, Garan H, Ruskin JN. Serious adverse effects of amiodarone. *Clin Cardiol* 7:131–137, 1984.

Morady F, et al. Long-term efficacy and toxicity of high-dose amiodarone therapy for ventricular tachycardia or ventricular fibrillation. *Am J Cardiol* 53:975–979, 1983.

Morady F, et al. Intravenous amiodarone in the acute treatment of recurrent symptomatic ventricular tachycardia. *Am J Cardiol* 51:155–159, 1983.

Mostow ND, et al. Amiodarone: Intravenous loading for rapid suppression of complex ventricular arrhythmias. *J Am Coll Cardiol* 4:97–104, 1984.

Naccarelli GV, et al. Amiodarone: Risk factors for recurrence of symptomatic ventricular tachycardia identified at electrophysiology study. *J Am Coll Cardiol* 6:814–821, 1985.

Nademanee K, et al. Amiodarone in refractory life-threatening ventricular arrhythmias. *Ann Intern Med* 98:577–584, 1983.

Nicklas JM, et al. Prospective, double-blind, placebo-controlled trial of low-dose amiodarone in patients with severe heart failure and asymptomatic ventricular ectopy. *Am Heart J* 122:1016–1021, 1991.

Podrid PJ, Lown B. Amiodarone therapy in symptomatic sustained refractory atrial and ventricular tachyarrhythmias. *Am Heart J* 101:374–379, 1981.

Raeder EA, Podrid PJ, Lown B. Side effects and complications of amiodarone therapy. *Am Heart J* 109:975–983, 1985.

Remme WJ, et al. Hemodynamic effects and tolerability of intravenous amiodarone in patients with impaired left ventricular function. *Am Heart J* 122:96–103, 1991.

Rosenbaum MB, et al. Clinical efficacy of amiodarone as an antiarrhythmic agent. *Am J Cardiol* 38:934–944, 1976.

Rotmench HH, Belhassen B, Swanson BN. Steady state serum amiodarone concentrations: Relationships with antiarrhythmic efficacy and toxicity. *Ann Intern Med* 101:462–469, 1984.

Saksena S, et al. Clinical efficacy and electropharmacology of continuous intravenous amiodarone infusion and chronic oral amiodarone in refractory ventricular tachycardia. *Am J Cardiol* 54:347–352, 1985.

Shannon JA, Hammill SC, Gersh BJ. Predictive value of early electrophysiologic testing in determining long-term outcome with amiodarone treatment in patients with sustained ventricular tachycardia. *Mayo Clin Proc* 66:1114–1119, 1991.

Sobol SM, Rakita L. Pneumonitis and pulmonary fibrosis associated with amiodarone treatment: A possible complication of a new antiarrhythmic drug. *Circulation* 65:819–824, 1982.

The place of amiodarone in cardiology today (Symposium). *Br J Clin Pract* 40(Suppl 44):1–163, 1986.

Toivonen L, Kadish A, Morady F. A prospective comparison of class IA, B and C antiarrhythmic agents in combination with amiodarone in patients with inducible sustained ventricular tachycardia. *Circulation* 84:101–108, 1991.

Veltri EP, et al. Amiodarone in the treatment of life-threatening ventricular tachycardia: Role of Holter monitoring in predicting long term clinical efficacy. *Am J Coll Cardiol* 6:806–813, 1985.

Veltri EP, et al. Results of programmed electrical stimulation and long term electrophysiologic effects of amiodarone therapy in patients with refractory ventricular tachycardia. *Am J Cardiol* 55:375–379, 1985.

Waxman HL, et al. Amiodarone for control of sustained ventricular tachyarrhythmia: Clinical and electrophysiologic effects in 51 patients. *Am J Cardiol* 50:1066–1074, 1982.

Weinberg BA, et al. Five-year follow-up of 589 patients treated with amiodarone. *Am Heart J* 125:109–121, 1993.

Wellens HJJ, et al. A comparison of the electrophysiologic effects of intravenous and oral amiodarone in the same patient. *Circulation* 69:120–124, 1984.

Wilson JS, Podrid PJ. Side effects from amiodarone. *Am Heart J* 121:158–171, 1991.

Winkle RA. Amiodarone and the American way. *J Am Coll Cardiol* 6:822–824, 1985.

Zipes DP, Prystowsky EN, Heger JJ. Amiodarone: Electrophysiologic actions, pharmacokinetics and clinical effects. *J Am Coll Cardiol* 3:1059–1071, 1984.

Unclassified Type 1 Antiarrhythmics
Bhandari AK, et al. Electrophysiologic evaluation of moricizine in patients with sustained ventricular tachyarrhythmias: Low efficacy and high incidence of proarrhythmia. *PACE* 16:1853–1861, 1993.

CAST II Investigators. Effect of the antiarrhythmic agent moricizine on survival after myocardial infarction. *N Engl J Med* 327:227–233, 1992.

Chazov EI, Shugushev KK, Rosenshtraukh LV. Ethmozin: I. Effects of intravenous drug administration on paroxysmal supraventricular tachycardia in the ventricular preexcitation syndrome. *Am Heart J* 108:475–482, 1984. II. Effects of intravenous drug administration on atrio-ventricular nodal reentrant tachycardia. *Am Heart J* 108:483–489, 1984.

Chiale PA, Przybylski J, Halpern MS. Comparative effects of ajmaline on intermittent bundle branch block and the Wolff-Parkinson-White syndrome. *Am J Cardiol* 39:651–657, 1977.

Chiale PA, et al. Electrocardiographic changes evoked by ajmaline in chronic Chagas' disease without manifest myocarditis. *Am J Cardiol* 49:14–20, 1982.

Chiale PA, et al. Usefulness of the ajmaline test in patients with latent bundle branch block. *Am J Cardiol* 49:21–26, 1982.

Clyne C, Estes NAM, Wang PJ. Moricizine. *N Engl J Med* 327:255–260, 1992.

Connolly SJ, et al. Clinical efficacy and electrophysiology of imipramine for ventricular tachycardia. *Am J Cardiol* 53:516–521, 1984.

Damle R, et al. Efficacy and risks of morcizine in inducible sustained ventricular tachycardia. *Ann Intern Med* 116:375–381, 1992.

Giardina EGV, Bigger JT. Antiarrhythmic effect of imipramine hydrochloride in patients with ventricular premature complexes without physiological depression. *Am J Cardiol* 50:172–179, 1982.

Giardina EGV, et al. The electrocardiographic and antiarrhythmic effects of imipramine hydrochloride at therapeutic plasma concentrations. *Circulation* 60: 1045–1052, 1979.

Giardina EGV, et al. Effect of imipramine and nortriptyline on left ventricular function and blood pressure in patients treated with arrhythmias. *Am Heart J* 109:992–998, 1985.

Mann DE, et al. Electrophysiologic effects of ethmozin in patients with ventricular tachycardia. *Am Heart J* 107:674–679, 1984.

Marshall JB, Forker AD. Cardiovascular effects of tricyclic antidepressant drugs: Therapeutic usage, overdose, and management of complications. *Am Heart J* 103:401–414, 1982.

Morganroth J. Safety and efficacy of a twice-daily dosing regimen for moricizine (ethmozine). *Am Heart J* 110:1188–1192, 1985.

Obayashi K, et al. Cardiovascular effects of ajmaline. *Am Heart J* 92:487–496, 1976.

Podrid PJ, et al. Ethmozin, a new antiarrhythmic drug for suppressing ventricular premature complexes. *Circulation* 61:450–457, 1980.

Powell AC, et al. Electrophysiologic response to moricizine in patients with sustained ventricular arrhythmias. *Ann Intern Med* 116:382–387, 1992.

Pratt CM, et al. Efficacy and safety of moricizine in patients with congestive heart failure: A summary of the experience in the United States. *Am Heart J* 119:1–7, 1990.

Pratt CM, et al. Ethmozine suppression of single and repetitive ventricular premature depolarizations during therapy: Documentation of efficacy and long-term safety. *Am Heart J* 106:85–91, 1983.

Schlarovsky S, et al. Paroxysmal atrial flutter and fibrillation associated with preexcitation syndrome: treatment with ajmaline. *Am J Cardiol* 48:929–933, 1981.

Seaborg SM, Cowan MD. Moricizine-induced proarrhythmia. *Clin Cardiol* 15:866–867, 1992.

Singh SN, et al. Effect of moricizine hydrochloride in reducing chronic high-frequency ventricular arrhythmia: Results of a prospective, controlled trial. *Am J Cardiol* 53: 745–750, 1984.

Tschaidse O, et al. The prevalence of proarrhythmic events during moricizine therapy and their relationship to ventricular function. *Am Heart J* 124:912–916, 1992.

Other Antiarrhythmics

Belhassen B, Pelleg A. Adenosine triphosphate and adenosine: Perspectives in the acute management of paroxysmal supraventricular tachycardia. *Clin Cardiol* 8:460–464, 1985.

Belhassen B, Pelleg A. Electrophysiologic effects of adenosine triphosphate and adenosine on the mammalian heart: Clinical and experimental aspects. *J Am Coll Cardiol* 4:414–424, 1984.

Berne RM, DiMarco JP, Belardinelli L. Dromotropic effects of adenosine and adenosine antagonists in the treatment of cardiac arrhythmias involving the atrioventricular node. *Circulation* 69:1195–1197, 1984.

Camm AJ, Garratt CJ. Adenosine and supraventricular tachycardia. *N Engl J Med* 325:1621–1629, 1991.

DiMarco JP, et al. Adenosine: Electrophysiologic effects and therapeutic use for terminating paroxysmal supraventricular tachycardia. *Circulation* 68:1254–1263, 1983.

DiMarco JP, et al. Adenosine for paroxsymal supraventricular tachycardia: Dose ranging and comparison with verapamil. *Ann Intern Med* 113:104–110, 1990.

DiMarco JP, et al. Diagnostic and therapeutic use of adenosine in patients with supraventricular tachyarrhythmias. *J Am Coll Cardiol* 6:417–425, 1985.

Favale S, et al. Effect of adenosine and adenosine-5′-triphosphate on atrioventricular conduction in patients. *J Am Coll Cardiol* 5:1212–1219, 1985.

Freilich A, Tepper D. Adenosine and its cardiovascular effects. *Am Heart J* 123:1324–1328, 1992.

Garratt CJ, et al. Effects of intravenous adenosine on antegrade refractoriness of accessory atrioventricular connections. *Circulation* 84:1962–1968, 1991.

Garratt CJ, et al. Comparison of adenosine and verapamil for termination of paroxysmal junctional tachycardia. *Am J Cardiol* 64:1310–1316, 1989.

Hood MA, Smith WM. Adenosine versus verapamil in the treatment of supraventricular tachycardia: A randomized double-crossover trial. *Am Heart J* 123:1543–1549, 1992.

Lerman BB. Response of nonreentrant catecholamine-mediated ventricular tachycardia to endogenous adenosine and acetylcholine. *Circulation* 87:382–390, 1993.

Lerman BB, Belardinelli L. Cardiac electrophysiology of adenosine. *Circulation* 83:1499–1509, 1991.

Wilber DJ, et al. Adenosine-sensitive ventricular tachycardia. *Circulation* 87:126–134, 1993.

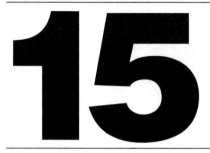

Controversies in Arrhythmia Management— I. The Noninvasive Approach

Philip J. Podrid

Of the options available for the treatment of patients with serious or symptomatic arrhythmia—pharmacologic therapy with an antiarrhythmic drug, surgery, catheter ablation, or an implantable device—pharmacologic therapy is often used first. Nonpharmacologic therapies such as catheter ablation utilizing radiofrequency energy, arrhythmia surgery, or an implantable device are very effective approaches and for some arrhythmias and in some patients are preferred. Thus, there is a growing use of radiofrequency ablation as primary and "curative" therapy for supraventricular tachyarrhythmias that involve the atrioventricular node or an accessory pathway and of implantable defibrillators in patients with serious ventricular tachyarrhythmias. However, it remains uncertain if such methods are better than or preferable to pharmacologic therapy or if they should be used in only certain patients. There are as yet no definite comparative data regarding pharmacologic and nonpharmacologic therapy of arrhythmias, but there are some suggestive data about long-term outcome. Despite the growing use of nonpharmacologic techniques, antiarrhythmic drug therapy still has an important role, and for many patients it is the first approach to management. Although there is still controversy about the best methods for drug selection (invasive versus noninvasive), recent data can provide assistance.

I. **Initial approach to therapy.** Often this approach is pharmacologic, and generally if the patient fails to respond to antiarrhythmic agents, nonpharmacologic approaches are used. However, even when surgery, ablation, or an implantable device is preferred or is necessary, pharmacologic therapy with an antiarrhythmic drug is often still required and the majority of patients receiving nonpharmacologic therapy (up to 70% in some reports) will require an antiarrhythmic drug to reduce the frequency of the clinical arrhythmia, suppress other arrhythmias (such as nonsustained ventricular tachycardia or atrial fibrillation) that may result in device discharge, or slow the rate of the arrhythmia, making it more amenable to termination with overdrive pacing and precluding the need for high-energy defibrillation.

There are a number of antiarrhythmic drugs available, each one unique, and there is no way to predict the response to an agent based on the effect of another drug. Nor are there any reliable guidelines for the selection of an effective and safe agent, because there is nothing about the electrophysiologic actions of the drug, its pharmacologic properties, the nature and extent of the underlying heart disease, or the etiology of the clinical arrhythmia that provides helpful information in drug selection. There are several ways that a drug may be selected for the individual patient, and all involve the administration of the agent:

1. Empiric therapy is not justified if some end point for drug activity is necessary to establish a beneficial or harmful effect of the agent.
2. Relief of symptoms may be an appropriate end point when the only reason for therapy is symptom relief. In such cases, the persistence of the arrhythmia may not be important if symptoms are abolished. However, potentially serious arrhythmia often causes no symptoms.
3. Drug blood levels do not predict drug efficacy, nor do they necessarily correlate with toxicity. Therefore, they are not helpful for establishing drug action, but rather confirm patient compliance and adequate drug absorption.
4. Interval changes on the ECG are commonly seen with the antiarrhythmic drugs and represent an effect of the drug on the myocardium. However, these changes do not correlate with drug efficacy.
5. The signal-averaged ECG provides information useful for risk stratification of certain groups of patients but is not helpful in the evaluation of antiarrhythmic drug effect.

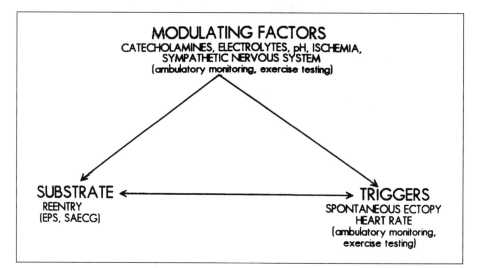

Fig. 15-1. Interrelationship of substrate, triggers, modulating factors, and role of invasive and noninvasive methods. (EPS = electrophysiologic study; SAECG = signal-averaged ECG.)

    6. Noninvasive ambulatory monitoring and exercise testing provide objective informa- tion about drug efficacy based on the suppression of spontaneous arrhythmia [1, 2].
    7. Invasive electrophysiologic testing provides objective information about drug effica- cy based on the induction of clinical arrhythmia [3, 4].

II. Drug selection: Invasive versus noninvasive methods. The only two reliable methods for evaluation of antiarrhythmic drugs and selection of an effective agent are noninva- sive and invasive methods. Although these two approaches are based on vastly different concepts, both are useful methods for the selection of an antiarrhythmic drug. Indeed, each provides important data, which are complementary, regarding the occurrence of serious ventricular or supraventricular arrhythmia and its prevention.

    A. Arrhythmogenesis. This involves three separate but interrelated concerns. (Fig. 15-1):

        1. An abnormal substrate, the myocardium, which as a result of damage caused by some disease process has heterogeneous electrophysiologic properties that promote arrhythmogenesis, the most common mechanism being reentry. The potential for the substrate to generate and sustain an arrhythmia—its stabili- ty, excitability, or irritability—can best be evaluated by electrophysiologic testing.
        2. Triggers that interact with the abnormal substrate, activating or initiating the mechanisms for arrhythmia, resulting in the occurrence of the clinical arrhyth- mia. Such triggers include spontaneous ectopic beats or change in heart rate. Ven- tricular ectopic beats, particularly runs of nonsustained ventricular tachycardia (VT) (three sequential ectopic beats), may also serve as markers for the ability of the substrate to generate a sustained arrhythmia; they are indicators of poten- tially active reentrant circuits. Hence, nonsustained VT is possibly a self-limited form of a sustained VT and may indicate the potential for a sustained ventricular tachyarrhythmia resulting from a reentrant circuit. Under appropriate circum- stances a nonsustained episode may become a sustained arrhythmia. These trig- gers, spontaneous ectopy, are best evaluated with extended ambulatory monitor- ing and exercise testing.
        3. Many modulating factors such as inputs from the autonomic nervous system, cat- echolamine levels, electrolytes, pH changes, and ischemia, which can alter the electrophysiologic properties of the myocardium and its ability to generate and sustain an arrhythmia. These factors can also alter the triggers, that is, change the frequency of spontaneous ectopy, or affect heart rate. These modulating fac- tors are highly variable, changing instantaneously, unpredictably, and frequently throughout the day and from day to day. They are best evaluated with extended

ambulatory monitoring and exercise testing; electrophysiologic testing, which is performed at only one point in time, is generally less helpful.

The interaction among these three factors, and possibly others, explains the unpredictability and sporadic occurrences of a clinical arrhythmia. It would seem reasonable that using both invasive and noninvasive methods would maximize the ability to identify a drug or combination of drugs that effectively prevent the recurrence of arrhythmia.

B. Choosing the method. The two approaches for drug selection have unique strengths and weaknesses (Tables 15-1 and 15-2). It is, however, the limitations of the techniques that primarily influence the method chosen by the physician.

   1. Noninvasive approach. Perhaps the most important limitation associated with noninvasive ambulatory monitoring is the random variability of spontaneous arrhythmia [5]. It is now well established that the presence, type, and frequency of ventricular arrhythmia vary from hour to hour and day to day—in some patients, tremendously (Fig. 15-2). Such variability is of particular concern when evaluating antiarrhythmic drugs since it can hinder the ability to distinguish between a true drug effect and a random change. In order to use ambulatory monitoring for drug selection, spontaneous ventricular arrhythmia must be frequent and reproducibly present from day to day so as to establish reliably that a change in arrhythmia is a result of the intervention. Arrhythmia must be of a high density and of repetitive forms; particularly nonsustained VT must be reproducibly present. Such forms are likely indicators of active reentrant circuits, and their suppression suggests that the electrophysiologic properties of the reentrant circuit have been altered, and its ability to generate a reentrant arrhythmia has been eliminated.

   Another concern is the definition of drug efficacy. Although a certain percentage reduction in arrhythmia frequency constitutes an antiarrhythmic effect, this may not be the same as efficacy for preventing a sustained arrhythmia. Other

Table 15-1. Noninvasive techniques

Strengths	Weaknesses
Widely available	Requires high density of arrhythmia
Easily performed	Frequent complex forms must be present
Inexpensive (relatively)	Arrhythmia must be reproducibly present
Can be repeated as often as necessary	No uniform criteria for drug efficacy
Results easy to interpret	Different criteria for drug effect (VPB
Normal physiologic changes evaluated	suppression) vs. drug efficacy
Can follow patients over time as substrate changes	(prevention of sustained arrhythmia)

VPB = ventricular premature beats.

criteria, which include arrhythmia reduction and elimination of repetitive

Table 15-2. Invasive techniques

Strengths	Weaknesses
Arrhythmia variability unimportant	Morbidity and mortality
Can document and expose clinical arrhythmia as necessary	Costly
	Requires special training and equipment
Useful for localizing arrhythmogenic area	Definition of drug efficacy uncertain
May expose certain groups of patients at risk for sudden death	Many patients not inducible
	Meaning of nonclinical arrhythmia uncertain
	Normal physiologic changes not accounted for
	Reproducibility a concern
	Studies not routinely repeated
	Changes in substrate occurring over time— not evaluated

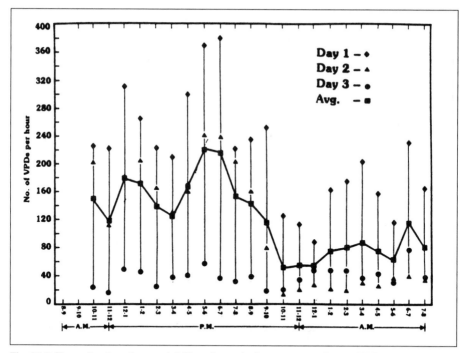

Fig. 15-2. Example of random variability of ventricular premature beats (VPBs) in a patient with coronary artery disease. Presented is the hourly frequency of VPBs during 3 sequential days of ambulatory monitoring in the absence of any intervention. There is a marked difference in VPB frequency over the 3-day period. (From J Morganroth et al. Limitations of routine long-term electrocardiographic monitoring to assess ventricular ectopic frequency. *Circulation* 58:408, 1978.)

arrhythmia, particularly nonsustained VT, have been associated with freedom from recurrence. Suppression of repetitive arrhythmia may be a noninvasive marker for changes in the ability of the substrate to generate and sustain a reentrant arrhythmia.

Despite these limitations, ambulatory monitoring and exercise testing have a number of important strengths:

Noninvasive methods are widely available, easily performed, and can be repeated frequently.

Any symptoms suggesting arrhythmia recurrence can be assessed promptly, and the effect of a new drug or a change in drug dose can be evaluated immediately. The results are easy to interpret.

The many physiologic changes or modulating factors such as electrolyte and pH changes, ischemia, and catecholamines that affect arrhythmia occurrence and interact with antiarrhythmic drug action can be evaluated over an extended period of time, permitting a longer duration of observation.

It must also be remembered that the substrate itself is a moving target and its electrophysiologic properties constantly changing, a result of the progressive nature of the underlying disease process. Monitoring and exercise testing offer attractive approaches to evaluate, over time, the influence that treatment and progressive disease-related changes have on arrhythmogenesis.

2. **Invasive approach.** A strength of invasive electrophysiologic testing is that it eliminates concerns about the random changes of spontaneous arrhythmia since the arrhythmia of interest is what is induced in the laboratory using programmed premature stimulation—the clinical, presenting arrhythmia. For sustained arrhythmias that are sporadic, infrequent, and unpredictable, electrophysiologic testing is necessary for their provocation and to identify a drug that is effective for suppression. If nonpharmacologic therapy is a preferred or neces-

sary approach, electrophysiologic testing is essential for localizing the site of arrhythmia origin (using mapping) or evaluating an implantable device.

Although a very valuable tool, electrophysiologic testing has a number of important limitations:

These methods are costly and require hospitalization.

There is an associated morbidity and mortality, although this is low.

Special equipment and training are necessary for performing these studies and evaluating the results.

This testing is carried out at only one point in time and does not provide any reliable information about the important effects of the many random and variable modulating factors that influence arrhythmogenesis and antiarrhythmic drug action. The underlying disease process itself progresses, and hence the substrate and its electrophysiologic properties change over time. In general, electrophysiologic testing is not repeated routinely in follow-up, and these ongoing, progressive changes are not assessed.

For these reasons, there are concerns about the short- and long-term reproducibility of electrophysiologic testing. A number of investigators have reported that there may be significant differences in the mode of arrhythmia induction from one day to the next, as well as inconsistency in the ability to induce an arrhythmia (Table 15-3). Nonreproducibility has been reported when two baseline studies are compared and has also been observed when the effect of a drug is evaluated on two sequential days. This is not unexpected since the modulating factors that can alter substrate stablity and its electrophysiologic properties and drug effect are highly variable. Moreover, a significant number of patients, particularly those presenting with ventricular fibrillation (VF) or those with a cardiomyopathy, may not have arrhythmia induced, precluding the use of electro-

Table 15-3. Reproducibility of electrophysiologic tests

Study[a]	Number tested	Time between tests	% Reproducible
Livelli	22	3 days	59
Schoenfeld	8	15.6 months	50
Duff	18	5.3 days	60
Lombardi	43	2 days	58
Kudenchuck	114	1 day	83 (1–2 extrastimuli)[b] 78 (3 extrastimuli)[b] 73 (4 extrastimuli)[b]
McPherson	66	3 days	95 (1–2 extrastimuli)[b] 56 (3 extrastimuli)[b]
Ferrick (on drug therapy)	64	3 days	77
Kudenchuk (on drug therapy)	49	3 days	71 55 (same drug levels) 82 (disparate drugs levels)

[a]Livelli FD, et al. Reproducibility of inducible ventricular tachycardia [Abstract]. *Circulation* 66:II–585, 1982; Schoenfeld MH, et al. Long-term reproducibility of responses to programmed cardiac stimulation in spontaneous ventricular tachyarrhythmias. *Am J Cardiol* 54:564–568, 1984; Duff HJ, et al. Lack of reproducibility of inducible ventricular tachycardia over time [Abstract]. *Circulation* 68:III–244, 1980; Lombardi F, et al. Daily reproducibility of electrophysiologic test results in malignant ventricular arrhythmia. *Am J Cardiol* 57:96–101, 1986; McPherson CA, Rosenfeld LE, Batsford WD. Day to day reproducibility of responses to right ventricular programmed electrical stimulation: Implications for serial drug testing. *Am J Cardiol* 55:689–694, 1985; Kudenchuk PJ, et al. Reproducibility of arrhythmia induction with intracardiac electrophysiologic testing: patients with clinical sustained ventricular tachyarrhythmias. *J Am Coll Cardiol* 7:819–828, 1986; Ferrick KJ, et al. Reproducibility of electrophysiologic testing during antiarrhythmic therapy for ventricular arrhythmia secondary to coronary artery disease. *Am J Cardiol* 69:1296–1299, 1992; Kudenchuk PJ, et al. Day-to-day reproducibility of antiarrhythmic drug trials using programmed electrical extrastimulus technique for ventricular tachyarrhythmias. *Am J Cardiol* 66:725–730, 1990.
[b]Number of extrastimuli to induce arrhythmia.

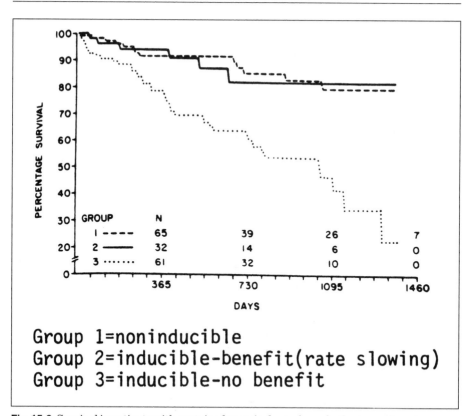

Group 1=noninducible
Group 2=inducible-benefit(rate slowing)
Group 3=inducible-no benefit

Fig. 15-3. Survival in patients with sustained ventricular tachyarrhythmias undergoing electrophysiologic studies for antiarrhythmic drug selection. The survival of group 1 patients (no arrhythmia induced) and group 2 patients (arrhythmia induced but at a slower rate as a result of drug) is identical. Mortality was high in group 3 patients who had no benefit from drug. (From TJ Waller et al. Reduction in sudden death and total mortality by antiarrhythmic therapy evaluated by electrophysiologic testing. *J Am Coll Cardiol* 10:83, 1987.)

physiologic testing. Another concern is the induction of a nonclinical arrhythmia, which has an uncertain meaning. While sustained monomorphic VT is considered to be a reliable and important end point, the importance of polymorphic VT, VF, or even nonsustained VT remains questionable. While these arrhythmias are often considered nonspecific, their significance likely depends on the nature of the underlying heart disease and type of presenting arrhythmia. This is of even greater concern during the evaluation of antiarrhythmic drugs because it is uncertain if the induction of such nonclinical arrhythmia represents a nonspecific response or a change (aggravation) of arrhythmia as a result of the drug, that is, arrhythmia aggravation.

Another important concern is the definition of drug efficacy. The inability to provoke a previously induced sustained ventricular tachyarrhythmia is the goal of drug therapy and the accepted criterion for drug efficacy. If achieved, the arrhythmia recurrence rate and sudden death mortality are significantly reduced. However, antiarrhythmic drug therapy only infrequently prevents arrhythmia induction, and overall only about 30–40% of patients respond to antiarrhythmic drugs when this definition is used. In several studies, other definitions of drug efficacy were employed, particularly slowing of the rate of the induced VT [6, 7]. When this end point is achieved, sudden death mortality is significantly reduced and is identical to that reported when the definition of drug efficacy is noninducibility [6] (Fig. 15-3). The arrhythmia recurrence rate is still high, however, although the arrhythmia is nonfatal. It is possible that for patients who present with VT that has not caused sudden death, a slowing of the tachycardia rate may be acceptable if the goal of therapy is the prevention of sudden death and prolongation of life rather than prevention of all recurrences. For survivors of out-of-hospital sudden death, particularly when due to VF, slowing of a VT rate may not be an acceptable criterion of drug effect and only noninducibility considered reliable.

C. **Studies of methods.** Although these two approaches for the selection of antiarrhythmic drug have their unique strengths and weaknesses, physicians over the years have depended on only one method, and there have been advocates for both approaches. Many studies have reported an improved outcome and a reduction in sudden death mortality when an effective antiarrhythmic drug is selected by either noninvasive ambulatory monitoring and exercise testing or with invasive electrophysiologic testing. The majority of these studies have employed electrophysiologic testing, and it has been felt, therefore, that the data favor an electrophysiologic approach to drug selection. However, this opinion was not based on any controlled studies in which these two methods were compared.

One small study reported by Mitchell and coworkers involved 52 patients who were randomized to drug selection by either electrophysiologic testing or ambulatory monitoring [8]. Sudden death mortality was equally low in both groups, but nonfatal arrhythmia recurrences were more frequent in those undergoing ambulatory monitoring.

Recently reported was the Electrophysiologic Study Versus Electrocardiographic Monitoring (ESVEM) trial, which enrolled patients presenting with VT or VF who had spontaneous ventricular ectopy documented on ambulatory monitoring (>10 ventricular premature beats/hour) and sustained ventricular arrhythmia induced by electrophysiologic testing [9]. Of the 486 eligible patients enrolled, 244 had drug selection guided by ambulatory monitoring and 242 patients underwent electrophysiologic testing for drug evaluation. Seven antiarrhythmic drugs (imipramine, mexiletine, pirmenol, procainamide, quinidine, propafenone, and sotalol) were administered in random fashion. Patients were discharged on an agent that was effective based on suppression of spontaneous ectopy on ambulatory monitoring or noninducibility with electrophysiologic testing.

Of the 244 patients in the Holter monitored group, 188 (77%) responded to an antiarrhythmic drug; 108 of 242 patients (45%) in the electrophysiologic study group responded. Thus, 296 patients were discharged on an effective drug and followed long term. The primary end point of the study was all arrhythmic recurrences, but also sudden death mortality, total mortality, and cardiac mortality were examined.

After a 6-year follow-up, the outcome of patients in the two limbs was identical in regard to each end point evaluated (Fig. 15-4, Table 15-4). However, it took less time to identify an effective drug when ambulatory monitoring was used compared with electrophysiologic testing (10 days vs. 25 days, $p < .0001$). The number of trials in which drugs were effective was greater when assessed noninvasively compared with invasive electrophysiologic testing (38% vs. 15%) and the number of patients in whom an effective drug was identified was higher when ambulatory monitoring was used (77% vs. 45% for electrophysiologic testing). Another surprising finding was that each of the antiarrhythmic drugs was equally effective when evaluated by ambulatory monitoring (45% vs. 67% response rate) (Table 15-5) [10]. When electrophysiologic testing was used, the response rate was also equivalent (Table 15-5) for all drugs (10% vs. 26%), except for sotalol, which was effective in 35% of patients ($p < .001$ compared to other drugs).

Although the ESVEM data confirm the value of both approaches and the equivalent outcome regardless of method used, there have been several criticisms of this study. The most important one concerns the protocol for electrophysiologic testing, which used two extrastimuli delivered at the right ventricular apex for evaluation of drug effect. If the patient did not have arrhythmia induced, stimulation was performed at the right ventricular outflow tract, and if necessary, three extrastimuli were added at the right ventricular apex. During drug evaluation, the protocol necessary to induce arrhythmia in control was repeated. A major criticism therefore relates to the use of only two extrastimuli at the right ventricular apex if this was the induction protocol during the baseline study. Current protocols use three extrastimuli at the apex, regardless of the number used baseline. A second concern is the patient population entered into the study; 73% presented with sustained VT, and only 22% had VF. The remaining 5% had syncope, felt to be due to an arrhythmia, and had VT induced. Despite these criticisms, for the evaluation and therapy of patients with sustained VT or VF who have frequent and reproducible spontaneous arrhythmia on ambulatory monitoring and a sustained ventricular arrhythmia

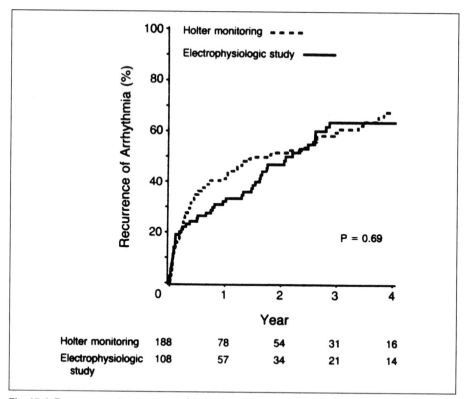

Fig. 15-4. Recurrence of arrhythmia in Electrophysiologic Study Versus Electrographic Monitoring. Patients who had electrophysiologic-guided drug selection are compared to those undergoing Holter monitoring. Recurrence of arrhythmia is identical in the two groups. (From JW Mason for the ESVEM Investigators. A comparison of seven antiarrhythmic drugs in patients with ventricular tachyarrhythmias. *N Engl J Med* 329:445, 1993.)

Table 15-4. Electrophysiologic study versus electrocardiographic monitoring (ESVEM)

	Percentage experiencing arrhythmic events		
	Total group ($N = 297$)	Holter monitor ($N = 189$)	Electrophysiologic study ($N = 108$)
Arrhythmic death	18	15	22
Cardiac arrest	12	13	10
Sustained ventricular tachycardia			
Direct current cardioversion	30	32	27
Drug terminated	8	8	8
Spontaneous termination	18	18	16
Syncope	6	7	4
Nonsustained ventricular tachycardia (>15 beats)	8	7	10
Torsades de pointes	2	1	4

induced by electrophysiologic testing, either approach can be used. When spontaneous ectopy is absent, electrophysiologic testing is necessary.

III. **Risk assessment: Noninvasive versus invasive.** A major concern is the primary prevention of sudden cardiac death by identifying the patient at high risk and intervening with an antiarrhythmic drug determined to be effective. One important group at increased risk for sudden death includes patients with a recent myocardial infarction. Among such patients, the group at highest risk are those who have spontaneous runs of nonsustained VT documented on ambulatory monitoring, especially when left ventricular dysfunction, generally considered to be a left ventricular ejection fraction (LVEF) below 40%, is also present (Table 15-6). Patients at lowest risk have LVEF above 40% and no runs of nonsustained VT. While the presence of nonsustained VT on an ambulatory monitor identifies a high-risk group, it is not helpful for exposing the individual patient at risk. However, when such arrhythmia occurs in association with other noninvasively obtained abnormalities such as left ventricular dysfunction, late potentials on a signal-averaged ECG, absent heart rate variability, and Q–T interval prolongation, risk stratification is improved.

Electrophysiologic testing has also been utilized for risk stratification in postinfarction patients (Table 15-7). A few trials have reported that the induction of arrhythmia with electrophysiologic testing identifies a high-risk patient. However, the majority of studies have reported that electrophysiologic testing is not predictive of outcome in patients after a myocardial infarction. Thus, unlike ambulatory monitoring, electrophysiologic testing has little, if any, value for risk stratification post–myocardial infarction.

Another group at high risk for sudden death are patients with a cardiomyopathy and congestive heart failure. Although data are contradictory, several larger studies have reported a significant association between nonsustained VT documented on ambulatory monitoring and an increased risk for sudden death in these patients, particularly those with type II and III congestive heart failure (Table 15-8). In patients with type IV congestive failure, death is often due to progressive heart failure or a bradyarrhythmia, and the presence of nonsustained VT may not be predictive of sudden or cardiac death. It is also likely that the importance of nonsustained VT is related to the etiology. When coronary artery disease is the cause, this arrhythmia may be of prognostic importance; its significance is questionable when the cardiomyopathy is nonischemic or idiopathic. The role of electrophysiologic testing for risk stratification and prognosis has been reported by a few studies that have involved only a small number of patients (Table 15-9). However, most of these studies have reported that electrophysiologic testing is of little value for identifying the patient with a cardiomyopathy who is at risk for sudden death.

While ambulatory monitoring has a role for risk stratification of patients after a myocardial infarction and in those with a cardiomyopathy—that is, nonsustained VT identifies a patient at a higher risk for sudden death—there are no data that suppression of this arrhythmia will reduce sudden death mortality in these patients. In many

Table 15-5. Drug efficacy in the electrophysiology study versus electrocardiographic monitoring trial

Drug	Number tested	N (%) with adverse effects	Efficacy (%)	
			Holter monitor	Electrophysiologic study
Imipramine	71	43	45	10
Mexiletine	162	27	67	12
Pirmenol	84	23	55	19
Procainamide	116	24	50	26
Propafenone	160	26	48	14
Quinidine	116	24	59	16
Sotalol	196	16	56	35
p value			.347	< .001 (sotalol compared to other drugs)

trials, antiarrhythmic drugs or placebo as randomly administered to all patients after an acute myocardial infarction, and none reported any benefit from antiarrhythmic drugs. However, these trials did not involve arrhythmia suppression, and hence the role of antiarrhythmic drugs cannot be established. However, the Cardiac Arrhythmia Suppression Trial (CAST) did randomize patients with documented ventricular arrhythmia to placebo or an antiarrhythmic drug (encainide, flecainide, or moricizine) determined to be effective for arrhythmia suppression based on ambulatory monitoring [11]. This study was halted prematurely when it was observed that mortality, primarily due to sudden death, was significantly increased in patients receiving encainide or flecainide compared to placebo. Moricizine was not implicated, and the study continued (CAST II), with patients randomized to moricizine or placebo. However, moricizine was subsequently reported to be associated with a higher mortality compared to placebo. This was a disturbing trend, although not statistically significant. However, it should be emphasized that the patients entered into CAST would be considered low risk; only 20% of patients had runs of nonsustained VT, and in only 10% was there more than one run/24 hours. Moreover, the average LVEF of patients in CAST was 39%, and in 52% of patients it was above 40%. Importantly, the low mortality in the placebo groups (3%) is identical to the mortality reported by the many post–myocardial infarction trials among patients without left ventricular dysfunction or nonsustained VT (see Table 15-6). This also suggests that CAST primarily involved low-risk patients.

It seems clear that some antiarrhythmic drugs may be harmful when administered to postinfarction patients who have frequent ventricular premature beats, but this may not be true of all drugs. Several studies have randomized post–myocardial infarction patients to amiodarone or placebo, and each one reported an improved survival in the group receiving amiodarone. Additionally, it is uncertain if antiarrhythmic drugs administered to the high-risk patient—the postinfarction patient with reduced LVEF

Table 15-6. Ventricular arrhythmia after myocardial infarction

Study[a]	Number tested	Duration of monitoring (hr)	Follow-up (mo)	Sudden death (%)	
				No complex VPBs[b]	Complex VPBs
Bigger	820	24	12	12	36
Kotler	160	6	36	20	60
Moss	978	6	36	4	15
Mukharji	388	24	14	3	16
Rappaport	139	24	12	6	34
Ruberman	1739	1	42	8	25
Vismara	64	20	26	11	30
Schultz	81	24	7	0	28
Andresen	1741	24	24	4	15

[a]Bigger JT, Fleiss JL, Rolnitzky LM. The multicenter post-infarction research group. Prevalence, characteristics and significance of ventricular tachycardia detected by 24-hour continuous electrocardiographic recordings in the late hospital phase of acute myocardial infarction. *Am J Cardiol* 58:1151–1160, 1986; Kotler MN, et al. Diagnostic significance of ventricular ectopic beats with respect to sudden death in the late post infarction period. *Circulation* 47:959, 1973; Moss AJ, et al. Ventricular ectopic beats and their relation to sudden and non-sudden cardiac death after myocardial infarction. *Circulation* 60:998–1003, 1979; Mukharji J, et al. The MILIS Study Group Risk Factors and sudden death following acute myocardial infarction: Two year follow-up. *Am J Cardiol* 54:31–36, 1984; Rappaport E, Remedios P. The high risk patient after recovery from myocardial infarction: Recognition and management. *J Am Coll Cardiol* 1:391, 1983; Ruberman W, et al. Ventricular premature complexes and sudden death after myocardial infarction. *Circulation* 64:297–303, 1981; Vismara LA, Amsterdam EA, Mason DT. Relation of ventricular arrhythmias in the late hospital phase of acute myocardial infarction to sudden death after hospital discharge. *Am J Med* 59:6–12, 1975; Schultz RA, Strauss HW, Pitt B. Sudden death in the year following myocardial infarction. Relation to ventricular premature contractions in the late hospital phase of left ventricular ejection fraction. *Am J Med* 62:192–199, 1977; Andresen D, et al. Importance of quantitative analysis of ventricular arrhythmias for predicting the prognosis in low risk post myocardial infarction patients. European Infarction Study Group. *Eur Heart J* 11:529, 1990.
[b]VPB = ventricular premature beats.

Table 15-7. Electrophysiologic studies in patients after myocardial infarction

Study[a]	Number of patients	Follow-up (mos)	Number inducible	Number with arrhythmia	Non-inducible	Number with arrhythmia	Electro-physiologic study prognostic
Hamer	70	12	12 (17)	5 (33)	58 (83)	5 (9)	Yes
Richards	165	12	38 (23)	13 (21)	127 (77)	3 (2)	Yes
Marchlinski	46	18	10 (22)	1 (6)	36 (78)	5 (14)	No
Waspe	50	23	17 (34)	7 (41)	33 (61)	0 (0)	Yes
Roy	150	10	35 (23)	2 (6)	115 (72)	2 (2)	No
Santarelli	50	11	33 (46)	0 (0)	27 (54)	0 (0)	No
Breithardt	132	15	61 (46)	10 (16)	71 (54)	3 (4)	Yes
Bhandari	45	12	20 (44)	2 (10)	35 (56)	1 (3)	No
Gonzales	84	20	19 (23)	0 (0)	65 (77)	4 (6)	No
Kowey	187	18	119 (64)	25 (21)[b]	68 (36)	20 (29)	No
	979		364 (36)	65 (18)	615 (65)	43 (7)	

Note: Figures in parentheses are percentages.

[a]Hamer A, et al. Prediction of sudden death by electrophysiologic studies in high risk patients surviving acute myocardial infarction. *Am J Cardiol* 50:223, 1982; Richards DA, et al. Ventricular instability: A predictor of death after myocardial infarction. *Am J Cardiol* 51:75, 1983; Marchlinski FE, et al. Identifying patients at risk of sudden death after myocardial infarction: Value of the response to programmed stimulation, degree of ventricular ectopic activity, and severity of left ventricular dysfunction. *Am J Cardiol* 52:1190, 1983; Waspe LE, et al. Prediction of sudden death and spontaneous ventricular tachycardia in survivors of complicated myocardial infarction. Value of the response to programmed stimulation using a maximum of three ventricular stimuli. *J Am Coll Cardiol* 5:192, 1985; Roy D, et al. Programmed ventricular stimulation in survivors of an acute myocardial infarction. *Circulation* 72:487, 1985; Santarelli P, et al. Ventricular arrhythmia induced by programmed ventricular stimulation after acute myocardial infarction. *Am J Cardiol* 55:391, 1985; Breithardt G, Borggrefe M, Haerten L. Role of programmed ventricular simulation and non invasive recording of ventricular late potentials for the identification of patients at risk of ventricular tachyarrhythmias after acute myocardial infarction. In Zipes D, Jalife J (eds). *Cardiac Electrophysiology and Arrhythmia.* New York: Grune & Stratton; Bhandari AJ, et al. Frequency and significance of induced sustained ventricular tachycardia or fibrillation two weeks after acute myocardial infarction. *Am J Cardiol* 56:737, 1985; Gonzales R, et al. Programmed electrical stimulation of the heart does not identify patients at high risk post myocardial infarction [abstr]. *Circulation* 40:II–19, 1984; Kowey P, Waxman HL, Greenspon A. Value of electrophysiologic testing in patients with previous myocardial infarction and nonsustained ventricular tachycardia. *Am J Cardiol* 65:594, 1990.

[b]Sustained ventricular tachycardia in 65 (35%) and nonsustained ventricular tachycardia in 54 (29%).

and nonsustained VT—will decrease sudden death mortality; no study to date has evaluated this group of patients.

The role of antiarrhythmic drug therapy in patients with nonsustained VT and cardiomyopathy is also uncertain because placebo-controlled antiarrhythmic studies are lacking. There are a few small, uncontrolled trials that have suggested benefit, and data regarding amiodarone are promising but not conclusive. Several ongoing studies involve the use of antiarrhythmic drug therapy, primarily amiodarone, in such patients.

IV. **Supraventricular tachycardia: Invasive versus noninvasive.** Supraventricular tachycardia (SVT), including AV nodal reentrant tachycardia (AVNRT) or AV reentrant tachycardia (AVRT) associated with an accessory pathway, is sporadic and unpredictable in occurrence. Unlike the situation with ventricular tachyarrhythmias, there does not appear to be a correlation between the presence, frequency, and repetitiveness of spontaneous atrial arrhythmia and the occurrence of a sustained SVT, although studies have not addressed this issue.

A. **Noninvasive method.** In general, ambulatory monitoring has a limited role in the evaluation and management of patients with paroxysmal SVT, although infrequently exercise testing may be of benefit, particularly when SVT is related to exertion or an elevated catecholamine level. If SVT occurs often and is associated with minor symptoms, drug therapy can be given empirically, with efficacy defined as freedom from recurrence evaluated noninvasively (symptoms, ambulatory, or transtelephonic monitoring). Such an approach may be effective since these arrhythmias are generally not life threatening. In some cases, a loading dose of an antiarrhythmic drug (or combination of drugs) can be given for an episode of SVT, and if the arrhythmia terminates within 1½–3 hours, the drug is felt to be effective.

Table 15-8. Prognostic significance of nonsustained ventricular tachycardia in patients with congestive heart failure

Study*	Number of patients	Follow-up (mo)	Prognosis of sudden death
Huang	35	34	No
Wilson	77	12	No
Meinertz	74	11	Yes
Von Olshausen	60	12	No
Holmes	43	14	Yes
Chakko	43	16	Yes
Unverferth	61	12	Yes
Costanzo-Nordin	55	16	No
Follansbee	19	19	Yes
Gradman	295	16	Yes
Keogh	137	10	Yes

*Huang SK, Messer JV, Denes P. Significance of ventricular tachycardia in idiopathic dilated cardiomyopathy: Observation in 35 patients. *Am J Cardiol* 51:507–512, 1983; Wilson JR, et al. Prognosis in severe heart failure: Relation to hemodynamic measurements and ventricular ectopic activity. *J Am Coll Cardiol* 2:403–410, 1983; Meinertz T, et al. Significance of ventricular arrhythmias in idiopathic dilated cardiomyopathy. *Am J Cardiol* 53:902–907, 1984; Von Olshausen K, et al. Ventricular arrhythmias in idiopathic dilated cardiomyopathy. *Br Heart J* 51:195–201, 1984; Holmes JR, et al. Milrinone in congestive heart failure: Observations in ambulatory arrhythmias (abst). *Circulation* 70:II–11, 1984; Chakko CS, Gheorghiade M. Ventricular arrhythmia in severe heart failure: Incidence, significance and effectiveness of antiarrhythmic therapy. *Am Heart J* 109:497–504, 1985; Unverferth DV, et al. Factors influencing the one-year mortality of dilated cardiomyopathy. *Am J Cardiol* 54:147–152, 1984; Costanzo-Nordin MR, et al. Dilated cardiomyopathy: Functional status, hemodynamics, arrhythmias and prognosis. *Cath Cardiovasc Diag* 11:445–453, 1985; Follansbee WD, Michelson EL, Morganroth J. Unsustained ventricular tachycardia in ambulatory patients. Characteristics associated with sudden cardiac death. *Ann Intern Med* 92:741–747, 1980; Gradman A, et al. for the Captopril Digoxin Study Group. Predictors of total mortality and sudden death in mild to moderate heart failure. *J Am Coll Cardiol* 14:564–590, 1989; Keogh AM, Baron DW, Hickie JB. Prognostic guides in patients with idiopathic or ischemic dilated cardiomyopathy assessed for cardiac transplantation. *Am J Cardiol* 65:903, 1990.

Such "cocktail therapy" may be particularly helpful when SVT is infrequent and relatively well tolerated, producing only moderate symptoms.

This approach precludes the need for long-term drug therapy and may be an alternative to a more invasive treatment, such as radiofrequency ablation. However, an empiric approach does not provide any objective evidence that the drug is in fact effective. Electrophysiologic testing is therefore important in some patients for establishing drug effectiveness. It is essential when SVT occurs infrequently but is associated with severe symptoms. In such cases, empiric or cocktail therapy is not appropriate. It has been argued that since SVT is generally a benign arrhythmia, invasive methods are not essential. However, it seems obvious that such invasive studies, although not mandatory, do result in more rapid identification of an effective antiarrhythmic agent, precluding continued therapy with a drug that may be ineffective or even potentially harmful.

B. **Invasive method.** The role of electrophysiologic testing for SVT management has recently expanded with the increasing use of radiofrequency ablation of the AV node. This approach is said to be "curative" of SVT. However, radiofrequency ablation is associated with some risks, albeit infrequent. There is the potential for complete heart block, catheter-induced complication, and possible excessive x-ray exposure. Moreover, long-term follow-up of patients is not yet available. The recurrence rate of SVT or occurrence of other arrhythmias is not well established. It is not yet certain if ablation is preferable to antiarrhythmic therapy because there are no controlled trials comparing these two therapeutic modalities. It remains unknown if all patients with SVT should have AV nodal ablation or if it should be reserved for those refractory to or intolerant of drugs, those with severe symptoms, or those with SVT in association with an accessory pathway, particularly the Wolff-Parkinson-White (WPW) syndrome. In such patients, SVT may be associated with or precipitate atrial fibrillation, a potentially serious arrhythmia that can result in VF and sudden death. In reality, however, this risk is extremely low.

Table 15-9. Role of electrophysiologic studies in patients with cardiomyopathy and nonsustained ventricular tachycardia

Study[a]	Number with cardiomyopathy	Number inducible (%)	Follow-up (mo)	Prediction
Veltri	6	3 (50)	23	No
Sulpizi	9	5 (56)	29	No
Das	24	8 (33)	12	No
Poll	20	1 (5)	18	No
Gomes	10	?	30	Yes
Zheutlin	13	7 (54)	22	Yes[b]
Buxton	18 28 CAD	9 (50) 14 CAD	33	No
Hammill	53 25 idiopathic	1 idiopathic	50	No

CAD = coronary artery disease.
[a]Veltri EP, et al. Programmed electrical stimulation and long-term follow-up in asymptomatic, nonsustained ventricular tachycardia. *Am J Cardiol* 56:309–314, 1985; Sulpizi AM, Friehling TD, Kowey PR. Value of electrophysiologic testing in patients with nonsustained ventricular tachycardia. *Am J Cardiol* 59:841–845, 1987; Das SK, et al. Prognostic usefulness of programmed ventricular stimulation in idiopathic dilated cardiomyopathy without symptomatic ventricular arrhythmias. *Am J Cardiol* 58:998–1000, 1986; Poll DS, et al. Usefulness of programmed stimulation in idiopathic dilated cardiomyopathy. *Am J Cardiol* 58:992–997, 1986; Gomes JA, et al. Programmed electrical stimulation in patients with high-grade ventricular ectopy: Electrophysiologic findings and prognosis for survival. *Circulation* 70:43–51, 1984; Zheutlin TA, et al. Programmed electrical stimulation to determine the need for antiarrhythmic therapy in patients with complex ventricular ectopic activity. *Am Heart J* 111:860–867, 1986; Buxton AE, et al. Prognostic factors in nonsustained ventricular tachycardia. *Am J Cardiol* 53:1275, 1984; Hammill SC, et al. Influence of ventricular function and presence or absence of coronary artery disease on results of electrophysiologic testing for asymptomatic nonsustained ventricular tachycardia. *Am J Cardiol* 65:712–728, 1990.
[b]Only noninducibility predictive.

The use of ablation in asymptomatic patients with a WPW pattern on the ECG who have never experienced arrhythmia is controversial. Indeed, the majority of patients with a WPW pattern on the ECG do not have arrhythmia, and these patients do not require pharmacologic or nonpharmacologic therapy. It is well established that not infrequently the WPW pattern resolves over time, a result of age-related changes in the electrophysiologic properties of accessory pathway, particularly prolongation of refractoriness and slowing of conduction.

V. **Management of patients with life-threatening ventricular arrhythmia: Pharmacologic versus nonpharmacologic (device) therapy.** Although ESVEM has provided important comparative data regarding the methods for evaluating antiarrhythmic drugs, a more recent debate about therapy for serious ventricular arrhythmia has focused on the issue of pharmacologic versus nonpharmacologic therapy, primarily the use of the implantable cardioverter-defibrillator (ICD).

Several large series have reported an impressively low yearly sudden death mortality (2–3%) associated with the use of the ICD [12]. Unfortunately, none of these were randomized studies in which the outcome of patients with an ICD was compared to those receiving pharmacologic therapy. There have been attempts to compare the outcome with an ICD with that achieved from pharmacologic therapy, but such studies have been retrospective, comparing two different populations of patients, treated at different points in time and by different investigators.

In a study from one institution, reported by Newman and coworkers, the outcome of 60 patients with an ICD was compared to 120 patients receiving amiodarone [13]. As expected, the sudden death mortality was lower in the ICD group (5% vs. 10%). However, nonsudden death cardiac mortality, which accounted for the major difference in total mortality, was also less in the ICD group (12% vs. 38%), suggesting that these patients were less sick and had less severe heart disease. Despite this probable difference in patient groups, the survival benefit in the ICD group dissipated over time and by 3 years there was no significant difference in total mortality between the two groups (Fig. 15-5).

In a few studies, the actual sudden death rate associated with the ICD was compared to a projected mortality—the mortality rate had the ICD not been present. The projections were based on analysis of the time to the first "appropriate shock"—ICD discharge associated with syncope or symptoms suggesting a ventricular tachyarrhythmia. Using this approach, the assumption made is that the ICD discharge resulted from a ventricular tachyarrhythmia that, in the absence of the ICD, would have resulted in death. However, this is not a valid assumption since it is well established that what is considered an "appropriate shock" may be a result of a symptomatic supraventricular tachyarrhythmia or nonsustained VT that terminated spontaneously but still resulted in a discharge. Even if the cause were a sustained ventricular arrhythmia, this might not have resulted in death. Moreover, it has been reported that the frequency of sustained ventricular tachyarrhythmias is increased after ICD implantation. Hence, the arrhythmia (and ICD discharge) might not have occurred in the absence of the ICD.

Another concern is that although the ICD has reduced sudden death mortality, it may not have any substantial impact in reducing total cardiac mortality. This was suggested by the previously mentioned study in which there was no difference in overall survival at three years [13] (see Fig. 15-5). However, a number of other investigators have also reported this finding. Indeed, Kim and coworkers have emphasized this point, suggesting that by reporting only sudden death mortality in patients with the ICD, the impact on mortality resulting from this technology is overestimated [14]. Other causes of death directly attributable to the device must be considered, including operative and perioperative mortality, which has been as high as 3%. Also included must be other arrhythmia-related deaths such as pulmonary and neurologic complications from recurrent cardiac arrest. Finally, other causes for cardiac death must be considered, among them, progressive congestive heart failure, myocardial infarction and ischemia, bradycardia, and asystole (Fig. 15-6). Thus, the question that needs to be answered is not whether the ICD can effectively terminate a sustained ventricular tachyarrhythmia and prevent sudden death, for this is well established and not arguable; rather, the important issue is whether the ICD can reduce overall mortality among survivors of sudden death compared with the best medical therapy [15]. The patient experiencing a sustained VT or sudden death who is a candidate for the ICD frequently has far advanced heart disease and significant left ventricular dysfunction. Although sudden death may be prevented, these patients will have a high cardiac and total mortality, a result of other cardiac causes, especially progressive congestive heart failure. Many studies reporting the

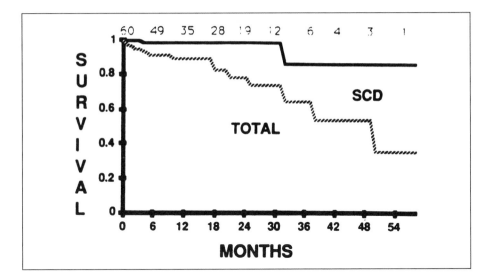

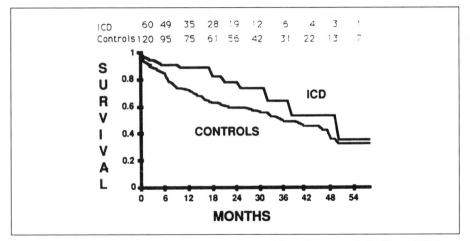

Fig. 15-5. Survival of 60 patients receiving an implantable cardioverter-defibrillator (ICD). **A.** Shows sudden cardiac death (SCD) and total mortality. **B.** Shows total mortality in the ICD group compared to a control group of 120 patients treated with amiodarone. (From D Newman et al. Survival after implantation of the cardioverter defibrillator. *Am J Cardiol* 69:899, 1992. Reprinted with permission.)

long-term follow-up of sudden death survivors have observed that only 20–68% die suddenly. Moreover, not all of these sudden deaths are due to a recurrent ventricular tachyarrhythmia; some are the result of bradycardia or asystole. Moreover, there is no certainty that the ICD will be effective for reverting all tachyarrhythmias. It is estimated, therefore, that the reduction in total mortality attributable to the ICD will be below 33%.

There have been a number of nonrandomized studies suggesting that the ICD does not reduce total mortality. Choue and coworkers reported the survival of 229 patients resuscitated from sudden death who were treated medically and 68 who received an ICD [16]. At 1, 2, 3, and 4 years, the sudden death mortality was, respectively, 8%, 11%, 13%, and 18% in the medical group and 3%, 6%, 9%, and 17% in the ICD group (p = N.S. at all time periods). Total mortality at each time period was no different between the medical and ICD groups (17%, 24%, 28%, and 33% in the medical group and 11%, 17%, 22%, and 33% in the ICD group). Crandale and coworkers studied 194 patients with sudden cardiac death who did not have arrhythmia induced by electrophysiologic stud-

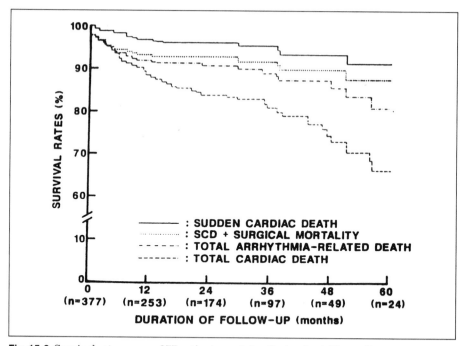

Fig. 15-6. Survival rates among 377 patients receiving the implantable cardioverter-defibrillator (ICD). Shown are sudden cardiac death (SCD), SCD and surgical mortality, total arrhythmia-related death, and total cardiac death. As seen, SCD mortality is low but underestimates the impact of the ICD on overall outcome. (From SG Kim et al. Influence of left ventricular function on survival and mode of death after implanter defibrillator therapy. *Am J Cardiol* 72:1263, 1993. Reprinted with permission.)

ies [17]. Of the 39 patients with LVEF below 30%, 22 received an ICD, and 17 were treated medically. There was no difference in sudden death at 1 and 2 years (6% and 15% vs. 20% and 20%, ICD vs. no ICD) or total mortality (14% and 22% vs. 25% and 25%, ICD vs. no ICD). Among the 139 patients with LVEF below 30%, 73 patients received an ICD, and 66 did not. While sudden death at 1 and 2 years was lower in the ICD group compared to the medical group (0% and 0% vs. 5% and 8%, $p = .02$), there was no difference in total mortality (4% and 4% vs. 5% and 10%, ICD vs. no ICD).

Finally, there are preliminary results from a randomized trial carried out in Hamburg, Germany (CASH) [18]. In this study, sudden death survivors were randomized to therapy with amiodarone, metoprolol, propafenone, or an ICD. In a preliminary report the sudden death mortality was 8.8%, 11.4%, 11.4%, and 0%, respectively, while all-cause mortality was 14.7%, 14.3%, 20.0%, and 14.3%, respectively. There was no significant difference in mortality among any group, except for the propafenone limb, and this drug has been eliminated from the study.

Additionally, the data from ESVEM suggest that antiarrhythmic drugs do reduce sudden death mortality. While it has been argued that the first-year sudden death rate was high at 7%, it was 18% at 6 years, or 3%/year, a rate that compares favorably with the sudden death mortality reported with the ICD. The nonfatal recurrence rate in ESVEM was high despite drug therapy (38% at 1 year and 68% at 6 years); however, the ICD does not prevent arrhythmia recurrence either, but rather, like antiarrhythmic drugs, it prevents death resulting from the arrhythmia.

Given the absence of comparative survival data between patients treated pharmacologically or with an ICD, there is now an ongoing NIH-sponsored trial known as AVID (antiarrhythmic drug versus implantable defibrillator). This study is randomizing patients with VT or VF to therapy with an implantable defibrillator or to an antiarrhythmic drug (amiodarone or sotalol). The primary end point in this study is total mortality. Other issues being addressed are mode of death, quality of life, and cost-effectiveness of the two approaches.

VI. Managing patients with ventricular arrhythmia: A proposal. The concerns and the results of the large arrhythmia studies have resulted in the following proposal for the management of patients with ventricular arrhythmia. **For patients who have frequent episodes of nonsustained VT associated with symptoms or for those without symptoms but who are felt to be at risk for sudden cardiac death** (those with underlying heart disease), therapy can be guided noninvasively based on the suppression of this spontaneous arrhythmia.

For the **patient presenting with sustained VT,** pharmacologic therapy is the first approach. **If the episodes of sustained tachycardia are frequent or if there is a high density of ventricular arrhythmia, primarily runs of nonsustained VT, which is stable and reproducible,** either ambulatory monitoring and exercise testing or electrophysiologic studies can be used for drug selection. It is possible that by using both techniques, drug selection can be enhanced and outcome improved, although either approach alone appears effective. **If episodes are infrequent and spontaneous ectopy is absent,** electrophysiologic testing is essential. In such patients drug efficacy is defined as the inability to induce an arrhythmia. Slowing of the tachycardia rate as a result of the antiarrhythmic agent may also be considered an indicator of drug efficacy if the goal is prevention of sudden death rather than prevention of all recurrence of arrhythmia. If no drug is effective (noninducibility or rate slowing is not achieved) or if there is a serious, symptomatic recurrence on drug therapy, options include the ICD or amiodarone. Amiodarone may be preferred for patients with severely reduced left ventricular function and congestive heart failure in whom nonarrhythmic cardiac mortality is substantial.

When the patient presents with out-of-hospital sudden death, both invasive and noninvasive methods are used to select an antiarrhythmic drug so as to maximize drug efficacy. In such patients, noninducibility is the goal, and tachycardia rate slowing may not be a reliable end point. If arrhythmia remains inducible (regardless of rate) and the patient has normal left ventricular function or only mild to moderate dysfunction, an ICD is the preferred therapy. If there is significant left ventricular dysfunction, amiodarone may be a reasonable option.

As with other areas of cardiology, the treatment of patients with ventricular tachyarrhythmia continues to evolve based on the results of large clinical trials and clinical experience. In the future, therapy will likely be based on which approach offers the best overall survival, is the most cost-effective, and offers the best quality of life for the patient.

References

1. Graboys TB, et al. Long-term survival of patients with malignant ventricular arrhythmia treated with antiarrhythmic drugs. *Am J Cardiol* 50:437–443, 1982.
2. Vlay SC, Kallman CH, Reid PR. Prognostic assessment of survivors of ventricular tachycardia and ventricular fibrillation with ambulatory monitoring. *Am J Cardiol* 54: 87–90, 1984.
3. Wilber DJ, et al. Out-of-hospital cardiac arrest: Use of electrophysiologic testing in the prediction of long-term outcome. *N Engl J Med* 318:19–24, 1988.
4. Swerdlow CD, Winkle RA, Mason JW. Determinants of survival in patients with ventricular tachyarrhythmia. *N Engl J Med* 308:1436–1439, 1983.
5. Morganroth J, et al. Limitations of long-term electrocardiographic monitoring to assess ventricular ectopic frequency. *Circulation* 58:408–414, 1978.
6. Waller TJ, et al. Reduction in sudden death and total mortality by antiarrhythmic therapy evaluated by electrophysiologic drug testing: Criteria of efficacy in patients with sustained ventricular tachyarrhythmia. *J Am Coll Cardiol* 10:83–89, 1987.
7. Borggrefe M, Trampisch HJ, Breithardt G. Reappraisal of criteria for assessing drug efficacy in patients with ventricular tachyarrhythmias: Complete versus partial suppression of inducible arrhythmias. *J Am Coll Cardiol* 12:140–149, 1988.
8. Mitchell LB, et al. A randomized clinical trial of the noninvasive and invasive approaches to drug therapy of ventricular tachycardia. *N Engl J Med* 317:1681–1687, 1987.
9. Mason JW, for the Electrophysiologic Study versus Electrocardiographic Monitoring Investigators. A comparison of electrophysiologic testing with Holter monitoring to predict antiarrhythmic drug efficacy for ventricular tachyarrhythmias. *N Engl J Med* 329:445–451, 1993.
10. Mason JW, for the ESVEM Investigators. A comparison of seven antiarrhythmic drugs

in patients with ventricular tachyarrhythmias. *N Engl J Med* 329:452–458, 1993.

11. CAST Investigators. Preliminary report: Effects of encainide and flecainide on mortality in a randomized trial of arrhythmia suppression after myocardial infarction. *N Engl J Med* 321:406–412, 1989.

12. Winkle RA, et al. Long-term outcome with the automatic implantable cardioverter-defibrillator. *J Am Coll Cardiol* 13:1353–1361, 1989.

13. Newman D, et al. Survival after implantation of the cardioverter defibrillator. *Am J Cardiol* 69:899–903, 1992.

14. Kim SG, et al. Benefits of implantable defibrillators are overestimated by sudden death rates and better represented by the total arrhythmic death rate. *J Am Coll Cardiol* 17:1587–1592, 1991.

15. Connolly SJ, Yusef S. Evaluation of the implantable cardioverter defibrillator in survivors of cardiac arrest: The need for randomized trials [Editorial]. *Am J Cardiol* 69:959–962, 1992.

16. Choue CW, et al. Survival rates of patients with malignant ventricular arrhythmias: Comparison of medical therapy versus implantable defibrillator therapy. *Circulation* 84(suppl II):II–21, 1991.

17. Crandall BG, et al. Implantable cardioverter-defibrillator therapy in survivors of out-of-hospital sudden cardiac death without inducible arrhythmias. *J Am Coll Cardiol* 21:1186–1192, 1993.

18. Siebels J, et al. and the CASH Investigators group. The Cardiac Arrest Study Hamburg (CASH): Preliminary results [abstr]. *Circulation* 86(suppl I):I–535, 1992.

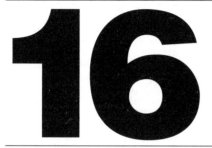

Controversies in Arrhythmia Management—II. The Invasive Approach

Lou-Anne M. Beauregard,
Andrea M. Russo, and
Harvey L. Waxman

I. Indications. The basis for the electrophysiologic approach to arrhythmia management has been that most arrhythmias are reentrant in mechanism and can be induced and terminated with programmed electrical stimulation, thereby allowing study of the arrhythmia in the electrophysiology laboratory. Whereas the initial role of electrophysiologic evaluation was diagnosis and assessment of drug efficacy, the evolution of ablative techniques has transformed a diagnostic tool into an interventional one.

Patient selection and the design of the electrophysiologic protocol depend on the type of arrhythmia being evaluated. For example, the patient with supraventricular tachycardia most likely to benefit from electrophysiologic evaluation is one in whom the arrhythmia can be diagnosed and ablated with radiofrequency catheter ablation techniques in one session, thereby eliminating the need for lifelong antiarrhythmic therapy and conserving resources. Other patients who may benefit, both diagnostically and therapeutically, are those whose arrhythmia is refractory to conventional drug therapy and has resulted in severe symptoms, syncope, or cardiac arrest (Table 16-1). In these patients, a combination of ablation and electrophysiologically guided drug therapy may be appropriate.

Ambulatory ECG monitoring is useful for the detection of supraventricular tachycardias and provides information about mechanism. Due to the episodic nature of these arrhythmias, ambulatory monitoring is rarely helpful in assessing therapy. However, these techniques can be used to document the cause of symptoms in patients with palpitations, thereby directing the course of therapy. An algorithm for management of supraventricular tachycardia is presented in Fig. 16-1.

Traditionally, patients with well-tolerated sustained ventricular tachycardias (VTs) were referred for electrophysiologic evaluation after failure of either empiric therapy or therapy guided by noninvasive monitoring. Contemporary management of these patients now involves early electrophysiologic evaluation to determine suitability for radiofrequency ablation and also identification of those patients who are not optimal candidates for drug therapy and should receive an antitachycardia/antifibrillatory device. Although electrophysiologic evaluation can be used to select pharmacologic therapy, this is less frequently done now, due to the availability of other, nonpharmacologic options.

While some investigators have advocated therapy guided by Holter monitoring in patients with VT or cardiac arrest, up to 25% of these patients will have infrequent ventricular premature beats (VPBs) on Holter monitoring. Because of major day-to-day variation in arrhythmia frequency, assessment of drug efficacy by Holter monitoring is impossible in this subset. In addition, few investigators have clearly documented the utility of this approach. A long-term study, Electrophysiologic Study Versus Electrocardiographic Monitoring (ESVEM), has been recently completed to evaluate whether ambulatory monitoring is sufficient to guide therapy in patients with VT compared to electrophysiologic study. (This study is discussed in **III.B.**)

In some cases, patients with refractory VT may be candidates for surgery. In this situation, preoperative electrophysiologic evaluation is utilized to induce the ventricular tachyarrhythmia and perform endocardial mapping for localization. Since catheter endocardial mapping correlates well with intraoperative mapping, the preoperative data can be used to identify the area of resection if stable VT cannot be induced in the operating room. As newer modalities of catheter-based ablation for VT are developed, such as microwave energy and laser therapy, these may be directly applied during electrophysiologic evaluation.

The precise role of invasive electrophysiologic evaluation for risk stratification of patients with depressed left ventricular function and previous myocardial infarction is under investigation. It is known that these patients are at higher risk for sudden death, presumed in most cases to be due to ventricular tachyarrhythmias. However, it is not known whether electrophysiologic testing can identify patients at higher risk. As the Cardiac Arrhythmia Suppression Trial (CAST) demonstrated, empiric therapy with type 1C agents may be detrimental. Currently, the Multi-Center Unsustained Tachycardia Trial (MUSTT) is evaluating the role of electrophysiologic testing in patients with depressed left ventricular function, previous infarction, and nonsustained VT. Using electrophysiologic testing to identify a group at presumed higher risk, patients with inducible sustained ventricular tachyarrhythmias are randomized to electrophysiologically guided therapy or no specific antiarrhythmic therapy. The study will test the hypothesis that electrophysiologic testing **does** identify a high-risk subset and that early intervention may decrease sudden death mortality.

Similarly, it is unknown what the role of electrophysiologic testing is in patients with cardiomyopathy and nonsustained VT. Holter monitoring, ejection fraction, and signal averaging may identify high-risk groups in both patients with myopathy and those with prior infarction, but ambulatory monitoring for pharmacologic efficacy may or may not be adequate to demonstrate reduction in arrhythmic risk. A suggested algorithm for management of patients with VT is presented in Fig. 16-2.

Electrophysiologic studies are indicated in the evaluation of patients with syncope of unknown cause if clinical history, physical examination, neurologic evaluation, and noninvasive testing are unrevealing. Electrophysiologic evaluation can help to uncover sinus node, atrioventricular (AV) node, or His-Purkinje system dysfunction and test for the presence of VT or supraventricular tachycardia as the cause of syncope. In addition, patients with conduction disease can be evaluated for His-Purkinje system reserve, allowing an estimate of the likelihood of imminent progression of the disease to complete heart block.

Selected patients with organic heart disease, including mitral valve prolapse, hypertrophic or congestive cardiomyopathy, and sarcoid heart disease, with documented VT may benefit if a sustained arrhythmia can be induced. For example, in patients with no apparent heart disease, right ventricular outflow tract or idiopathic left VTs may occur. In these patients, the automatic VT can be cured with radiofrequency catheter ablation, often avoiding the need for lifelong antiarrhythmic therapy. About 5% of patients with sustained VT have bundle branch reentrant VT, which can be identified by electrophysiologic testing and treated with catheter ablation. Patients with arrhythmogenic right ventricular dysplasia may have identification of an appropriate drug regimen by electrophysiologic testing. The role of noninvasive techniques in the management of these patients is not clear.

Noninvasive techniques are more appropriate to evaluate arrhythmias in patients with complex ectopy and normal hearts or in asymptomatic patients with coronary artery disease, patients with frequent VPBs, and possibly patients with nonischemic heart disease and nonsustained VT. In these patients, who are asymptomatic from their arrhythmia, therapy may well be guided by ambulatory monitoring and no therapy or an empiric trial of an antiarrhythmic agent considered. Current trials are evaluating the empiric use of amiodarone in some subgroups of patients, with encouraging results in terms of long-term survival and efficacy in arrhythmia control.

Table 16-1. Indications for invasive electrophysiologic testing

Supraventricular tachycardia
Associated with syncope or cardiac arrest
Refractory to conventional agents
Define mechanism of symptomatic arrhythmia with intent to ablate

Ventricular tachycardia (VT)
Associated with syncope or cardiac arrest
Tolerated VT refractory to conventional agents
Diagnosis of wide-complex arrhythmia
Preoperative/preablation evaluation and mapping with intervention
Selection of patients at high risk following infarction

Syncope
Patients with nondiagnostic noninvasive procedures

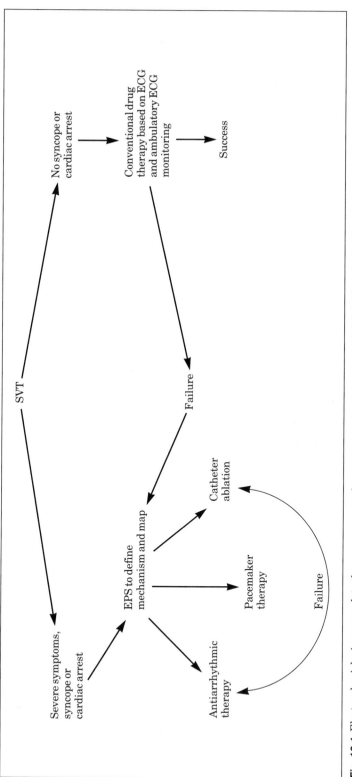

Fig. 16-1. Electrophysiologic approach to the management of supraventricular tachycardia (SVT). (EPS = electrophysiologic study.)

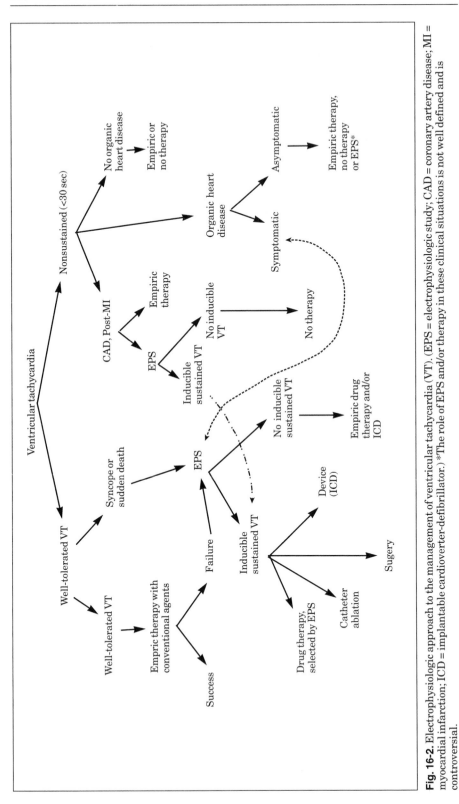

Fig. 16-2. Electrophysiologic approach to the management of ventricular tachycardia (VT). (EPS = electrophysiologic study; CAD = coronary artery disease; MI = myocardial infarction; ICD = implantable cardioverter-defibrillator.) *The role of EPS and/or therapy in these clinical situations is not well defined and is controversial.

In summary, with the recent developments in catheter-based intervention in patients with both supraventricular and ventricular arrhythmias, there has been a shift in focus of electrophysiologic testing from diagnosis and assessment of drug efficacy to cure or amelioration of symptoms. The noninvasive approach can be used to identify patients and select those for whom electrophysiologic testing may be of most benefit but is not always adequate to assess continued therapy.

II. **Methods.** Patients who are selected for electrophysiologic study should have an appropriate preliminary examination to document the clinical arrhythmia and extent of heart disease. It is important to be able to reproduce the clinical arrhythmia in the electrophysiology laboratory. Thus, identification of clinical arrhythmias by 12-lead ECG and Holter monitoring is helpful in patients with both supraventricular and ventricular arrhythmias. Patients who have ventricular tachyarrhythmias should have an assessment of ventricular function and extent of ischemic heart disease, either noninvasively, using radionuclide angiography, echocardiography, and stress testing, or by cardiac catheterization. Cardiac catheterization should be performed in most patients with suspected coronary artery disease, as the extent of such disease should be determined and angina controlled, either medically or surgically, before programmed electrical stimulation. If ischemia plays a role in the genesis of the arrhythmia, it may well respond to antianginal therapy or bypass surgery. In selected patients, right ventricular angiography or transesophageal echocardiography may be appropriate to evaluate right ventricular function.

The electrophysiologic study is conducted in the following manner. Multipolar electrode catheters are placed by the percutaneous transfemoral approach to positions in the high right atrium and the right ventricle and across the septal leaflet of the tricuspid valve to record the His bundle electrogram. A catheter is frequently placed in the coronary sinus from the internal jugular or subclavian vein. For left ventricular mapping, an arterial sheath is placed in the femoral artery and an additional mapping catheter in the left ventricle (see Chap. 12). Additional catheters may be placed for ablation as needed, through either the venous or arterial approach. For routine electrophysiologic testing, systemic anticoagulation is rarely required, but for prolonged intravascular procedures, such as ablation, full heparinization is customary.

Routinely, sinus node, AV node, and His-Purkinje system function are evaluated using atrial pacing and programmed electrical stimulation. The type of evaluation performed is determined by the goal of the procedure. For example, electrophysiologic testing of patients with supraventricular tachycardias requires a great deal of individualization. In patients with the Wolff-Parkinson-White syndrome, ventricular pacing and extrastimulation are often performed before atrial stimulation to avoid precipitation of atrial fibrillation by atrial pacing. In addition, detailed mapping of the coronary sinus to localize the bypass tract is performed. If intervention is the goal, more detail is required than if the patient is to be followed on pharmacologic therapy. Atropine or isoproterenol may facilitate the initiation of supraventricular tachycardias, by mimicking endogenous changes in sympathetic and parasympathetic tone.

The evaluation of VT is more standardized. Ventricular tachycardia induction is attempted using ventricular extrastimulation at two or more right ventricular pacing sites, usually the right ventricular apex and outflow tract. Several pacing cycle lengths are used, from 600–400 msec, and up to three extrastimuli are delivered to initiate VT. Extrastimulation in sinus rhythm and rapid ventricular pacing may increase the yield of VT. On occasion, isoproterenol is administered to facilitate initiation of VT by enhancing automaticity and uncovering parasystole. In addition, by improving conduction and shortening refractoriness in the tissue between the pacing site and the site of reentry, isoproterenol may also help to induce reentrant arrhythmias. Traditionally, invasive serial electropharmacologic testing is performed by completing a baseline study of antiarrhythmic agents, followed by repeat testing on either intravenous (IV) or oral antiarrhythmic therapy. If sustained VT cannot be induced on an individual agent, it has been shown that this agent will have substantial long-term efficacy. Previous serial testing involved multiple drugs and multiple combinations of available antiarrhythmic agents; current practice is to test antiarrhythmic agents in a class-specific manner and decide whether the response is adequate or if ablation or device therapy is indicated.

The site of earliest endocardial activation in VT may be localized by mapping the left ventricle during sustained VT. Results of this mapping have been correlated with those of endocardial mapping under direct vision at the time of surgery. Some groups have suggested that regions of continuous diastolic electrical activity or fractionated electrograms in sinus rhythm correlate with the site of origin of VT. If endocardial mapping in sinus rhythm or VT fails, activation mapping by left ventricular pacing may localize the arrhythmia.

Radiofrequency catheter ablation can be performed using similar endocardial mapping for atrial tachycardia, atrial flutter, AV nodal reentrant tachycardia, and tachycardia associated with an accessory pathway. For AV nodal reentrant tachycardia, two techniques have been described: radiofrequency ablation of the slow or fast pathway. Slow-pathway ablation is preferred, since the risk of complete heart block is much less than that following ablation of the fast pathway. In cases of refractory atrial fibrillation, radiofrequency ablation of the AV conduction system can be performed. This can most often be accomplished from the right side of the heart, but occasionally left-sided ablation of the His bundle is required. New techniques of modification of AV junction input to control ventricular response in atrial fibrillation are under investigation, and may accomplish the same goal of rate control without the need for permanent pacing. Ablation of the accessory pathway in the Wolff-Parkinson-White syndrome can be performed with a high degree of success in most pathway locations. Anteroseptal, posteroseptal, and right free-wall pathways are somewhat more difficult than pathways in other locations and are associated with a slightly lower success rate. Whereas left-sided pathways are usually ablated from the retrograde transaortic approach, and right-sided pathways from a venous approach, the course of posteroseptal pathways is more variable and ablation may actually be performed from within the coronary sinus or a branch of the coronary sinus.

III. Choice of drugs

A. **Supraventricular tachycardia.** In the case of the common forms of supraventricular tachycardia—AV nodal reentry and those associated with Wolff-Parkinson-White syndrome—there is a growing trend to favor catheter ablation over pharmacologic therapy. This is due to the young age group usually affected, the long-term toxicities of the drugs, and the limited efficacy of pharmacotherapy.

Treatment of supraventricular tachycardia is based on the ability of drugs to prolong atrial, AV nodal, retrograde, and antegrade pathway refractoriness or conduction or to suppress automaticity. For acute drug testing, IV verapamil (0.5 mg/kg to a total dose of 10 mg), or propranolol hydrochloride (0.1–0.15 mg/kg) may be given to assess effects on AV nodal reentry. Verapamil, digitalis, and propranolol most often slow conduction in the antegrade pathway of the common type of AV nodal reentrant tachycardia. The effects of these agents may in part, however, be overridden by enhanced sympathetic tone. In contrast, the type 1A antiarrhythmic agents (procainamide, quinidine, disopyramide) more often prolong refractoriness of the retrograde pathway, thereby inhibiting initiation of AV nodal reentrant tachycardia, and are less susceptible to changes in autonomic tone. Procainamide 1 g IV may be given followed by attempts to initiate the tachycardia.

In the Wolff-Parkinson-White syndrome, the type of clinical tachycardia often determines the type of antiarrhythmic therapy necessary. For orthodromic supraventricular tachycardia (conduction down the AV node and up the accessory pathway), AV nodal blocking drugs may be effective in preventing recurrences of paroxysmal supraventricular tachycardia. In cases of Wolff-Parkinson-White syndrome associated with atrial fibrillation with a rapid ventricular rate, only drugs that act directly on the accessory pathway will prove effective.

In patients with Wolff-Parkinson-White syndrome, drugs are often selected that act on both anterograde and retrograde function of the accessory pathway. Ideally, an antiarrhythmic agent that is totally effective in blocking conduction of the accessory pathway will prevent paroxysmal supraventricular tachycardia as well as atrial fibrillation with a rapid rate. Unfortunately, currently available agents are not this effective. More often there is some prolongation of the refractory period, with continued inducibility of arrhythmias. The type 1A (procainamide, quinidine and disopyramide), type 1C (flecainide and propafenone), and type 3 drugs (sotalol, amiodarone) are most effective in prolonging refractoriness and slowing conduction over the accessory pathway.

Following baseline electrophysiologic study, antiarrhythmic medications can be given IV with immediate electrophysiologic testing or orally with electrophysiologic testing after steady state is reached, to determine clinical efficacy. There seems to be a fairly good correlation between the effects of these agents in the electrophysiologic laboratory and subsequent clinical outcome.

For some patients with supraventricular tachycardia, so-called cocktail therapy may be appropriate. In this situation, the patients take episodic drug therapy to terminate an acute episode but are not on chronic suppressive therapy. To be suitable for this type of treatment, a patient should have infrequent and well-tolerated arrhythmias.

B. Ventricular tachycardia. Serial electrophysiologic testing with multiple conventional agents is time-consuming, costly, and difficult for the patient and family. Studies previously showed concordance of response to multiple agents predicted with acute administration of procainamide. However, other studies have questioned this result, and with the development of new type 1C and type 3 antiarrhythmic agents, the type of testing may not have predictive value. Mason et al. recently reported results from the ESVEM study and found a higher predicted success rate of therapy with sotalol, a type 3 agent, compared to a variety of type 1 agents, based on both electrophysiologic testing and ambulatory monitoring [1]. This suggests an expanding role for type 3 agents in VT management. The study also raised the question whether electrophysiologic testing was necessary in the subset of patients with frequent complex ectopy, as there was a good correlation of predicted efficacy by noninvasive means with that of invasive means. This study had significant limitations, however. Of 2103 patients considered, only 1005 patients were eligible for study entry. Of these, 141 had insufficient ectopy on ambulatory monitoring to be randomized, 349 did not have reproducibly initiated VT, and 29 did not meet either criterion. Thus, only 23% of those enrolled actually entered the study. Of these, 188 had drug efficacy predicted by ambulatory monitoring and 108 by electrophysiologic testing. There was a similar incidence of arrhythmic death, cardiac arrest, and VT in both groups where drug efficacy was predicted. The overall arrhythmic mortality in this study was 10% at 1 year and 20% at 4 years in patients with effective drug therapy. The methodology used to predict drug efficacy, however, was limitation of the extrastimulation protocol to that which had been effective at baseline, and not pursuing a more aggressive protocol while on an antiarrhythmic drug. This approach is somewhat controversial and may tend to overestimate drug efficacy. The study concluded that of all antiarrhythmic agents, sotalol was most effective in preventing arrhythmia recurrence and arrhythmic death. Nevertheless, the results of the study did not allow a determination of whether noninvasive or invasive pharmacologic management of VT is preferable.

Amiodarone, which is probably the most successful agent for control of recurrent sustained VT, was not considered in the ESVEM trial. Amiodarone is classified as a type 3 antiarrhythmic agent but has multiple other effects. In addition to prolonging refractoriness and slowing conduction, amiodarone has been reported to have an antifibrillatory effect. When series from a variety of investigators of amiodarone therapy are combined, of a total of 435 patients taking daily maintenance doses of 200–1200 mg, the overall success rate in controlling VT evaluated after 1–2 weeks of therapy was 51%. The drug was ineffective in 43% of patients, and the remaining 6% had a partial response. The efficacy of amiodarone assessed 7–10 days after initiation of therapy is somewhat controversial, as the electrophysiologic effect may not reach its peak until several weeks after initiation of therapy. The inducibility of sustained VT in patients receiving amiodarone therapy may also not correlate with long-term success of the agent. In several series, long-term survival has been reported despite inducibility of VT after amiodarone loading. However, patients who have rapid VT induced while taking amiodarone may be more likely to have a poorly tolerated arrhythmia recurrence and benefit from implantation of an automatic defibrillator.

The evaluation of amiodarone effect by following VPB suppression on Holter monitoring may not correlate well with clinical efficacy. Meaningful suppression of VPB frequency during amiodarone therapy may correlate with drug success; however, many patients do not have serious ventricular ectopy or a change in the ventricular ectopy while taking amiodarone, and in these patients the long-term success of amiodarone cannot be correlated with objective data.

The utility of IV amiodarone for rapid control of malignant arrhythmias is controversial. Some recent reports, including one from the authors, have demonstrated excellent clinical response in patients with recurrent refractory ventricular arrhythmias who receive high-dose oral loading of amiodarone [2]. In all patients taking amiodarone, careful follow-up with chest x rays, liver and thyroid function studies, ophthalmologic evaluation, and other routine tests are recommended because of the multiple toxicities and drug interactions associated with long-term use of amiodarone.

IV. Choice of devices

A. Supraventricular tachycardia. Available devices for control of arrhythmias include patient-activated and automatic antitachycardia pacemakers. In many of these cases, where antitachycardia pacing might have been appropriate, radiofrequency catheter ablation is now the treatment of choice for permanent cure of the arrhythmia. In rare cases, including patients with drug-refractory supraventricular tachycardia in whom ablation is not feasible or not successful, antitachycardia pacing may be an option.

The use of a device to control supraventricular tachycardia necessitates full electrophysiologic evaluation for efficacy of the device and repeated stimulation studies to ensure that there is no unintentional precipitation of atrial fibrillation by the pacing modality chosen. Patient-activated units require a high degree of patient reliability in that the activator (radiofrequency or magnet) must be carried all the time and is subject to manipulation by the patient and the possibility that the patient may use the device inappropriately at home. Automatic antitachycardia pacemakers may be selected if the patient has hemodynamic collapse from the arrhythmia or is not reliable enough to use a patient-activated device.

Modalities that may be selected for control of supraventricular tachycardias include underdrive pacing, scanning pacemakers, or burst pacing. There is a limited role for continuous overdrive pacing to suppress supraventricular arrhythmias, some of which are presumed to be automatic in origin. The rates required for continuous overdrive suppression of an arrhythmia are poorly tolerated, and this does not pose a viable long-term solution to an arrhythmic problem.

B. Ventricular tachycardia. The use of pacemakers alone for control of VT is more limited than for supraventricular tachycardia. Complex interactions between the device selected and antiarrhythmic agents may make pacemaker therapy more or less effective. The patient must be fully tested in the electrophysiologic laboratory for reliable termination of the tachycardia with either underdrive or overdrive (burst) pacing and lack of acceleration of VT or degeneration into ventricular fibrillation (VF). The major limitation of pacing for VT is acceleration of the rate resulting in cardiac arrest, which in one series occurred in 43% of patients. Previously, antitachycardia pacemakers were often implanted in conjunction with backup automatic defibrillators to treat arrhythmias resulting from acceleration or degeneration of VT. With currently available devices, this is no longer necessary.

Realistic device therapy for life-threatening ventricular arrhythmias is provided by automatic implantable cardioverter-defibrillators. The first-generation devices were capable of responding to rate and/or morphology (probability density function) and were committed, nonprogrammable devices. The second-generation devices were programmable for several functions, including rate cutoff, initial shock energy, and delay to first shock. These devices were also committed once the device started to charge. Only investigational second-generation devices had a reconfirmation algorithm.

Third-generation devices have recently been approved and offer the choices of monophasic or biphasic waveforms (some units), backup bradycardia pacing, and one or more antitachycardia algorithms, including low-energy cardioversion, and high-energy defibrillation. These devices also contain data logging, which provides information about shock delivery and stored electrograms, and they offer the option of noninvasive electrophysiologic testing to ensure device function. Nonthoracotomy implantation is now also possible, allowing implantation of these devices in patients who are otherwise not optimal for thoracotomy implantation. Despite significant improvements, third-generation devices are still capable of inappropriate or problematic shocks, often for nonventricular tachyarrhythmias. Other complications include death, infections, superior vena caval thrombosis, lead dislodgement, and malfunction. The types of malfunction include hermeticity loss, breakdown of the gaseous dielectric within the device, misdirection of the battery-testing pulse toward the patient, and random component failure. False-positive discharges have occurred, generally because of fractured leads or miscounting of the heart rate, but have become less of a problem with increased experience with these devices.

Automatic defibrillators have proven efficacy in prolonging sudden death–free survival, although they do not alter survival from the underlying heart disease. In the case of sudden death survivors, use of a defibrillator as primary therapy with or without electrophysiologic testing has been advocated by many investigators.

Patients who have devices for control of arrhythmias still need follow-up to ensure device efficacy, and if concurrent pharmacotherapy is undertaken, device function must be reassessed. Drugs alter both the cycle length of the tachycardia and often its conduction pathway, and they may also raise or lower the defibrillation threshold. These factors must be considered in antiarrhythmic drug selection in patients with automatic defibrillators.

V. **Choice of surgery.** Traditional surgical therapy has been replaced by catheter ablation for patients with medically refractory supraventricular arrhythmias and in some patients with VTs. Surgery may still be an option in some patients with VT, especially those with large left ventricular aneurysms who may need coronary artery bypass surgery or for management of congestive heart failure. Recently the Maze procedure has been used to maintain sinus rhythm in patients with medically refractory atrial fibrillation.

A. **Supraventricular tachycardia.** Supraventricular tachycardias are often amenable to radiofrequency catheter ablation at low risk to the patient. Surgery has thus been largely supplanted by catheter techniques.

Techniques have been described to control patients with sinus tachycardia, sinus node reentrant tachycardia, atrial tachycardia, and atrial flutter, using radiofrequency ablation. While the success rates for these arrhythmias are lower than those for AV nodal reentry or Wolff-Parkinson-White syndrome, early results are nevertheless encouraging.

Catheter ablation for modification of AV nodal conduction in AV nodal reentry has been demonstrated to be successful in control of recurrent paroxysmal AV nodal reentrant tachycardia. Two-thirds of patients with paroxysmal supraventricular tachycardia who have no evidence of preexcitation during sinus rhythm have AV nodal reentry as the culprit arrhythmia. Fast-pathway ablation is associated with a 5–6% incidence of complete heart block, and therefore most investigators prefer slow-pathway modification. Slow-pathway modification may require more complex mapping and have a higher recurrence rate. However, experienced operators can achieve a very high success rate with an extremely low risk of damage to the AV node or His-Purkinje system.

Multiple surgery series have demonstrated high efficacy with low morbidity and mortality associated with the surgical interruption of accessory pathways. There is still a rare need for surgical interruption when radiofrequency ablation is unsuccessful. With either the transseptal technique or the retrograde transaortic approach, the success rate is well over 90% for most pathways when performed by experienced operators, with a very low recurrence rate.

Atrioventricular junctional or His bundle ablation has become an accepted method of treating medically refractory atrial fibrillation. Originally, direct current shock ablation was used in this situation, with successful development of complete heart block but an apparent increase in sudden death rate. While radiofrequency ablation results in a smaller lesion, catheter stability during atrial fibrillation often makes right-sided ablation untenable, and a left-sided approach can be used with good success. It does not appear that the increased risk of sudden death seen with direct current shock ablation occurs following radiofrequency application, perhaps due to the smaller size of the lesion. This procedure requires permanent backup ventricular pacing.

Atrial flutter and atrial tachycardias have been ablated successfully using radiofrequency techniques. While the success rates for these arrhythmias are lower than those for AV nodal reentry and Wolff-Parkinson-White syndrome–related arrhythmias, early results are encouraging.

Complications of radiofrequency catheter ablation are small and include the immediate complications of vascular access, cardiac perforation, pericarditis, stroke, infection, and thromboembolism. A significant procedurally related complication occurs in less than 1% of patients. Theoretical long-term complications of the significant radiation exposure, often to a young patient, scarring of coronary arteries adjacent to the ablation site, and the possibility of arrhythmogenicity from the lesions created remain to be evaluated.

B. **Ventricular tachycardia.** Surgical techniques were first applied to VT in the late 1960s, when simple aneurysmectomy was used for treatment of medically refractory VT. Over the course of the next few years, two techniques were used: encircling endocardial ventriculotomy and subendocardial resection. Encircling endocardial ventriculotomy involves a transmyocardial incision sparing only the epicardial vessels and pericardium around the border zone of the myocardial infarction. Subendocardial resection involves resection of endocardium, subendocardium, and some myocardium at the site where activation mapping indicates the earliest site during VT. This results in removal of the arrhythmogenic focus. Cryosurgery and laser applications have been used with either of these techniques to eliminate the arrhythmogenic focus. Both subendocardial resection and encircling ventriculotomy result in serious perioperative morbidity and mortality because of impaired left ventricular function and prolonged bypass time, and use of these procedures has decreased in recent years. Patients selected for either of these surgical techniques must undergo extensive preoperative catheter mapping and intraoperative endocardial or epicardial mapping.

Despite the success in cure of arrhythmias in mapping-guided surgery, mapping requires time spent in a hemodynamically unstable arrhythmia on normothermic bypass, increasing morbidity and mortality. Damage to papillary muscles from endocardial resection and traumatic ventricular septal defects produced by septal incisions with the encircling endocardial ventriculotomy technique may occur. Cryosurgery may have an application in many patients in whom the planned area of excision for either technique involves the papillary muscles or the high, proximal septum and may afford an option for completing surgery that might otherwise be inadequately performed. Cryosurgical techniques result in the same kind of hemodynamic embarrassment as encircling endocardial ventriculotomy, and this should be recognized. It is possible that the most effective surgery involves combinations of all these techniques. Due to the hemodynamic complications of these procedures, most patients undergo device implantation rather than surgery to control VT.

Small numbers of patients have been treated with transthoracic direct current shock catheter ablation for VT. Endocardial mapping was performed to identify the site of endocardial breakthrough of the tachycardia, and a shock of 100–400 joules delivered to this site. If there were multiple morphologies of VT, each could be mapped and ablated in the same manner. The major complications of this procedure have been heart failure and refractory arrhythmias, presumed due to the direct current shock effects on the myocardium, myocardial rupture, and thromboembolism. Transcoronary chemical ablation has also been attempted when the artery supplying the tachycardia circuit is patent and can be identified. This technique is successful in small numbers of patients but not always possible.

Currently, multiple centers are evaluating and developing better mapping techniques and energy sources for ablation of VT. Due to the complexity of the reentry circuit, localizing the area of slow conduction and energy penetration into this region has proved difficult. It is probable that the technique will gain wider application in the next few years. Catheter tip design and alternative energy sources, including microwave energy, are being investigated.

For one form of VT, bundle branch reentry, radiofrequency catheter ablation of the right bundle eliminates the tachycardia circuit with a great deal of success. Successful ablation has also been performed in patients with right ventricular outflow tract tachycardias and idiopathic left ventricular tachycardia. Even in patients with VT successfully treated with catheter ablation, many investigators advocate prophylactic defibrillator implantation.

In summary, surgical techniques for VT yielded an acceptable degree of success but were associated with considerable patient morbidity and mortality. Current devices and use of the nonthoracotomy approach to implant defibrillators have resulted in a decreasing number of patients referred for surgery. The application of catheter ablation techniques may permit selected patients to undergo direct ablation of the arrhythmia, but long-term studies are needed to ensure its success and assess the morbidity and mortality expected from the procedure.

VI. Chronic follow-up. The gold standard for patients with symptomatic sustained supraventricular tachycardia (SVT) or VT is lack of recurrence of the clinical arrhythmia on therapy. Patients may be followed for assessment of arrhythmia recurrence with Holter monitoring, intermittent transtelephonic monitoring, and drug level assays. Many patients with control of their clinical arrhythmia may continue to have atrial premature beats, VPBs, or even nonsustained arrhythmias without symptoms. These do not usually require a change in management.

VII. Advantages and disadvantages of electrophysiology studies. Electrophysiologic testing should be regarded as a diagnostic aid and a therapeutic tool. In fact, it is quite different from and complementary to noninvasive techniques. It may be the only tool available to differentiate wide-complex SVT from VT. In addition, it can help to diagnose the mechanism of SVT and differentiate automatic from reentrant SVT and VT. Drug efficacy can be reliably predicted by electrophysiologic testing and has been shown to correlate with long-term prognosis in several series. While the results of ESVEM suggest that there may be a greater role for drug selection using noninvasive means, many patients with lethal ventricular arrhythmias do not have sufficient ambient ectopy to guide therapy. In addition, ESVEM did not directly compare results with amiodarone therapy to other agents, nor did it consider directly the role of devices in managing the study group. The overall mortality statistics in both groups where drug efficacy was predicted were disappointingly high. In large part, the high mortality in the group with electrophysiologically guided therapy may be due to the electrophysiologic protocol chosen, which was unaggressive and not commonly applied. In many ways, ESVEM did not clarify the appropriate relationship between therapy guided by electrophysiologic testing and that guided by noninvasive means. While electrophysiologic testing may overpredict drug failure for patients with VT, once a "successful" drug has been identified, patient survival has been repeatedly shown to be improved.

Electrophysiologic testing is the only way to predict the efficacy of an antiarrhythmic device or a pacemaker or to cure an arrhythmia therapeutically by radiofrequency catheter ablation. Electrophysiologic techniques may be more cost-effective over the long term in the management of many arrhythmia cases, resulting in fewer hospitalizations for arrhythmia recurrence and less expenditure for diagnosis and therapy. In addition, reduction in long-term health care cost has been demonstrated with catheter ablative techniques compared to surgical ablation for supraventricular tachyarrhythmias. A similar reduction in long-term health care costs may be demonstrated for the use of automatic cardioverter-defibrillators, although the initial cost of these devices is high.

The major disadvantage of electrophysiologic testing has been the adverse psychologic consequences of repeated invasive testing (see Chap. 20). Previously, the tests were conducted at a referral center with specialized equipment and personnel with expertise in the diagnosis and evaluation of arrhythmias. Now there is greater regional availability of electrophysiologic testing. Thus the patient no longer has to spend a large amount of time for his or her workup away from home or family.

Several factors raise serious questions about the sensitivity and specificity of the results of electrophysiologic testing: (1) There are day-to-day variations in arrhythmia inducibility. (2) Stimulation protocols vary from center to center, which influences the inducibility of arrhythmias. (3) More vigorous protocols may produce more false-positive arrhythmias. (4) Different investigators use different end points for a positive or negative study, with some groups reporting nonsustained tachycardia as an unsuccessful end point and others including only sustained clinical arrhythmias. This technique may not always identify high-risk patients, particularly among those who have suffered a cardiac arrest and have structurally normal-appearing hearts.

VIII. Advantages and disadvantages of noninvasive techniques. The major advantages of noninvasive techniques for the study of arrhythmias are availability in most hospitals, patient preference of noninvasive techniques over invasive studies, and outpatient workup and therapy in selected patients. However, given the modern direction of antiarrhythmic therapy with devices and ablation, and the lack of evidence that treatment of asymptomatic patients with arrhythmias is worthwhile, it seems that the role of noninvasive management has lessened.

The only patients who can be safely managed with noninvasive testing are those with well-tolerated recurrent sustained VT in whom there is a high level of frequent ambient activity to judge the efficacy of noninvasive therapy. Alternatives for therapy in these patients include electropharmacologically guided therapy with electrophysiologic testing, implantation of a pacemaker-defibrillator device, and radiofrequency ablation or surgical correction.

Other disadvantages of noninvasive techniques are day-to-day variability in arrhythmia frequency, inability to treat some patients because of the absence of significant ambient ventricular ectopy, and paucity of evidence that using noninvasive techniques results in acceptable outcomes. In addition, noninvasive techniques for assessment of arrhythmias limit the options to drug therapy only; ablation, antitachycardia devices, or surgery cannot be utilized.

In summary, electrophysiologic testing with programmed electrical stimulation represents a modality by which arrhythmias may be studied and optimal therapy selected. Noninvasive techniques may be used concurrently to supplement information about frequency of ventricular or supraventricular ectopy and daily occurrence of clinical arrhythmias. The two methods should be considered comlementary for the design of an appropriate treatment plan in a given individual rather than as alternative modalities.

References

1. Mason JW, et al. A comparison of electrophysiologic testing with Holter monitoring to predict antiarrhythmic-drug efficacy for ventricular tachyarrhythmias. *N Engl J Med* 329:445–451, 1993.
2. Russo AM, et al. Oral amiodarone loading for the rapid treatment of frequent, refractory, sustained ventricular arrhythmias associated with coronary artery disease. *Am J Cardiol* 72:1395–1399, 1993.

Bibliography

Cohen TF, et al. Radiofrequency catheter ablation for treatment of bundle branch reentrant ventricular tachycardia: Results and long-term follow-up. *J Am Coll Cardiol* 18:1767–1773, 1991.

Cox JL, Gallagher JJ, Ungerleider RM. Encircling endocardial ventriculotomy for refractory ischemic ventricular tachycardia: IV. Clinical indications, surgical technique, mechanism of action and results. *J Thorac Cardiovasc Surg* 83:865–872, 1982.

de Buitleir M, et al. Reduction in medical care cost associated with radiofrequency catheter ablation of accessory pathways. *Am J Cardiol* 68:1656–1661, 1991.

Echt DS, et al. Mortality and morbidity in patients receiving encainide, flecainide or placebo: The Cardiac Arrhythmia Suppression Trial. *N Engl J Med* 324:781–788, 1991.

Ezri M, et al. Electrophysiologic evaluation of syncope in patients with bifascicular block. *Am Heart J* 106:693–697, 1983.

Ferguson D, et al. Management of recurrent ventricular tachycardia: Economic impact of therapeutic alternatives. *Am J Cardiol* 53:531–536, 1984.

Harken AH, Horowitz LN, Josephson ME. The surgical treatment of ventricular tachycardia. *Ann Thorac Surg* 30:499–508, 1980.

Hartzler GO. Electrode catheter ablation of refractory focal ventricular tachycardia. *J Am Coll Cardiol* 2:1107–1113, 1985.

Herling IM, Horowitz LN, Josephson ME. Ventricular ectopic activity after medical and surgical treatment for recurrent sustained ventricular tachycardia. *Am J Cardiol* 45: 633–639, 1980.

Horowitz LN, Josephson ME, Kastor JA. Intracardiac electrophysiologic studies as a method for the optimization of drug therapy in chronic ventricular arrhythmia. *Prog Cardiovasc Dis* 23:81–98, 1980.

Jackman WM, et al. Catheter ablation of accessory atrioventricular pathways (Wolff-Parkinson-White syndrome) by radiofrequency current. *N Engl J Med* 324:1605–1611, 1991.

Josephson ME, et al. Role of catheter mapping in the preoperative evaluation of ventricular tachycardia. *Am J Cardiol* 49:207–220, 1982.

Kadish AH, et al. Amiodarone: Correlation of early and late electrophysiologic studies with outcome. *Am Heart J* 112:1134–1140, 1986.

Karagueuzian HS, et al. Appropriate diagnostic studies for sinus node dysfunction. *PACE* 8:242–254, 1985.

Kuck K-H, et al. Successful catheter ablation of human ventricular tachycardia with radiofrequency current guided by an endocardial map of the area of slow conduction. *PACE* 14:1060–1071, 1991.

Lee MA, et al. Catheter modification of the atrioventricular junction with radiofrequency energy for control of atrioventricular nodal reentry tachycardia. *Circulation* 83: 827–835, 1991.

McPherson CA, Rosenfeld LE, Batsford WP. Day-to-day reproducibility of responses to right ventricular programmed electrical stimulation: Implications for serial drug testing. *Am J Cardiol* 55:689–695, 1985.

Morady F, et al. Clinical characteristics and results of electrophysiologic testing in young adults with ventricular tachycardia or ventricular fibrillation. *Am Heart J* 106:1306–1314, 1983.

Platia EV, Vlay SC, Reid PR. A comparison of the predictive value of programmed electrical stimulation and Holter monitoring in patients with malignant ventricular arrhythmias. *Am J Cardiol* 49:928, 1982.

Platia EV, et al. Sensitivity of various extrastimulus techniques in patients with serious ventricular arrhythmias. *Am Heart J* 106:698–703, 1983.

Powell AC, et al. Influence of implantable cardioverter-defibrillators on the long-term prognosis of survivors of out-of-hospital cardiac arrest. *Circulation* 88:1083–1092, 1993.

Ross DL, et al. Comprehensive clinical electrophysiologic studies in the investigation of documented or suspected tachycardias: Time, staff, problems and costs. *Circulation* 61:1010–1016, 1980.

Ruskin JN, DiMarco JP, Garan H. Out-of-hospital cardiac arrest: Electrophysiologic observations and selection of long-term antiarrhythmic therapy. *N Engl J Med* 303:607–613, 1980.

Ruskin JN, et al. Antiarrhythmic drugs: A possible cause of out-of-hospital cardiac arrest. *N Engl J Med* 309:1302–1306, 1983.

Siebels J, et al. ICD versus drugs in cardiac arrest survivors: Preliminary results of the Cardiac Arrest Study Hamburg. *PACE* 16:552–558, 1993.

Waspe LW, et al. Prediction of sudden death and spontaneous VT in survivors of complicated myocardial infarction: Value of the response to programmed stimulation using a maximum of three ventricular extrastimuli. *J Am Coll Cardiol* 5:1292–1301, 1985.

Waxman HL, et al. Amiodarone for control of sustained ventricular tachyarrhythmia: Clinical and electrophysiologic effects in 51 patients. *Am J Cardiol* 50:1066–1074, 1982.

Waxman HL, et al. The response to procainamide during electrophysiologic study for sustained ventricular tachyarrhythmias predicts the response to other medications. *Circulation* 67:30–37, 1983.

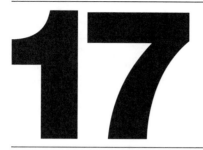

17

Pacemakers, Pacemaker-Mediated Tachycardias, and Antitachycardia Pacemakers

James A. Reiffel
and Henry M. Spotnitz

Permanent pacemakers have evolved remarkably from their rudimentary beginnings in the 1950s. Increasing capabilities, flexibility, and reliability; prolonged battery life; decreasing size; and the ability to nearly mimic normal physiology have provided great convenience for the patient. Programmability and telemetric capabilities have improved the level of care that can be administered. At the same time, enormous complexity has been introduced by the proliferation of programmable functions, manufacturers, and models and multiple unique programmers and routines. Antitachycardia devices have been fruitfully developed, while pacemaker-mediated arrhythmias have added to the variety of issues to deal with. The rising cost of pacemakers and the high frequency of pacemaker insertion in the United States have led to attempts to limit costs to the health care system by defining specific acceptable indications for pacing and appropriate guidelines for the use of the more expensive pacemakers and leads. In this chapter, we shall touch on several of the factors that underlie current pacemaker choices, complexities, and complications.

I. **Classification and international coding.** Pacemakers can be classified according to whether leads are inserted by thoracotomy (epicardial) or transvenously (endocardial) and according to which chambers are paced and sensed. The response to sensed events, programmability, and telemetric and antiarrhythmic capabilities are also important coding properties. The most important property of a permanent pacemaker in the international classification is the functional algorithm. These algorithms are described by a five-letter code defined in 1981 [1], which is abbreviated to three letters in common usage. The codes are set out in Table 17-1. The first letter of the code defines the chamber paced, the second letter the chamber sensed, and the third letter the way in which the sensing data are used (Fig. 17-1). The fourth letter refers to the capacity of the pacemaker to respond to activity; the fifth letter, to antiarrhythmic capabilities. However, the fifth letter is only infrequently stated in practice.

A VVI pacemaker paces and senses in the right ventricle. The sensed electrogram inhibits the pacing impulse if the patient's intrinsic heart rate is faster than a programmed value (Fig. 17-2). A DVI pacemaker is similar to a VVI, except that with a DVI both the atrium and the ventricle are paced sequentially, with a physiologic atrioventricular (AV) delay (Fig. 17-3). This increases stroke volume in correctly selected patients. A DDD ("universal") pacemaker paces and senses in both the atrium and ventricle. This allows almost normal physiologic function. The DDD pacemaker can also usually be programmed to perform in any of the known modes of pacemaker function, from VOO to VAT (see Table 17-1). The great versatility of the DDD unit is obtained at a cost of $2000–3000 over other pacemaker types. A VVIR pacemaker senses and paces in the ventricle, and it changes the paced rate in response (rate responsiveness) to a sensor-derived indicator of physiologically appropriate heart rate. An AAIR unit functions analogously in the atria. Such sensors may be triggered by chest wall muscle activation, movement, minute ventilation, temperature, changes in Q–T intervals, dp/dt, chemosensors, surrogates for catecholamine levels, or the like [2]. A DDDR pacemaker, the most versatile mode available, senses and paces in both the atrium and ventricle, and, in addition, it can respond to an activity sensor as above. Thus, the ventricular rate can be programmed to follow the atrial rate or the sensor-driven rate, whichever is more appropriate at a given instant. Such rate-responsive devices return chronotropic competence to patients with AV block or sick sinus syndrome and thereby provide improved activity tolerance. At present, multiple types of rate-responsive, non-P-wave sensing sensors are not available in any single pacemaker.

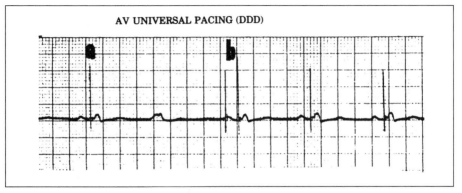

Fig. 17-1. Example of DDD pacing modes. Two of the three common pacing patterns inherent to DDD pacing are illustrated. In the beat labeled *a*, the pacemaker senses atrial activity and paces the right ventricle after an appropriate physiologic interval (VAT pacing). The subsequent ventricular premature beat (VPB) (not labeled) is appropriately sensed by the pacemaker, which does not fire. At *b*, the pacemaker reverts to its DVI mode because the interval between the VPB and the paced ventricular depolarization will exceed 1 second if the pacemaker does not fire (lower pacer rate set at 60 beats/minute). The patient's intrinsic P wave is concealed in the atrioventricular (AV) interval at *b*. The remaining beats in the sequence are VAT mode function. (Table 17-1 explains pacemaker code.)

II. **Indications for the considerations in temporary pacing.** Temporary pacing is most commonly utilized for transient control of bradyarrhythmias that are symptomatic or potentially life threatening (Table 17-2). Dual chamber temporary pacing is occasionally utilized for hemodynamic support in the presence of a junctional or ventricular rhythm. Pacing is continued until the conditions producing the arrhythmia have been corrected or until permanent pacing has been elected and established. Temporary pacing may also be utilized to increase the safety of general anesthesia or cardiac catheterization in patients with a risk of severe bradycardia but without an arrhythmic potential requiring permanent pacing.

Reversible bradycardia requiring temporary pacing is most commonly associated with acute myocardial infarction and with drug therapy (especially in the setting of underlying sinus node dysfunction or AV conduction disease). Common examples of offending agents are digitalis, type 1A or 1C antiarrhythmic agents (especially with underlying His-Purkinje dysfunction), beta blockers, diltiazem or verapamil, severe electrolyte imbalance, lithium, antidepressant medications, and sympatholytic antihypertensive agents. Combination drug therapy considerably increases the risk. Inferior myocardial infarction is particularly likely to be associated with transient complete heart block requiring only temporary pacing, whereas complete heart block with anteroseptal myocardial infarction, even if only transient, usually indicates a need for

Table 17-1. Pacemaker code

Chambers paced	Chambers sensed	Response to sensing	Rate response	Arrhythmia response
V: Ventricle	V	T: Triggered	R: Changes	B: Bursts
A: Atrium	A	I: Inhibited	rate in	N: Normal
D: Dual (V + A)	D	D: Triggered	response to	rate
	S	or inhibited	a sensor	competition
S: Single	O: None	R: Reverse		S: Scanning
(V or A)		O		E: External
				activation

Paces if intrinsic rate exceeds rate limit.
Source: From V Parsonnet, S Furman, NPD Smyth, A revised code for pacemaker identification. *PACE* 4:400, 1981.

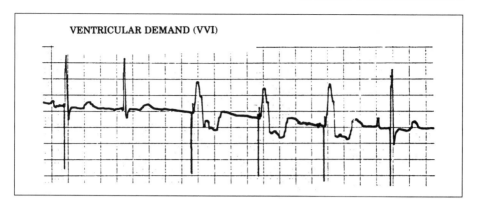

Fig. 17-2. Example of VVI pacing mode. Pacemaker stimuli are not related to P waves. Paced beats are characterized by widening of the QRS complex. Appropriately sensed spontaneous beats are also present. (Table 17-1 explains pacemaker code.)

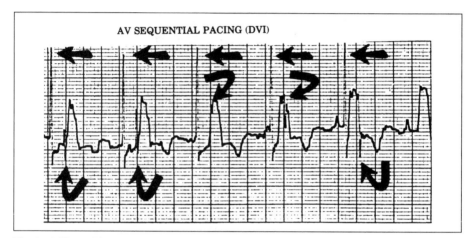

Fig. 17-3. Normal function and peculiarities of committed DVI pacing. The vertical pacing spikes *(horizontal arrows)* are electrical stimuli delivered through the atrial pacing wire. Each atrial stimulus must be followed by a ventricular pacing spike in this committed pacing mode. The curved arrows beneath the isoelectric line identify ventricular stimuli, which are appropriately timed in the first two beats in the series. In the beats identified by the curved arrows above the isoelectric line, the ventricular stimulus is delivered into the QRS complex and would ideally be inhibited, as in standard VVI pacing. (Table 17-1 explains pacemaker code.)

temporary followed by permanent pacing. Inferior myocardial infarction requires temporary pacing in the setting of symptomatic bradycardia or escape ventricular ectopy. Anteroseptal myocardial infarction requires temporary pacing in the same settings but also prophylactically for new multifascicular bundle branch block. Cardiac surgery may also be associated with sinus bradycardia, sinus arrest, or transient complete heart block, particularly aortic or mitral valve replacement or correction of congenital heart disease (e.g., endocardial cushion defects or transposition of the great vessels). Temporary pacing is not indicated for asymptomatic bundle branch block, even if trifascicular, or simply as prophylaxis for general anesthesia, except in ischemic heart disease. Temporary pacing may also be employed to prevent tachyarrhythmias that result from preceding bradyarrhythmias or pauses, or to treat by overdrive suppression or other programmed stimulation techniques, already established tachycardias, such as paroxysmal supraventricular tachycardia (PSVT), some atrial flutters, and some ventricular tachycardias (VTs).

Temporary pacing can be established by insertion of temporary transvenous electrode catheters induced from jugular, subclavian, and femoral veins, as well as from veins of the upper extremity. The antecubital vein approach carries the lowest risk of hemorrhage or pneumothorax. Temporary pacing is usually single chamber but may be dual chamber if AV sequential contraction is needed for improved hemodynamics. Temporary epicardial wires or permanent wires with temporary percutaneous lead extenders can be placed at the time of cardiac surgery. Pacing kits are available for direct insertion of right ventricular pacing wires by percutaneous transthoracic needle puncture in emergencies (see Chap. 2).

III. **Indications for permanent pacing.** Because of the economic and social implications of frequent use of permanent transvenous pacing and because some aspects of clinical pacing remain controversial [3], the indications for permanent pacing have been subjected to increased scrutiny. As a result of activity by medical review panels and insurance carriers, recommendations for permanent transvenous pacing have recently become more rigidly defined [4] (Table 17-3).

Table 17-2. Indications for temporary pacing

Emergency arrhythmia control (e.g., bradycardia with symptoms)

Prophylaxis
    Coronary care (e.g., anteroseptal myocardial infarction
       with new bundle branch block)
    Cardiac catheterization
    Surgery
    Drug trials

Permanent pacemaker failure

Bradycardia following heart surgery

Diagnostic studies

Simulation of permanent pacing (for effects on hemodynamics and symptoms)

Research studies

Source: Modified from DW Escher, The use of cardiac pacemakers. In E Braunwald (ed), *Heart Disease: A Textbook of Cardiovascular Medicine*. Philadelphia: Saunders, 1980.

Table 17-3. Indications for permanent pacing

Accepted, in symptomatic patients
Atrioventricular (AV) block
    Complete (third-degree)
    Incomplete (second-degree)
       Mobitz I
       Mobitz II
    Incomplete with 2:1 or 3:1 block
Sinus node dysfunction (symptomatic)
    Sinus bradycardia
    Sinoatrial block, sinus arrest
    Bradycardia-tachycardia syndrome

Controversial
In symptomatic patients
    Bifascicular intraventricular block and syncope
    Hypersensitive carotid sinus syndrome
In asymptomatic patients
    Alternating bundle branch block
    Mobitz II
    Type II AV block and bundle branch block following myocardial infarction
    Congenital AV block

Source: Modified from AMA Council on Scientific Affairs, The use of cardiac pacemakers in medical practice. *JAMA* 254:1952, 1985.

Irreversible bradycardia causing symptoms of cerebral ischemia or congestive heart failure is the primary indication for permanent transvenous pacing. Complete heart block, which may be acquired or congenital, persistent or intermittent, is an accepted indication for permanent pacing in the presence of symptoms. Symptomatic second-degree heart block also requires permanent pacing, including Mobitz types I and II. Symptomatic sinus node dysfunction, including sinus bradycardia, sinus arrest, sinus exit block, and the bradycardia-tachycardia syndrome, is also an acceptable indication for pacing.

Practical problems center on proving an association between the patient's symptoms and the underlying arrhythmias, particularly in the elderly patient with sinus bradycardia and intermittent syncope or "presyncope." Electrophysiologic evaluation may be especially useful in demonstrating a causal relation between arrhythmias and symptoms or in formally documenting previously unrecognized disease of the cardiac conduction system. However, electrophysiologic evaluation (see Chap. 12) should be utilized for these purposes only if ambulatory ECG monitoring (see Chap. 10) fails to document a relationship between symptoms and a dysrhythmia or a dysrhythmia in and of itself severe enough to warrant pacing.

Somewhat controversial indications for transvenous pacing include bifascicular block with syncope (without Mobitz II or complete heart block) and asymptomatic congenital heart block. Electrophysiologic studies are particularly useful in evaluating the former. Also controversial, but less so, is transient complete heart block or Mobitz II block with bundle branch block after myocardial infarction. Asymptomatic alternating bundle branch block and primary Mobitz II block are still controversial to some; however, most would consider them accepted indications for pacing. Hypersensitive carotid sinus syndrome is an accepted indication for pacing if an association of the bradycardia with syncope can be demonstrated.

Blue Cross and Blue Shield of New York, one of the largest U.S. local carriers, will not reimburse the cost of pacemaker insertion for syncope of undetermined cause, various forms of asymptomatic first-degree heart block, asymptomatic sinus node dysfunction, or asymptomatic forms of type I second-degree heart block (AV Wenckebach). Asymptomatic second-degree heart block is acceptable if an ECG or electrophysiologic study demonstrates an "infra-Hisian" block. Most authorities would also suggest permanent pacing for patients with His-Purkinje disease who have inducible sub-Hisian block with fixed-rate atrial pacing in the physiologic range or with an H–V interval greater than 100 msec, since these patients frequently progress to complete heart block. Pharmacologic stress with a type 1 agent, such as 10 mg/kg intravenous (IV) procainamide, may be used in place of atrial pacing in this diagnostic role. Some believe the same is true for patients with an H–V interval longer than 75–80 msec. Permanent pacing is not indicated, however, in asymptomatic patients with lesser degrees of H–V prolongation or in asymptomatic patients with sinus bradycardia, even with sinus rates below 40 beats/minute [5].

It is readily apparent from reviewing these issues that individual clinical problems will not always be well handled by general guidelines or insurance carrier regulations. Individual judgments and appropriate decisions must be made based on the best clinical and electrophysiologic data available. On the other hand, it is also apparent that justifying these decisions to the insurance carriers may be even more difficult than arriving at a good clinical decision. Physicians must document their decisions carefully and anticipate a difficult battle in attempting to obtain reimbursement for pacemaker insertions recommended in these controversial areas.

IV. **Physiology of pacing.** The examination of patients undergoing permanent cardiac pacing has revealed considerable information about the electrophysiologic and hemodynamic effects of rhythm disturbances and pacemakers [6, 7]. Bradycardia at heart rates of 40 or below is often associated with decreased cardiac output and decreased mean arterial BP. Right and left ventricular end-diastolic volume and pressure increase. The decrease in heart rate usually exceeds the fall in cardiac output, causing stroke volume and pulse pressure to increase. Systemic resistance also tends to increase. In a recumbent patient, a sudden decrease in heart rate from a normal 72 to a rate of 30–40 in complete heart block may be well tolerated without syncope or apparent change in level of consciousness. In the upright patient, the same events are usually associated with profound hypotension and syncope (Stokes-Adams attacks) or presyncope. In patients with a poor escape rhythm, prolonged loss of consciousness or death may ensue, and patients are subject to injury resulting from sudden, uncontrolled collapse. Chronically, heart block may be relatively well tolerated, and patients born with congenital complete heart block may be asymptomatic.

The institution of fixed-rate atrial or ventricular pacing usually restores cardiac output to basal levels. Cardiac output can increase with exercise in patients with fixed heart rates, because stroke volume is augmented by increased venous return. This may occur less readily, however, in patients with impaired ventricular function where the Starling mechanism may be impaired. On the other hand, cardiac output increases to a greater extent during exercise if heart rate increases normally, which confirms the impression that potentiation of heart rate during exercise is important physiologically [8]. DDD or VAT pacing (see **V**) allows the ventricularly paced rate to increase with exercise in response to a physiologically increasing atrial rate. However, the optimum heart rate and the physiologic response to variable heart rate are not always predictable in patients with organic heart disease. DDDR pacing would achieve the same goal in patients with chronotropic sinus node incompetence. VVIR pacing may be used when only ventricular pacing is needed and VAT pacing is not possible. Ideally, the physiologic effects of rate variation would be determined before pacemaker implantation in patients with abnormal cardiac function, but this is not always practical.

In addition to rate-related phenomena, atrial-synchronous or dual chamber pacing provides additional hemodynamic benefit because sequential AV contraction potentiates diastolic ventricular filling, via the atrial "kick." That is, synchronous atrial contraction increases end-diastolic volume, which may increase ventricular stroke volume by 10–20%. Conversely, initiation of permanent asynchronous ventricular pacing has been thought to be responsible for the "pacemaker syndrome," in which the decrease in stroke volume produced by asynchronous pacing is thought to produce symptoms attributable to decreased cardiac output and to cannon a waves. This is most profound when ventriculoatrial (VA) conduction is present and each atrial contraction falls on closed AV valves. Use of a physiologic AV delay rather than one unusually long or short has also been shown to help maximize cardiac output during pacing. Rate-responsive AV delays (decreasing AV with increasing atrial rate) have begun to appear as options in some units.

V. Modes of pacing. Current understanding of the physiology of pacing strongly influences views of appropriate pacemaker selection. In 1995, preferred permanent pacemaker modes are VVI, DDD, and rate-responsive variants. These modes, as well as pacing modes more popular in the past [9], are briefly described.

AOO and VOO pacemakers, capable only of asynchronous pacing of atrium or ventricle at a fixed rate, were popular early in the history of transvenous pacing because of electronic simplicity. These modes subsequently have proved to have serious disadvantages in patients with competitive intrinsic heart rates and are unnecessarily limited in useful life because pacing is continuous, even when it is not required. AAT and VVT pacemakers function by discharging during the absolute atrial or ventricular refractory period in patients with competitive rates; function is similar to AOO and VOO pacers when rates are not competitive. The advantage of this arrangement is that the theoretical risk of inducing arrhythmias by pacemaker stimulation during vulnerable periods in the atrium or ventricle is avoided. Also, the pacemaker cannot be inappropriately inhibited, regardless of external sources of interference. Practically, however, the potential benefits of these pacemakers have been obviated by improvements in pacemaker technology. As a result, AAT and VVT pacemakers appear awkward electrophysiologically and wasteful of battery charge. AAT or VVT pacing, however, is sometimes used transiently as one means of assessing pacemaker sensing function. VAT pacemakers, when introduced, were potentially very attractive because they allow ventricular pacing synchronous with atrial contraction. The principal difficulties interfering with their popularity in the past were unreliable atrial sensing, instability of atrial electrodes, lack of physician confidence in complex pacing devices, and a lack of programmable functions that could compensate for minor degrees of lead dysfunction or alterations in intrinsic cardiac rhythm. As these issues were overcome, the VAT pacemaker has evolved into the more versatile DDD model.

VVI pacing has been extremely popular over the past two decades. VVI pacemakers are simple and relatively inexpensive. The system consists of a single ventricular lead, which is usually unipolar but may be bipolar or ambipolar. The generator is programmed to a predetermined heart rate and repetitively fires at a cycle length appropriate to maintain that rate. If an R-wave impulse is detected at a cycle length shorter than that programmed into the generator, the generator is inhibited from firing, and the timing "clock" recycles to time zero (see Fig. 17-2). The same pacemaker generator type may be applied to AAI pacing, which is useful for sinus bradycardia with intact AV conduction. AAI is a much less popular mode of pacing, because P-wave sensing is less reliable chronically than R-wave sensing and because sinus node dysfunction may be followed by AV conduction disturbances during the evolution of conduction system disease. Most current VVI models are programmable for rate, R-wave sensitivity, and pulse width. Some are programmable for pulse amplitude as well. When available, rate-responsive features (VVIR) may also be programmed on and off. These programmable features provide overwhelming benefits to both patient and physician, to such an extent that we no longer implant pacemakers that are not programmable. The availability of telemetry as an option is of less consistent utility. Telemetry can provide information regarding changes in lead impedance, battery life, pacing frequency, and arrhythmias. However, the benefits of these features for most pacemaker patients are unproved, and their inclusion as an extra cost option is often not justifiable at present.

DVI pacers were very similar in function to VVI models. The principal difference is in the addition of an atrial lead, which is used for atrial pacing. The atrial stimulus is delivered first, separated from the ventricular stimulus by a predetermined physiologic delay. The benefit of this generator is in maintenance of the atrial kick, which may avoid the pacemaker syndrome in susceptible individuals. The principal disadvantage of this pacing mode is that many of the DVI pacers were committed pacers, which means that once the atrial stimulus has been initiated, the ventricular stimulus cannot be inhibited. For patients with intrinsic rates close to the pacemaker rate, ventricular stimulation in committed DVI units may result in the frequent appearance of ventricular pacing spikes during the QRS complex (see Fig. 17-3). The practical impact of this phenomenon is frequent calls from house officers concerned with pacemaker malfunction, sensing failure, and other such problems. The theoretical risk of induction of ventricular fibrillation as the result of an R-on-T phenomenon did not lead to practical problems in extensive clinical use. This is apparently due to the relatively low amplitude of pacemaker discharges. In patients with myocardial ischemia or other critical illnesses, decreases in fibrillation threshold may occur, increasing the possibility that pacemaker-induced fibrillation may occur. Because of atrial nonsensing and therefore asynchronous atrial pacing, precipitation of atrial tachyarrhythmias was also a concern with DVI pacers. In some DVI pacemakers, the ventricular stimulus could be inhibited by a sensing function capable of detecting spontaneous R waves that occur during the programmed AV interval. These DVI pacers are termed **noncommitted**. DVI pacing has essentially become antiquated with the advent of DDD units.

The DDD pacemaker has been referred to as the universal pacemaker because of its great versatility. The pacemaker utilizes atrial and ventricular leads (unipolar in most models) for both sensing and pacing. In the DDD mode, the pacemaker function depends on the patient's intrinsic atrial rate. If the atrial rate is less than the lower limit of the pacemaker, DVI pacing results. However, most DDD pacemakers will be inhibited from delivering a ventricular stimulus if an R wave is detected during the period of pacemaker AV delay; that is, the pacemaker is not committed. If the atrial rate is between the lower and upper programmed rate limits of the pacemaker, it functions in the VAT mode, that is, as an atrial-tracking pacemaker in which a ventricular stimulus is delivered after an appropriate delay following each sensed atrial P wave in the absence of spontaneous AV conduction at a P–R less than the programmed AV interval. If the atrial rate exceeds the upper rate limit of the pacemaker, ventricular pacing no longer follows the atrial rate in a 1:1 ratio. Most commonly a Wenckebach pattern is established, or the pacemaker returns to an analogue of the VVI mode, with ventricular stimuli delivered at a programmable "fallback" rate.

The potential Achilles heel of the DDD pacemaker lies in difficulties with chronic P-wave sensing. P-wave amplitude is intrinsically smaller than R-wave amplitude, and exploration within the right atrium in search of higher amplitudes is usually much less rewarding than in the right ventricle. As a result, the P-wave sensitivity of the DDD pacemaker must frequently be increased (by reprogramming) to achieve reliable function. The pacemaker, if unipolar as many DDD units are, can become vulnerable to being triggered or inhibited inappropriately by myopotentials from muscles of the chest and upper extremities. An additional problem in DDD (and DVI) units is the possibility of **crosstalk,** in which the atrial pacing stimulus is sensed by the ventricular lead, resulting in inappropriate inhibition of the ventricular stimulus. (This problem is avoided with committed DVI pacing.) This problem is dealt with by the presence of a short **blanking period** in which R-wave sensing is inhibited simultaneously with the atrial pacing spike (about 10 msec). In addition, most DDD units have a period of **safety**

pacing during the AV delay of the pacemaker. If a sensed event is detected during the latter interval, the pacemaker will deliver an R-wave stimulus rather than be inhibited, but the AV delay will be reduced to around 100–120 msec. This reduced AV delay warns the physician that inappropriate sensing may be occurring and prevents pacing on the T wave of a ventricular premature beat (VPB), if one should fall in the AV interval. An additional problem is presented in patients with VA conduction in whom the pacemaker may inadvertently participate as a short-refractory antegrade-conducting bypass tract, resulting in a paroxysmal supraventricular tachycardia analogous to Wolff-Parkinson-White syndrome.

In addition to DDD function, DDD pacemakers can be reprogrammed to function in AOO, VOO, DOO, VVI, DVI, and VAT modes. Specialized programming can be utilized to customize the pacemaker to peculiarities of the specific electrophysiology of patients with arrhythmias and lead systems that are less than optimal. However, much of this programming is complex and potentially hazardous and should be carried out by physicians with considerable understanding of the interactions of the parameters involved.

Essential to the proper function of DDD pacemakers is the reliable operation of complex, ultraminiaturized integrated circuits. Not only is the reliability of these circuits remarkable, but they also afford a great deal of customized versatility, providing such functions as telemetry, arrhythmia detection, and, in some instances, the ability to track an externally applied stimulus. This last function is very useful in patients who require serial electrophysiologic testing for ventricular arrhythmias, since the pacemaker system itself can be used for programmed ventricular stimulation. All this versatility is expensive, however. DDD pacemakers generally cost $2000–3000 more than VVI pacemakers. It can be anticipated that market pressures will force prices down substantially in the future, particularly for DDD pacers. Also expensive are nuclear pacemakers, powered by decay of radioactive isotopes, but their 40-year lifetime may be beneficial to selected patients.

One additional problem in DDD pacing is the effect of atrial tachyarrhythmias, in which the rapid atrial rhythm provokes a rapid ventricular response. One approach to this problem was the development of DDI pacing, the combination of AAI and VVI. In DDI, the absence of a spontaneous P wave results in atrial pacing at the pacemaker's escape interval. The presence of spontaneous atrial activity inhibits atrial pacing. There is no triggered ventricular response (VAT) to an atrial event. The absence of a spontaneous QRS results in ventricular pacing at the pacemaker's escape interval. The presence of spontaneous ventricular activity inhibits ventricular pacing. Because there is no ventricular triggered pacing specifically in response to atrial activity, there is no fixed AV interval; thus, the hemodynamics may not be quite as physiologic as with DDD pacing. When employed in patients with sinus node disease, DDI pacing ensures the prevention of atrial pauses, thereby perhaps minimizing pause-related atrial tachyarrhythmias, while at the same time not generating rapid ventricular rates should atrial tachyarrhythmias develop.

VI. **Single versus dual chamber pacing.** Patients most likely to benefit from dual chamber pacing are those with low-compliance left ventricles, particularly with hypertrophy owing to chronic hypertension or aortic stenosis, or patients with left ventricular (LV) failure owing to factors other than low heart rate without massive LV dilatation. The use of dual chamber pacing in patients with atrial fibrillation is not beneficial since atrial stimulation is of no hemodynamic significance. Persistent atrial tachyarrhythmias of all types probably contraindicate DDD pacing. Intermittent atrial tachyarrhythmias mandate a low upper tracking rate and/or mode switching. The merits of DDD pacing are probably most relevant to patients who are young and vigorous and can profit from maximum potentiation of cardiac output during exercise. For patients who are referred for transvenous pacing as protection against syncope during periods of intermittent sinus bradycardia or intermittent heart block, single chamber pacing in the VVI mode, with the pacemaker programmed to a rate below the patient's usual intrinsic heart rate, may serve best. This arrangement prolongs pacemaker battery life, minimizes competition, and is most economical in terms of hardware, physicians' fees, and complexity of follow-up care. Dual chamber pacing may also be valuable in advanced congestive heart failure.

VII. **Lead systems.** Lead characteristics include the number of wires, the number of electrodes in contact with the myocardium (unipolar, bipolar), the surgical approach (endocardial or epicardial), and the means of fixation (passive or active). Initially, lead design was a serious problem. Hazards including lead dislodgement, fracture, and cardiac perforation all occurred. Chronically, pacing thresholds, current drain, and sensing amplitude were frequently a source of difficulty. More recently, lead designs have improved for both epicardial and endocardial approaches, so that conductor lead fractures and cardiac injury by permanent pacing wires are rarely seen. Improvements are due to more durable materials, better contact geometry, and more flexible lead shafts. One recent problem has been insulation fracture in some bipolar polyurethane leads, which can result in compromised pacemaker performance due to oversensing.

Lead tips have been redesigned to minimize surface area and charge requirements for pacing while retaining excellent sensing characteristics. Steroid-eluting tips can improve pacing thresholds substantially in the first year of lead function. Permanent epicardial wires are now often designed in a corkscrew configuration, allowing the active surface of the lead to be physically screwed into the myocardium, and avoiding sutures. For patients who require pacemaker insertion during open heart surgery, an endocardial approach is useful, allowing positive-fixation leads to be inserted into the right ventricle and/or atrium through a small, strip-away introducer during cardiopulmonary bypass. This provides improved lead function and reduced pericardial fibrosis compared to epicardial leads, also simplifying removal of pacemaker leads in the rare event of infection.

For transvenous leads, fixation devices include plastic hooks or wedges (tines) that hook trabeculae of the right ventricle or atrium. A successful alternative is a miniature corkscrew, which anchors directly into the myocardium. In our experience, the rate of transvenous lead dislodgement was about 10% with standard leads, 7% with passive fixation, tined leads, and is currently 1% using positive fixation, fixed-screw leads. Improved tip fixation allows the shaft of the lead to be very flexible, since lead stiffness is of diminished importance for maintaining position. The lead is stiffened during insertion with a stylet to improve handling, with the stylet removed after lead positioning. Confidence about lead security allows pacing from locations that would provide inadequate stability with standard lead designs. In our experience, these locations are the outflow tract of the right ventricle, distal branches of the coronary sinus, and anterior and lateral surfaces of the right atrium. We have been able to achieve stable transvenous pacing in infants as small as 3 kg while leaving an atrial lead loop to allow for growth. Finally, we are able to offer pacemaker insertion via ambulatory surgery for patients who have dependable escape rhythms.

Currently, we do not recommend epicardial pacemaker leads except in some patients undergoing epicardial internal cardioverter-defibrillator (ICD) insertion, patients with atrial or ventricular septal defects, and patients in whom an endocardial approach is not possible for mechanical reasons. Thresholds and durability appear superior by the endocardial approach, and the operation is better tolerated by the patient. The relative merits of unipolar and bipolar pacing are a matter of individual preference. Unipolar generators are smaller and simpler; unipolar leads are smaller and more flexible. The smallest designs will pass through a 6 or 7 French introducer. Benefits of bipolar systems include reduction of myopotential interference with sensing and less spurious pacing of the chest wall, phrenic nerve, or diaphragm.

VIII. Pacemaker insertion. The chance of infection during pacemaker insertion is minimized through the use of systemic and local antimicrobials, and the field is draped so that it is isolated from flora exhaled or expectorated by the patient. Access for surgery and fluoroscopy can be provided while the patient's comfort is maintained and the patient's face is uncovered. After appropriate skin preparation, wide infiltration with 1% lidocaine (without epinephrine) produces adequate anesthesia. Systemic medication that may produce confusion, lack of cooperation, or depression of respiration or BP is minimized. General anesthesia is preferable for patients under the age of 18. Elderly, demented, uncooperative patients who require pacemaker insertion to maintain life are a difficult management problem. Expert anesthesia help is required for such patients; general anesthesia may be necessary, with increased risk. The use of restraints in such patients following surgery may result in struggling and pacemaker lead displacement.

Surgically, we prefer a cephalic vein cutdown via a horizontal, 5-cm incision below the left clavicle. In obese females, an incision parallel to the deltopectoral groove over the course of the cephalic vein is advantageous. An effective cautery is essential for hemostasis. The cautery must be bipolar to prevent inhibition or damage to temporary or permanent pacemakers. If the cephalic vein is too small to accept a pacemaker lead, we introduce a flexible guide wire centrally through the vein, followed by a strip-away introducer. For most pacemakers, we employ a fixed-screw unipolar lead, which passes through a 7 French introducer. After removing the obturator and inserting the pacing lead, the guide wire is reintroduced through the introducer before stripping away the introducer. This provides venous access for a second introducer, if needed. If the cephalic vein is too small for two leads, the second lead can be inserted by direct puncture of the subclavian vein, using a 7 French introducer. The first pacemaker lead serves as a radiologic guide to the location of the subclavian vein, and the puncture is accordingly performed under fluoroscopy. Using this approach, we have performed 500 consecutive pacemaker insertions without a complicating hemothorax or pneumothorax.

Leads are inserted under fluoroscopic guidance. To minimize perforation hazards in the most apical aspect of the right ventricle in elderly patiens, we pull the stylet 5 cm back before rotating the lead to achieve fixation. Apical cardiac perforation, occasionally observed fluoroscopically before adopting this expedient, has not recurred in more than 200 subsequent pacemaker insertions. Alternatively, leads can be placed in a myriad of other useful locations away from the extreme apex, where the myocardium is often extremely attenuated. Interestingly, we have not observed or suspected atrial perforation with positive fixation leads, and we have not seen ventricular perforation in infants or children.

Measurement of pacing thresholds should be confirmed during coughing and deep inspiration to ensure that electrical properties are stable during excursion of the diaphragm. These maneuvers also confirm that the leads are physically secure, and patients should be encouraged to cough as vigorously as possible during this testing. It is also helpful to confirm that pacing and sensing thresholds are stable over time (5 minutes) immediately after fixation. With unipolar leads, testing at maximum (10 V) output of the analyzer should be done to rule out direct chest wall, diaphragmatic, or phrenic nerve stimulation. All lead testing should be performed after removal of the stylet.

Measurements at surgery include right ventricular R-wave amplitude and pacing threshold, which averaged 8 mV (R wave) and 0.6 V at 0.9 mA (pacing threshold) in a recent review of our experience. Measurement of R-wave amplitude in patients with complete heart block and a poor escape rhythm is hazardous and unnecessary. For dual chamber pacing, P-wave amplitude and pacing thresholds are also measured. These averaged 2.5 mV (P wave) and 1.4 V at 2.7 mA (pacing threshold) in our recent experience. Measurement of the intracardiac electrogram during DDD pacer insertion is a sensitive method for detection of VA conduction. We prefer to use pacemaker generators capable of transmitting real-time electrograms to aid with troubleshooting in the operating room. A quick and expedient method for proving P-wave adequacy for dual chamber pacing if electrograms are not available is to set the P-wave sensitivity to 2 mV, the AV delay to 125 msec, and the lower rate to 40. The generator is then connected to the leads. If each P wave is followed immediately by a ventricular pacing spike, a P-wave amplitude of at least 2 mV is confirmed. This effectively eliminates far field sensing as a concern when a dual chamber, unipolar pacemaker is being inserted in a pacemaker-dependent patient on temporary ventricular pacing. In patients in complete heart block (only), atrial capture can be confirmed by pacing the atrium at 120–150 beats per minute while observing the atrial wall or atrial lead tip fluoroscopically for characteristic movement.

In most patients, we remove temporary pacing wires at the time of surgery to facilitate postoperative ambulation and management. We no longer employ a pressure dressing, but hemostasis is meticulously reviewed before closure. Heparin anticoagulation is stopped the night before surgery, and it is not resumed for at least 48 hours postoperatively. The morbidity and mortality of pacemaker surgery should be minimal, but problems that should be anticipated include lead-triggered arrhythmias, angina or myocardial infarction, air embolism, and Stokes-Adams attacks caused by lead-induced mechanical bundle branch (septal) trauma or inadvertent inhibition of a temporary pacemaker during lead threshold testing with a pacing system analyzer. Additional problems may include hemothorax, pneumothorax, loss of patient cooperation, tamponade due to cardiac perforation by temporary or permanent leads, and venous anomalies, including left superior vena cava and obstruction of the innominate veins or superior vena cava. Serious postoperative problems include infection, lead displacement, exit block, and hematoma formation in the pacemaker pocket.

IX. Follow-up. Permanent pacemakers are not permanent but are subject to battery depletion. Threshold or electrogram changes with time may affect sensing or capture. Fractures of lead conductors or insulation or lead displacement also may cause pacemaker dysfunction. Acute or chronic pacemaker infections or pocket erosions may occur. Accordingly, the patient with a permanent pacemaker requires regular postimplant follow-up. Clinical experience with specific battery and lead types and projected battery life based on laboratory data is used to estimate life expectancy for individual pacemakers. The frequency of postimplant follow-up evaluations is based on these data and projections.

Follow-up evaluation can be performed by pacemaker clinics in an implanting physician's hospital or office, by transtelephonic ECG monitoring, or by some combination of these. Appropriateness of demand mode function, the rate during demand mode pacing, and the rate of the pacer when converted to asynchronous mode for the "magnet test" are part of all follow-up tests. Holter monitoring may be necessary to detect some pacemaker malfunctions. Application of a magnet to many current pacemaker generators triggers a "threshold margin test," which reduces pulse width 25–50% to test the safety margin for pacing. Many current pacemakers have a built-in capacity for safe and expeditious measurement of pacing threshold and sensing characteristics. However, these tests should be carried out only by individuals who understand how to maintain patient safety and comfort during these tests.

If sensing or pacing function is abnormal, reprogramming may be adequate. Reprogramming of sensitivity can correct under- or oversensing. Reprogramming of pulse width or amplitude can correct loss of pacing or threshold changes. We prefer a 100% safety margin for pacing output over threshold requirement. Alternatively, lead repositioning may be indicated. Conversion from a unipolar to a bipolar system may be necessary in response to myopotential inhibition not corrected by increasing pacemaker sensitivity. Once chronic thresholds have been achieved, testing will frequently reveal that generator output is far in excess of pacing requirements. Reprogramming to reduce pulse width to the minimum value consistent with safety may extend battery life under these circumstances. Whether patients with both defibrillator and DDD pacemaker implants should be provided with magnets for pacemaker testing is of concern, since improper use of the magnet could inadvertently turn off the ICD.

The response to decreasing battery charge in some early pacemakers was an acceleration of heart rate. Currently, pacemaker rate decreases in most models with declining battery charge. When an unprogrammed decrease in spontaneous or magnet rate (usually >6 beats/minute) indicates exhaustion of one battery cell, most manufacturers recommend elective generator replacement.

In past years, lead function was also evaluated during follow-up in pacemaker clinics, primarily by examination of the configuration of the pacer spike on a rapid sweep storage oscilloscope. This is now accomplished in many units via telemetric interrogation of the pacemaker. Such interrogation, which varies in detail from unit to unit, can provide information on battery status and lead status. In some units, additional information, such as the number of paced beats since the last inquiry or the presence of spontaneous arrhythmias, can also be ascertained from memory chips in the pacer. Regardless of the specifics, it should be kept in mind that the main feature of follow-up is identification of impending pacer failure before a symptomatic emergency.

In addition, patients are encouraged to transmit their ECG transtelephonically at any time symptoms occur. Such transmissions are generally covered by third-party carriers, as are the follow-up evaluations when they are on the frequency schedule that is preapproved for the specific pacer mode and battery type being utilized. In addition, in response to pacemaker-generated tachycardias, changes in spontaneous rhythm, or both, the pacing mode may also have to be reprogrammed. Gross pacemaker malfunctions owing to electrical failure are exceedingly rare in current models. However, pacemakers can be severely disabled by direct current cardioversion. If this occurs, proper function can sometimes be restored by reprogramming. For life-threatening pacemaker malfunctions that necessitate neutralizing the pacemaker, the alternatives are programming to minimize rate, amplitude, and pulse width or surgically dividing the leads. Conversion to a fixed-rate mode by taping a magnet to the skin over the generator can also be helpful in special circumstances, but this will render some units subject to reprogramming by spurious electrical signals that otherwise would be ignored.

An important problem for pacemaker recipients is how to handle electrocautery when sugical procedures are planned by surgical teams inexperienced with pacemakers. Recently we observed complete and irreversible destruction of the output of a VVI pacemaker by unipolar cautery utilized for hip replacement surgery. Fortunately, proper medical care avoided injury to the patient, who was pacemaker dependent. In the past, taping a magnet over the generator was frequently employed to "protect" pacemaker patients during the use of unipolar cautery. This measure is currently viewed as inadequate, not only because of the rare possibility that pacemaker output will be permanently destroyed by the cautery but also because many current designs, particularly

DDD designs, do not maintain VOO or DOO function for more than a few seconds under the influence of a magnet. Optimally, unipolar cautery should always be avoided in a pacemaker patient in favor of bipolar or no cautery. If unipolar cautery must be used, the pacemaker should be reprogrammed to the VOO or DOO mode until surgery is completed. In addition, if the patient is pacemaker dependent, temporary pacing or isoproterenol for maintenance of heart rate should be available.

X. **Pacer-mediated tachycardias: Mechanisms, termination, and prevention.** In current pacemaker usage, the term **pacemaker-mediated tachycardia** (PMT) is usually used to denote a specific AV tachycardia associated with VDD and DDD pacemakers, in which VA conduction results in an atrially sensed event that initiates ventricular stimulation (after the present AV delay), which is then followed by VA conduction, an atrially sensed event, another ventricular stimulus, and so on [10, 11] (Fig. 17-4). In a more general sense, however, pacemaker-mediated tachycardia refers to any tachycardia that the pacemaker plays a role in generating.

Historically, the first form of PMT was a variety of pacemaker failure called the "runaway pacemaker," in which the pacing rate increased in association with battery failure. Since such events are no longer the property of currently available pacemakers, we do not consider the runaway pacemaker any further.

Generally, pacemaker-mediated tachycardias may result from the absence of or alterations in sensing, from adversely timed pacing, or even from normal functioning of a pacemaker according to its preset or programmed parameters [10–30]. These mechanisms are discussed below within the context of several pacemaker modes. Before considering each pacemaker mode, however, certain common themes should be examined. In doing so, data provided in Chaps. 3, 6, 8, 9, and 12 concerning cardiac electrophysiologic properties should be kept in mind.

In the susceptible myocardium (which does not exist in all patients), critically timed electrical stimuli can precipitate tachyarrhythmias. This concept, in fact, underlies the utility of clinical electrophysiologic testing in which patients with arrhythmic symptoms are assessed for tachycardia induction and patients with induced tachycardias undergo therapeutic trials with the goal of achieving noninducibility. Most patients with clinically occurring tachyarrhythmias can have their arrhythmia induced, while few if any patients without spontaneous tachyarrhythmias will have arrhythmias precipitated (except with protocols that are far more aggressive than the stimulation sequences likely to be encountered with permanent pacemakers). In some patients, either single premature stimuli (especially if they are placed early in the relative refractory period of the stimulated chamber) or underdrive pacing are adequately stressful to induce the target arrhythmia.

Consequently, in patients prone to tachycardias, as determined from their history or as a result of the natural evolution of their underlying illness, electrical stimuli from implanted devices may trigger tachyarrhythmias. This is most likely to occur when a chamber is paced but not sensed (appropriately or at all) (see Fig. 17-4). It may also occur in a chamber that is stimulated in the trigger mode, but the triggering event is inappropriate. It is also important to recall that the conditions that render a cardiac chamber vulnerable to the induction of a tachycardia may vary. One may be at greater risk for fibrillation during ischemia or hypoxemia, for example, than in the stable or baseline state. Or one may generate the appropriate dispersion of refractoriness or conduction delay necessary for the initiation of reentry only after successive short cycles or after abrupt changes in cycle length, as when a short cycle follows a longer cycle. This has implications for the role of hysteresis as a tachycardia risk or for the risk of a pacemaker that senses properly during normal sinus rhythm (NSR) but does not reliably sense VPBs.

A. **AOO, VOO, and DOO modes.** In the asynchronous AOO, VOO, and DOO modes, pacemaker stimuli are generated at a fixed rate with no relationship to the spontaneous cardiac rhythm. If the myocardium is vulnerable and is activated by an appropriately timed stimulus, a tachyarrhythmia (fibrillation or flutter more often than monomorphic tachycardia) may occur [13, 27]. Depending on the chamber stimulated, the arrhythmia may be atrial or ventricular. Although AOO, VOO, and DOO pacing modes are rarely used today, such modes are often initiated during management testing as is utilized during pacemaker follow-up, and thus the risk does exist for most patients with implanted pacemakers.

The specific risk of tachyarrhythmia induction, however, is related not only to the presence and timing of a pacemaker stimulus but to the magnitude, polarity, and width of the pacemaker stimulus and characteristics of the myocardium as well.

Although the risk of tachycardia induction is greater with increasing current, regardless of the pacemaker mode, we have raised the point during the discussion of AOO and VOO pacing because it is a lesson that was learned early in the era of asynchronous pacing.

To keep the problem in perspective, when VOO pacing was commonly employed, precipitation of ventricular tachyarrhythmias was infrequent, probably because the fibrillation or tachycardia threshold is usually much higher than the energy actually delivered by the pulse generator.

B. **AAI pacing.** With AAI pacing, which is used infrequently clinically except in selected patients with sinus node dysfunction, atrial pacing is inhibited when a spontaneous atrial event is sensed. Thus, the risk of stimulus generation during the atrial vulnerable period is minimal. If an atrial event is not sensed, however, a stimulus may be emitted during atrial vulnerability. The major factor underlying atrial nonsensing is too low an amplitude of the atrial electrograms. Poor atrial signals are relatively common in patients with sick sinus syndrome.

C. **VVI pacing.** With VVI pacing, ventricular pacing is inhibited when a spontaneous ventricular event is sensed. Unlike the atrium, ventricular electrogram amplitudes are rarely too small to provide adequate triggers for sensing. Thus, inappropriate stimulation during the ventricular vulnerable period is rare, and VVI pacing has been remarkably free of inadvertent tachycardia precipitation. However, if the patient has VPBs that are not sensed though sinus rhythm is (usually because of an alteration in the activation vector at the implanted electrode or electrodes such that the VPB electrogram has a more perpendicular orientation and therefore lower amplitude), ventricular tachyarrhythmias can be precipitated. Such sensing problems are somewhat less likely to occur with unipolar than bipolar systems.

D. **DVI pacing (of historical interest).** From the ventricular standpoint electrically, DVI pacing is analogous to VVI pacing, and thus the likelihood of ventricular tachyarrhythmia initiation is low. From the atrial standpoint, however, there is atrial stimulation without atrial sensing (see Fig. 17-4). Thus, asynchronous atrial pacing is present. Accordingly, as with AOO pacing, the risk of precipitating atrial tachyarrhythmias, most commonly atrial fibrillation or flutter, has been more than theoretical [11]. This risk plus the lack of rate responsiveness via P-wave sensing are the two major reasons DVI pacers have been replaced by DDD units. One advantage of the newer mode of DDD pacing is the availability of both atrial and ventricular sensing, which is associated with a reduced likelihood of precipitation of atrial fibrillation as compared to DVI pacing.

Yet another tachycardic risk also existed with certain DVI units. In committed DVI units, that is, those in which a ventricular pulse is generated once an atrial pulse is, regardless of whether spontaneous AV conduction results in a spontaneous QRS before completion of the pacemaker AV delay, the pacemaker's ventricular spike could fall on or after the native QRS (see Fig. 17-4). If the spontaneous AV conduction interval is short, the QRS is not prolonged, and the pacemaker AV delay is sufficiently long, the paced ventricular spike could fall on the ST–T segment following the QRS and initiate a ventricular tachyarrhythmia. This was even more likely to occur if a spontaneous VPB occurred after atrial activity but before AV conduction ensued, thereby moving the native QRS even earlier with respect to the committed ventricular pacing spike.

E. **Atrially synchronous ventricular pacing.** In VAT pacing, a ventricular stimulus is triggered in response to an atrially sensed event. Because VPBs are not sensed in this mode, there is the potential for ventricular stimulation (as a normal response to a sinus P wave or an atrial premature beat) during the vulnerable period following the VPB. Thus, ventricular tachyarrhythmias may be precipitated. In addition, with VAT pacing, another type of pacemaker-mediated tachycardia becomes evident. In response to a spontaneous atrial tachycardia, the ventricular rate will rise because of ventricular triggering by the atrial events. Thus, atrial tachycardia, flutter, or fibrillation will result in a rapid ventricular response, limited only by rate limits programmed into or refractoriness properties of the pacemaker. Similarly, if artifact (such as electromagnetic interference of myopotentials) or T waves or the QRS itself is sensed by the atrial channel and interpreted as atrial activity, tachycardiac ventricular responses will ensue [15–17].

In practicality, like DVI, VAT pacing is more of historic than realistic interest, but it should be understood as a learning model. Because of the concerns about precipitation of such tachycardias, VDD and DDD pacing has replaced VAT pacing when ventricular stimulation in response to atrial activity is needed. Moreover, for all

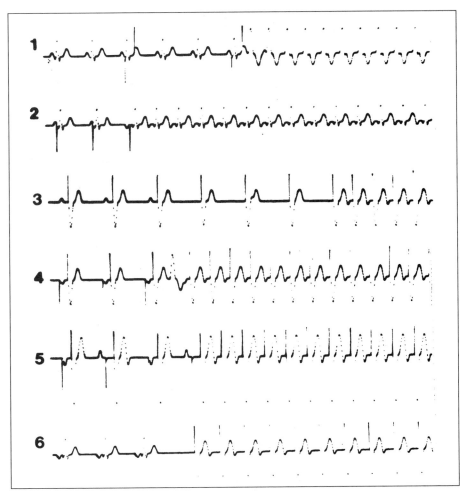

Fig. 17-4. Six examples of pacemaker tachycardias. (*1*) Tracing from a committed DVI unit in which a ventricular stimulus that falls on the T wave of a spontaneous QRS induces ventricular tachycardia. (*2*) Tracing from a noncommitted DVI unit in which an atrial stimulus that falls on a spontaneous P wave induces paroxysmal supraventricular tachycardia. (*3*) Tracing from a patient with sinus bradycardia and a VDD unit in which a pacer-mediated ("endless-loop") tachycardia is initiated once the timing relationship between ventricular pacing and sinus bradycardia allows retrograde atrial activation to follow ventricular stimulation. (Note the small inverted P waves immediately after the termination of the T waves in the last five complexes.) (*4*) Tracing from a patient with a DDD unit in which a ventricular premature beat (VPB) with retrograde atrial conduction initiates an endless loop tachycardia. The postventricular atrial refractory period is 250 msec; the ventriculoatrial (VA) conduction time following the VPB, 260 msec. (*5*) Tracing from a DDD unit that fails to sense properly in the atrium. The long P–R interval preceding the fourth ventricular stimulus provides time for enough recovery in the atrioventricular conduction system to allow VA conduction to occur after this ventricular paced complex and an endless loop tachycardia to ensue. (*6*) Tracing showing the initiation of endless-loop tachycardia by a ventricularly paced complex that is not preceded by atrial activity but that is associated with VA conduction. (This pacer is in the VDD mode.) (Table 17-1 explains pacemaker code.) (Courtesy Cordis Corp.)

such units—VAT, VDD, and DDD alike—it has become the practice to create a long refractory period after atrial sensing, so that short atrial cycle lengths (shorter than the pacemaker refractory period) cannot be consecutively sensed, thereby preventing a life-threateningly rapid ventricular response. A refractory period of 400 msec after an atrially sensed event, for example, will prevent the pacer from responding at a rate over 150 beats/minute. Hence, atrial flutter (cycle length 200 msec), for example, would result in a 2:1 rather than a 1:1 ventricular response. A tachycardiac ventricular rate, yes, but devastating, no. Similarly, programming an upper limit to the number of pulses the pacemaker will generate will also limit the overall ventricular response to rapid atrial rates. In many VDD and DDD units, certain values of atrial refractoriness and upper rate limits, when combined, will result in a Wenckebach type of sequence, which avoids abrupt 2:1 blocking but still limits the overall ventricular rate. To achieve this result, the upper rate limit in milliseconds must be longer than the atrial refractory period in milliseconds. In still other pacemakers, reversion to VVI pacing (often at gradually decreasing rates) automatically occurs when the atria go faster than the upper tracking rate of the atrially triggered pacemaker. This response, called **fallback**, also prevents unduly rapid ventricular rates during atrial tachyarrhythmias. With the advent of DDDR units, a low upper tracking rate can be programmed, with the expectation that sensor-driven activity rate will supersede when the P-wave tracking rate has been exceeded. Alternatively, some DDDR units have "automatic mode switching" where preset atrial rate or regularity criteria will cause reversion from P-wave tracking to sensor-driven pacing, thus avoiding rapid ventricular pacing in response to atrial tachyarrhythmias, such as atrial fibrillation. Finally, in rate-responsive units (AAIR, VVIR, DDDR, and the like), artifactual stimulation of the sensor can also result in unduly rapid responses for the physiologic state.

F. Atrioventricular reentrant pacemaker-mediated tachycardia in atrially triggered ventricularly paced pacemakers (endless-loop tachycardias). The term *pacemaker-mediated tachycardia* is most commonly used today to refer to a particular type of tachycardia that can occur in association with dual chamber, atrially sensing pacemakers when VA conduction is intact. It is an AV tachycardia that is analogous to the form of paroxysmal supraventricular tachycardia using a bypass tract (anomalous pathway) for its retrograde limb and the normal AV conduction system for its antegrade limb. Hereafter, in this chapter, *PMT* will specifically denote this type of tachycardia [10, 11, 16–25, 28].

Pacemaker-mediated tachycardia depends on atrial activation via VA conduction following ventricular stimulation while the atrial channel is nonrefractory. The atrial event thus being sensed initiates a subsequent paced ventricular response, which is followed by another retrograde atrial depolarization, and so on indefinitely. These PMTs have been referred to as endless-loop tachycardias (see Fig. 17-4). Thus, for endless-loop PMT to occur, the following must all exist:

1. A dual chamber pacemaker with atrial sensing and ventricular pacing.
2. Intact VA (retrograde) conduction.
3. Retrograde atrial activation falling outside the pacemaker's atrial refractory period.

The cycle length of this tachycardia will be the sum of the programmed AV interval, the VA interval, and that portion of the QRS interval that occurs between the onset of the QRS and the onset of atrial activation (generally the entire QRS). The tachycardia cannot be faster than the upper rate limit of the pacemaker and is typically at or near it. Because VA conduction is more likely to be intact in patients whose pacemakers are implanted for sick sinus syndrome than in those whose pacemakers are implanted for AV block [12, 18, 31], the frequency of endless-loop PMT is different in these two conditions. Most commonly, PMT is initiated by a VPB. Less frequently, it is initiated by a spontaneous or paced QRS that follows a long P–R interval or by a paced QRS initiated in response to an artifact sensed by the atrial channel. In each circumstance, no P wave exists immediately before the initiating ventricular event, and therefore spontaneous atrial myocardial refractoriness that follows atrial events and may limit retrograde atrial activation is not present.

Endless-loop PMT can be terminated in any of several ways [12, 18, 21, 23, 24, 28, 29]:

1. Transiently changing the pacing mode by application of a magnet (to the DOO mode, for example) so that atrial sensing no longer occurs.

2. Transiently reprogramming the pacemaker's atrial sensitivity, its total atrial refractory period, or its postventricular atrial refractory period (PVARP) so that atrial depolarization cannot be sensed.
3. Transiently increasing or decreasing the upper rate limit markedly with or without shortening the AV interval.
4. Carotid sinus massage (if VA block is induced).

Similarly, it also follows that endless-loop PMT can be prevented in several ways:

1. At a preimplant evaluation, retrograde VA conduction is assessed with multiple-rate ventricular pacing or decremental ventricular premature stimulation during NSR and atrial or AV sequential pacing. The longest value of VA conduction time is then determined and the PVARP is programmed to exceed the VA conduction time if possible (Fig. 17-5). Because a long PVARP will limit the upper tracking rate of the pacemaker, thereby rendering it less physiologically responsive to increases in sinus rate with activity, some manufacturers have built their dual chamber pacers in such a way that one value of PVARP is chosen for ventricularly paced complexes that are preceded by atrial activity (as in sinus rhythm with AV sequential pacing) while another, longer PVARP is chosen (either programmably or by automatic extension of the prior PVARP by the pacer) in response to QRS complexes that are not preceded by atrial activity (such as VPBs).
2. The programmed AV interval can be shortened so that there is less time for recovery of atrial responsiveness before retrograde atrial activation would occur.
3. The pacemaker can be built with an algorithm that causes the unit to withhold one ventricular pacing impulse if a preset number of atrially triggered ventricular paced cycles have occurred **exactly** at the upper rate limit of the pacemaker. Intermedics, Inc., has taken this approach.
4. Antiarrhythmic drugs may be added (or transcatheter ablation tried) to attempt to induce VA block. (In an analogous vein, in patients who have not experienced PMT but who require antiarrhythmic drugs, drugs that are not likely to cause VA conduction delay should be chosen first.)
5. The pacing mode can be changed or the atrial sensitivity altered so that retrograde atrial activation is not sensed. (The latter may or may not affect sensing of NSR, depending on the relative amplitudes of the atrial electrogram with sinus complexes and with retrograde atrial activation.)
6. A single atrially paced complex could be placed as soon as the pacemaker senses a ventricular complex without an immediately preceding P wave (such as a VPB). This isolated paced atrial complex would not conduct to the ventricles or be followed by ventricular pacing and would render the atrium refractory to retrograde activation from the VPB.
7. The use of activity sensors to end PMT via mode switching.

Regardless of the approach taken, effectiveness requires interruption of one of the three conditions necessary for the genesis of endless-loop PMT.

Finally, reprogramming is also necessary to terminate and prevent another, though rare, type of pacemaker-associated tachycardia, which is analogous to "triggered automaticity" arrhythmias [19]. In this tachycardia, spontaneous ectopy initiates self-perpetuating rapid DOO pacing. This occurs only in selected pacemaker models and only if the lower rate limit minus the AV interval (in milliseconds) is less than the upper rate limit (in milliseconds).

XI. **Antitachycardia pacemakers.** Just as electrical impulses of proper timing, sequence, energy, and location can initiate reentrant arrhythmias, so can they terminate them [12, 32–54] (Figs. 17-6 through 17-8). Programmed premature, overdrive, or burst stimulation in appropriate circumstances can initiate atrial or ventricular flutter or fibrillation, or sinoatrial, atrial, AV nodal, AV reciprocal, or ventricular tachycardia. Once initiated, fibrillation cannot be terminated by programmed stimulation at pacemaker energy levels, while flutter may be and reentrant tachycardias often can be.

In order to understand the termination of such arrhythmias by implanted antitachycardia pacemakers [46, 47], it is important to review briefly the conditions that allow reentry to be sustained.

A sustained reentrant tachycardia can be thought of as a continuously advancing wave front whose course of depolarization traverses the same closed pathway over and over again. Such continuous preexcitement of the same pathway cannot occur unless the rate at which the depolarizing wave front proceeds is such that adequate

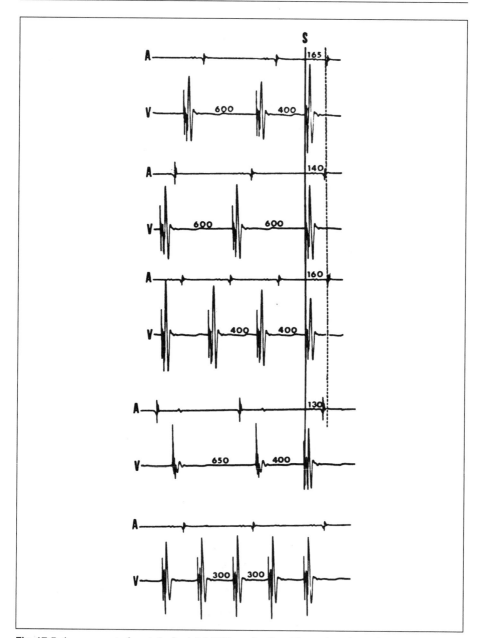

Fig. 17-5. Assessment of ventriculoatrial (VA) conduction. Five pairs of atrial (A) and ventricular (V) electrograms are shown. The solid line labeled S runs vertically through the last ventricularly paced beat in each of the top four pairs, while the dotted line is dropped vertically from the onset of retrograde atrial activation in the top pair of tracings. In the top pair, the right ventricle is being paced at a fixed cycle length of 600 msec for eight beats (the last two of which are shown), after which a ventricular premature stimulus is given at a coupling interval of 400 msec. In the second pair down, pacing is at a fixed cycle length of 600 msec for eight beats (the last three of which are shown), and no premature stimulus is given. The third pair is the same as the second except that ventricular pacing is at a fixed cycle length of 400 msec (the last four beats are shown). In the fourth pair, a premature ventricular stimulus with a coupling interval of 400 msec is placed in sinus rhythm, i.e., after sequential atrial and then ventricular depolarization. In the fifth pair, the ventricles are (continued)

time exists for the fibers at the continuously shifting tail of activated tissue to repolarize and recover excitability before the depolarizing wave front reaches them again. Repolarization must be relatively quick and propagation of the wave front must be relatively slow (because of slow conduction velocity or a long pathway).

Termination of such an arrhythmia, whether pharmacologically, electrically, or spontaneously, requires that the delicate balance between conduction and refractoriness within the circuit be altered. Electrical stimuli can achieve such a goal, provided there is an excitable gap of tissue (repolarized and therefore responsive cells) between the head of the depolarizing wave front and the refractory cells at its tail. If the depolarizing wave front reaches cells at its tail precisely as they recover responsiveness, no excitable gap exists.

When an excitable gap is present, an electrically stimulated impulse can reach and depolarize the fibers from this portion of the loop. If the stimulated impulse reaches these cells at a time when it cannot propagate around the loop (owing to incomplete recovery of excitability of cells ahead of it in the loop), the reentrant arrhythmia will terminate because the spontaneous wave front will now collide with fibers depolarized by the electrical stimulus and forward propagation will stop. This is a mechanism by which an antitachycardia pacemaker may terminate a reentrant tachycardia.

For the stimulated impulse of the antitachycardia pacemaker to be effective, however, an excitable gap must exist, and the impulse must reach those cells during this interval of time. Protective entrance block (physiologic or anatomic) around the focus, impaired conduction toward the focus, or refractoriness of tissues between the pacemaker site and the reentrant loop may prevent this goal from being achieved. The closer the pacing focus is to the tachycardia pathway, the more likely it is to be effective. Active fixation leads may be of significant assistance in this regard. Unlike PSVT, however, in most cases of VT, the site of the loop is not known.

Since refractoriness properties of the normal His-Purkinje system and myocardium are rate related (refractory periods being shorter with shorter drive cycle lengths), limitations imposed by interposed refractory tissue can be overcome to some extent by using a series of rapid pacing bursts or progressive shortening of the coupling interval of one or more extrastimuli rather than single stimuli with a fixed coupling interval as the attempted mode of termination. High delivered energy is also sometimes more effective.

Generally, in our experience, the faster the tachycardia is, the less likely it is to be responsive to termination by pacing techniques. Whether this is because at shorter cycle lengths no adequate excitable gap can exist or whether it is due to inadequate time for recovery of repolarization of tissue interposed between the loop and the pacemaker is not usually known.

Some tachycardias, especially the faster ones, and especially those from the ventricle, also have a tendency to be accelerated by rapid pacing or by multiple premature stimulation techniques that fail to convert them [12, 39, 45]. This tendency suggests that these stimuli are effective in altering the conduction properties, refractoriness, or pathway size of the loop even if they do not effect the precise conditions necessary to terminate the tachycardia. Such accelerated tachycardias commonly reveal an alteration in morphology as well and are typically less well tolerated hemodynamically and symptomatically. Fibrillation may ensue. For this reason, free-standing antitachycardia pacing is rarely used in the ventricles. Rather, antitachycardiac pacing features are incorporated into devices with backup defibrillation capacities.

Let us now examine some of the specific pacing sequences that have been utilized most commonly in tachycardia pacemakers. Specific references to brands and models are not detailed; this chapter is meant to be a review of methods and theory, not a

---

Fig. 17-5 (continued) being paced at a fixed cycle length of 300 msec. Note that the VA conduction time is 165 msec in the top pair, 140 msec in the second, 160 msec in the third, and 130 msec in the fourth. There is no VA conduction with the more rapid pacing in the bottom pair. Thus, VA conduction in this patient, as in most others, is slower with premature stimuli placed during ventricular pacing than during atrioventricular sequential activation and is slower at more rapid pacing rates than at slower ones. Thus, an assessment of VA conduction depends on the stimulation technique being utilized. This must be kept in mind during preimplant assessment (see text). While the differences are small in this normal subject, such differences can be magnified in patients with underlying conduction abnormalities.

product endorsement, and is not meant to be limited by the current availability of some units, in some countries.

A. **Underdrive.** Underdrive pacing is the simplest and least effective antitachycardia technique. In its basic form, it is merely asynchronous AOO, VOO, or DOO pacing. The technique assumes that an impulse emitted at a fixed rate that is asynchronous with respect to the tachycardia rate will, if an adequate number of cycles pass, cause stimuli to fall so as to scan all of diastole. If an appropriately timed single stimulus from the chosen pacing site is capable of terminating the tachycardia, this technique should work if adequate time is given. Some or all of the conditions detailed above, however, usually prevent such impulses from reaching the reentrant loop at a vulnerable period of time, if at all. The simplest approach to effecting this method is to implant a standard AAI, VVI, or DVI pacemaker and have the patient apply a magnet (thereby converting it to asynchronous pacing) at the time of symptoms.

B. **Dual demand.** Dual demand pacing is a simple modification of standard demand mode pacing in which a standard AAI, VVI, DVI, or DDD unit is modified so that either a specified bradycardic rate or a specified tachycardiac rate activates fixed-rate pacing (see Fig. 13-6). The tachycardia may initiate asynchronous underdrive pacing at the same pacing rate that a bradycardia would, or a more rapid rate response to a tachycardia may be chosen, depending on the pacemaker used. In some, when DVI pacing is chosen, sequential paced cycles have progressively shorter AV intervals.

Underdrive or dual demand pacing with short or decremental AV intervals may be particularly effective with AV reciprocating tachycardias associated with bypass tracts.

C. **Overdrive.** The term **overdrive pacing** has been used in two contexts. In one, **overdrive** means pacing at a rate faster than (thus "over") rather than slower than ("under") the rate of the tachycardia. The rate and duration of such pacing varies according to the particular arrhythmia and from patient to patient, but typically it is for short (such as eight-beat) salvos at rates faster than the tachycardia or for salvos long enough to achieve apparent capture of the chamber electrocardiographically. When short runs of pacing at rates much faster (>30 beats/minute) than the tachycardia are used, the term **burst pacing** is often employed (Figs. 17-7 and 17-8). Burst pacing usually utilizes successive intervals of equal length, but in some pacer models, successively incrementing or decrementing intervals may be chosen. Similarly, in most models, the bursts are always at a fixed, preprogrammed rate, but in some the rate is automatically adaptive; that is, the burst cycle length is a fixed percentage of the tachycardia cycle length (e.g., 70–90%). In some, the burst train starts at a fixed coupling interval to the sensed tachycardiac complex, while in others the pacer may automatically increment or decrement the coupling interval of successive trials of bursts, termed **scanning bursts.** Bursts and rapid overdrive must be used with caution in patients with preexcitation and short bypass tract refractory periods and in patients with documented flutter or fibrillation, because of the high risk in such patients of the induction of rapid arrhythmias.

The units may be patient activated or may activate automatically in response to the tachycardia. Among the patient-activated units are those in which the implanted unit consists of only an induction coil, without battery or complex circuitry, and the patient activates the device with an external radiofrequency transmitter held against the skin over the implanted receiver. Thus, battery changes need be made only to the external unit (standard 9-V batteries), and the implanted unit is quite small. In others, the patient activation serves to activate overdrive pacing by the implanted pacemaker at a preselected rate, or triggered mode pacing in response to external stimulation sensed on the skin surface. The latter units have short (200-msec) refractory periods (programmable) and can be used to follow external stimuli to induce or terminate tachycardias as well. Thus, they can be used for noninvasive electrophysiologic testing (which might be considered yet another type of PMT). Such units can follow all sequences of external stimuli, and therefore such triggered pacing is not limited to overdrive stimulation.

In its other context, **overdrive pacing** means atrial or ventricular pacing during sinus rhythm at rates designed to prevent the appearance of atrial or ventricular ectopy that might serve to trigger a tachycardia. Since rate-related changes in conduction and refractoriness may affect the ability to initiate reentry, such overdrive may be effective even though the paced rate is typically much less than the rate of the tachycardia it is designed to prevent.

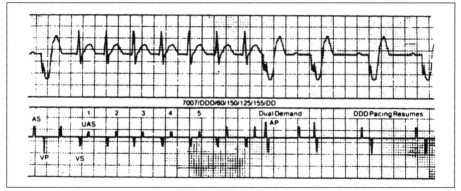

Fig. 17-6. Paroxysmal supraventricular tachycardia terminated by dual demand pacing. The pacer is activated by a tachycardia (once the recognition rate limit is exceeded) and then by a bradycardia (less than the lower rate limit of this DDD unit). UAS = unused atrial sensed; AS = atrial sensed; VP = ventricular paced; VS = ventricular sensed; AP = atrial paced. Table 17-1 explains pacemaker codes.) (Reprinted with permission of Medtronic, Inc. Copyright Medtronic, Inc., 1985.)

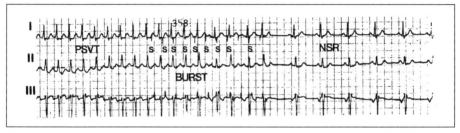

Fig. 17-7. Burst pacing to terminate paroxysmal supraventricular tachycardia (PSVT). Shown are electrocardiogram leads I, II, and III. PSVT is terminated by a burst of atrial stimuli (S) generated by a patient-activated radiofrequency device (see text), after which normal sinus rhythm (NSR) returns.

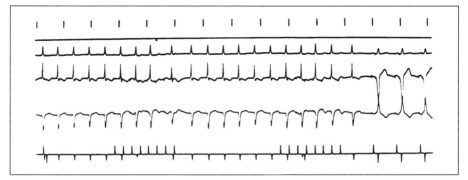

Fig. 17-8. Tachycardia termination by atrial burst pacing. In this patient, a Medtronic, Inc., 2008 pacer (with backup DVI pacing) terminated paroxysmal supraventricular tachycardia with automatic activation of its atrial burst sequence. (Shown are time lines, three electrocardiogram leads, and a marker channel.) The lower rate limit of this unit was 70 beats/minute; the upper, 100 beats/minute; and the atrioventricular interval, 150 msec. (Table 17-1 explains pacemaker code.) (Reprinted with permission of Medtronic, Inc. Copyright Medtronic, Inc., 1985.)

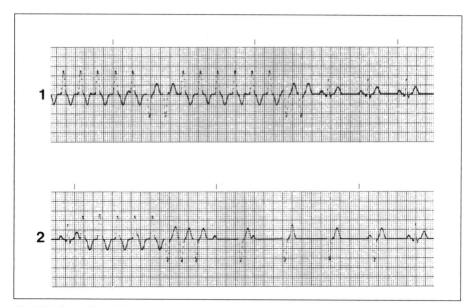

Fig. 17-9. Scanning. (*1*) Pairs of ventricular premature stimuli are placed repeatedly during ventricular tachycardia (VT) with the coupling intervals between the pair and the VT QRS varied so as to scan ventricular diastole. The last pair occurs at a time that allows the tachycardia to be broken (see text). The scan decrement interval is 30 msec. (*2*) Three-beat burst pacing is used to terminate a ventricular tachycardia. This automatic antitachycardia pacer has bradycardia backup pacing, as is exemplified by the first four complexes after the tachycardia. The burst cycle length is 260 msec. (Courtesy Cordis Corp.)

D. **Premature stimulation.** Other approaches to antitachycardia pacing employ premature stimuli coupled to the tachycardiac impulse. They may involve single or sequential (usually two) impulses. The coupling interval from the tachycardiac complex to the first stimulus or between successive stimuli may be incremented or decremented (the specifics varying with different units) but changes progressively until the tachycardia stops or all settings have been tried. The possible combinations are almost endless.

The most advanced of such units start with single stimuli, increment or decrement them by a series of preprogrammed intervals, and, if the tachycardia does not stop, repeat the sequence with pairs of stimuli, independently changing the interstimulus and tachycardia-to-first-stimulus intervals. The initial coupling interval may be determined by an absolute millisecond value or as a percentage of the tachycardia cycle length. This type of antitachycardia pacemaker is known as a **scanning pacemaker** because it scans the tachycardia with sequentially changing stimuli (Fig. 17-9). In the most sophisticated of such units, the effective intervals of stimuli are committed to memory and are the first intervals tried at the next tachycardia recurrence.

E. **Trains.** In the trains mode, ultra-rapid bursts (cycle lengths as short as 10 msec) are used. The bursts begin during myocardial refractoriness and extend toward the T wave until one response is produced. Thus, they achieve capture with the shortest possible coupling interval that could exist for a single premature complex. In some respects they resemble single prematures or underdrive pacing, but the risk of acceleration or fibrillation may be greater with trains.

F. **Additional considerations.** Not all tachycardias are equally responsive to termination by pacing techniques, and not all techniques are equally effective in terminating most tachycardias. Although for any given tachycardia in any given patient the efficacy and safety of different pacing techniques must be individually assessed, certain general behavior characteristics are evident [12, 45]. For the most part, the slower a reentrant tachycardia is, the more responsive it will be to termination by pacing techniques and the less likely it will be accelerated by them. In addition, the more "aggressive" the stimulation mode used for termination (i.e., faster drive rates, shorter coupling intervals, more premature stimuli), the greater will be the efficacy for termination and the risks of acceleration or of fibrillation induction. To some extent, these two observations are linked, as the slower tachycardias usually do not require very aggressive protocols for termination. Unfortunately, nonreentrant tachycardias and the effect of cardiac drugs on properties of conduction and refractoriness make the empiric application of these generalizations somewhat unpredictable in many patients. Therefore, in each patient, when preimplant testing is performed, one usually assesses the less noxious (less aggressive) modalities first and reserves the more aggressive ones for last. Before permanent antitachycardia pacing is instituted for a given tachycardia, it must be documented that the pacing mode chosen is reliable and does not provoke dangerous acceleration or fibrillation. More than 20 trial runs are typically tried once a seemingly effective mode is chosen by preliminary trials. Conversely, before concluding that a tachycardia is resistant, several stimulation patterns, sites, or rates must be tried. Even results that appear to be reliably reproducible in the laboratory may be less so over time, as the effects of posture, autonomic balance, other therapy, and disease course may all have an influence.

Finally, brief mention must be made of one limitation of antitachycardia pacemakers: the somewhat imperfect recognition criteria of the algorithms used by the automatic units [48, 49]. Since automatically activated units do not require patient initiation or interaction for their activation, they must automatically recognize a tachycardia in order to self-initiate their pacing sequence. Currently all the algorithms for such automatic activation involve rate criteria (attainment of a cycle length shorter than a recognition threshold and maintenance of it for some defined number of cycles). In atrially sensing units, however, this alone will not distinguish among different types of tachyarrhythmias or even between pathologic tachycardias and rapid sinus tachycardia. In the ventricles it will not distinguish among different ventricular tachyarrhythmias or between ventricular and conducted supraventricular tachycardias. Other criteria are therefore used. Not yet available is an assessment of VA dissociation or activation sequencing during the tachycardia. This would be most useful. The additional features commonly available, however, include the abruptness of onset, the stability of cycle length, and the duration of stable cycle length. Sinus tachycardia is usually neither abrupt nor absolutely regular. The use of multiple rate criteria for different tachycardias or multielectrode vector analysis of the activation wave front, however, which would be better yet, has not been perfected. Assessing irregularity and QRS width has been used (by the implantable defibrillator; see Chap. 18) for the recognition of fibrillation, but the differentiation of ventricular fibrillation from atrial fibrillation with aberration is currently impossible. Thus, the patient with multiple types of tachycardias, which may require different pacing modes for termination or may not all be responsive to pacing, presents a serious problem to the application of antitachycardia pacing.

Similarly, the risk of hemodynamic deterioration or death from tachycardia acceleration or fibrillation presents a major limitation in the eyes of most electrophysiologists to antitachycardia pacing alone, at least for ventricular tachyarrhythmias. For this reason, the application of antitachycardia pacing approaches for ventricular tachyarrhythmias has reached fruition only in its marriage with automatic cardioverter-defibrillator units.

References

1. Parsonnet V, Furman S, Smyth NPD. A revised code for pacemaker identification. *PACE* 4:400, 1981.
2. Dodinot B. Rate-responsive cardiac pacing. *Ann Cardiol Angeiol* (Paris) 39:597, 1990.
3. Selzer A. Too many pacemakers. *N Engl J Med* 307:183, 1982.
4. AMA Council on Scientific Affairs. The use of cardiac pacemakers in medical practice. *JAMA* 254:1952, 1985.
5. Scheinman MM, et al. Value of H–Q interval in patients with bundle branch block and the role of prophylactic permanent pacing. *Am J Cardiol* 50:1316, 1982.
6. Buckingham TA, Janosik DL, Pearson AD. Pacemaker hemodynamics: Clinical implications. *Prog Cardiovasc Dis* 34:347, 1992.
7. Lemke B, et al. Aerobic capacity in rate modulated pacing. *PACE* 15:1914, 1992.
8. Kruse IK, et al. A comparison of the acute and long-term hemodynamic effects of ven-

tricular inhibited and atrial synchronous ventricular inhibited pacing. *Circulation* 65: 846, 1982.

9. Escher DW. The Use of Cardiac Pacemakers. In E Braunwald (ed), *Heart Disease: A Textbook of Cardiovascular Medicine.* Philadelphia: Saunders, 1980.

10. Johnson CD. Endless loop tachycardia. *PACE* 7:20, 1984.

11. Furman S, Fisher JD. Endless loop tachycardia in an AV universal (DDD) pacemaker. *PACE* 5:486, 1982.

12. Medina R, Michelson EL. Update on cardiac pacemakers: Description, complications, indications, and followup. In LS Dreifus (ed), *Cardiac Arrhythmias: Electrophysiologic Techniques and Management.* Philadelphia: Davis, 1985. Pp 177–213.

13. Sawton E. Artificial pacing and sinus rhythm. *Br Heart J* 27:311, 1965.

14. Furman S, Cooper JA. Atrial fibrillation during A-V sequential pacing. *PACE* 5:133, 1982.

15. Levander-Lindgren M, Pehrssan SK. Occurrence and significance of arrhythmias associated with atrial-triggered ventricular pacing. *PACE* 7:628, 1984.

16. Furman S. Arrhythmias of dual chamber pacemakers. *PACE* 5:469, 1982.

17. Bathen J, Gundersen T, Farfang K. Tachycardias related to atrial synchronous ventricular pacing. *PACE* 5:471, 1982.

18. DenDulk K, Lindemans F, Wellens HJJ. Management of pacemaker circus movement tachycardias. *PACE* 7:346, 1984.

19. Seltzer JP, Levine PA, Watson WS. Patient-initiated autonomous pacemaker tachycardia. *PACE* 7:961, 1984.

20. VanGelder LM, Elgamal MIH. Myopotential interference inducing pacemaker tachycardia in a DVI programmed pacemaker. *PACE* 7:970, 1984.

21. Weber H, Schmitz L, Hellberg K. Pacemaker-mediated tachycardias: A new modality of treatment. *PACE* 7:1010, 1984.

22. Rozanski JJ, Blankstein RL, Lister JW. Pacer arrhythmias: Myopotential triggering of pacemaker mediated tachycardia. *PACE* 6:795, 1983.

23. Harthorne JW, Eisenhauer A, Steinhaus DM. Pacemaker-mediated tachycardias: An unresolved problem. *PACE* 7:1140, 1984.

24. Levine PA. Post ventricular atrial refractory periods and pacemaker mediated tachycardias. *Clin Prog Pacing Electrophysiol* 1:394, 1983.

25. DenDulk K, et al. Pacemaker-related tachycardias. *PACE* 5:476, 1982.

26. Freedman RA, Rothman MT, Mason JW. Recurrent ventricular tachycardia induced by an atrial synchronous ventricular inhibited pacemaker. *PACE* 5:490, 1982.

27. Tommaso C, Belie N, Brandfonbrener B. Asynchronous ventricular pacing: A rare cause of ventricular tachycardia. *PACE* 5:561, 1982.

28. Akhtar M, et al. Pacemaker mediated tachycardia: Underlying mechanisms, relationship to ventriculoatrial conduction characteristics, and management. *Clin Prog Electrophysiol Pacing* 3:90, 1985.

29. Lau CP, et al. The use of implantable sensors for the control of pacemaker mediated tachycardias: A comparative evaluation between minute ventilation sensing and acceleration sensing dual chamber rate adaptive pacemakers. *PACE* 15:34, 1992.

30. Fahraeus T, Lassvik C, Sonnhag C. Tachycardias initiated by automatic antitachycardia pacemakers. *PACE* 7:1049, 1984.

31. Hayes DL, Furman S. Atrioventricular and ventriculoatrial conduction times in patients undergoing pacemaker implant. *PACE* 6:38, 1983.

32. Osborn M, Holmes DR Jr. Antitachycardia pacing. *Clin Prog Electrophysiol Pacing* 3:239, 1985.

33. Greene HL, et al. Termination of ventricular tachycardia by programmed extra stimuli from an externally activated permanent pacemaker. *PACE* 5:434, 1982.

34. Luderitz B, et al. Therapeutic pacing in tachyarrhythmias by implanted pacemakers. *PACE* 5:366, 1982.

35. Solti F, et al. Refractory supraventricular reentry tachycardia treated by radiofrequency atrial pacemaker. *PACE* 5:275, 1982.

36. Kerr CR, et al. Use of Electrical Pacemakers in the Treatment of Ventricular Tachycardia and Ventricular Fibrillation. In LS Dreifus (ed), *Cardiac Arrhythmias: Electrophysiologic Techniques and Management.* Philadelphia: Davis, 1985. Pp 215–237.

37. Luceri RM, Costellanos A, Myerberg RJ. Implantable devices for the treatment of cardiac arrhythmias. *Cardiol Clin* 3:113, 1985.

38. Zipes DP, Heger JJ, Prystowsky EN. Pacing and transvenous cardioversion to control tachyarrhythmias. *Cardiol Clin* 1:341, 1983.

39. Jentzer JH, Hoffman RM. Acceleration of ventricular tachycardia by rapid overdrive pacing combined with extra stimuli. *PACE* 7:922, 1984.

40. Crick JCP, Way B, Sowton E. Successful treatment of ventricular tachycardia by physiological pacing. *PACE* 7:949, 1984.
41. Fisher JD, et al. DDD/DDT pacemakers in the treatment of ventricular tachycardia. *PACE* 7:173, 1984.
42. German LD, Strauss HC. Electrical termination of tachyarrhythmias by discrete pulses. *PACE* 7:516, 1984.
43. Bertholet M, et al. Clinical experience with implantable devices for control of tachyarrhythmias. *PACE* 7:548, 1984.
44. Medina-Ravell V, et al. Management of tachyarrhythmias with dual chamber pacemakers. *PACE* 6:333, 1983.
45. Fisher JD, et al. Comparative effectiveness of pacing techniques for termination of well tolerated sustained ventricular tachycardia. *PACE* 6:915, 1983.
46. Reid PR, Mower M, Mirowski M. Pathophysiology of ventricular tachyarrhythmias amenable to electric control. *PACE* 7:505, 1984.
47. Fisher JD, et al. Mechanism for the success and failure of pacing for termination of ventricular tachycardia: Clinical and hypothetical considerations. *PACE* 6:1094, 1983.
48. Arzbaecher R, et al. Automatic tachycardia recognition. *PACE* 7:541, 1984.
49. Jenkins J, et al. Tachycardia detection in implantable antitachycardia devices. *PACE* 7:1273, 1984.
50. Porterfield JG, et al. Experience with three different third-generation cardioverter defibrillators in patients with coronary artery disease of cardiomyopathy. *Am J Cardiol* 72:301, 1993.
51. Bardy GH, et al. A prospective randomized repeat-crossover comparison of antitachycardia pacing with low-energy cardioversion. *Circulation* 87:1889, 1993.
52. Newman D, Dorian P, Hardy J. Randomized controlled comparison of antitachycardia pacing algorithms for termination of ventricular tachycardia. *J Am Coll Cardiol* 21: 1413, 1993.
53. Gross JN, et al. The antitachycardia pacing ICD: Impact on patient selection and outcome. *PACE* 16:165, 1993.
54. Wietholt D, et al. Clinical experience with antitachycardia pacing and improved detection algorithms in a new implantable cardioverter defibrillator. *J Am Coll Cardiol* 21: 885, 1993.

18

Internal Cardioverter-Defibrillators

Stephen C. Vlay

There has been an explosion of knowledge and technology in internal cardioverter-defibrillators (ICDs). The devices have become more sophisticated and have multiple programmability. Features include antitachycardia pacing, bradycardia pacing, low-energy cardioversion, and high-energy defibrillation. They may now be implanted without thoracotomy. Currently three manufacturers have FDA-approved devices and more are expected to follow.

The problem of sudden cardiac death (SCD) resulted in the development of a device by Mirowski and colleagues in the late 1960s, with initial reports in the 1970s and the first human implantation in 1980 (Fig. 18-1). The limitations of antiarrhythmic drug therapy, recently amplified by data from the Cardiac Arrhythmia Suppression Trial (CAST) study, provide further support for a nonpharmacologic approach. Arrhythmia surgery is restricted to those who have discrete aneurysms and is usually not performed in those with diffuse aneursymal ventricles.

I. **The electrodes.** Originally, Mirowski conceived of a single endocardial electrode to sense and to shock, but technical limitations resulted in a system with a spring electrode at the junction of the superior vena cava (SVC) and right atrium (RA) and another patch electrode over the left ventricular (LV) apex. In addition, two epicardial sensing electrodes were needed. Utilization of two patch electrodes became common. The most recent innovation has permitted a return to a single lead in the right ventricular (RV) apex, with proximal and distal shocking electrodes and also with sensing electrodes.

Bipolar electrodes are used for sensing, pacing, cardioversion, and defibrillation. Today the preferred approach is nonthoracotomy. Systems have a bipolar sensing electrode to sense and in some units also to pace the ventricle. In some of the new endocardial systems, the sensing electrodes are combined in one unit. In some of the older systems, either an individual bipolar endocardial sensing electrode or two epicardial screw-in electrodes were used. Dual chamber pacing capability is currently unavailable. Sensing is usually performed by rate counting. The probability density function (PDF), still available on some older devices but no longer recommended, monitors the amount of time spent at the isoelectric line of the ECG to differentiate chaotic activity from regular rhythms. Probability density function was associated with some problems. High-amplitude P waves could be sensed as QRS complexes (double counting), and postdefibrillation ST–T wave changes made rhythm identification difficult. In some cases, the morphology of the ventricular tachycardia (VT) might not meet the PDF criteria, even though the rhythm was VT.

Defibrillating electrodes are available in various forms. Endocardial electrodes are of the cylindrical coil type, while epicardial and subcutaneous electrodes are of the patch or array variety. The traditional anode was a spring coil electrode positioned at the SVA-RA junction. The cathode was a rectangular patch positioned over the left ventricular apex. Some patients received two patch electrodes, in an attempt to cover more surface area. Today many patients are able to use the proximal and distal electrodes of an endocardial electrode alone. This lead is inserted via cephalic or the subclavian vein and the connector end tunneled subcutaneously to the abdominal pocket. New tunnelers reduce the risk of injuring the electrode during the tunneling process. If the defibrillation threshold is high, a subcutaneous patch electrode may be inserted at the left lateral chest wall. There is a new array-type electrode that involves three fingerlike electrodes that are individually tunneled into the subcutaneous tissue. Other manufacturers have devices that utilize an individual electrode in the RV and a second in the RA or coronary sinus. Varying configurations are available, depending on the device. For patients undergoing thoracotomy for an additional procedure, it is still possible to implant two to

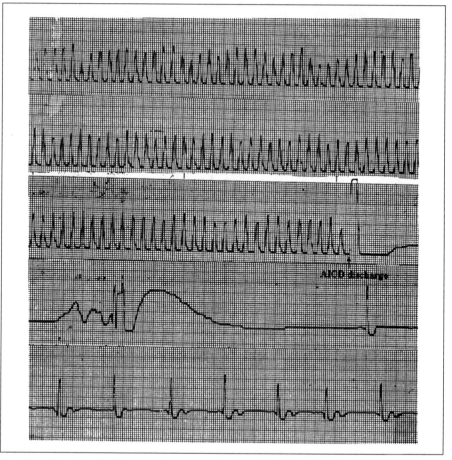

Fig. 18-1. This historic Holter monitor tracing depicts the first electrophysiologic test of the initial automatic implantable defibrillator (AID) in the first patient with the device (February 22, 1980). After induction of ventricular flutter at a rate greater than 300 beats/minute, the AID sensed and recognized the arrhythmia, charged, and defibrillated approximately 23 seconds after onset. Note the initial recovery bradyarrhythmia.

three epicardial patch electrodes to form the defibrillator system, although this may increase difficulty if aortocoronary bypass is necessary again in the future. The polarity of the electrodes is no longer restricted to the original proximal anode and distal cathode configuration. Recently reverse polarity (distal anode–proximal cathode) has been used with success. With multiple electrodes, various combinations are tested at the time of implant. Newer devices can program polarity noninvasively.

II. **The generator.** The pulse generator contains the sensing circuitry and battery to which the electrodes are connected. The units have lithium batteries that are able to deliver either monophasic or biphasic (depending on the manufacturer and the device) pulses across the defibrillating electrodes. The monophasic wave form is a truncated exponentially decaying pulse with a 65% tilt. One newer device uses sequential pulsing with two capacitors firing in rapid succession. The biphasic wave form is created by switching the output polarity of a single capacitor during its discharge. The biphasic wave form usually results in a lower defibrillation threshold and is the preferred wave form in most patients.

Depending on the device and its programmability, either antitachycardia pacing, low-energy cardioversion, or high-energy defibrillation is delivered. Cardioversion or defibrillation discharges are synchronized to the onset of ventricular depolarization

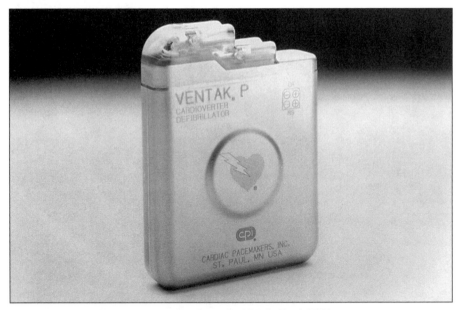

Fig. 18-2. VENTAK P pulse generator. (Courtesy CPI, St. Paul, MN.)

detected locally through the rate detector lead. The unit then reanalyzes the rhythm and, if the malignant arrhythmia persists, will deliver the next programmed therapy, up to a preset number of attempts. Battery size is the limiting factor in the size of the unit. Studies of smaller-size generators have demonstrated successful implantation of pulse generators in the pectoral area. Investigational devices utilize the generator as one of the electrodes (active can). Battery longevity with most units is expected to be within the range of 3–5 years. The more the features of the unit are used, the shorter is the time to replacement. The actual size and shape of the different units vary with the manufacturer. Since there are differences, the currently available devices will be described by manufacturer.

The generator is implanted in a subcutaneous pocket in the left (sometimes right) paraumbilical area. Newer units can be implanted subpectorally. The electrodes, which have been subcutaneously tunneled into this same region, are connected to the head of the device. After activation by a programmer or a ring magnet, the ICD becomes operational and will be able to sense and deliver the programmed therapies. If a malignant ventricular tachyarrhythmia occurs, the ICD should recognize it within 5–15 seconds and start therapy. This sequence should enable termination of the VT or ventricular fibrillation (VF) within 30 seconds of onset in most cases. If the arrhythmia persists, the device recycles for another attempt. If the arrhythmia is terminated, the ICD is reset and restarts its monitoring function.

III. **Review of devices by manufacturer.** The FDA has strict guidelines for manufacturers of ICDs and does not allow release of information about products before formal approval. In the following section, some of the newer devices are mentioned for informational purposes only. This information is important to physicians who have referred patients for ICD therapy and in whom these investigational devices have been implanted as part of clinical trials.

A. **CPI.** CPI purchased the automatic implantable cardioverter-defibrillator (AICD) from the original manufacturer, Intec. It has the longest experience with the manufacture and follow-up of implantable defibrillators. CPI has a variety of devices available and some new models expected to be available shortly, after FDA approval (Figs. 18-2, 18-3, and 18-4).

CPI units utilize a truncated exponential wave form with constant energy ("fixed tilt"). The amount of delivered energy is a function of the initial and terminal voltages and is independent of the impedance of the lead system. CPI used a monophasic wave form for its units until the P2 and PRx III models, which utilize a biphasic wave form.

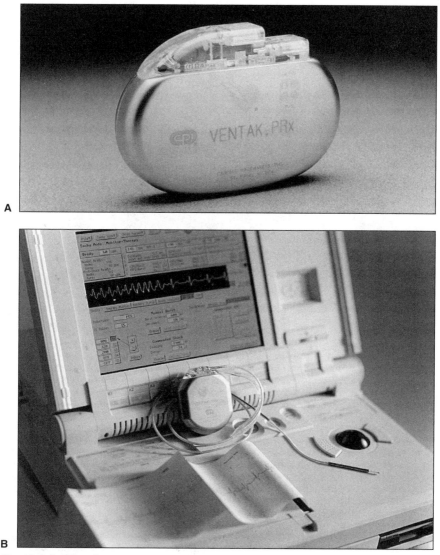

Fig. 18-3. A. PRx pulse generator (tiered therapy device). (Courtesy CPI, St. Paul, MN.)
B. VENTAK PRx III pulse generator. ENDOTAK electrode and CPI model 295D programmer
recording monitor. This CPI tiered therapy device was released in May 1995 and may be
implanted subpectorally. (Courtesy CPI, St. Paul, MN.)

Automatic gain control is used for arrhythmia detection. After an event is sensed,
the automatic gain control filters cardiac signals and adjusts the next sensitivity
point according to the amplitude of the previous R wave.

Application of a ring magnet over the reed switch of the ICD results in audible
tones synchronous with the patient's heartbeat. If the magnet is applied for 30 seconds, the device is inactivated, resulting in a continuous audible tone. Reactivation
occurs after another 30 seconds and the return of audible tones synchronous with
the heartbeat. The features are programmable on the newer units.

The basic unit was the **VENTAK 1550,** which had the ability to sense VT or VF and
deliver a high-energy shock—either 26 or 30 joules for the first shock and 30 joules
for up to four succeeding shocks. The rate was programmable from 125–200
beats/minute. Probability density function was programmable on and off. There was

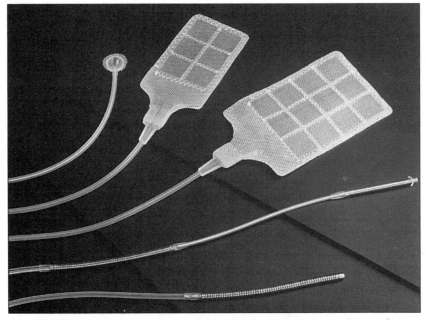

A

Fig. 18-4. A. CPI electrodes. *From top*: epicardial sensing electrode, small epicardial patch, large epicardial patch, ENDOTAK, spring coil. (Courtesy CPI, St. Paul, MN.)

a nonprogrammable first shock delay of 2.5 seconds to ensure that the arrhythmia was sustained before charging. Telemetry provided information on the charge time and lead impedance during the last discharge, as well as a summary of the shock counts. These included the number of first shocks, second through fifth shocks, total patient shocks, and test shocks.

The pulse generator was 10.1 cm × 7.6 cm × 2.0 cm in dimension, 145 cc in volume, and 235 g in weight. It had lithium batteries in a titanium case. It was replaced by the high-energy unit, the **VENTAK 1555,** that has the same specifications, except that only one energy level, 35 joules, is available.

The **VENTAK P 1600** provides a system that allows low-energy cardioversion with energies programmable from 0.1 joule to 30 joules. The unit is otherwise similar to the VENTAK 1550, except that the first shock delay is programmable from 2.5–10 seconds, which may avoid delivery of therapy to patients who have only nonsustained VT (see Fig. 18-2).

The **VENTAK PRx 1700/1705** is a tiered therapy device that provides tachycardia sensing, antitachycardia pacing, low-energy cardioversion (0.1–34 joules up to two attempts), high-energy defibrillation (34 joules for the third through fifth attempts), and both backup (VVI) and postshock (independent of bradycardia pacing or ATP) pacing. The unit has rounded edges with dimensions of 6.8 cm (7.5 cm for 1705) × 10.7 cm × 2.4 cm. The weight is 220 g (230 g for 1705) and the volume 130 cc (140 cc for 1705). It also uses lithium batteries in a titanium case. Antitachycardia pacing is programmable with 1–30 attempts of 1–30 pulses, varying coupling intervals, and either decremental burst (fixed interval between pulses) or ramp (decreasing intervals between pulses) pacing. Telemetry provides summary information for the most recent 128 therapy attempts. The therapy history data include time of detection, cycle length of the tachycardia, detection criteria met, the zone of the therapy, therapy used, success of therapy, whether the arrhythmia accelerated, and the posttherapy cycle length (see Fig. 18-3).

The **VENTAK P2 1625** provides tachycardia sensing, low-energy cardioversion, high-energy defibrillation (up to 34 joules), noninvasive induction (burst pacing, fibrillation induction), programmable wave form (biphasic or monophasic), and both postshock pacing and bradycardia (VVI) pacing. Telemetry includes stored and real-time intracardiac electrograms, as well as pacing and shocking lead impedance. In addition, it features automatic capacitor reformation. This unit has rounded edges

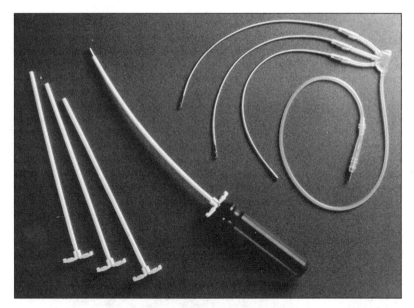

B

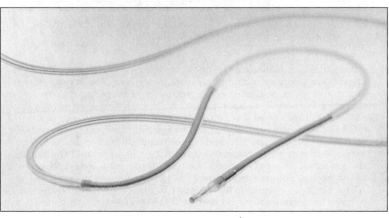

C

Fig. 18-4 (continued) **B.** ENDOTAK SQ array electrode—subcutaneous array electrode. Courtesy CPI, St. Paul, MN.) **C.** ENDOTAK DSP lead. An investigational endocardial electrode that is being designed to be more flexible and easier to manipulate into the RV apex. (Courtesy CPI, St. Paul, MN.)

with dimensions of 7.5 cm × 10.7 cm × 2.4 cm. The weight is 233 g and the volume 144 cc. It has lithium batteries in a titanium case.

The **VENTAK PRx II 1710/1715** (investigational) provides tachycardia sensing, antitachycardia pacing, low-energy cardioversion (starting at 0.1 joule), high-energy defibrillation (up to 34 joules), noninvasive induction, biphasic wave form, stored annotated R–R intervals and electrograms, and both postshock and bradycardia (VVI) pacing. Telemetry includes episode number, data, time, detection criteria met, average rate (pre- and posttherapy), type and zone of therapy, success of therapy, charge times, and impedance. Stored electrograms (up to 2.5 minutes) from the shocking electrodes are available. This unit has rounded edges with dimensions of 7.2 cm (7.5 cm for 1715) × 10.7 cm × 2.4 cm. The weight is 230 g (233 g for 1715) and the volume 143 cc (144 cc for 1715). It has lithium batteries in a titanium case.

The **VENTAK PRx III 1720/1725,** released in May 1995, probably will replace all other CPI models. It is the smallest of all CPI units, weighing 179 g with a volume of 97 cc (105 cc for 1725) and dimensions of 8.7 cm (9.0 cm for 1725) × 7.4 cm × 2.1 cm. It may be implanted in a subpectoral or abdominal pocket. The PRx III may be pro-

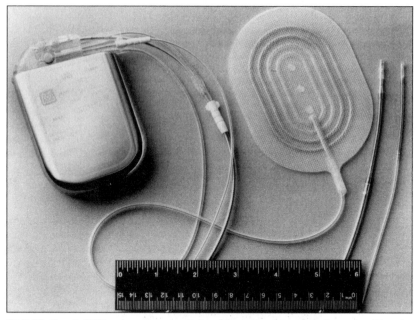

Fig. 18-5. Medtronic PCD pulse generator, epicardial and endocardial electrodes. (Reprinted with permission from Medtronic, Inc. © Medtronic, Inc., 1994.)

grammed either biphasic or monophasic, either reverse or standard polarity, and has the other features of a tiered therapy device. It can detect two different VT zones and one VF zone, delivering either antitachycardia pacing, low energy cardioversion, or defibrillation as appropriate for the arrhythmia detected. Capacitors are automatically reformed every 60 days. Extensive telemetry is provided. The PRx III has both VVI pacing and post-shock VVI pacing. Electrophysiologic testing can be performed noninvasively through the system. Up to five shocks can be delivered with the first two programmable from 0.1 to 34 joules and the remaining three shocks factory preset at 34 joules. Similar to other units, it has lithium batteries in a titanium case. The expected longevity is 4 years.

The variety of features in the various CPI units reflects the advances in technology made by each successive generation of cardioverter defibrillators. The latest have the advantages of biphasic shocks, extensive computerization and programmability.

B. Medtronic. The first Medtronic device was called the **Pacer-Cardioverter-Defibrillator** (PCD). The model 7217B had the following capabilities: (1) automatic detection of VT and delivery of pacing or cardioversion therapies; (2) automatic detection of VF and delivery of defibrillation therapies; (3) backup VVI pacing; (4) noninvasive electrophysiologic study stimulation; and (4) telemetry of parameters, event data, status, and ventricular electrograms (Fig. 18-5). The newer model (Jewel) is more compact and has been implanted in the pectoral region (Fig. 18-6). Newer investigational versions of the ICD utilize the actual case (active can) of the pulse generator as one of the electrodes.

The Medtronic PCD uses stored energy with the joules applied dependent on the impedance and pulse width (a variable energy device). When energy is delivered, termination of capacitor discharge is determined by a preestablished pulse width interval. The wave form is a monophasic truncated exponential pulse delivered over dual or triple electrode configurations. The pulse generator has a lithium battery and titanium shield. The dimensions are $101 \times 70 \times 20$ mm with a weight of 197 g and a displacement volume of 113 cc. The epicardial electrode system consists of two to three epicardial patch electrodes with two myocardial pacing/sensing electrodes. The endocardial system consists of a tripolar screw-in electrode for the right ventricle (usually the apex or distal septal wall) and a nonfixed unipolar electrode placed in varying positions in the superior vena cava. A third subcutaneous patch electrode can also be added if necessary.

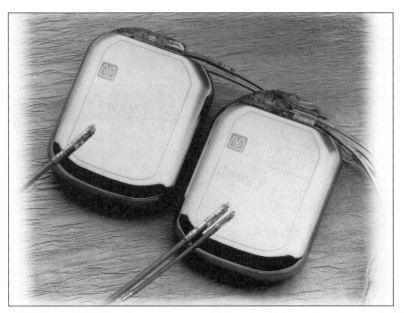

Fig. 18-6. Medtronic JEWEL pulse generator and electrodes. This smaller generator has been implanted in the pectoral area. (Reprinted with permission from Medtronic, Inc. © Medtronic, Inc., 1994.)

Ventricular tachycardia is recognized by interval length determined by the number of consecutive VT intervals and a specific tachycardia detection interval. In addition, two optional criteria include onset as determined by change in cycle length and stability or variability of interval length. Options for VT termination include adaptive burst and adaptive ramp pacing and cardioversion. Ventricular fibrillation is recognized by variations in ventricular depolarization amplitudes and intervals. The PCD uses an auto-adjusting sensitivity threshold function to minimize sensing of a t wave.

Burst therapy consists of a train of 1–15 sequences of 1–15 pulses at **equal** interstimulus intervals delivered in the VVI mode. Redetection of the VT episode is required before the next sequence can be delivered. Burst therapy can be adapted to the rate of the tachycardia and delivered as a percentage of the measured R–R interval. The R–R interval of each succeeding sequence is decremented or shortened from the previous sequence.

Ramp therapy consists of a train of 1–15 sequences of 1–15 pulses with **decreasing** interstimulus intervals delivered in the VVI mode. Redetection is again required before the next sequence can be delivered. Ramp therapy also can be adapted to the rate of the tachycardia and delivered as a percentage of the measured R–R interval. The R–R interval of each succeeding sequence is decremented or shortened from the previous sequence.

Cardioversion therapy consists of a synchronized cardioversion pulse that can be delivered as a single pulse or as two pulses either simultaneously or sequentially. The single pulse is delivered over one pathway from the anode to the cathode. Simultaneous delivery involves two pulses delivered simultaneously from each of two anodes to the common cathode. Sequential delivery involves the same pathways as for simultaneous delivery, but the second pulse is delivered 0.2 msec after the first.

Defibrillation therapy consists of a high-energy defibrillation pulse delivered over the same pathways as for cardioversion therapy.

The programmable parameters include **pulse width** (2.0–8.1 msec), **energy** (0.2–34 joules for the first two therapies and 10–34 joules for therapies 3 and 4), and **pathways** (single, simultaneous, or sequential).

Programmable parameters of VVI pacing include rate (30–90 ppm), pulse width (0.03–1.59 msec), sensitivity (0.3–2.4 mV), amplitude (2.8–5.4 V), and refractory periods (320–480 msec).

The **battery life** is dependent on how often and how many of the features of the device are used. The projected longevity for a unit with a monthly 34-joule charging frequency and 100% pacing is 3.4 years. If pacing occurs only 15% of the time, the longevity is predicted to be 4.2 years. The elective replacement indicator is when the telemetered battery voltage is 4.97–4.74 V.

Positioning a magnet or programming head over the PCD closes a reed switch and suspends automatic VT/VF detection and therapy capabilities but does not affect bradycardia pacing or result in VOO pacing.

The manufacturer recommends 3-month follow-up visits and device interrogation including conditioning of the high-energy capacitors and pacing threshold determinations every 3 months until the battery voltage falls below 5.25 V. Then the test should be performed monthly until replacement. Interrogation of the device provides a summary of the events since the last visit. The real-time endocardial electrogram can be visualized at the time of interrogation.

The Medtronic JEWEL model 7219D is the smallest ICD currently approved by the FDA. The volume is 83 cc (89 cc for models 7219B and E) and the dimensions are 8.8 cm (9.5 cm for 7219B and E) × 6.3 cm × 1.8 cm (1.9 cm for 7219B and E). The weight is 132 g (139 g for 7219B and E). The JEWEL can be implanted subpectorally.

The features of the JEWEL include a choice of wave forms (biphasic or monophasic), programmable polarity, and automatic capacitor formation. Two detection zones for VT and one for VF are programmable. Therapy includes antitachycardia pacing, low energy cardioversion, and defibrillation. VVI pacing is available. Antitachycardia pacing algorithms include burst, ramp, and decremental ramp. Up to four shocks can be delivered for VT or VF.

Noninvasive EPS can be performed with up to triple extrastimuli. For defibrillation threshold testing, VF can be induced by the delivery of a shock on the t wave as well as with 50 Hz bursts. The device has stored electrograms, intervals, and markers. If pacing is not utilized, the projected longevity is 6 years. Pacing if needed and frequent shocks will shorten the time to elective replacement.

The Medtronic JEWEL has replaced the PCD and offers the advantages of biphasic wave form, extensive programmability, and therapy options. Its small size has resulted in the ability to confine the surgery to the upper chest, similar to a permanent pacemaker. The programmer is also one of the smallest in the industry.

C. **Ventritex.** The Ventritex device is called the **Cadence** model V-100 tiered therapy defibrillator. It has the following features: (1) detection of tachyarrhythmias, (2) antitachycardia pacing, (3) cardioversion therapy, (4) defibrillation therapy, and (5) backup bradycardia pacing. The device uses automatic gain control (Fig. 18-7). The model V-110 is smaller in size (Fig. 18-8). Nonthoracotomy Ventritex leads are being evaluated (Fig. 18-9, p. 409). The FDA has approved the use of a hybrid defibrillating system using CPI Endotak electrodes and Ventritex Cadence pulse generators. This combination is one of the most frequently implanted systems today.

The dimensions of the V-100 device are 9.72 × 8.21 × 2.36 cm. It has a weight of 240 g and a displacement of 145 cc. It contains lithium batteries in a titanium case. The dimensions of the V-110 C are 9.3 × 7.6 × 2.1 cm. The weight is 198 g and the displacement volume 132 cc. The case and the batteries are of the same material. The investigational Cadet model will be small enough to implant in the pectoral region.

Ventricular fibrillation detection is based on a programmed rate criterion. **Ventricular tachycardia detection** is based on both programmed rate criterion and a programmable number of intervals.

High-voltage therapy is programmable in terms of voltage (100–750 V for the first two shocks, 750 V for all subsequent), wave form (either biphasic or monophasic truncated exponential wave form), and pulse width (3.0–12.0 msec for monophasic and 3.0–10.0 msec positive phase + 1.0 − 10.0 msec negative phase for biphasic).

Antitachycardia pacing may be autodecremental or burst pacing, either fixed or rate adaptive. The minimum burst cycle length is programmable from 150–600 msec in increments of 5 msec. The number of stimuli in each burst is programmable from 2–20 and the number of bursts from 1–15.

Bradycardia pacing is available with programmable parameters including rate (25–90 ppm), pulse amplitude (1.0–10.0 V), pulse width (0.10–2.0 msec), and mode (VVI or OFF).

This device has a **noninvasive stimulation mode** for inducing arrhythmias for testing and can deliver up to four extrastimuli or induce fibrillation by burst pacing (20–50 msec).

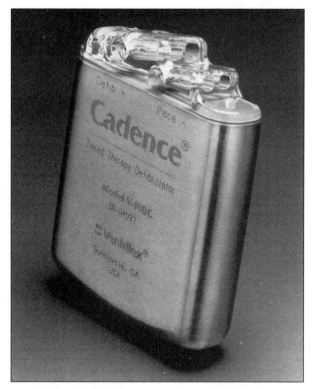

Fig. 18-7. Ventritex Cadence V-100 pulse generator (tiered therapy device). (Courtesy Ventritex Inc., Sunnyvale, CA.)

The **magnet mode** allows the application of a magnet to close the reed switch and prevent delivery of tachyarrhythmia therapy. Unlike other devices, it will be inactive only as long as the magnet is over the unit. Bradycardia pacing and noninvasive stimulation are unaffected by magnet application.

The Cadence device provides for **automatic charging of the high-voltage capacitors** to 500 V if a period of 6 months passes without charging for therapy. This energy is not dumped but decreases gradually with time. Very little voltage is left after 10 minutes.

Telemetry provides a summary of the parameters, charging history, as well as stored electrograms of the events sensed and treated (Fig. 18-10, p. 410). The excellent quality of the stored endocardial electrograms facilitates interpretation of events that resulted in tachycardia therapy.

The Ventritex programmer is easy to use and the software is user friendly, making interrogation and programming simple and straightforward.

D. **Choice of ICD.** Each one of the latest sophisticated tiered therapy ICDs described above, the CPI PRx III, the Medtronic JEWEL, and the Ventritex Cadence, provides adequate protection against sustained VT or VF. Each device differs from its competitors in a variety of ways. Differences include the type of information available from telemetry, the size and shape of the generator and programmer, the number of options for therapy (including the number of shocks), the options for noninvasive EPS, the different options for pacing, the need for follow up, the ease of programming (user-friendlier software), the availability of different electrodes, as well as the service the company provides.

Each center and each physician will take all of these factors into consideration. Therapy will also be tailored to the individual needs of the patient. It will be necessary for physicians to be familiar with all of these devices since one will encounter patients who were implanted at another center. Survival of the patient and longevity of these new devices are now being reassessed.

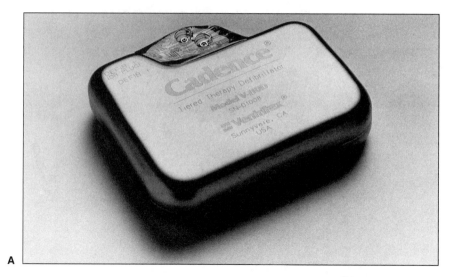

A

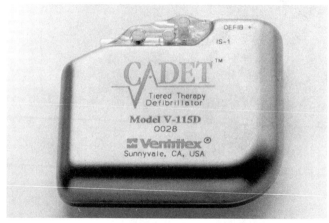

B

Fig. 18-8. A. Ventritex V-110 pulse generator (smaller-size tiered therapy device). (Courtesy Ventritex Inc., Sunnyvale, CA.) **B.** The Ventritex Cadet ICD is a small ICD (130 g, 73 cc) that will be suitable for implantation in the pectoral area. This device is investigational. (Courtesy Ventritex Inc., Sunnyvale, CA.)

    E. Other manufacturers. Only the three manufacturers already noted have FDA-approved devices. Others have products in clinical trials including Telectronics (Guardian), Intermedics (Res-Q), and Siemens-Pacesetter (Siecure), which may be available in the near future.

IV. Impact of the ICD. Survival data from the Johns Hopkins Hospital and Stanford University Hospital conclusively demonstrated that survival in individuals at high risk of recurrent VF or VT and treated with the AICD was far superior to that in patients treated with other modalities. In fact, as the device was improved (from the automatic implantable defibrillator [AID] to the AICD), survival also improved. The initial device had a 1-year mortality from VT or VF of 8.5% (total mortality from all causes 22.9%) (Fig. 18-11). A subsequent comparison between AID (original device) and AICD (modified device) patients revealed 1-year arrhythmic mortalities of 10.6% and 2%, respectively (with total mortalities of 26% and 16.6%, respectively). The subsequent experience of the Stanford group with the "rate-only" device (which uses heart rate as the only criterion, not PDF, for triggering discharge) revealed a 1-year arrhythmic mortality of 1.8% (Fig. 18-12, p. 411). Pooled data revealed 1-year arrhythmic mortalities for the original AID of 11.9% (37 patients), for the AICD of 1.9% (209 patients), and for the

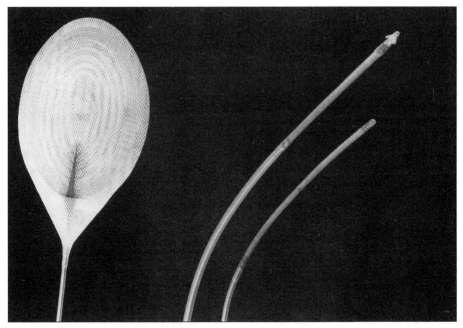

Fig. 18-9. Ventritex TVL transvenous lead system and patch electrode (investigational). (Courtesy Ventritex Inc., Sunnyvale, CA.)

AICD rate-only device of 1.3% (95 patients). As Mirowski indicated in 1985, traditional mortality for similar patients ranged from 27–66%, which highlights the markedly favorable impact of this device on mortality [1]. A study from the University of Pennsylvania by Grimm et al. in 241 patients revealed survival rates from arrhythmic death to be 97%, 89%, and 83% at 1, 3, and 5 years, respectively [2]. Cumulative survival from all-cause mortality was 84%, 62%, and 57% for the same time period. A low left ventricular ejection fraction (LVEF) (<30%) was the best predictor of survival. Saksena and Camm published combined actuarial survival curves [3] (Fig. 18-13, p. 412). There is an early contribution of cardiac nonsudden death and a later contribution of noncardiac death. As of January 1, 1995, more than 45,000 units have been implanted worldwide. Significant predictors of a poor outcome even with the device include severe congestive heart failure with a low ejection fraction, the need for multiple cardiac surgical procedures, and failure of multiple antiarrhythmic drugs. Dr. Kim from Montefiore Hospital warned in a series of articles that while sudden death rates seem dramatically low in patients with ICDs, the total cardiac death rates are higher [4–6]. Part of the problem stems from the way the data are analyzed. The exclusion of surgical mortality, definitions of nonsudden arrhythmic deaths, hypothetical death rates in patients receiving "appropriate" shocks, and possible misclassification of events may potentially favor the beneficial effect of the ICD. While he does not argue that ICD therapy does prolong life in patients with recurrent VT/VF, he cautions to assess the data carefully, compare ICD to other therapies, and look at the total mortality as the end point.

V. **Patient selection.** The criteria for consideration of an ICD have been relaxed since the initial clinical trials in 1980. Initially patients selected had survived two cardiac arrests (not associated with acute myocardial infarction [MI]), at least one of which occurred while undergoing antiarrhythmic drug therapy. Both conventional and investigational antiarrhythmic drugs had failed in most of these patients. There is no question that this group was a high-risk subset of the population at risk who were fortunate enough to be resuscitated multiple times and whose arrhythmias were resistant to drug therapy. These patients merited aggressive measures. But what about the 300,000–500,000 individuals who die suddenly every year and are not resuscitated? These are persons who might derive the most benefit from such a device, especially if they are relatively young, have no overt heart disease, and are otherwise healthy. Certainly, we cannot implant devices in the entire population. We must guard against an abuse of technology.

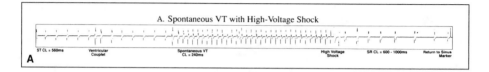

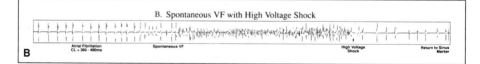

Fig. 18-10. Stored electrograms from Ventritex Cadence ICD. **A.** Spontaneous ventricular tachycardia (VT) cycle length (CL) 240 msec sensed and terminated by a high-voltage shock. **B.** Spontaneous ventricular fibrillation (VF) sensed and terminated by a high-voltage shock. **C.** Noninvasive induction of sustained VT cycle length 360 msec sensed and terminated by antitachycardia pacing (ATP) therapy. (Courtesy Ventritex Inc., Sunnyvale, CA.)

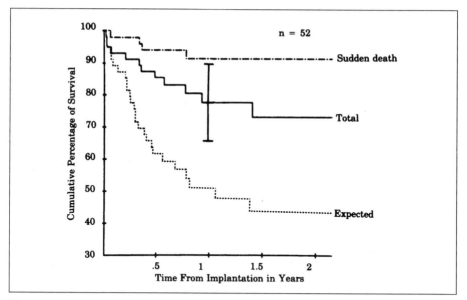

Fig. 18-11. Life table analysis of patients with the automatic defibrillator. The upper curve (*broken line*) indicates sudden cardiac death (SCD) caused by ventricular tachycardia or ventricular fibrillation. The middle curve indicates total survival (i.e., including death from other causes). The lower curve represents the predicted estimate of SCD without the defibrillator. (From M Mirowski et al., Mortality in patients with implanted automatic defibrillators. *Ann Intern Med* 98:586, 1983.)

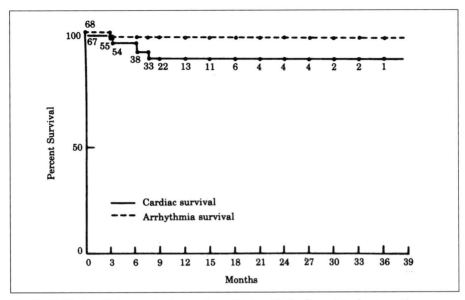

Fig. 18-12. Kaplan-Meier survival curve for patients with the five original automatic implantable defibrillator and 72 rate-sensing devices. (From DS Echt et al., Clinical experience, complications and survival in 70 patients with the automatic implantable cardioverter defibrillator. *Circulation* 71:294, 1985.)

While ICDs are lifesaving, they are also costly, to both the individual patient and the health care system. Nevertheless, there is a valid argument for attempting to identify a subset of individuals at very high risk of VT or VF who have not yet manifested their fatal arrhythmia. Some of these issues will be settled after the completion of several trials now in progress. They include the CABG-PATCH, Multicenter Automatic Defibrillator Implantation Trial (MADIT), and the Multicenter Unsustained Tachycardia Trial (MUSTT).

A task force of the American College of Cardiology and the American Heart Association on Assessment of Diagnostic and Therapeutic Cardiovascular Procedures (Committee on Pacemaker Implantation) provided a set of indications in 1991 [7]:

Type I indications: Conditions for which there is general agreement that the device should be implanted.

Type II: A divergence of opinion in which the device is frequently used by some and others question its necessity.

Type III: General agreement that the device should not be implanted.

Note that these indications were recommended before the advent and availability of the new tiered therapy devices. In the future these indications may be expanded.

Type I indications include:

1. One or more documented episodes of hemodynamically significant VT or VF in a patient in whom electrophysiologic study (EPS) and ambulatory ECG monitoring cannot be used to predict efficacy of therapy accurately.
2. One or more documented episodes of hemodynamically significant VT or VF in a patient in whom no drug was found to be effective or no drug currently available and appropriate was tolerated.
3. The patient who remains inducible into hemodynamically significant VT or VF at EPS despite the best available drug therapy or despite surgery or catheter ablation if drug therapy has failed.

Type II indications include:

1. One or more documented episodes of hemodynamically significant VT or VF in a patient in whom drug efficacy testing is possible. Many physicians utilize this indication due to the undesirability of antiarrhythmic drugs (short- and long-term adverse effects, inconvenience, expense).

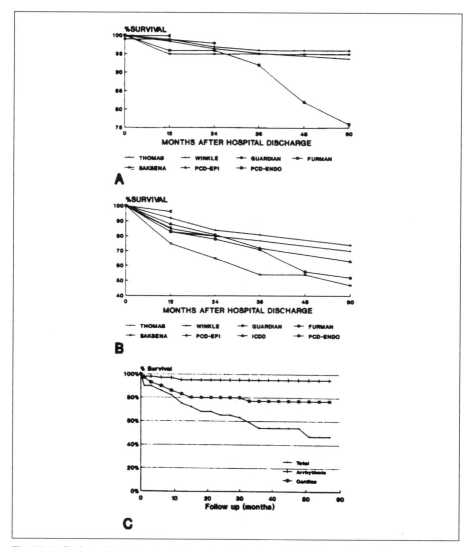

Fig. 18-13. Eight published actuarial survival data charts for implantable cardioverter-defibrillator (ICD) recipients after hospital discharge. Three individual centers at the extremes of clinical outcome data are shown: Winkle, Furman, and Saksena. Two multicenter registries—one manufacturer based (Thomas) and one hospital based (ICDD)—are included. Three recent multicenter trials of pacemaker-defibrillator—Telectronics Guardian and Medtronic PCD with epicardial (EPI) or endocardial (ENDO) leads—are also shown. **A.** Survival from sudden death. **B.** Total survival. **C.** Total, cardiac, and nonsudden death and later contribution of noncardiac death to the mortality. (Reprinted with permission from S Saksena, AJ Camm, Implantable defibrillators for prevention of sudden death. *Circulation* 85:2316–2320, 1992.)

2. Recurrent syncope of undetermined origin in a patient with hemodynamically significant VT or VF induced at EPS in whom no effective or no tolerated drug is available or appropriate.

Type III indications include:

1. Recurrent syncope of undetermined cause in a patient without inducible tachyarrhythmias.
2. Arrhythmias not due to hemodynamically significant VT or VF.
3. Incessant VT or VF (the ICD would continuously fire).

The North American Society of Pacing and Electrophysiology published a similar set of guidelines, but they differ in that they do not mention that the VT must be hemodynamically significant [8]. Additional considerations may include patients with the prolonged Q–T syndrome and selected patients with hypertrophic cardiomyopathy and sustained ventricular arrhythmias. Patients in whom VT or VF is related to acute myocardial infarction, transient electrolyte abnormalities, or drug toxicity are not candidates for device therapy.

Furthermore, some patients should not be offered ICD therapy: those with psychological conditions who would not be able to adapt to this type of therapy, those with a short life expectancy due to terminal illness, and those with incessant VT due to their poor prognosis and continuous triggering of the ICD if sinus rhythm is restored intermittently. Patients with frequent long runs of nonsustained VT would also trigger frequent ICD discharges. If the VT is hemodynamically stable and shorter than the upper limit of delay time before the ICD charges, ICD therapy may be a consideration. However, the caveat is that the duration of nonsustained VT is not always predictable and frequent ICD shocks may not be tolerable.

VI. **Evaluation.** Patients who are candidates for an ICD are those with malignant ventricular tachyarrhythmias who deserve the complete assessment recommended for any survivor of sudden cardiac arrest. The evaluation should include ambulatory monitoring, stress testing, and echocardiography and/or radionuclide angiography as appropriate, as well as invasive evaluation with cardiac catheterization and electrophysiologic testing.

Cardiac catheterization is necessary to determine whether any adjunct cardiovascular surgical procedure is indicated to improve the overall cardiac status of the patient. Is the patient a candidate for angioplasty (PTCA) or coronary artery bypass graft (CABG) surgery? Is there an indication for valve replacement? Does the patient have a discrete left ventricular aneurysm? If the patient already has had cardiac surgery, are the bypass grafts patent and the prosthetic valves functioning? What is the ejection fraction? Is the overall left ventricular function too poor to consider endocardial resection or cardiac surgery? Should the ICD be implanted at the time of bypass surgery or after surgery by the nonthoracotomy approach?

Electrophysiologic testing is necessary to identify the native arrhythmia and to determine whether it can be suppressed by antiarrhythmic drugs. Next, if the arrhythmia is not suppressed by drugs, have the drugs administered changed the rate of the tachycardia? The physician must decide whether long-term therapy with a particular agent is desired, as changes may occur not only in the rate of the VT but also in the defibrillation threshold. These factors will have a bearing on the selection of the generator.

VII. **Selection of the ICD generator and lead system.** The selection will depend on the patient's clinical arrhythmia. If it is VF or a fast VT or flutter, the therapy needed is one that delivers high energy—a "shock box." This patient may not need antitachycardia pacing and probably not the low-energy cardioversion. Patients who will benefit most from these features have a slower VT and usually one that is better tolerated hemodynamically. Nevertheless, these options are present in most of the newer devices, particularly those with the biphasic wave form. **The longer the patient is in a life-threatening arrhythmia, the more difficult it is to terminate it.** Thus, spending minutes with antitachycardia pacing in a hypotensive patient with a rapid VT may not only prolong effective therapy but also further compromise the patient hemodynamically and decrease the success rate of the eventual shock. Most devices have programs that automatically proceed to high-energy defibrillation if the arrhythmia is prolonged.

For patients who can benefit from antitachycardia pacing, manufacturers will have a variety of programmable ramp or burst pacing algorithms to use in tachycardia termination. The patient will require repeat EPS after implant to test the ability of the selected algorithm to terminate the VT successfully. If that fails, the next programmable feature will be low-energy cardioversion or high-energy defibrillation based on the clinical arrhythmia. There is a **limited amount of time that the physician should allow the arrhythmia to continue before delivering definitive therapy.** It is not unreasonable to expect that all of these features, with minor variations, will be available from all manufacturers in the near future.

The next consideration will be whether the device can or should be implanted by the nonthoracotomy approach or implanted at the time of other indicated cardiac surgery. This decision may dictate the use of a particular device or combination since not all manufacturers have FDA-approved nonthoracotomy electrodes available with their systems.

The defibrillation threshold depends on the underlying cardiac substrate. In addition to having an impact on nonthoracotomy versus thoracotomy approaches, it may dictate the use of a particular system that has the capability of delivering biphasic energy wave forms. Biphasic energy delivery may result in lower defibrillation thresholds, as described by Saksena et al., and may be particularly useful in patients with the endocardial lead system [9].

VIII. Programming. Arrhythmia recognition is accomplished by rate criteria. It is critical to know the rate of the clinical arrhythmia. If the patient has a VT rate of 160 beats/minute and the ICD cutoff rate is 175 beats/minute, the device will not recognize the rhythm as VT. This patient should have an ICD with a cutoff rate of 150–155 beats/minute.

Antitachycardia pacing has been an important advance for patients who have arrhythmias that respond to pacing. In one study by Wieholt et al., ATP was able to terminate 91% of hemodynamically stable VTs effectively and appropriately [10]. Bardy et al. found similar rates of tachycardia conversion with ATP and low-energy cardioversion [11].

For patients who require high-energy defibrillation, the ICD must be able to provide a 10-joule safety margin over the defibrillation threshold. This safety margin is important since progression of disease or the administration of antiarrhythmic drug therapy may later increase the defibrillation threshold (DFT). If the energy delivered is ineffective in terminating the ventricular tachyarrhythmia, the electrode configuration or polarity must be changed or a different wave form (e.g., biphasic vs. monophasic) selected. The inability of the delivered energy to terminate VT or VF cannot always be related to cardiac size, LV dysfunction, or nature of the underlying problem. Certain antiarrhythmic drugs increase the defibrillation threshold. Solutions in individual patients have included correcting hypokalemia, changing antiarrhythmic drug therapy, changing the lead systems, or using a **high-energy** ICD, which will deliver up to 36 joules. To be certain that the implanted electrodes are effective in terminating the arrhythmia, careful testing at the time of surgery is imperative.

IX. Surgical approach: Thoracotomy versus nonthoracotomy. The choice of surgical approach is determined by the procedures contemplated: ICD alone, or with CABG, valve replacement, endocardial resection, or aneurysmectomy. Severe left ventricular dysfunction is usually not a contraindication to ICD implantation; however, it may place additional procedures such as aneurysmectomy and subendocardial resection, valve replacement, or CABG at very high risk. These issues are discussed further in Chap. 19.

Today the preferred approach is nonthoracotomy. The electrode is inserted through the cephalic or subclavian vein and advanced to the right ventricle. Some systems require a second electrode in the right atrium or superior vena cava. The connector ends of the electrodes are tunneled subcutaneously to an abdominal pocket or left in a pectoral pocket. If the defibrillation threshold is high, a subcutaneous electrode (patch or array) is added.

The thoracotomy approach is usually used today only if the patient is undergoing other indicated cardiac surgery. (Even so, most surgeons may prefer placing a nonthoracotomy electrode after the patient has recovered from surgery.) Median sternotomy is the approach used during aortocoronary bypass or when the placement of two apical patch electrodes is needed. If the patient previously underwent median sternotomy, lateral thoracotomy may be preferable because of the scar tissue. The addition of the subcutaneous patch or array electrode to the endocardial electrode has eliminated the need for most of these approaches. The surgeon may elect lateral thoracotomy in certain patients with massive cardiomegaly. Care must be taken at the time of surgery not to injure new or existing bypass grafts or epicardial coronary arteries. The surgeon must decide in which order to perform additional procedures. If subendocardial resection is contemplated, it is usually performed first. Usually it is guided by intraoperative electrophysiologic mapping. Ventricular tachycardia is induced by standard programmed electrical stimulation techniques, with the surgeon holding the exploding electrode. Occasionally standard techniques will not be able to reproduce the results found in the electrophysiology laboratory when the patient is under anesthesia and the endocardium is exposed after cardiotomy. Alternating current may be used to induce the arrhythmia. Since there is only a limited time available for intraoperative mapping, the surgeon may decide to proceed with resection, guided by the mapping previously performed in the electrophysiology laboratory, if the arrhythmia cannot be induced at the time of surgery.

After mapping, the heart is cooled and cardioplegic solution is applied for myocardial preservation. Endocardial resection is performed by surgical stripping, cryoablation, or laser techniques, which are particularly useful in areas that cannot be easily resected (e.g., around the papillary muscle). Once the endocardial resection has been completed, the cardiotomy is repaired with resection of discrete aneurysm if necessary; CABG surgery is performed if necessary.

After the anastomoses are completed, attention is directed to the implantation of the patch electrode (or electrodes). The patch electrode is usually sutured directly on the left ventricular apex. The position of the spring electrode (if used) at the junction of the superior vena cava and right atrium is verified. If epicardial screw-in leads are used, they are placed within 1–2 cm of each other on the proximal left ventricular lateral wall. The leads from the spring electrode, patch electrode, and sensing electrodes are then tunneled subcutaneously to the generator pocket, which was created subcutaneously in the left paraumbilical area.

Thoracotomy may not be necessary or desirable in certain patients. Two alternative procedures were developed to implant the apical patch electrode. The first was the **subxiphoid approach** developed by Watkins (1982). The pericardium is opened anteriorly via a subxiphoid incision. The rectangular patch electrode is advanced into the pericardial sac so that its long axis is parallel to the diaphragm, anteriorly, and then pushed laterally to the apex. The patch is sutured to the cut edge of the pericardium. The **subcostal approach** developed by Lawrie (1984) provides good access to the left ventricle. The tunneling of the electrode leads to the generator pocket is the same as described above. Some investigators are looking into thoracoscopic approaches.

X. Defibrillation threshold measurements. Defibrillation threshold measurements are performed at the time of implantation to verify that the system will be able to terminate VT or VF. If the DFT is very high, the standard ICD generators may not provide sufficient energy, and therefore the system must be modified. Repositioning the electrodes, using additional electrodes, redirecting the direction of the energy pulses (i.e., changing the polarity), using different wave forms, or choosing a high-energy unit are the available options.

Defibrillation threshold measurements are performed utilizing an external cardioverter-defibrillator (ECD) or other type of high-voltage system (HVS) (Fig. 18-14). DFT may also be measured using the new tiered therapy ICD. Signals are analyzed from both the defibrillating electrodes and the bipolar sensing electrodes to verify that they are of sufficient amplitude and good quality. Pacing threshold is determined. The arrhythmia is then induced. Winkle et al. make the point that VF should always be induced even if the native arrhythmia is VT since the potential exists for a cardioversion impulse to convert VT to VF [12]. One must be certain that the next pulse will terminate VF. Some centers use alternating current to induce VF as little time is necessary for this type of induction. Once the arrhythmia is induced, the ECD or HVS is used to terminate it (Fig. 18-15, pp. 418–419). It is necessary to perform the test more than once to determine the threshold. For example, an initial test with 15 joules may terminate VF. The test is then repeated with 10 joules. If VF persists, the VF is then immediately terminated with a rescue shock of 25–40 joules. The defibrillation threshold is between 10 and 15 joules. Several tests should be performed with 15 joules to be certain that it will reproducibly terminate VF. Some electrophysiologists may prefer to start with a low energy and try successive shocks with increasing energy until defibrillation is successful. One must always be prepared to defibrillate the heart directly with an external defibrillator should the ECD fail to restore sinus rhythm. **Several successful attempts must be accomplished before a DFT is established.**

Once the energy requirement is ascertained, the appropriate ICD generator is removed from its sterile package and connected to the electrodes in the generator pocket

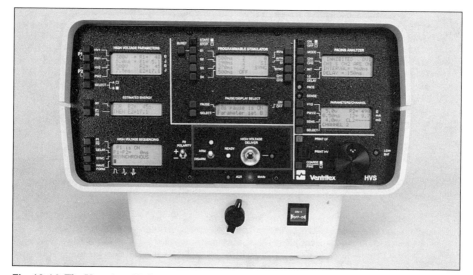

Fig. 18-14. The Ventritex High Voltage Stimulator HVS-02 is used to evaluate defibrillation threshold and pacing threshold at the time of implantation. Its features include a pacing analyzer, a programmable stimulator, and a high-voltage cardioverter-defibrillator. (Courtesy Ventritex Inc., Sunnyvale, CA.)

by the surgeon. An ICD test is then performed to be certain that the ICD itself will be able to terminate the arrhythmia. It is activated by the programmer using the wand. Ventricular fibrillation is induced, usually via the noninvasive mode of the ICD. If the induced arrhythmia spontaneously terminates and is not sustained, the test is repeated. Ventricular fibrillation is again induced, the ICD senses the arrhythmia, delays to be certain it is a sustained arrhythmia, charges, and delivers the pulse (Fig. 18-16, p. 420). Once some ICDs have charged, they are committed to delivering the pulse, either to the patient or internally. After the ICD is functioning properly, the connections are again checked for tightness and the pocket closed. Since many surgeons may use an electrocautery, the device is deactivated for closure and reactivated before leaving the operating room.

XI. **Postoperative follow-up of the ICD patient.** Further testing depends on the clinical situation. A formal EPS may be desirable for the patient who has undergone arrhythmia surgery (i.e., subendocardial resection) or the one in whom alteration of the drug regimen is contemplated. The surgeon may insist on a certain time interval before further testing, particularly if the patient has undergone aneurysmectomy. A repeat study is indicated, in particular, for the individual with marginal DFTs at the time of implant (Fig. 18-17, p. 421). For patients who receive units with antitachycardia pacing, only the ability to defibrillate successfully is tested at the time of implantation. Further electrophysiologic testing is necessary to determine the most appropriate pacing algorithms and program them. In addition, for patients receiving an endocardial shocking electrode, it is considered prudent to test the ability of the system to terminate VF several days after the initial implantation, to be certain that the electrode has not moved.

Once it is determined that the ICD function is adequate, further follow-up is necessary on an outpatient basis to monitor battery life. Testing is accomplished noninvasively with the programmer, which measures the time required to charge the capacitors and displays this information along with the number of pulses previously delivered. Depending on the system chosen, a wide variety of other information is available, particularly with units that have the capability to store the electrograms the unit recognized as VT/VF and treated (Fig. 18-18). Some of the newer units have the ability to recharge the capacitors automatically completely every 2 to 6 months, avoiding the need for frequent outpatient visits. Nevertheless, there is often a medical indication for regular visits in patients with serious arrhythmias, serious underlying heart disease, who are taking a variety of medications. For systems in which the pulse generator requires capacitor formation and charge times, these tests should be performed at the intervals recommended by the manufacturer. Generator life depends on the number of pulses delivered to the patient during episodes of arrhythmia and the number of tests performed. Each test depletes the generator of one pulse. Other factors that contribute to the life include the time the ICD has been activated (i.e., the monitoring time), the energy setting of the particular unit (how much energy is delivered), and the performance of other functions, particularly bradycardia pacing. It is imperative to know when the battery is reaching the end of its life so that the patient is not jeopardized by suffering a clinical arrhythmia without sufficient energy in the ICD to terminate it. Consequently the **elective replacement indicator** (ERI) was devised to determine when the energy reserve has fallen to 10% of its original capacity. At this point, arrangements should be made for elective replacement. Each manufacturer provides individual indicators of time to elective replacement.

XII. Potential complications of the implantation procedure. Despite the need for a major or minor surgical procedure to implant the ICD, complications have been relatively minimal. Now with the nonthoracotomy endocardial electrode approach, the aftermath of thoracotomy has been largely avoided. Additional complications not present with the original systems include lead dislodgement, hematoma at the subcutaneous patch electrode site, fracture of the subcutaneous patch electrode, and cardiac perforation by the endocardial electrode. Perhaps the most common finding among patients who receive an epicardial patch electrode is a transient pericardial rub in the immediate postoperative period, which usually resolves spontaneously. Accumulation of sterile fluid in the generator pocket (seroma) is occasionally noted. The fluid is usually resorbed without need for further treatment. Local tenderness may occur at the surgical site, as is seen with any other surgical wound.

The major concern is infection. In the original Hopkins report on 112 patients, infection occurred in six patients (four related to the generator pocket). Two required removal of the ICD system, while the other four responded to antimicrobials. Other complications related to the surgical procedure included postoperative bleeding and one death caused by perforation of the subclavian vein by a polyethylene central catheter. A list of other potential complications is summarized in Table 18-1 (p. 422). Almost all are uncommon except for pericarditis (if an epicardial patch is used) and seroma in the generator pocket.

XIII. Problems related to the ICD
  A. Component malfunction. In any sophisticated electronic device, component malfunction is a possibility. A number of technical problems did occur with the earlier models, one of which was premature battery depletion, necessitating early replacement of the generator, but few resulted in serious injury to the patient.
  B. Spurious discharges. One problem associated with the ICD was the inability to record the rhythm responsible for the discharge. Thus, unless the patient was monitored during the arrhythmia and discharge, only a presumptive diagnosis of the arrhythmia was possible. With the telemetry now available on certain systems, the precise determination of the reason for activation is available. If the shock is appropriate, the termination sequence, either antitachycardia pacing or low- or high-energy cardioversion, can be validated. If inappropriate, further investigation is performed. Patients with a fast heart rate will satisfy the criteria once the rate cutoff is satisfied. Often the patient with atrial fibrillation may develop a rapid ventricular response if an intercurrent illness or stress is present. Either the rate cutoff will have to be adjusted or a negative chronotropic or dromotropic drug to slow the maximal heart rate will be necessary. If there is a problem with the sensing electrode, it will have to be replaced. Insulation breaks or even a loose set screw can cause inappropriate sensing and discharge. Inappropriate discharges are undesirable; they are painful and result in adverse psychological reactions. Inappropriate discharges do occur in a small percentage of cases, as reported by most studies.
  C. Interference from permanent pacemakers. At this time the ICD does not have dual chamber pacing capability, only VVI bradycardia pacing. In certain units, constant bradycardia pacing will prematurely deplete the pulse generator. For these patients, an independent pacemaker may be a wise choice. Many ICD patients have impaired ventricular function and would benefit from dual chamber pacing. Patients with bradyarrhythmias or heart block requiring pacing must have a **bipolar** pacing electrode and generator if they are to receive an ICD for VT or VF. The unipolar lead may result in high-amplitude signals that may be sensed as sinus rhythm by the ICD. Thus, if the patient has VT and the permanent pacemaker is not inhibited but continues to discharge, there is the possibility that the ICD would sense the

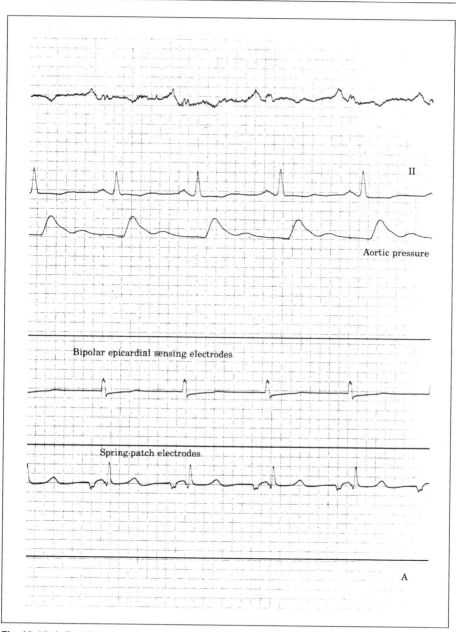

Fig. 18-15. A. Baseline recording of surface leads I and II, aortic pressure, and the automatic internal cardioverter-defibrillator (AICD) electrodes (*bipolar epicardial sensing* and *spring-patch electrodes*).

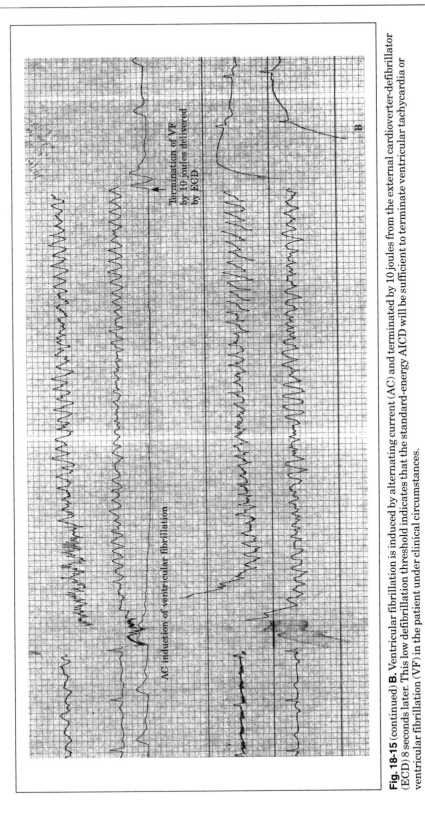

Fig. 18-15 (continued) **B.** Ventricular fibrillation is induced by alternating current (AC) and terminated by 10 joules from the external cardioverter-defibrillator (ECD) 8 seconds later. This low defibrillation threshold indicates that the standard-energy AICD will be sufficient to terminate ventricular tachycardia or ventricular fibrillation (VF) in the patient under clinical circumstances.

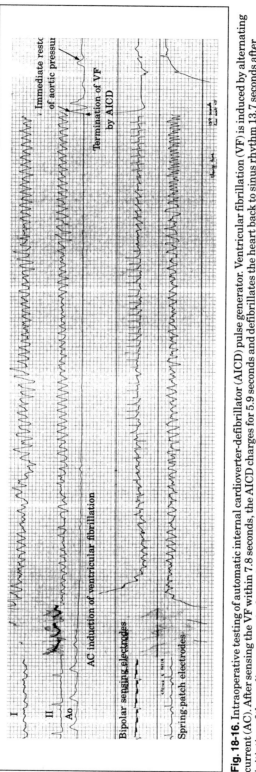
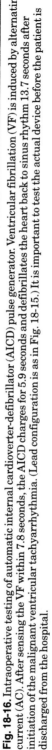

Fig. 18-16. Intraoperative testing of automatic internal cardioverter-defibrillator (AICD) pulse generator. Ventricular fibrillation (VF) is induced by alternating current (AC). After sensing the VF within 7.8 seconds, the AICD charges for 5.9 seconds and defibrillates the heart back to sinus rhythm 13.7 seconds after initiation of the malignant ventricular tachyarrhythmia. (Lead configuration is as in Fig. 18-15.) It is important to test the actual device before the patient is discharged from the hospital.

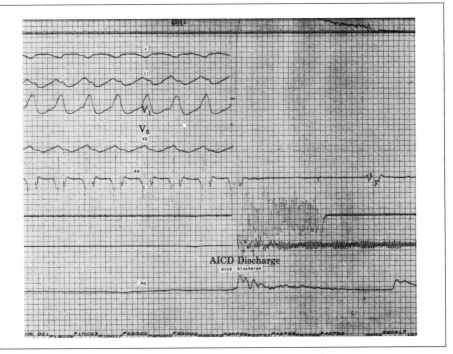

Fig. 18-17. Termination of ventricular tachycardia by automatic internal cardioverter-defibrillator (AICD). The leads recorded are I, II, V_1, and V_5 (surface); right ventricle (RV) (endocardial); and aortic pressure (Ao). After recognition of the monomorphic ventricular tachycardia by the AICD, charging, and discharging, sinus rhythm is restored. Note the immediate restoration of aortic pressure after AICD discharge.

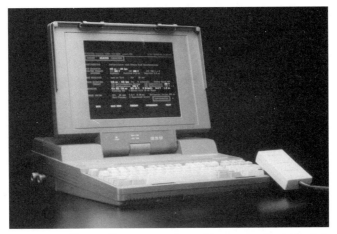

Fig. 18-18. The Ventritex PR-1500 Programmer is used to program Ventritex internal cardioverter-defibrillators. The programmer is portable, has touch screen control and a color display. (Courtesy Ventritex Inc., Sunnyvale, CA.)

pacemaker discharge but not the VT. In addition, the pacemaker electrodes should be placed in a position as far as possible from the ICD sensing electrodes. Since many patients undergo transtelephonic monitoring of their pacemakers, which includes the self-application of a magnet over the pacemaker generator, one must be careful to keep the pacemaker magnet away from the ICD generator. If the magnet is placed over the ICD generator, there is a possibility of inactivating certain devices. Some DDDR pacemakers may revert to a unipolar mode if the patient receives a defibrillatory shock. Other DDDR pacemakers are protected and remain bipolar. It is imperative to be aware of this information when selecting a permanent pacemaker.

D. **Modification of the arrhythmia and defibrillation thresholds by antiarrhythmic drugs.** Antiarrhythmic drugs may modify the rate of the VT. Commonly this may be seen as a dose response. As more drug is administered, the VT rate may become slower and slower, until the VT is completely suppressed. If it is not suppressed and the patient receives an ICD, one must be certain that the VT rate is faster than the cutoff rate of the ICD. Some drugs may result in a faster VT. One of the original AID patients had a VT rate of 187 beats/minute when the arrhythmia occurred, which was not sensed by the device. After switching to tocainide, the VT rate was 250 beats/minute when it broke through drug therapy and was sufficient to trigger the device. Thus, it is sometimes possible electropharmacologically to alter the tachycardia to the patient's advantage.

Table 18-1. Reported potential complications of internal cardioverter-defibrillator (ICD) implantation

---

Mortality
Acute myocardial infarction ⎫
Congestive heart failure ⎬ Related to severity of underlying
Cardiogenic shock ⎭ heart disease
Vascular tear
Coronary artery erosion caused by patch

Morbidity
Cardiac
    Pericarditis[a]
    Pericardial tamponade
    Bradyarrhythmia after ICD discharge requiring pacemaker

Pulmonary
    Atelectasis
    Pneumonia
    Pneumothorax
    Pulmonary embolus

Vascular
    Subclavian vein thrombosis
    Cerebrovascular accident after conversion of atrial fibrillation
    Hemorrhage requiring transfusion

Local
    Skin erosion
    Seroma in generator pocket
    Infection in generator pocket

Device
    Lead fracture
    Lead migration
    Misdirect[b]
    Inappropriate discharge during supraventricular tachycardia
    Replacement of generator due to premature battery depletion

---

[a]Almost all patients with an epicardial patch electrode will experience even a minor degree of pericarditis. All the other complications listed are uncommon.
[b]Charge delivered to patient rather than internally during magnet test.

Recent data have indicated that antiarrhythmic drugs may alter the defibrillation threshold. Antiarrhythmic drugs that may increase the DFT and necessitate higher energy for successful termination of VT or VF include amiodarone, encainide, flecainide, propafenone, and lidocaine, among others. If these alterations interfere with the function of the ICD, substitution of another antiarrhythmic drug may be necessary. Sotalol has not been shown to increase DFT.

E. **Exacerbation of the arrhythmia.** Ventricular tachycardia can be modified not only by drugs but also by pacing or cardioversion. This phenomenon is familiar to every electrophysiologist who has attempted overdrive pacing of induced VT. Occasionally the tachycardia accelerates or degenerates into VF. For this reason, antitachycardia pacemakers without backup defibrillator capability were abandoned. Even during electrical cardioversion, there is a similar risk of exacerbating the arrhythmia. One of the initial reports on the implantable transvenous cardioverter described cardioversion of the VT resulting in atrial fibrillation. Further spontaneous episodes of VT were recognized and cardioverted, but shock caused VF. The ability of the ICD to resense and deliver more shocks will deliver effective therapy to an accelerated VT or VF.

XIV. **Psychosocial aspects of the automatic internal cardioverter-defibrillator.** There are a number of aspects of arrhythmia management, including medical, surgical, and other technical factors, but one that cannot be neglected is the psychosocial needs of the patient and family. This topic is discussed in detail in Chaps. 20 and 21. Initially, when the ICD was investigational, the patients viewed this device with some skepticism. Most of the patients had few other options, therapy with antiarrhythmic drugs having failed while symptomatic arrhythmias continued. Once the ICD was implanted, however, their outlook on life changed dramatically, becoming hopeful once again. They derived a tremendous sense of security from the ICD, knowing that if the arrhythmia recurred, they would be rescued. One can only speculate on what relationship this form of anxiety reduction may have on the incidence of arrhythmias, but the relationship of neural influence on the heart is recognized.

What does the patient sense when the ICD discharges? If the patient has a hemodynamically compromising arrhythmia, collapses, and immediately loses consciousness, there is no sensation of the discharge. In fact some patients are not even certain, once they regain consciousness, if the ICD fired. One patient described a dream that the ICD fired. Interrogation of the unit confirmed a discharge, and Holter monitoring demonstrated recurrent arrhythmias. If the patient is conscious, the reaction to the discharge may be very subjective. Some patients note very little discomfort and are barely aware that the device fired. Some patients report a very noticeable and sometimes painful shock. Most patients describe a somewhat uncomfortable or unpleasant internal twitch or shock. Psychologically, they are disappointed that they had recurrence of the arrhythmia but also glad to be alive. Patients with frequent discharges find them not only annoying but disconcerting. This situation requires revision of the antiarrhythmic regimen.

XV. **Economic impact of the automatic internal cardioverter-defibrillator.** The cost of the treatment is a factor that cannot be ignored. One of the key factors that the ICD adds to the management of malignant ventricular arrhythmias is the safety net or backup if primary treatment fails. The patient will be rescued even if out of the hospital. Hospitalization time for patients with refractory VT at one time was as long as 6 weeks (and often longer). The ability to implant an electronic rescue device earlier in the treatment of refractory VT or VF may shorten initial hospitalizations. This is particularly relevant during the health care crisis and emphasis on short length of stay. In addition, if a patient has an out-of-hospital episode of VT or VF that is successfully treated with the ICD, it may not always be necessary to hospitalize him or her. Certainly if there are frequent discharges, revision of the antiarrhythmic regimen may be best performed in a monitored situation.

A conservative estimate of the cost to the patient and insurance carrier of initial evaluation and treatment, hospitalization, cardiac catheterization, repeated EPSs, cardiac surgery, and the ICD itself is $50,000–65,000. O'Donoghue et al. pointed out that earlier intervention with the ICD may be more cost-effective than proceeding with serial drug testing and may even compare favorably as a therapy [13]. If the patient is able to return to a productive life, this procedure may become even more cost-effective, perhaps more so than coronary bypass surgery. In the initial Stony Brook report of ICD patients, all five who were working before the problem with VT or VF returned to work full- or part-time. The four who were retired remained active. Over the past 14 years, this experience has continued.

XVI. Driving. Loss of consciousness while operating a motor vehicle, even for 15 seconds, whether driving at 55 mph on the highway or at 20 mph in a residential area, may result in tragedy. Thus, even if an ICD restores a regular rhythm, an accident may occur. Consequently physicians usually instruct their VT/VF patients not to drive. Patients should be told that it is the rhythm disorder, not the ICD, that results in the restriction.

The restriction on driving for patients with VT or VF can be devastating, not only in terms of employment but even in activities of daily living. The recommendations of O'Donoghue and Platia merit consideration by the electrophysiology community [14]. For patients who have syncope or cardiac arrest due to arrhythmia, driving is prohibited. If there are no events or if the ICD terminates arrhythmias without symptoms, the restriction is reevaluated after 6–12 months. No restriction is placed if the patient has VT without hemodynamic compromise and if the ICD terminates the arrhythmia without symptoms. One concern, however, is that the patient may not always have the same arrhythmia and also that tiered therapy devices may accelerate an otherwise stable arrhythmia, which then becomes symptomatic. The issue of driving is being addressed in a conference sponsored by the American Heart Association and the North American Society for Pacing and Electrophysiology and hopefully will result in a policy statement or general guidelines.

XVII. Current strategies in arrhythmia management with the ICD. Once the ICD is implanted, there are a number of options to consider. One may elect to continue the current antiarrhythmic drug regimen, reduce it, or eliminate it. In choosing any of these options, one must weigh the individual characteristics of the patient, the potential toxicity of the antiarrhythmic drugs, and the frequency of the arrhythmic episodes. Perhaps the best example of a patient in whom drug therapy could be discontinued is one who underwent subendocardial resection of a tachycardia zone at the time of ICD surgery and was rendered noninducible during electrophysiologic testing (or perhaps required a more potent stimulation technique to induce VT). This patient has less chance of recurrence and would be rescued by the ICD if it occurred. At that time, further drug therapy could be considered.

Patients who are taking an antiarrhythmic drug with potential long-term toxicity, such as amiodarone, may reduce the chance of an adverse reaction, while still deriving partial benefit, if the dosage is reduced. If the patient develops frequent episodes of VT or VF requiring multiple discharges, the drug regimen must be improved since the ICD battery will become depleted and the discharges may be uncomfortable.

The impact of tiered therapy devices remains to be seen. Not all patients benefit from antitachycardia pacing. Nevertheless, if antitachycardia pacing converts most episodes of VT to normal sinus rhythm and cardioversion terminates those that persist, there may be less reliance on antiarrhythmic drug therapy. In addition, with few high-energy discharges necessary by the ICD, battery life will be prolonged. The continued efficacy of antitachycardia pacing in individual patients remains to be determined, particularly if the substrate and arrhythmia change.

XVIII. Future strategies. New ICD systems have antitachycardia and bradycardia pacing capability, internal memory, smaller size, extensive noninvasive programmability, and telemetry. It is no longer necessary for major surgery to implant leads. The most desirable features for the next generation will be smaller size and increased longevity. One may anticipate a further increase in the utilization of the ICD, perhaps implanting some prophylactically in patients stratified as high risk, and hope for a decline in the incidence of sudden cardiac death.

Many have participated in the development of the automatic ICD: physicians, nurses, staff, and patients. Nevertheless, a debt of gratitude is owed to the physician who had the foresight, fortitude, and determination to pursue his dream, the ICD, from its conception to successful utilization in patients with devastating arrhythmias: Dr. Michel Mirowski.

References

1. Mirowski M. The automatic implantable cardioverter-defibrillator: An overview. *J Am Coll Cardiol* 6:461–466, 1985.
2. Grimm W, Flores B, Marchlinski FE. Shock occurrence and survival in 241 patients with implantable cardioverter-defibrillator therapy. *Circulation* 87:1880–1888, 1993.
3. Saksena S, Camm AJ. Implantable defibrillators for prevention of sudden death. *Circulation* 85:2316–2321, 1992.
4. Kim SG. Management of survivors of cardiac arrest: Is electrophysiologic testing obsolete in the era of implantable defibrillators? *J Am Coll Cardiol* 16:756–762, 1990.
5. Kim SG. Implantable defibrillator therapy: Does it really prolong life? How can we prove it? *Am J Cardiol* 71:1213–1218, 1993.
6. Kim SG, et al. Influence of left ventricular function on outcome of patients treated with implantable defibrillators. *Circulation* 85:1304–1310, 1992.
7. American College of Cardiology and American Heart Association. Task Force on Assessment of Diagnostic and Therapeutic Cardiovascular Procedures. *J Am Coll Cardiol* 18:1–13, 1991.
8. North American Society of Pacing and Electrophysiology. *PACE* 14:969–979, 1991.
9. Saksena S, et al. Prospective comparison of biphasic and monophasic shocks for implantable cardioverter-defibrillators using endocardial leads. *Am J Cardiol* 70:304–310, 1992.
10. Wietholt D, et al. Clinical experience with antitachycardia pacing and improved detection algorithms in a new implantable cardioverter-defibrillator. *J Am Coll Cardiol* 21:885–894, 1993.
11. Bardy GH, et al. A prospective randomized repeat-crossover comparison of antitachycardia pacing with low-energy cardioversion. *Circulation* 87:1889–1896, 1993.
12. Winkle RA, Stinson EB, Echt DS. Practical aspects of automatic cardioverter defibrillator implantation. *Am Heart J* 108:1335–1346, 1984.
13. O'Donoghue S, et al. Automatic implantable cardioverter-defibrillator: Is early implantation cost effective? *J Am Coll Cardiol* 16:1258–1263, 1990.
14. O'Donoghue S, Platia, EV. Economic consequences of ICD implantation. In GV Naccarelli, EP Veltri (eds), *Implantable Cardioverter Defibrillators*. Boston: Blackwell Scientific, 1993. Pp 268–283.

Bibliography

Bardy GH, et al. An effective and adaptable transvenous defibrillation system using the coronary sinus in humans. *J Am Coll Cardiol* 16:887–895, 1990.

Bardy GH, et al. Implantable transvenous cardioverter-defibrillators. *Circulation* 87:1152–1168, 1993.

Bardy GH, et al. A simplified single-lead unipolar transvenous cardioversion-defibrillation system. *Circulation* 88:543–547, 1993.

Bardy GH, et al. Clinical experience with a tiered-therapy multiprogrammable antiarrhythmia device. *Circulation* 85:1689–1698, 1992.

Brooks R, Torchiana D, Vlahakes GJ. Successful implantation of cardioverter-defibrillator systems in patients with elevated defibrillation thresholds. *J Am Coll Cardiol* 22:569–574, 1993.

Brodman R, et al. Implantation of automatic cardioverter-defibrillators via median sternotomy. *PACE* 7:1363–1369, 1984.

Cannon DS. A critical appraisal of indications for the implantable cardioverter defibrillator (ICD). *Clin Cardiol* 15:368–372, 1992.

Dreifus LS, et al. Guidelines for implantation of cardiac pacemakers and antiarrhythmia devices. *J Am Coll Cardiol* 18:1–13, 1991.

Echt DS, et al. Clinical experience, complications and survival in 70 patients with the automatic implantable cardioverter/defibrillator. *Circulation* 71:289–296, 1985.

Epstein AE, et al. Clinical characteristics and outcome of patients with high defibrillation thresholds. *Circulation* 86:1206–1216, 1992.

Estes NAM (ed). *The Implantable Cardioverter Defibrillator: A Comprehensive Text.* New York: Marcel Dekker, 1994.

Fogoros RN, et al. Efficacy of the automatic implantable cardioverter-defibrillator in prolonging survival in patients with severe underlying cardiac disease. *J Am Coll Cardiol* 16:381–386, 1990.

Hook BG, et al. Implantable cardioverter-defibrillator therapy in the absence of significant symptoms. *Circulation* 87:1897–1906, 1993.

Jung W, et al. Effects of chronic amiodarone therapy on defibrillation threshold. *Am J Cardiol* 70:1023–1027, 1992.

Kim SG. Benefits of implantable defibrillators are overestimated by sudden death rates and better represented by the total arrhythmic death rate. *J Am Coll Cardiol* 17: 1587–1592, 1991.

Lawrie GM, Griffin JC, Wyndham CRC. Epicardial implantation of the automatic implantable defibrillator by left subcostal thoracotomy. *PACE* 7:1370–1374, 1984.

Lehmann MH, Saksena S. Implantable cardioverter defibrillators in cardiovascular practice: Report of the policy conference of the North American Society of Pacing and Electrophysiology. *PACE* 14:969–979, 1991.

McCowan R, et al. Automatic implantable cardioverter-defibrillator implantation without thoracotomy using an endocardial and submuscular patch system. *J Am Coll Cardiol* 17:415–421, 1991.

Meissner MD, et al. Ventricular fibrillation in patients without significant structural heart disease: A multicenter experience with implantable cardioverter-defibrillator therapy. *J Am Coll Cardiol* 21:406–412, 1993.

Mirowski M, et al. Termination of malignant ventricular arrhythmias with an implanted automatic defibrillator in human beings. *N Engl J Med* 303:322–324, 1980.

Mirowski M, et al. The automatic implantable defibrillator: New modality for treatment of life-threatening ventricular arrhythmias. *PACE* 5:384–401, 1982.

Mirowski M, et al. Mortality in patients with implanted automatic defibrillators. *Ann Intern Med* 98:585–588, 1983.

Mirowski M, Reid PR, Mower MM. Clinical performance of the implantable cardioverter-defibrillator. *PACE* 7:1345–1350, 1984.

Mower MM, Reid PR, Watkins L. Automatic implantable cardioverter-defibrillator structural characteristics. *PACE* 7:1331–1337, 1984.

Naccarelli GV, Veltri EP (eds). *Implantable Cardioverter Defibrillators.* Boston: Blackwell Scientific Publications, 1993.

Porterfield JG, et al. Experience with three different third generation cardioverter-defibrillators in patients with coronary artery disease or cardiomyopathy. *Am J Cardiol* 72:301–304, 1993.

Reid PR, et al. Clinical evaluation of the internal automatic cardioverter-defibrillator in survivors of sudden cardiac death. *Am J Cardiol* 51:1608–1613, 1983.

Reid PR, Griffith LSC, Mower MM. Implantable cardioverter-defibrillator: Patient selection and implantation protocol. *PACE* 7:1338–1344, 1984.

Saksena S, et al. Endocardial pacing, cardioversion and defibrillation using a braid endocardial lead system. *Am J Cardiol* 71:834–841, 1993.

Troup PJ, Chapman PD, Olinger GN. The implanted defibrillator: Relation of defibrillating lead configuration and clinical variables to defibrillation threshold. *J Am Coll Cardiol* 6:1315–1321, 1985.

Vlay SC. Defibrillation threshold testing: Necessary but evil? *Am Heart J* 117:499–504, 1989.

Vlay SC. The automatic internal cardioverter defibrillator: Comprehensive clinical followup, economic and social impact: The Stony Brook experience. *Am Heart J* 112: 189–194, 1986.

Watkins L, et al. Automatic defibrillation in man: The initial surgical experience. *J Thorac Cardiovasc Surg* 82:492–500, 1981.

Watkins L, et al. Implantation of the automatic defibrillator: The subxiphoid approach. *Ann Thorac Surg* 34:515–520, 1982.

Watkins L, et al. The treatment of malignant ventricular arrhythmias with combined endocardial resection and implantation of the automatic defibrillator: Preliminary report. *Ann Thorac Surg* 37:60–66, 1984.

Watkins L, et al. Surgical techniques for implanting the automatic implantable defibrillator. *PACE* 7:1357–1362, 1984.

Winkle RA, Stinson EB, Bach SM. Measurement of cardioversion/defibrillation thresholds by a truncated exponential waveform and an apical patch-superior vena cava spring electrode configuration. *Circulation* 69:766–771, 1984.

Winkle RA, et al. The automatic implantable defibrillator: Local ventricular bipolar sensing to detect ventricular tachycardia and fibrillation. *Am J Cardiol* 52:265–270, 1983.

Zipes DP, et al. Early experience with an implantable cardioverter. *N Engl J Med* 311:485–490, 1984.

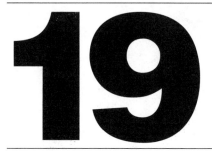

Surgical Treatment of Cardiac Arrhythmias

Eric Taylor, Jr.
and Levi Watkins, Jr.

Sudden cardiac death continues to account for two-thirds of the annual cardiac mortality. Improved resuscitative efforts have resulted in a growing population of survivors, many of whom remain at risk of recurrent arrest. Modern techniques of electrophysiologic assessment have facilitated identification of this high-risk group. While tremendous strides have been made in the surgical treatment of these patients, it is important to point out that modalities such as radiofrequency catheter ablation have made equally important progress, with a heavy impact on surgical interventions. This chapter reviews the current surgical approaches to major cardiac arrhythmias.

I. **Supraventricular arrhythmias.** This section reviews the surgical management of four types of supraventricular tachycardia: Wolff-Parkinson-White syndrome, automatic atrial tachycardia, atrioventricular nodal reentry tachycardia (AVNRT), and atrial fibrillation. Of note, some of the most successful applications of radiofrequency ablation have occurred in the area of supraventricular arrhythmias.
   A. **Wolff-Parkinson-White syndrome.** The underlying pathology of accessory pathway arrhythmias is ventricular preexcitation resulting from the presence of accessory atrioventricular connections [1–3]. The goal of surgery is to interrupt these abnormal pathways while maintaining normal physiologic conduction [4–6].
      1. **Indications for surgery**
         a. Patients with 1:1 conduction and rapid ventricular response.
         b. Patients refractory to medical therapy and catheter ablation.
      2. **Preoperative assessment**
         a. **Surface electrocardiography.** Electrocardiography may demonstrate evidence of preexcitation and delta waves.
         b. **Cardiac catheterization.** Routine cardiac catheterization is usually not necessary.
         c. **Electrophysiologic testing.** Electrophysiologic testing is essential in determining the anatomic location and number of the accessory pathways.
      3. **Operative procedure**
         a. **Direct surgical interruption of Kent bundles.** After standard sternotomy, epicardial mapping is undertaken. If preexcitation is present and stable, the mapping can be done in sinus rhythm. If not, atrial pacing is used to stimulate tachycardia, which is then mapped. Usually intraoperative mapping correlates well with the preoperative data. In patients with septal pathways, right atrial endocardial mapping is performed in addition to the epicardial mapping. Occasionally pacing and attempts to induce tachycardia result in hypotension; in such cases, we advise cannulation and the initiation of cardiopulmonary bypass.

         Left free-wall pathways are approached via the left atrium. An incision is made just above the anulus posterior to the mural leaflet of the mitral valve (Fig. 19-1). Care is taken to avoid the circumflex marginal artery and the coronary sinus. The incision is carried through the atrial wall down to the epicardial reflection. Superficial myocardial fibers attached to the anulus are also divided. The anular incision and atriotomy are closed in a continuous fashion (Fig. 19-2). The heart is rewarmed and weaned from cardiopulmonary bypass. Postoperative electrophysiologic assessment is then performed. The ECG is examined for evidence of preexcitation. Antegrade and retrograde pacing should no longer induce tachycardia. The Wenckebach phenomenon usually occurs with pacing.

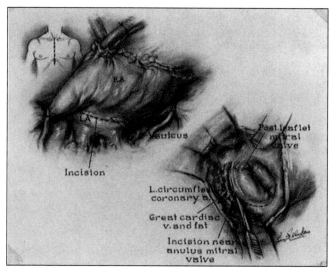

Fig. 19-1. Supraanular incision posterior to mural leaflet of mitral valve for interruption of left free-wall pathway.

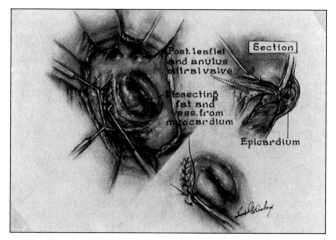

Fig. 19-2. Dissection of epicardial fat and superficial myocardial fibers attached to anulus.

Successful division of accessory pathway occurs in 95% of patients with free-wall connection and 80% of those with septal locations. Operative mortality is 1–2%.

    b. Cryoablation. Successful cryoablation of accessory pathways has been achieved [7–9]. In the operative procedure the site of earliest ventricular activation is cooled to −60°C for 90 seconds with a cryoprobe. The advantages of the procedure are that surgical dissection is minimized.

B. Automatic atrial tachycardia. This is an uncommon arrhythmia that accounts for 2–3% of supraventricular tachycardia in adults and 10% in children [10]. The underlying mechanism seems to be due to either a single extranodal automatic focus or heightened automaticity of the sinoatrial node [11]. Historically, this arrhythmia has been less amenable to surgery because it cannot be electrically induced with programmed stimulatory techniques. Recently, the development of innovative surgical techniques has made it possible to treat refractory automatic atrial tachycardia.

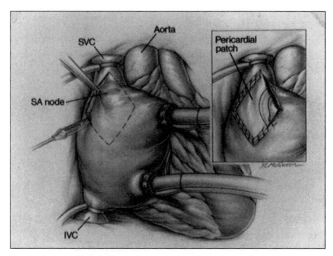

Fig. 19-3. Excision of sinoatrial node and surrounding tissue with pericardial repair. (SA = sinoatrial; SVC = superior vena cava; IVC = inferior vena cava.) (Courtesy of Dr. Lowe, Duke University, Durham, NC.)

1. **Indications.** Patients are symptomatic and refractory to medical therapy.
2. **Preoperative assessment**
   a. **Surface electrocardiogram.** Electrocardiogram may show incessant, narrow-complex supraventricular tachycardia. In patients with increased automaticity of the sinus node, the ECG may demonstrate homogeneous P waves, whereas in that arising from a single extranodal focus, the ECG tends to show a morphologically different P wave from that seen during sinus rhythm.
   b. **Cardiac catheterization.** Cardiac catheterization is not usually necessary.
   c. **Electrophysiologic testing.** Mapping is utilized to identify the site of ectopic activity and also to exclude AVNRT or concealed extranodal bypass tracts.
3. **Operative procedure**
   a. Treatment for increased automaticity of the sinus node consists of excision of the sinus node and placement of a pericardial patch (Fig. 19-3).
   b. Treatment of chronic ectopic atrial tachycardia is dependent on the ectopic site. Essentially, the surgical procedure consists of excision of the area surrounding the ectopic focus. Defects are then repaired by oversewing them or using a rotation flap (Fig. 19-4). Areas difficult to excise are treated with cryoablation.

      The surgical treatment of automatic atrial tachycardia has a reported success rate of 87% [12].
C. **Atrioventricular nodal reentry tachycardia.** This arrhythmia is the most common type of supraventricular tachycardia, constituting 63–87% [11–15]. Until recently the only effective treatment for refractory atrioventricular (AV) nodal tachycardia was surgical ablation of the His bundle [6]. This method, although successful, results in another problem, heart block. Consequently, other methods were sought to interrupt the reentry circuit responsible for the tachycardia without blocking normal AV conduction.
   1. **Indications for surgery.** Patients with symptomatic AVNRT refractory to medical therapy and radiofrequency catheter ablation are candidates.
   2. **Preoperative evaluation**
      a. **Surface electrocardiogram.**
      b. **Electrophysiologic testing** usually demonstrates evidence of AVNRT.
   3. **Operative procedure.** Reentrant circuits may be interrupted with cryosurgical interruption or with surgical skeletonization of the AV node.
      a. **Cryosurgical interruption** [16]. The principal objective of the procedure is to ablate as much of the perinodal tissue as possible without causing permanent AV conduction block. The approach is median sternotomy. Under normothermic cardiopulmonary bypass and during atrial pacing with constant monitor-

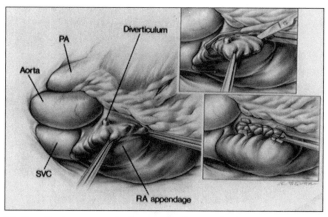

Fig. 19-4. Atrial diverticulum representing ectopic focus, which is excised and oversewn. (SVC = superior vena cava; RA = right atrial; PA = pulmonary artery.) (Courtesy of Dr. Lowe, Duke University, Durham, NC.)

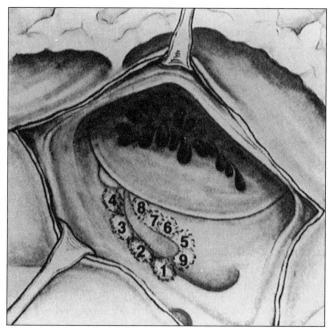

Fig. 19-5. Right atrial view of triangle of Koch and surrounding cryolesions.

ing of AV nodal conduction, nine separate cryolesions (−60°C for 2 minutes) are placed at selected sites around the triangle of Koch in the lower right atrial septum (Fig. 19-5). This effectively ablates most of the perinodal tissue without causing permanent damage to the AV node.

b. **Skeletonization of the AV node** [17]. The principal objective of this procedure is to dissect the node from most of the atrial inputs with the intent of altering perinodal substrate and averting reentry. The surgical approach is median sternotomy. After right atriotomy, the exposed AV node is dissected free from surrounding tissue (Fig. 19-6). On completion of AV node skeletonization, the superficial and posterior atrial inputs to the node are separated. The deep atrial inputs are left intact.

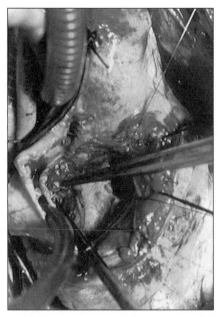

Fig. 19-6. Right atrial septal wall has been mobilized and atrioventricular node skeletonized (pointed out by forceps). (Courtesy of Dr. Guiraudon, London, Ontario, Canada.)

D. **Atrial fibrillation.** Atrial fibrillation is a frequently encountered arrhythmia that is secondary to a number of cardiac and noncardiac disease processes. This dysrhythmia is characterized by its ECG pattern of chaotic atrial activation associated with reentry mechanism. The arrhythmogenic substrate is diffuse, involving the entire atria without a single discrete lesion. Electrophysiologic mapping during atrial fibrillation has revealed complex and variable macroreentrant pathways. Current therapy has three principal objectives: (1) restoration of sinus rhythm, (2) control of ventricular response, and (3) prevention of stroke and embolic complications. Currently, two operative approaches are available to treat atrial fibrillation: the Maze and the corridor procedures [18–26].

1. **Indications.** Surgical candidates are patients with general intolerance of the arrhythmia or patients in whom there is drug intolerance. Patients who have experienced cerebral thrombolic events can also be candidates.

2. **Preoperative evaluation**
   a. **Surface electrocardiography.** The ECG documents atrial fibrillation.
   b. **Cardiac catheterization** demonstrates the presence of coronary or valvular heart disease.
   c. **Electrophysiologic testing.** This may reveal the presence of sinus node dysfunction.

E. **Operative procedures**
   1. **The Maze operation** [24–27]. The principal objectives of this surgery are to restore sinus rhythm and atrial contraction. In performing the Maze procedure, routine median sternotomy is used, and moderate systemic hypothermia is employed. The Maze procedure abolishes atrial fibrillation by strategically positioning multiple atriotomies close enough together to prevent the development of large macroreentrant circuits characteristic of atrial fibrillation. Over 5 years, approximately 100 patients have undergone the Maze procedure, with a cure rate of 99%. It is important to note that pacer therapy was required in 42% of these patients. Most of the patients who required pacer therapy had preoperative sinus node dysfunction. In the patients without sinus node dysfunction, only five of six required pacing.
   2. **The corridor procedure** [18–23]. This procedure consists of the construction and electrical exclusion of an atrial corridor. The corridor is fashioned from horseshoe-type incisions in the left and right atrial walls. Nine of 11 patients have

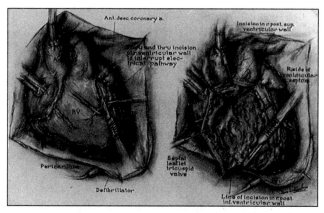

Fig. 19-7. Right ventricular disconnection. Longitudinal ventriculotomy extending from pulmonary anulus to tricuspid anulus.

been successfully treated with this operation. Postoperative pacing is required in approximately 50% of patients.

II. **Right ventricular arrhythmias.** The underlying disease of right ventricular arrhythmias consists of right ventricular dysplasia, cardiomyopathy, or both. Islands of diseased tissue surrounded by viable myocardium provide a substrate for reentry.
  A. **Right ventricular disconnection**
    1. **Indications.** Medical refractory tachycardia.
    2. **Preoperative assessment**
      a. **Echocardiography.** Echocardiography typically demonstrates a dilated, hypocontractile right ventricle. The left ventricle is usually normal.
      b. **Cardiac catheterization.** Cardiac catheterization is done to assess the coronary pathology and usually confirms the echocardiography.
      c. **Electrophysiologic testing.** Electrophysiologic testing typically demonstrates polymorphic ventricular tachycardia, often originating in the right ventricle or outflow tract.
    3. **Operative procedure** [28]. After standard sternotomy with individual cannulation of the superior vena cava and inferior vena cava, cardiopulmonary bypass is begun. Normothermia is maintained to facilitate epicardial mapping. The procedure is performed on the beating, nonworking heart. A longitudinal ventriculotomy in the anterior right ventricle is made parallel to the interventricular septum. It is extended superiorly to the pulmonary artery anulus then inferiorly to the tricuspid valve anulus (Fig. 19-7). The posterior wall of the right ventricle is incised from the endocardial surface. Cryolesions are placed at the pulmonary valve and tricuspid valve anuli, completing the isolation. The ventricle is then repaired in a single-layered fashion (Fig. 19-8).
    Although right ventricular disconnection is limited in use, arrhythmia control has been without fail, and no operative mortality has been reported.

III. **Left ventricular arrhythmias.** The most common cause of ventricular tachycardia and fibrillation is coronary artery disease and its complications, left ventricular aneurysm formation and myocardial fibrosis. The underlying pathophysiologic mechanism in these arrhythmias is believed to reflect interventricular reentry with circuits including endocardial scar. Myocardial ischemia may also play a role. Currently operative procedures are designed to interrupt or ablate reentrant tachycardia [29].
  A. Endocardial resection guided by endocardial mapping
    1. **Indications**
      a. Patients with medically refractory ventricular tachycardia are candidates.
      b. The arrhythmia must be clearly defined by programmed electrical stimulation.
    2. **Preoperative assessment**
      a. **Cardiac catheterization.** Cardiac catheterization is performed to determine the extent of coronary artery disease. Ventriculography also permits assessment of regional wall motion, which is important in determining operative

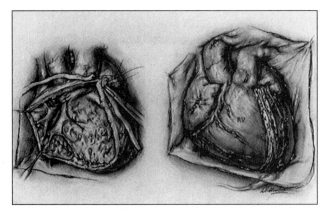

Fig. 19-8. Repair of right ventriculotomy.

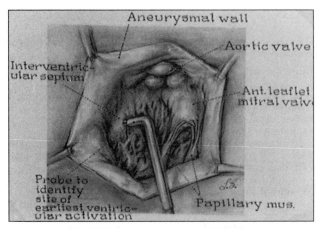

Fig. 19-9. Left ventriculotomy and hand-held probe used for endocardial mapping.

risk. Candidates with active remaining wall segments have relatively low risk independent of aneurysmal size.

   b. **Electrophysiologic testing.** Programmed electrophysiologic stimulation determines the presence or absence of sustained ventricular tachycardia. In addition, catheter endocardial mapping localizes the site of origin of the ventricular myocardium. Mapping is important because it may localize this site to the septal border, which is unperturbed by conventional aneurysmectomy.

3. **Operative procedure** [29–31]. After sternotomy and standard cardiac cannulation, cardiopulmonary bypass is instituted. Normothermia is maintained to facilitate intraoperative endocardial mapping. The aneurysm is opened, and sustained ventricular tachycardia is induced using programmed electrical stimulation (Fig. 19-9). After determining the site of earliest ventricular activation, the heart is cooled at 25°C and arrested with potassium cardioplegia. The endocardium is widely resected at this site (Fig. 19-10). Any additional endocardial scar is also resected. Aneurysmectomy is then done, and coronary artery bypass grafting is performed when indicated. In the event ventricular tachycardia cannot be induced or if rapid deterioration to ventricular fibrillation occurs, blind endocardial resection of the entire endocardial scar is performed, taking into account the preoperative information.

   The operative mortality of this procedure is 5%. The success rate in controlling the arrhythmia ranges from 80–90%.

B. **The internal cardioverter-defibrillator (ICD).** The ICD is a totally implantable device that provides continuous cardiac monitoring and automatic cardioversion

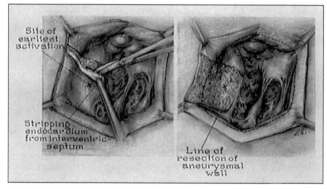

Fig. 19-10. Septal focus of earliest ventricular activation and surrounding endocardial resection.

and defibrillation for individuals at high risk of malignant ventricular arrhythmias [32–38]. In recent years, enormous technological progress has been made in this modality, and new third-generation defibrillators are now available.

There are currently several models manufactured by Cardiac Pacemakers Incorporated, Ventritex, and Medtronic (see Chap. 18). The model generally referred to in this chapter is the CPI device. The device consists of an intravenous lead system connected to a generator currently implanted in an abdominal pocket. The current lead system is referred to as the Endotak system and consists of a sensing electrode and two defibrillation coils, all in a single intravascular lead. The cathode is represented by the distal coil located in the right ventricular apex, and the anode is a proximal coil located in the right atrium. Polarity can be reversed, as well. In the event of failure of the intravenous lead, a subcutaneous patch is available to supplement lead configurations. The standard double-patch system is used when the Endotak system is not successful.

The pulse generator is encased in titanium and hermetically sealed. It is powered by lithium batteries that last approximately 24–36 months and are capable of discharging greater than 200 discharges. In addition to cardioversion and defibrillation, the current models, the PRx I and PRx II, have the capacity of VVI pacing and postshock pacing. The PRx II is equipped with event markers and stored electrograms. (See Chap. 18 for a description of the latest model.) Biphasic and monophasic wave forms are also options. The device is totally programmable.

The ICD system detects malignant ventricular arrhythmias by the rate detection capability. Essentially, upon occurrence of malignant tachyarrhythmias, the ICD senses it within 5–15 seconds, charges the capacitor in another 5–10 seconds, and delivers a shock.

1. **Indications.** Most patients have survived cardiac arrest or have inducible ventricular tachycardia.
2. **Preoperative assessment**
   a. **Cardiac catheterization.** Conventional cardiac catheterization is performed to establish the presence and extent of cardiac disease.
   b. **Electrophysiologic testing.** Electrophysiologic testing is done to evaluate the inducibility and drug responses.
3. **Operative procedures.** The introduction of the nonthoracotomy lead system has dramatically affected the surgical technique for ICD implantation. Currently, the Endotak lead system is placed in the right ventricular apex under fluoroscopic control. In the operating room, this lead is tested for pacing and defibrillation threshold. After satisfactory testing of this lead, a subcutaneous pocket is placed in the left periumbilical area. The lead is then tunneled to the subcutaneous pocket and connected to the generator. The entire system is then tested.
4. **Results.** Recent evidence indicates that the Endotak lead system utilizing the nonthoracotomy lead was successfully implanted in 100% of 832 patients when combined with biphasic wave forms [39]. In 87% the lead only was successful. Consequently, the nonthoracotomy Endotak lead system has supplanted the other surgical techniques for ICD implantation. We now reserve the subxiphoid and the anterior thoracotomy techniques for use only when there is failure of the

nonthoracotomy lead [35]. Median sternotomy is still used for combined proce-dures [39]. Video-assisted thoracotomy is also available in situations when the lead-only attempt results in failure. In the future, smaller devices and subpec-toral implantation will be available.

References

1. Bellet S. *Clinical Disorders of the Heart Beat* (3rd ed), Philadelphia: Lea & Febiger, 1971. P 506.
2. Gallagher JJ, et al. Epicardial mapping in the Wolff-Parkinson-White syndrome. *Circulation* 57:854, 1978.
3. Chung KY, Walsh TJ, Massie E. Wolff-Parkinson-White syndrome. *Am Heart J* 69:1–8, 1965.
4. Sealy WC, Gallagher JJ. The surgical approach to the septal area of the heart based on experiences with 45 patients with Kent bundles. *J Thorac Cardiovasc Surg* 79:542, 1978.
5. Sealy WC. The evolution of the surgical methods for interruption of right free wall Kent bundles. *Ann Thorac Surg* 36:29, 1983.
6. Guiraudon GM, et al. Surgical repair of Wolff-Parkinson-White syndrome: A new closed-heart technique. *Ann Thorac Surg* 37:67–71, 1984.
7. Guiraudon GM, et al. Closed-heart technique for Wolff-Parkinson-White syndrome: Further experience and potential limitations. *Ann Thorac Surg* 42:651–657, 1986.
8. Klein GJ, et al. Surgical correction of the Wolff-Parkinson-White syndrome in the closed heart using cryosurgery: A simplified approach. *J Am Coll Cardiol* 3:405–409, 1984.
9. Gallagher JJ, et al. Cryosurgical ablation of accessory atrioventricular connections: A method for correction of the pre-excitation syndrome. *Circulation* 55:471, 1977.
10. Wu D, et al. Clinical, electrocardiographic and electrophysiologic observations in patients with paroxysmal supraventricular tachycardia. *Am J Cardiol* 41:1045–1051, 1978.
11. Guiraudon GM, et al. Surgical treatment of supraventricular tachycardia: A five year experience. *PACE* 9:1376–1380, 1986.
12. Hendry PJ, et al. Surgical treatment for automatic atrial tachycardias. *Ann Thorac Surg* 49:253–260, 1990.
13. Wellens HJJ, Durrer D. The role of an accessory atrioventricular pathway in reciprocal tachycardia: Observations in patients with and without the Wolff-Parkinson-White syndrome. *Circulation* 52:58, 1975.
14. Farshidi A, et al. Electrophysiologic characteristics of concealed bypass tracts: Clinical and electrical correlates. *Am J Cardiol* 41:1052, 1978.
15. Sealy WC, Gallagher JJ, Kasell J. His bundle interruption for control of inappropriate ventricular responses to atrial arrhythmias. *Ann Thorac Surg* 32:429, 1981.
16. Cox JL, Holman WL, Cain ME. Cryosurgical treatment of atrioventricular node reen-trant tachycardia. *Circulation* 76:1329–1336, 1987.
17. Guiraudon GM, et al. Skeletonization of the atrioventricular node for AV node reen-trant tachycardia: Experience with 32 patients. *Ann Thorac Surg* 49:565, 1990.
18. Guiraudon GM, et al. Combined sinoatrial node atrioventricular isolation: A surgical alternative to His bundle ablation in patients with atrial fibrillation (Abstract). *Circulation* 75:III–220, 1985.
19. Guiraudon GM, et al. Early clinical results of corridor surgery for treatment of chronic atrial fibrillation (Abstract). *J Am Coll Cardiol* 12:111A 1988.
20. Guiraudon GM, et al. Surgery for Atrial Flutter, Atrial Fibrillation and Atrial Tachy-cardia. In DP Zipes, J Jalife (eds). Philadelphia: Saunders, 1990. P 915.
21. Leitch JW, et al. Sinus node-atrioventricular node isolation: Long term results with the corridor operation for atrial fibrillation. *J Am Coll Cardiol* 17:970, 1991.
22. Defauw JJAMT, et al. Surgical therapy of paroxysmal atrial fibrillation with the "corri-dor" operation. *Ann Thorac Surg* 53:564, 1992.
23. van Hemel NM, et al. Longterm results of the "corridor" operation: A surgical therapy for atrial fibrillation. *Circulation* 1992 (In press).
24. Cox JL, et al. The surgical treatment of atrial fibrillation. III. Development of a defini-tive surgical procedure. *J Thorac Cardiovasc Surg* 101:569, 1991.
25. Cox JL, et al. The surgical treatment of atrial fibrillation. II. Intraoperative electro-physiologic mapping and description of the electrophysiologic basis of atrial flutter and atrial fibrillation. *J Thorac Cardiovasc Surg* 101:406, 1991.

26. Ferguson TB, et al. The requirement for permanent pacemaker therapy following the Maze procedure for atrial fibrillation: Incidence and therapeutic indications. *PACE* 17(4):485, 1994.
27. Cox JL, et al. Successful surgical treatment of atrial fibrillation: Review and clinical update. *JAMA* 266:1976, 1991.
28. Cox JL, et al. Right ventricular isolation procedures for nonischemic ventricular tachycardia. *J Thorac Cardiovasc Surg* 90:212, 1985.
29. Josephson ME, Harken AH, Horowitz LN. Endocardial excision: A new surgical technique for the treatment of recurrent ventricular tachycardia. *Circulation* 60:1430, 1979.
30. Watkins L Jr., et al. The treatment of malignant ventricular arrhythmias with combined endocardial resection and the implantation of the automatic defibrillator: A preliminary report. *Ann Thorac Surg* 37:60–66, 1984.
31. Platia EV, et al. Treatment of malignant ventricular arrhythmias with endocardial resection and the implantation of the automatic implantable cardioverter-defibrillator.
32. Mirowski M, et al. Termination of malignant ventricular arrhythmias with an implanted automatic defibrillator in human beings. *N Engl J Med* 303:322–324, 1980.
33. Mirowski M, et al. The automatic defibrillator: New modality for treatment of life-threatening ventricular arrhythmias. *PACE* 5:384–401, 1982.
34. Mirowski M, et al. The automatic implantable cardioverter-defibrillator: An Overview. *J Am Coll Cardiol* 6:461–466, 1985.
35. Veltri EP, et al. Clinical efficacy of the automatic implantable cardioverter-defibrillator: Six-year cumulative experience. *Circulation* 74(Suppl):109, 1986.
36. Watkins L Jr, et al. Implantation of the automatic defibrillator: The subxiphoid approach. *Ann Thorac Surg* 34:515, 1982.
37. Watkins L Jr, et al. Automatic defibrillation in man: The initial experience. *J Thorac Cardiovasc Surg* 82:492–500, 1981.
38. Watkins L Jr, et al. Surgical techniques for implanting the automatic implantable defibrillator. *PACE* 7:1357–1362, 1984.
39. Nuezner J, Pitschner HF, Steinmetz F. 100% successful implantation of nonthoracotomy lead systems with biphasic cardioverter/defibrillator: European Multicenter results in 832 patients. *PACE* 17(4):79, 1994.

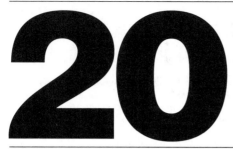

Neuropsychiatric Aspects of Arrhythmia Evaluation and Management

Gregory L. Fricchione
and Stephen C. Vlay

Sudden cardiac death (SCD), the leading single cause of mortality in the United States, accounting for 300,000 deaths annually, has been called the major challenge confronting contemporary cardiology [1, 2]. For reasons we examine in this chapter, part of this medical challenge is psychiatric.

A number of predisposing factors appear to operate in most cases of SCD. Myocardium, usually though not necessarily compromised by ischemic coronary artery disease, may be the substrate for electrical instability [1–3]. An acute stimulus or event may then initiate a life-threatening arrhythmia, usually in the form of ventricular tachycardia (VT) or ventricular fibrillation (VF) [4, 5]. It has thus been postulated that the electrophysiologic occurrence of VT or VF may be due to transient risk factors, and evidence has been accumulating that some of these risk factors may be related to CNS activity [4, 5]. Indeed some researchers have favored an expansion of study from the "heart as target to the brain as trigger" [1].

Psychiatric physicians are becoming more involved with the care and study of patients at risk for SCD. Survivors of out-of-hospital cardiac arrests, patients with postinfarction ventricular arrhythmias, and others are often seen in consultation while they are undergoing rigorous and often disturbing examinations. Complicated matters of therapeutic management arise, with modification of transient and chronic risk factors often a priority.

The purpose of this chapter is to familiarize cardiologists, general internists and practitioners, emergency room specialists, and psychiatrists coming into contact with these special patients with background information and recent developments in the psychiatric aspects of these life-threatening arrhythmias and their management.

I. Neurophysiology of sudden cardiac death and ventricular arrhythmias

A. **Role of the autonomic nervous system.** The role of the autonomic nervous system in SCD is important. If this role is better understood, the basic mechanisms leading to VT and VF may be elaborated, making preventive strategies more practical. It should be noted that structural lesions of the CNS such as subarachnoid hemorrhage, head injuries, cerebral ischemia, and tumors can lead to profound cardiac regulatory changes, resulting at times in VT or VF and SCD [6]. Some early studies found intracerebral hemorrhages in 5–8% of patients dying from SCD [6]. Parizel suggested that patients with intracranial hemorrhages be treated as aggressively for arrhythmia as are patients with acute myocardial infarctions [7].

B. **Central neural mechanisms in sudden cardiac death syndrome, ventricular tachycardia, and ventricular fibrillation.** While no structural lesions in the CNS have been related specifically to SCD syndrome, a growing body of evidence points to a contributory role for central neural mechanisms in the disorder. From animal studies, it is known that the cortical areas affecting cardiovascular function include the upper portion of the frontal lobe, the orbital cortex, the motor and premotor cortex, and the anterior part of the temporal lobe. Electrical stimulation in these areas can provoke ventricular premature beats (VPBs) [4, 5]. However, arrhythmias are more readily provoked from subcortical areas such as the hypothalamus [6]. If the posterior hypothalamus is stimulated in dogs with coronary artery occlusion, the incidence of VT is 10 times that in occluded dogs without stimulation. Stimulation and ablation studies of neural structures demonstrate that the efferent sympathetic pathway arises in the paraventricular nucleus of the hypothalamus, midbrain, and quadrigeminal bodies; traverses the ventrolateral medullary reticular formation, specifically the C1 adrenergic neurons; synapses in the intermediolateral cell column in the spinal cord; and arrives at the heart via stellate ganglia and cardiac sympathetic nerves [4–6, 8].

C. **Sympathetic nervous system activity.** The evidence that sympathetic nervous system activity predisposes to VT and VF is substantial. In animals, electrical stimulation of cardiac sympathetic fibers markedly lowers the vulnerable period threshold and, in the presence of myocardial ischemia, may result in VT or VF [4, 5]. The left stellate ganglion appears to be most important in this respect [5, 6]. The left stellate is the recipient of most of the afferent sympathetic reflex nerve fibers. Stimulation of the left stellate results in a prolonged Q–T interval and decreased VT threshold, while ablation increases VT threshold by 72%.

D. **Sympathetic-parasympathetic interaction.** When sympathetic activity is enhanced by thoracotomy or by direct stimulation of cardiac sympathetic fibers, a definite vagal antifibrillatory effect is noted [2]. Vagal stimulation seems to lower ventricular vulnerability indirectly by opposing increased adrenergic tone [3, 5]. After norepinephrine infusion, the vulnerable period threshold is markedly decreased, but if the vagus is stimulated, the threshold normalizes. The vagal effect is a muscarinic property that can be reversed by atropine. The principal site of vagal projection to the ventricle is the His-Purkinje system, where numerous sympathetic neurons are located. It may be that predilection for SCD reflects an adrenergic-cholinergic imbalance.

E. **Summary of evidence for a central neural mechanism in sudden cardiac death.** The evidence for autonomic nervous system involvement in SCD includes the following:

1. Autonomic stimulation, especially if the left side is overactivated, can lead to VT or VF.
2. Sympathetic activation reduces VF threshold in normal and particularly in ischemic myocardium.
3. Autonomic activity is closely connected to behavior that is under CNS modulation.
4. Psychological and social strain and environmental stimulation can give rise to abnormal autonomic flow.
5. Ventricular fibrillation threshold can be normalized after stress if the hypothalamus and descending pathways are destroyed.
6. Stress is associated with VT, VF, and SCD in animal studies as well as with the elevated incidence of SCD in human beings.

II. **Psychosocial stress, sudden cardiac death, and ventricular arrhythmias**
   A. **Animal studies.** What is the evidence that psychological stimuli can alter cardiac vulnerability and increase susceptibility to VT, VF, and SCD? Lown and colleagues in the 1970s employed a repetitive extrasystole technique (two-thirds of the electrical current required for VF induction) to show a 30–50% decrease in threshold in dogs exposed to aversive situations [4]. They were able to demonstrate in dogs with ischemia that repeated exposures to an aversive environment produced ventricular arrhythmias, while removal to a calm locale abolished them.
   B. **Patient experience.** Ventricular irritability can sometimes be diminished by reassurance, relaxation, or tranquilization. For example, interruption of recurrent VF by psychiatric interview has been reported [9]. The most striking evidence that sympathetic activity and stress together can be important in initiating VT or VF is seen in the long Q–T interval syndrome, which consists of a prolonged Q–T, congenital deafness, syncope, and VT or VF after emotional and physical stresses. It is thought to be related to an imbalance in sympathetic outflow to the heart with the left stellate ganglion predominating [5].
   C. **Psychological risk factors for SCD.** Efforts have been made to characterize those at risk for SCD using psychological variables (Table 20-1). While "there is no specific link between a given type of psychological derangement and cardiac arrhythmias," as pointed out by Regestein in 1975, there seems to be a relationship between psychosocial strain in general and SCD [4]. Studies have variously shown depression, anger, type A behavior, type B behavior, anxiety, and both acute and chronic stress to be correlated with SCD. It has also come to light that mental stress rivals physical exercise as a precipitate for myocardial ischemia, which in turn might lower the threshold for VT or VF [10].

III. **Psychosocial aspects of sudden cardiac death**
   A. **The cardiac patient in general.** Hackett and Cassem have described the psychological problems of cardiac patients [11]. These problems predominantly center around two mood states: depression and anxiety. Anxiety generally arises from the threat of

sudden death, while depression stems from the question of whether the patient can perform in his or her roles as a spouse, parent, and citizen. The patient who has had a myocardial infarction also generally experiences a sense of loss of a valued part of himself or herself such as strength, energy, or independence.

B. **The survivor of sudden cardiac death with ventricular tachycardia or ventricular fibrillation.** Treatment of patients with VT or VF requires attention to the multiple psychosocial aspects of the disease, in addition to the choice of antiarrhythmic drugs, surgical procedures, or pacemaker-defibrillator devices [2, 12]. Management of psychosocial stress in refractory VT or VF patients at risk for recurrent cardiac arrest has become an important aspect of their care, given the effects of stress on the CNS and its ability to trigger arrhythmias.

Table 20-1. Psychological studies of sudden cardiac death (SCD)

Reference	Summary
Greene et al., *Arch Intern Med* 129:725, 1972	Stress in over 50% of SCD victims was acute and involved a coexistence of depressive and arousal states
Bruhn et al., *J Psychosom Res* 18:187, 1974	In prospective study in patients with myocardial infarction (MI), elevated depression, pattern of joyless striving at work, and type A behavior correlated with SCD
Rahe et al., *Arch Intern Med* 133:221, 1974	Marked increase in life change units during the 6 months immediately before infarction or death, compared to same time interval 1 year earlier, particularly in SCD victims
Meyers and Dewar, *Br Heart J* 37:1133, 1975	Acute psychological stress was an important variable in SCD of 100 men, with 23 experiencing stress within 30 minutes of arrest, 40 within 24 hours
Rissanen et al., *Acta Med Scand* 204:389, 1978	Nineteen percent of patients with ventricular arrhythmias had acute stress before the event
Cebelin and Hirsch, *Hum Pathol* 11:123, 1980	Fifteen of 497 homicide deaths showed no evidence that actual trauma was cause of death; acute stress cardiomyopathy with ventricular fibrillation and SCD more likely in those 15
Cottington et al., *Psychosom Med* 42:567, 1980	Death of a close person only significant factor among 81 SCD victims, who were six times as likely to have lost someone close in preceding 6 months
Orth-Gomer et al., *Acta Med Scand* 207:31, 1980	Depressive emotional state was associated with severe ventricular arrhythmia in healthy men but not in men with ischemic disease; type A behavior by Jenkins Activity Survey was not correlated with higher incidence
Reich et al. *JAMA* 246:233, 1981	Twenty-five of 117 experienced stress within 24 hours of the onset of ventricular arrhythmias; in 17 instances, predominant affect was anger
Trichopoulos et al., *Lancet* 1:441, 1983	Subjects exposed to a natural disaster and stress without escape had a higher incidence of cardiac arrhythmias and sudden death
Katz et al., *Am J Med* 78:589, 1985	Greater anxiety, depression, and social alienation were prominent in arrhythmia patients without MI
Ahern et al., *Am J Cardiol* 66:59, 1990	Type B behavior, depression, lower pulse reactivity to challenge were post-MI risk factors for cardiac arrest

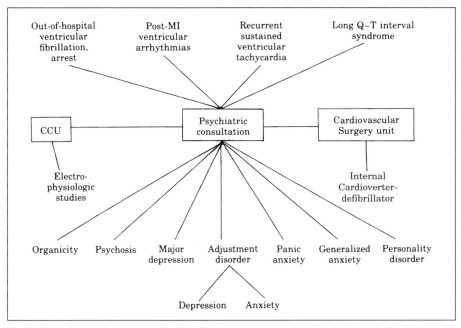

Fig. 20-1. Routes to psychiatric consultation and outcomes. (MI = myocardial infarction; CCU = coronary care unit.)

The individual who survives sudden cardiac arrest associated with the acute phase of myocardial infarction has little chance of recurrence. On the other hand, survivors of out-of-hospital VT or VF without myocardial infarction who have refractory arrhythmias are at high risk of a similar event. Refractory VT or VF patients have a 70–90% chance of clinical recurrence if a regimen capable of suppressing induction cannot be discovered in the electrophysiology (EP) laboratory [12, 13]. The mortality in the first year ranges from 25–40%, but in patients in whom VT suppression is accomplished during EP studies (EPS), it is reduced to 2–10%. Nevertheless, in addition to prolonged coronary care unit stays and invasive testing, these patients might confront their mortality in strikingly concrete terms. Often anxiety and depression result. These and other problems such as delirium and psychosis lead to psychiatric consultations in VT and VF patients (Fig. 20-1).

1. **Anxiety**
   a. **Presentation.** The patient with VT or VF experiences uncertainty and loss of a sense of control over destiny. Anxiety may result as the patient attempts to cope. It may present with certain physical signs and symptoms that challenge the clinician dealing with cardiac patients (Table 20-2). As with recent myocardial infarction (MI) patients, anxiety arises from the specter of sudden death. The intensity of this fear may be greater than in survivors of MI because of the likely discussion of sudden death potential during the early stages of VT and VF evaluation. Hypervigilance may emerge in some patients, along with a "time bomb" mentality. Dependence on monitors may arise, leading to separation anxiety when disconnection takes place. A sleep disturbance beyond the normal restlessness seen in patients in an intensive care unit may result from anxiety. Often a fear of going to sleep will be described, and this is occasionally related to the apprehension that "if I go to sleep, I'll need to be resuscitated," or "if I fall asleep I may not wake up." Some SCD patients have reported near-death experiences. These are usually soothing to patients but sometimes result in anxiety, which can be helped through verbalization and normalization of the experiences.
   Repeated cardioversion can result in fear that sometimes prevents completion of evaluation. In the EP laboratory, the induced sustained ventricular tachyarrhythmias may be paced back to sinus rhythm in 65–85% of cases,

depending on rate. Electrical cardioversion is necessary in the remaining cases. Patients are allowed to lose consciousness very briefly before shock, which, it is hoped, will make them amnesic for the event. Sometimes this is not feasible and the patient recalls the event, which sets up an aversive conditioning paradigm. The thought of further EP testing with the possibility of countershock may elicit a paniclike anxiety with palpitations, chest tightness, GI symptoms, hyperventilation, sweating, and other symptoms. This can progress to a phobic state, with the patient avoiding and refusing further tests. Nevertheless, prior frightening episodes of SCD outside the hospital are often sufficient incentives to make patients persist with EP evaluation until a treatment is found.

b. Management. Anxiety is often accompanied by increased sympathetic tone, which may increase the risk of VT or VF. Thus, there is an incentive to modulate the patient's anxiety through psychiatric intervention when necessary. Management of anxious patients with refractory VT may be instituted in four parts.

(1) The attending cardiologist provides clear information with an optimistic tone, while affording patients a glimpse of potential frustrations before resolution. Shared confidence and diminished apprehension of the unknown are usually achieved.

(2) The consulting psychiatrist provides supportive therapy designed to allow ventilation of the patient's concerns at his or her own pace, while helping to maintain and strengthen coping mechanisms. Adaptive denial such as the statement, "This hasn't really changed my life," should be left in place. Indeed, there are some patients capable of denying the objective danger of their illnesses. This denial becomes maladaptive when compliance with recommendations and treatment is disrupted, as when the patient says, "I'm not sick. I don't need these drugs. I'm leaving." Maladaptive denial needs to be addressed and altered if possible, sometimes using the leverage of family opinion.

(3) Anxiolytic medication can usually benefit these patients. Benzodiazepines such as diazepam, oxazepam, lorazepam, and alprazolam are the drugs of choice since their cardiotoxicity is minimal and their benefit-safety margin is advantageous. Indeed, diazepam has intrinsic antiarrhythmic properties occasionally effective even against refractory arrhythmias [14]. Buspirone is a nonbenzodiazepine anxiolytic with a good cardiac safety profile. It may take 2 weeks or so to see an effect, however. Beta-blocking medications have been known to lessen the peripheral manifestations of anxiety.

(4) Behavioral techniques, including relaxation response, hypnosis, and biofeedback, are taught to patients. A sense of self-control over anxiety can accompany proficiency in these techniques (Table 20-3).

For anxiety of the panic type characterized by discrete periods of apprehension or fear accompanied by symptoms such as dyspnea, choking sensations, dizziness or unsteadiness, unreal feelings, paresthesias, hot and cold flashes, trembling, sweating, faintness, and fear by dying or going crazy, alprazolam may offer a combination of safety and effectiveness [15].

Table 20-2. Physical signs and symptoms of anxiety

System	Signs and symptoms
Cardiac	Chest pain or tightness, palpitations, tachycardia, pallor, lightheadedness
Neurologic	Dizziness, faintness, headache, tremulousness, paresthesias, numbness, muscle tension
Gastrointestinal	Anorexia, "butterflies in stomach," nausea, vomiting, abdominal discomfort
Respiratory	Dyspnea, hyperventilation
Miscellaneous	Diaphoresis, dry mouth, flushing, sexual dysfunction, urinary frequency

Imipramine, a tricyclic antidepressant, and monoamine oxidase inhibitors (MAOI) such as phenelzine have also shown effectiveness in treating panic disorders but require special considerations [15] (Table 20-4). The selective serotonin reuptake inhibitors (SSRIs), such as sertraline, paroxetine, and fluoxetine, offer useful alternatives since they are not likely to lower the threshold for ventricular arrhythmia and have effectiveness in the management of panic disorder itself. One of the identified medications may need to be tried in panic states precipitated by exposure to a circumscribed phobic stimulus such as repeated EP study although often acute use of a benzodiazepine will suffice.

Table 20-3. Anxiety management and treatment

Informative sessions: information and confidence through frequent sessions with the cardiologist

Supportive psychotherapy: ventilation of concerns, clarification and strengthening of coping skills through sessions with the psychiatrist

Pharmacotherapy
  Benzodiazepines
    Diazepam 2–10 mg 2–4 times daily
    Oxazepam 10–30 mg 3 or 4 times daily. May be less likely than other drugs to cause paradoxical agitation
    Lorazepam 2–6 mg/day in divided doses. Not cleared by cytochrome P-450 system so will not accumulate when used in combination with drugs such as cimetidine. May have reasonably consistent absorption when given intramuscularly in the deltoid
    Alprazolam 0.5–4.0 mg/day in divided doses. Less likely than other drugs to cause depressed mood. Elderly men require only small doses for therapeutic effect
  Buspirone 5–10 mg 2–3 times daily
  Beta-blocking medications
Behavioral therapy
  Relaxation techniques: Jacobsen progressive relaxation, Benson relaxation response
  Hypnosis
  Biofeedback

Table 20-4. Treatment of panic anxiety

1. **Alprazolam:** 0.5–6.0 mg/day in divided doses. Alprazolam can be used safely in patients already taking type 1A antiarrhythmic drugs, in patients with impaired left ventricular performance, in patients with orthostatic hypotension, and in patients with preexisting bundle branch block (BBB). Long-term use requires slow taper to avoid withdrawal symptoms

2. **Selective serotonin reuptake inhibitors (SSRIs):** Sertraline (25 mg PO q A.M. to start), paroxetine (10 mg PO q A.M. to start), fluoxetine (10–20 mg PO q A.M. to start). These antidepressants are relatively safe for patients with ventricular arrhythmias. Monitor antiarrhythmic levels and digoxin levels because of SSRI inhibitory effects on cytochrome P-450 CYP2D6 enzymes

3. **Imipramine:** up to 300 mg/day. Can cause atrioventricular (AV) block; orthostatic hypotension, especially in the elderly; and reflex tachycardia. Can worsen ventricular arrhythmias as can other type 1A drugs. Can be used as a type 1A antiarrhythmic. Caution required, including hospital monitoring in patients with BBB at risk for AV block and in patients with ventricular tachycardia or ventricular fibrillation. Can be used only in patients not taking other type 1A drugs

4. **Monoamine oxidase inhibitors:** e.g., phenelzine 60–90 mg/day. Requires tyramine-free diet and attention to drug interactions to avoid hypertensive crisis; orthostatic hypotension is a common side effect. More investigation in this population would be helpful; in one study phenelzine shortened the Q–Tc interval but had no effect on P–R or QRS interval

2. Depression

a. Presentation. Depression may develop in patients with malignant ventricular arrhythmias. The depressed or demoralized mood seen in cardiac illness is often reactive—an adjustment disorder with depressed mood. It is marked by a maladaptive response within 3 months of the onset of a stressor. It is accompanied by the assumption that the disturbance will eventually disappear or lessen when the stressor ceases or a new level of adaptation is achieved. Adjustment disorders are often found in patients without history of psychiatric morbidity. The individual with malignant ventricular arrhythmias will worry primarily about the impact on the family and about employment and source of income. Will one become dependent on one's spouse? How will sexual performance be affected? Who will provide for the children and their education? Will the breadwinner's job be lost? In essence, as Hackett and Cassem have pointed out with cardiac patients in general, "Depression centers around the question of whether they can function successfully as a spouse, parent, and citizen" [11]. These self-doubts can only be answered with time, but they affect the ruminating patient daily while in the hospital undergoing examinations.

These patients, like those with other cardiac diseases, must come to terms with certain real and perceived losses. There is a loss of security, control, and independence, as well as a potential loss of role. Patients grieve for these lost qualities. Sometimes what is felt most strongly is the loss of the veneer of invulnerability people apply in their everyday lives. Depression or demoralization sets in, and patients may lose interest, energy, and ability to concentrate. They may become irritable and demanding, and feelings of hopelessness, helplessness, and worthlessness are at times present. In the evaluation of the arrhythmia, the patient encounters many frustrations if the selected drug fails or produces untoward side effects. Some patients feel culpable when they "fail the test." While appeals to the patient for patience are commonplace, helping him or her understand the necessity for testing, the potential risk and benefits, and the possibility of initial failures is important in avoiding a "giving up–given up state." Reassurance that some treatment will be sought no matter how long it takes is important.

The signs of depression often remit as progress is made toward treatment. Occasionally a major depression or autonomous depression arises, as set out in the *Diagnostic and Statistical Manual of Mental Disorders* [16], particularly in patients with previous psychiatric affective morbidity [17, 18]. It is characterized by the presence of at least five of the following symptoms during the same 2-week period, with at least one of the symptoms being either prominent dysphoric mood or loss of interest or pleasure: depressed mood, appetite disturbance and weight change, sleep disturbance, psychomotor agitation or retardation, anhedonia or loss of interest, loss of energy, feelings of worthlessness or excessive guilt, decreased concentration or indecisiveness, and suicidal ideation or attempt or recurrent thoughts of death. Psychosocial interventions alone are not sufficient for these patients. Some investigators feel that in medically ill patients, mood and cognitive symptoms are better indicators of major depression than are vegetative and somatic symptoms. It should be noted that physically ill patients with major depression have a poorer prognosis medically, and patients with recurrent VT may be at higher risk for SCD if they are also depressed. This point is supported by the finding that some patients with major depression have been found to have increased Q–T intervals. It has also been noted that some anorexia nervosa patients who die a sudden cardiac death have prolonged Q–T intervals.

b. Management. Adjustment disorder (reactive) depression can often be managed with supportive, educational psychotherapy and medications such as alprazolam. More traditional antidepressants often can be avoided, although they are effective for adjustment disorders with depressed mood. For patients with VT or VF who meet the criteria for major depression, cautious pharmacotherapy as well as psychotherapy is definitely indicated. Alprazolam has been reported to be effective not only for anxiety and panic attacks but also for depression in major depressive disorder, as well as adjustment disorder [19]. Alprazolam also has relatively minor cardiotoxicity, making it a reasonable first choice for adjustment disorder depression and of possible benefit in major depression (Table 20-5).

Tricyclic antidepressants (TCAs), though proved effective for depression, require more caution because of their considerable cardiac effects: orthostatic hypotension, reflex tachycardia, and conduction delay, particularly in the His-Purkinje system, reflected in lengthening of the P–R, QRS, and Q–T intervals [20]. In patients with preexisting bundle branch block, there is a risk of heart block with TCAs. In some cases, complete heart block may lead to SCD. Type 1A antiarrhythmic drugs may be arrhythmogenic and cause VT and VF and SCD. Thus, VT or VF patients can have an exacerbation of the underlying arrhythmia since TCAs are type 1A antiarrhythmic agents similar to quinidine, procainamide, and disopyramide. This exacerbation may be related to further prolongation of the Q–T interval, which is common in ventricular arrhythmias induced by type 1A drugs. One study, however, showed that antiarrhythmic agents contributed to the occurrence of cardiac arrest in 5 of 98 patients, but in none of these was Q–T interval prolongation noted [21]. These data raise the question whether some other poorly understood electrophysiologic mechanisms can also cause or exacerbate VT and VF.

On the other hand, imipramine is effective as a type 1A medication, and it can be used as an antiarrhythmic as well as an antidepressant in VT and VF patients with depression [22]. Nortriptyline has also been used. Imipramine treatment can be initiated in these patients while they are hospitalized in a telemetry unit. Other type 1A medication is usually tapered off. Prolonged simultaneous use of two type 1A antiarrhythmics may be deleterious [18]. In one study using imipramine as an antiarrhythmic, VT was suppressed in 50% of subjects given 150 mg/day or less in two doses 12 hours apart, whereas 50% of patients had VPBs suppressed at doses of less than 250 mg/day [22]. Follow-up Holter monitoring is obtained with patients maintained on an imipramine regimen. Patients with a Q–Tc interval greater than 0.440 second and a history of infarction deserve special caution when taking TCAs because of the increased risk of SCD owing to VT or VF with prolonged Q–Tc [23]. Another ECG marker, the QRS duration, may have some predictive value for ventricular arrhythmias. In TCA overdose patients, a QRS of 0.16 second was associated with a 50% incidence of ventricular arrhythmias [24]. Second-generation antidepressants such as maprotiline, trazodone, and amoxapine may increase ventricular ectopic activity. Caution and monitoring must accompany their use in patients with recurrent VT since experience with their use in this population is sparse. Antidepressants such as buproprion and the SSRIs are increasingly used as the antidepressants of first choice in this patient population because they are unlikely to precipitate tachyarrhythmias. Buproprion has been studied in the cardiac population, and it appears

Table 20-5. Treatment of depression

1. **Alprazolam:** 0.5–6.0 mg/day in divided doses. See Table 20-4. Works particularly well in patients with adjustment disorder with depressed mood. May also be effective in major depression. See text
2. **Selective serotonin reuptake inhibitors:** See Table 20-4
3. **Tricyclic antidepressants:** e.g., imipramine, up to 300 mg/day. Use a q12h dosage schedule to ensure antiarrhythmic activity. See Table 20-4. Effective in both adjustment disorder and major depression. See text
4. **Monoamine oxidase inhibitors:** e.g., phenelzine 60–90 mg/day in divided doses. See Table 20-4. See text
5. **Buproprion:** 225–450 mg/day in 75-mg divided doses. Start with 75 mg bid–tid and increase as tolerated every third day. Early clinical trials show little adverse cardiovascular or heart rhythm effects. May cause seizures. Would await more extensive clinical experience before using in patients with ventricular tachyarrhythmias
6. **Electroconvulsive therapy (ECT):** After ventricular tachycardia is controlled, ECT can be used cautiously. Must monitor for arrhythmias owing to increased sympathetic flow after seizure
7. **Behavior therapy:** possible role for cognitive behavior therapy in patients with milder depression

to be well tolerated [25]. The cardiac electrophysiologic effects of monoamine oxidase inhibitors are largely unstudied, although their hypotensive properties and ability to cause hypertensive crisis when mixed with tyramine-containing foods and certain medications are well documented [25]. More investigation of MAOI in depressed patients with ventricular arrhythmias would be welcome. In one study, phenelzine sulfate produced a significant shortening of the Q–Tc interval but had no effect on P–R or QRS intervals [26].

Cognitive behavior therapy may be tried in depressed VT and VF patients, especially if antidepressant medication is not tolerated. If the depression is severely disabling or life threatening, carefully monitored electroconvulsive therapy (ECT) may be required after the ventricular arrhythmia is controlled. The dangers of ECT are short-lived but include increased heart rate and BP, ECG changes such as increased P-wave amplitude and QRS and ST–T-wave changes, and atrial and ventricular arrhythmias [27].

3. **Delirium and psychosis.** On occasion severe agitation and psychotic behavior emerge, usually during treatment of patients with defects in sensorium or cognition or with histories of psychosis. A brief course of oral or parenteral haloperidol, usually in low doses, is considered a relatively safe and effective pharmacotherapy in the management of such cases.

In the canine model, VT threshold has not been found to be lowered by haloperidol. Phenothiazines, particularly thioridazine and chlorpromazine, have rarely been associated with onset or worsening of ventricular arrhythmias. Ventricular tachycardia and VF patients with manic-depressive illness who develop mania may be treated acutely with haloperidol or with lithium carbonate or both. Lithium occasionally causes conduction disturbances, including sinus node dysfunction, rare ventricular arrhythmia, and most often first-degree atrioventricular block. Thus, chronic psychiatric patients who also have VT or VF may need to have their medication stabilized in a monitored setting.

Many antiarrhythmics can produce a delirium similar to lidocaine toxicity. Quinidine, procainamide, disopyramide, mexiletine, tocainide, flecainide, lorcainide, and encainide may all occasionally be associated with CNS manifestations and mental status changes. Amiodarone is not yet reported to cause delirium. It can cause thyroid dysfunction, particularly hypothyroidism in the elderly, as well as peripheral neuropathy, headaches, sleep disturbance, and tremors. Propafenone, a bupropionlike antiarrhythmic, was recently reported to cause secondary mania in one patient.

IV. **Results.** For the patient with refractory VT, hospitalization for evaluation and treatment may last weeks or longer. When the EP studies are finished and a regimen is chosen, the individual usually feels relatively comfortable. Adaptive denial is retained, although patients frequently maintain an underlying apprehension that VT or VF will recur. However, if they remain healthy, over time apprehension recedes, allowing the patient to be active and more secure. The patient in whom complete suppression of VT and VF with drugs is accomplished through EPS is different from the patient with refractory disease who eventually requires implantation of a pacemaker and an internal cardiovertor-defibrillator (ICD). Here the treatment emphasis changes from prevention to prompt eradication. The defibrillator patient is aware that the arrhythmia may recur, but a sense of security emerges from the knowledge that the device will restore normal sinus rhythm. Although the ICD, which requires no active intervention, provides a good measure of security, the patient literally experiences a shock when it does discharge. The main reaction to this shock may be anxiety, and the patient may then anticipate repeated firings. His or her range of activity may shrink as a result of this vulnerability, until confidence can be rebuilt. With time and a concentration on the positive, most individuals make the necessary adjustments.

V. **Patient's viewpoint: A case report.** Mr. V. A. is a 52-year-old married investment banker with a history of MI and out-of-hospital cardiac arrest. After medical management of recurrent VT and VF failed, he underwent successful ICD implantation. He continues to work, commuting long distances by railroad, but notices that his exercise tolerance is lower. He was recently hospitalized for repeat EPS and for replacement of the ICD battery. The patient was originally seen by psychiatry during his first cardiac coronary unit stay for adjustment disorder, anxiety. Alprazolam as needed, supportive therapy, and relaxation techniques were helpful in managing his anxiety. This treatment regimen is repeated for depressed mood as well as anxiety during readmissions. Family meetings are held as needed, particularly at crisis points. Mr. V. A. was recently asked several questions related to his illness. These included his personal reactions to the recurrent ventricular arrhythmias, the EPS, and the ICD. Family changes were also discussed.

A. **Personal reactions.** The patient stated that the loss of health did bother him in several ways. Part of his attitude, he said, was a self-pitying "Why me?" feeling. The illness made him more self-concerned than he had ever been. He was also quite aware of sadness and depressed mood, centering around feelings of hopelessness, helplessness, and worthlessness: "I have the notion that I'm certainly not going to live 10 more years." "I'm not that good anymore at work. They decided to cut down on my responsibility, and then they decided against giving me a raise." He did feel he could now relax at work, however. "I'm also not that good at home anymore either." He felt he cannot do the same things he used to do about the house. "I'm like a pregnant woman about to go into labor when I work around the house now," he laughed. He also admitted to experiencing a "fear in the pit of my stomach" when he thinks about the arrhythmia. He denied being angry. "I just try to do my best," he said. "It's not that bad. I still enjoy life."

While this account has individual specific considerations, the common themes of grief over loss of role and vulnerability to early death clearly emerge. Nevertheless, this patient, like most others, has adjusted adaptively.

B. **Electrophysiologic studies.** Mr. V. A. was in the hospital this time for repeat EPS. During the EPS, he had an episode of VT and VF and was allowed to approach the loss of consciousness briefly. He imagined seeing his family gathered around him and hearing the cardiologist calling him and then countershocking him back to normal sinus rhythm. The most difficult part of the experience was, he said, "the feeling of loss of control when you start losing consciousness. I dread that feeling. It is the worst and it almost makes me not come to the hospital when I know an EP study is likely." "Getting shocked is not as bad," he reports. "It is like getting a shock from an electric socket but stronger."

Unusual perceptual experiences such as near-death phenomena may accompany VT or VF episodes even in the EP laboratory. This patient dreaded the process of losing consciousness more than the electrical cardioversion, which is perhaps uncharacteristic of these patients.

C. **Internal cardioverter-defibrillator.** Mr. V. A. saw his ICD as "insurance," as a "security blanket." "It would have been very hard to make the decision not to replace the battery if the EP study had been negative this time around. I think I'm relieved that now I know the battery needs to be put back in." At times the patient uses denial and does things without taking into account the ICD. However, most of the time he holds his hand over the power pack located in the left upper quadrant of the abdomen underneath the diaphragm to protect it, "like a pregnant lady." When he bangs it against something, it hurts, he explained.

The patient's increased security with an ICD is a common reaction; however, the device also serves as an ever-present reminder of the recurrent arrhythmia, which perhaps makes complete denial more difficult to achieve.

D. **Family relationships.** The patient has cherished a closer relationship with his wife. "I give her more attention and vice versa." His 15-year-old son seems to be "rebelling." "I know he loves me but right now it's a hidden love. He knows I'm weaker than I was; he answers back. Once when I was chasing him and arguing, the defibrillator went off!"

Because of shifts in the balances of power caused by illness, the family may be a source of strain at times. However, it also often represents a source of strong support for these patients.

VI. **The family**

A. **Adaptation.** The family of the patient with recurrent ventricular arrhythmia faces adaptive tasks similar to those of the patient. Family members, the spouse in particular, need to surmount the crisis of loss and change, which are accompanied by **anxiety** and **depression.** There may be feelings of **anger,** sometimes directed at the patient for getting sick. The family then may be faced with resultant **guilt** over their angry feelings. Questions surface. Will they lose their mate, parent, child? How will their lifestyle be changed? These questions, if expressed, should be handled calmly with understanding. **Ventilation** and **normalization** of the experience often is helpful.

As in other chronic illnesses, there is frequently an alteration in the **balance of power** between patient and spouse. It can lead to turmoil if not addressed. **Independency-dependency conflicts** may emerge in the patient, leading to family strug-

gles. Helping patients and families at "fed-up" **crisis points** seems to be crucial. In one case, the destabilizing stress of a medication side effect (aprindine-induced confusion), added to the stress of recurrent ventricular arrhythmia, increased the wife's need to take care of the patient. Considerable marital strain resulted. With a successful medication change and with couple and individual psychotherapy with patient and wife, an equilibrium was reestablished. Occasionally adjustment problems within the family surface only after discharge. A formerly tranquil domestic situation may become discordant. The opportunity to return for counseling or psychotherapy should be afforded the patient and the family.
   B. **Education.** On occasion **overconcern** on the part of the family may lead to excessive restrictions on the patient. In some cases, the individual may then become depressed, overly dependent, and too fearful even to carry out activities of daily living. With **education** by the physician, many of these problems may be overcome. Following are some crucial educational goals:

   1. The patient and family should understand the nature of the illness.
   2. Physical limitations, if any, should be delineated.
   3. Recommended activity should be clarified.
   4. The name, purpose, and potential side effects of medications should be understood.
   5. The operation and rationale of devices such as the ICD should be known.
   6. What to do in an emergency should be made clear and practiced. Family members are encouraged to learn cardiopulmonary resuscitation (CPR). In fact, the ability to perform CPR is more often reassuring than anxiety provoking since family members become more comfortable knowing what to do in an emergency. A plan to summon aid is important. In addition, the patient and family are taught the warning signs of a problem (e.g., recurrent dizzy spells) and instructed when to call the physician.

   This amount of information is a great deal to assimilate, particularly for families that are not medically oriented. Therefore, it is imperative that patient education begin immediately in the evaluation phase and continue as an ongoing feature with family involvement. Repetition and explanation in terms that the patient and family can grasp are keys to better understanding.

VII. **The physician and the electrophysiology team**
   A. **The cardiologist.** For the cardiologist, the most challenging psychosocial management issue is the patient's anxiety about his or her cardiac status and the EPS. Through patient education and physician awareness of emotional needs, confidence is established, strengthening the physician-patient relationship. If the patient lacks this confidence, he or she will be unable to endure the arduous, occasionally frustrating hospital stay and evaluation. Psychiatric intervention may also diminish anxiety.
      Another common psychosocial management problem for the cardiologist is excessive dependency after a successful regimen is found and the patient has been discharged from the hospital. Some patients may become alarmed at any minor symptom and call the cardiologist or visit the emergency room. Again, patient education is essential. Careful instruction in regard to symptoms requiring physician evaluation and medication side effects will help. Patient self-confidence and return to independent living must be fostered. Family support and understanding require cultivation. Thus, the cardiologist performing EPS must be skilled not only in electrophysiology and pharmacology but also in the ability to relate to the patient and family on a personal basis.
      Certainly not every cardiologist wants to perform EPS. It is in a way "flirting with death" to induce ventricular arrhythmias that may require cardioversion, even though EPS is recognized to be a safe procedure [28]. It is obvious that no one performs EPS without extensive training. By the time that training has been completed, the cardiologist looks at the procedure more objectively and with more familiarity.
      In addition to expertise, however, the cardiologist must have patience and a high frustration threshold. Successes are exhilarating and failure extremely discouraging, particularly because of the close relationship with the patient and the family.
   B. **The team.** Nurses play a key role in the care of the patient, especially in the EP laboratory during the EPS itself. Gentle nurturing, support, and conversation aid the patient through a potentially overwhelming experience. Nurses too may experience

to a lesser extent the anxiety, frustration, and depression of patients and families. Group support sessions and meetings of the technical and nursing staff along with the cardiologist and psychiatrist may be of some benefit in this regard.

VIII. **Summary.** Sudden cardiac death remains the single leading cause of cardiac mortality in the nation. It is most often the sequela of VT and VF. Transient risk factors including psychiatric states and psychosocial stresses mediated through the CNS may contribute to the electrophysiologic accidents of SCD. Cardiologic progress in the evaluation and management of malignant ventricular arrhythmia has been paralleled by challenging psychiatric treatment issues.

References

1. Lown B. Sudden cardiac death: The major challenge confronting contemporary cardiology. *Am J Cardiol* 43:313–328, 1979.
2. O'Nunain S, Ruskin J. Cardiac arrest. *Lancet* 341:1641–1647, 1993.
3. Lown B, Verrier R, Rabinowitz S. Neural and psychologic mechanisms and the problem of sudden cardiac death. *Am J Cardiol* 39:890–902, 1977.
4. DeSilva R. Central nervous system risk factors for sudden cardiac death. *Ann NY Acad Sci* 382:143–161, 1982.
5. Schwartz P, Stone H. The role of the autonomic nervous system in sudden coronary death. *Ann NY Acad Sci* 382:162–180, 1982.
6. Talman W. Cardiovascular regulation and lesions of the central nervous system. *Ann Neurol* 220:71–76, 1979.
7. Parizel G. On the mechanism of sudden death with subarachnoid hemorrhage. *J Neurol* 220:71–76, 1979.
8. Schwartz P, et al. The effect of antiarrhythmic drugs on life-threatening arrhythmias induced by the interaction between acute myocardial and sympathetic hyperactivity. *Am Heart J* 109:937–948, 1985.
9. Reich P, Gold P. Interruption of recurrent ventricular fibrillation by psychiatric intervention. *Gen Hosp Psychiatry* 5:255–257, 1983.
10. Rozanski A, et al. Mental stress and the induction of silent myocardial ischemia in patients with coronary artery disease. *N Engl J Med* 318:1005–1012, 1988.
11. Hackett T, Cassem E. Coping with cardiac disease. *Adv Cardiol* 31:212–217, 1982.
12. Fricchione GL, Vlay SC. Psychiatric aspects of patients with malignant ventricular arrhythmias. *Am J Psychiatry* 143:1518–1526, 1986.
13. Ruskin J, DiMarco J, Garan H. Out-of-hospital cardiac arrest: Electrophysiologic observations and selection of long term antiarrhythmia therapy. *N Engl J Med* 303:607–612, 1980.
14. Spracklem F, Chambers R, Schure V. Value of diazepam ("valium") in treatment of cardiac arrhythmias. *Br Heart J* 32:827–832, 1970.
15. Sheehan D. Current perspectives in treatment of panic and phobic disorders. *Drug Ther* 12:179–193, 1982.
16. American Psychiatric Association. *Diagnostic and Statistical Manual of Mental Disorders* (4th ed rev). Washington, DC: American Psychiatric Association, 1994.
17. Lloyd G, Cowley R. Distress or illness? A study of psychological symptoms after myocardial infarction. *Br J Psychiatry* 142:120–125, 1983.
18. Levenson J, Friedel R. Major depression in patients with cardiac disease: Diagnosis and somatic treatment. *Psychosomatics* 26:91–102, 1985.
19. Richels K, Feighner J, Smith W. Alprazolam, amitriptyline, doxepin and placebo in the treatment of depression. *Arch Gen Psychiatry* 42:134–141, 1985.
20. Glassman A, Bigger JT. Cardiovascular effects of therapeutic doses of tricyclic antidepressants. *Arch Gen Psychiatry* 38:815–820, 1981.
21. Ruskin J, et al. Antiarrhythmia drugs: A possible cause of out-of-hospital cardiac arrest. *N Engl J Med* 309:1302–1306, 1983.
22. Giardina E, Bigger JT. Antiarrhythmia effect of imipramine hydrochloride in patients with ventricular premature complexes without psychological depression. *Am J Cardiol* 50:172–179, 1982.
23. Schwartz P, Wolf S. QT intervals prolongation as predictor of sudden death in patients with myocardial infarction. *Circulation* 57:1074–1077, 1978.
24. Boehnert M, Lovejoy F. Value of the QRS duration versus serum drug level in predicting seizures and ventricular arrhythmias after an acute overdose of tricyclic antidepres-

sants. *N Engl J Med* 313:474–479, 1985.
25. Roose SP, et al. Cardiovascular effects of buproprion in depressed patients with heart disease. *Am J Psychiatry* 148:512–516, 1991.
26. Robinson D, et al. Cardiovascular effects of phenelzine and amitriptyline in depressed outpatients. *J Clin Psychiatry* 43 (Sec 2):8–15, 1982.
27. Fink, M. *Convulsive Therapy: Theory and Practice*. New York: Raven Press, 1979.
28. DiMarco J, Garan H, Ruskin J. Complications in patients undergoing cardiac electrophysiologic procedures. *Ann Intern Med* 97:490–493, 1982.

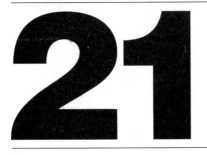

Counseling the Arrhythmia Patient and the Family

Linda C. Vlay

In the past ten years, the medical treatment of complex cardiac arrhythmia has become more intricate and better established. While there is still a role for antiarrhythmic drugs, sophisticated modalities such as tiered therapy ICDs (internal cardioverter-defibrillator) and radiofrequency catheter ablation are widely available and used frequently. Less well defined, but equally important, is the impact of both the potentially life-threatening arrhythmia and the treatment selected on the individual patient and family. There are several issues to consider: Are we altering quality of life and performance while preventing sudden cardiac death and prolonging life? What are the biopsychosocial effects experienced by the patient and family? What role do behavior and emotion play in the development and treatment of cardiac arrhythmia? How does one live with the diagnosis of cardiac arrhythmia?

These questions may not always be foremost in the practitioner's approach, but they are exceedingly important to the patient, family, and ultimately the management and outcome of cardiac arrhythmia. Counseling the patient and family with cardiac arrhythmia presents a new challenge for the health care practitioner who must utilize the disciplines of both medicine and psychiatry.

As the severity of cardiac arrhythmia ranges from benign to malignant, so do the emotional responses and symptomatology [1]. Patients with ventricular tachycardia (VT) may be asymptomatic or present with dizziness, dyspnea, or as a full cardiac arrest. Near-death experiences can alter the survivor's values, beliefs, and attitudes [2]. Ventricular premature beats can sometimes be extremely disconcerting and annoying and may even result in "fatigue." Patient reports of "skipped beats," "loud thumping," "a lump in the throat," fleeting "dizziness," and a "feeling of impending doom" are not uncommon. Supraventricular tachycardias such as atrial fibrillation with a rapid ventricular response, Wolff-Parkinson-White syndrome with reciprocating tachycardia, and other paroxysmal atrial tachycardias, may be perceived as a "racing heartbeat" or "dizziness" and can result in syncope. Onset can be sudden and frightening. These arrhythmias can be incapacitating at times. The unpredictable nature lends itself to feeling a loss of control. Emotions such as anger, anxiety, and hostility have been investigated as triggers of cardiac events by elicitation of a catecholamine surge and may also contribute to creation of an environment conducive to arrhythmia induction [3].

I. **Approaches to treatment.** In order to address the emotional component of the illness, and the issues raised above, the treatment approach must not be limited to medical aspects. The biopsychosocial approach may be the most appropriate choice of treatment as it takes into consideration both the biological responses and the human experience. This was first introduced by George Engel, who developed this integrated approach and challenged the pure biomedical model that separates the body and mind [4]. The biopsychosocial approach recognizes the interdependent relationships of the biological, psychological, individual, family, and community systems.

The fourth edition of the *Diagnostic and Statistical Manual of Mental Disorders* (DSM-IV) addresses psychological or behavioral factors affecting a medical illness [5]. These factors can adversely affect the course, treatment, and physiologic response of a medical illness. Furthermore, they can delay recovery, interfere with treatment recommendations, or precipitate symptoms by eliciting a stress-related physiological response (increased heart rate, elevated blood pressure, chest pain, arrhythmia). Compounding problems may include the presence of a major mental illness such as major depression or schizophrenia. Other variables may include psychological symptoms such as anxiety or depression; personality traits such as anger or hostility; coping styles such as "type A"; or maladaptive health behaviors such as a sedentary lifestyle, smok-

451

ing, or overeating. The inclusion of these factors in the DSM-IV adds to the body of evidence that the biological and psychosocial aspects of the patient are interdependent.

II. **Treatment strategies.** There are several strategies to choose from in treating the psychological needs of the patient and family with a medical illness.

A. **The family systems approach** is based on the Bowenian model. This model views the family as a system with multigenerational patterns of communication, relationships, and anxieties. A change involving one member of the family system affects individual members along with affecting the entire system. In medical family therapy, the focus is on the patterns within the family system and between the family system and medical community in response to the stressor, the medical illness (see III) [6–8].

B. **In cognitive-behavioral therapy** the goal is to replace the maladaptive behaviors and cognitive distortions that can result in psychosocial stress and illness. The patient learns to identify the environmental stimuli that evoke the maladaptive behavior. Faulty self-perception, irrational beliefs, and view of the world are challenged and modified. This can be accomplished with simple interventions such as teaching time management, anger control, assertiveness training, self-monitoring techniques, thought stopping of automatic negative thoughts, and teaching effective problem solving. The patient's core belief system is identified and slowly corrected in order to achieve a more adaptive behavioral and cognitive state. In the cardiac arrhythmia patient, an additional desired outcome is reduction of cardiovascular reactivity (decreased sympathetic and neurohumoral response). This can be done by elicitation of the relaxation response. According to Dr. Herbert Benson in his research assessing hypertension and the effects of behavioral relaxation exercises, the relaxation response is an "innate physiologic response that counters the effects of stress." He mentions four essential elements needed to perform this exercise [9]:

1. a quiet environment
2. a mantra, or mental device (word) that is repeated during the exercise
3. adoption of a passive attitude
4. a comfortable position

By using meditation and actively letting go of intrusive thoughts, the relaxation response can be evoked. Other relaxation exercises include transcendental meditation, yoga, visual imagery, and progressive muscle relaxation (PMR), which is isometric muscle squeezes and muscle relaxation. These exercises can be initiated in the hospital and the patient should be encouraged to perform these for 20 minutes twice a day.

Another strategy to consider as a stress management technique is therapeutic touch. Therapeutic touch is an ancient Western practice, "laying of the hands," reintroduced into nursing by Dr. Dolores Krieger in 1975. Therapeutic touch can be defined as a voluntary transfer of energy from a well person with an intent to heal to an ill person. It has been used in pain management [10], anxiety reduction [11], and also as a means to facilitate physiologic change and healing [12]. A recent study compared the effects of therapeutic touch and relaxation therapy on anxiety reduction [13]. In this study, both interventions resulted in significant anxiety reduction.

C. **Supportive therapy** deals with the here and now, which means the practitioner recognizes where the patient and the family are during the session and addresses those needs. Individual and family strengths are bolstered; healthy defenses are reinforced. Through active listening and empathy, supportive therapy can increase self-esteem and self-confidence. This in turn can positively affect illness outcome and is especially useful in patients who experience depression and adjustment disorders.

D. **Group therapy** may be especially therapeutic with families and patients with an ICD. According to Yalom, group therapy can produce the conditions for change through the "interplay of various guided human experiences" referred to as therapeutic factors [14]. Therapeutic factors such as instillation of hope, universality (we're all in the same boat), altruism, socialization, and group cohesiveness can be invaluable to a patient and family who have issues regarding surviving sudden cardiac death or implantation of an ICD device. Patients may have ambivalent feelings about the ICD. They fear that it will shock them, while at the same time they fear that it will fail and not deliver a shock. Patients have questions such as, "How will I know if I'm going to get a shock?"; "Will the shock hurt me?"; "Will it damage my heart?"; "Will I faint?"; "Why me?" More important, "Can I drive?" and "Will this shock me and my partner during sex?" Driving restrictions are of a concern to patients and families with ICDs and are currently under consideration by the medical community involved.

In our center, we organized a support group that I led. It later continued as a patient and family self-run group and serves as a source of support and socialization to ICD patients and families. At the completion of the original group sessions, I conducted an exit survey to elicit each member's opinion of the group. The results were favorable. Members stated that they found the sessions valuable and felt that the support group should be attended soon after ICD implantation. Members felt the group was friendly. They experienced a sense of universality, support, and cohesion. Didactic sessions about arrhythmia, medications, relaxation techniques, treatment modalities, and diet were included. These sessions helped correct misconceptions about arrhythmia and treatment. Themes arising during sessions included anger, isolation, frustration, depression, and fear of ICD discharge. Members expressed a realization of the importance of family support during their hospitalization. This small group served as a pilot for evaluation of the need and benefit of an ICD support group.

Therapy can be tailored using one or a combination of therapeutic approaches. Selection can be based on both the clinician's and patient's level of comfort, belief system, and commitment to change. Any and all of these different approaches require the practitioner to be caring, empathic, supportive, understanding, and trustworthy in order to foster the ability to create change if needed and to facilitate healing.

III. Facing chronic illness. Unless the cardiac arrhythmia was the result of an acute organic cause or was corrected permanently through surgery or radiofrequency catheter ablation, it is a condition that is potentially lifelong. It can be either stable or unstable, and may or may not be incapacitating. The degree of uncertainty of these illness characteristics can lead to anticipatory grief for the patient and family. Patients may have structural or organic heart disease associated with the cardiac arrhythmia. Because chronic illness can redefine and reshape one's world, identification of the presence or absence of illness chronicity is essential [15]. According to Dr. Arthur Kleinman in the *Illness Narratives* (1988), "chronic illness by definition cannot be cured, the goal should be to reduce the frequency and the severity of exacerbations, the family as well as the patient must learn to accept this treatment objective" [16].

A. Phases. Chronic illness can be categorized in three phases: crisis (acute), chronic, and terminal phases [17].

  1. Crisis phase. This phase occurs during the presenting hospitalization and is a period of uncertainty. During this phase, the practitioner should attend to the immediate physical needs of the patient and then begin to educate the family and patient about the arrhythmia. Depending on the arrhythmia, the patient and family will be faced with decisions regarding medications, diagnostic tests including electrophysiology study (EPS), and possibly interventions such as tiered therapy ICD, bradycardia pacemaker, cardiovascular surgery, and radiofrequency ablation. An electrophysiology study may be perceived by the patient and family as frightening, depending on how the test is explained or what prior knowledge they have. We find it helpful to give the patient and family written information prior to the procedure and then allow enough time for questions. Following the test, the response to arrhythmia induction and/or treatment options presented may be psychologically stressful. The patient who experienced external defibrillation during the EPS and may require further EPS is vulnerable to depression and anxiety reactions. Premorbid personality and psychological status, family dynamics and structure, and cognitive appraisal of the situation will influence the psychological response and adjustment and should be part of the baseline assessment during hospitalization. These factors will influence the ability to undergo diagnostic procedures and make sound decisions regarding medical therapy.

  During the crisis phase, the patient and family define the meaning of the illness. Responses often exhibited by patient and family include anger, anxiety, fear, denial, ambivalence, depression, and grief. These are related to losses of health, identity, control, sexuality, employment, role, and financial security, in addition to possible alterations of plans for the future. Some patients and loved ones have experienced a sudden death episode, or have been informed that they are at high risk for sudden death, and are facing mortality for the first time. Some are worried about increased dependence and reduction of autonomy [18].

Interventions for the crisis phase should focus on stabilizing the physical condition, provision of patient and family education, and psychological, emotional, and spiritual support. It is important to focus on patient and family strengths. The goal is a healthy illness acceptance, minimizing a negative appraisal of the situation. This can be fostered through support, empathy, active listening, and controlling symptoms to the extent possible. The practitioner should respect defenses needed by the patient and family at this stage such as denial. Maladaptive behaviors can be addressed after the acute phase. Empowerment can be developed by maintaining communication between family, patient, and health care providers with inclusion of all concerned in decisions regarding therapy. During this phase we often request a psychiatric liaison consult by a psychiatrist, psychologist, advanced practice psychiatric nurse, or psychiatric social worker along with pastoral support to assist the patient and family during this difficult period. Supportive therapy along with cognitive-behavioral stress management techniques such as relaxation exercises may be beneficial to the patient and family. Anxiolytic therapy may be necessary to allay dysfunctional anxiety.

2. **Chronic phase.** This phase takes place during recovery and rehabilitation. During this time patient and family move toward a return to normalcy. The illness definition continues to develop. The patient and family are faced with and begin to accept permanent change and may grieve for pre-illness losses such as health, role, employment, and sexuality. Family discord may arise. Family members are active in maintaining the well-being of the patient and are involved with caretaking issues as well as experiencing varied feelings of helplessness, anger, guilt, blame, and fears of their own. A communion (emotional bonding) of patient, family, friends, health care providers, and employer that is supportive and respective of the needs and desires of the patient while maintaining the morale of all involved is desirable. Interventions during this phase can include the development of agency in the patient and family, maintenance of interpersonal relationships, attention to the developmental issues of patient and family members, resolution of conflicts, removal of blame, continuation of education, psychological and spiritual support, and ongoing medical management.

Agency is defined as an active involvement in and commitment to one's care and choices with the illness and the health care system [7]. It instills a sense of control and empowerment. During this phase the patient and family may convey their illness definition as either a positive or negative cognitive appraisal. The term *cognitive* refers to the mental process of comprehension, judgment, memory and reasoning [5]. Cognitive appraisal is a process in which the significance of stressors is evaluated with respect to one's well-being. Negative cognitive appraisal of an illness has been identified as a predictor of less effective adjustment [19]. This suggests the use of cognitive reframing by minimizing negative appraisals rather than emphasizing and identifying the positive appraisals. Cognitive reframing is a process by which there is a change in appraisal due to new information. By reappraising the situation, it is thought that the patient gains control and thus minimizes the sense of harm, threat or loss.

In this phase, patients and families may manifest symptoms related to anger, anxiety, or depression. These may precipitate an arrhythmia event and should be assessed during outpatient follow-up visits. Patients may develop or continue to manifest maladaptive coping mechanisms such as denial, self-defeating behaviors, or noncompliance to treatment that may negatively affect their condition. Often patients and families use blame to control the outcome of the illness scenario. They may blame one another or blame the medical community. This is maladaptive and is an indication that the illness has not been accepted. Patients may somaticize during outpatient visits, complaining about unrelated symptoms. This is an expression of psychosocial distress and a mechanism used to externalize the illness. Referral to the appropriate psychiatric service will benefit the patient and family and facilitate the healing process. Therapy may be brief or may require a longer period of time, depending on the symptoms and willingness to participate in therapy. Patients may require antidepressant or anxiolytic medications.

3. **Terminal phase.** In this phase of a chronic illness, the patient may be approaching death, or the illness has actually been arrested and the patient and family face the adjustment from illness to recovery. During this phase, issues are related to separation, the mourning process, and unresolved conflicts. The patient

may need assistance in life review, saying goodbye, and expression and execution of final wishes.

The use of agency and communication is especially important to manage the dying patient. The patient and family often desire control over the death process. Issues regarding mechanical devices that would prolong death should be discussed. Learning to talk about death and watching a family member or significant other die are difficult tasks and require psychological and spiritual support.

IV. **Medical follow-up.** Ongoing outpatient medical follow-up of cardiac arrhythmia patients can be complex. Visits consist of interrogation of implanted devices such as bradycardia pacemakers and tiered therapy ICDs, along with assessment of the underlying cardiac disorder, arrhythmia status, response to treatment, and psychological adaptation. Antiarrhythmic medications require monitoring for compliance, side effects, and interactions with other medications. Patients and families utilize these visits to ask questions and express their feelings and fears about their condition. Fears may be manifested by the occurrence of phantom shocks (patient-reported shocks not validated on interrogation of the ICD), panic attacks, or nightmares. The visit itself may be a source of anxiety for the patient, bringing back to mind the traumatic experiences during hospitalization. Patients fear that they will receive bad news regarding their arrhythmia status. They fear the interrogation of the devices implanted. Often they exhibit hypertensive reactions, tremors, diaphoresis, and even phantom shocks during outpatient ICD visits. Practitioners need to convey a calm, empathic, nonthreatening attitude during clinic visits. Patients and families may need to share their experiences and worries with their medical practitioner in order to integrate and accept the condition.

Psychiatric referrals may be underutilized. It is important for the practitioner, the patient, and the family to know that the psychosocial stressors of a life-threatening arrhythmia are common. Furthermore, assistance is available and can be obtained through support groups or individual and family counseling by a psychiatrist, psychologist, advanced practice psychiatric nurse, or psychiatric social worker. Familiarity with cardiac disorders, cardiac arrhythmias, and treatment modalities is desirable for those treating this population of patients. Appropriate care delivered early may avoid or defuse a crisis occurring in the course of an illness that may delay medical treatment and recovery.

Most important to remember is that we are made up of both mind and body. Treating one without regard for the other may adversely affect morbidity and mortality.

References

1. Fricchione GL, Vlay LC, Vlay SC. Cardiac psychiatry and the management of malignant ventricular arrhythmias with the internal cardioverter defibrillator. *Am Heart J* 128: 1050–1059, 1994.
2. Greyson B. Varieties of near death experiences. *Psychiatry* 56:390–399, 1993.
3. Mittleman MA, et al. Triggering of myocardial infarction onset by episodes of anger. *Circulation* 89:936, 1994.
4. Engel GL. The clinical application of the biopsychosocial model. *American Journal of Psychiatry* 137:535–544, 1980.
5. American Psychiatric Association. *Diagnostic and statistical manual of mental disorders* (4th ed). Washington DC: APA, 1994.
6. Bowen M. *Family therapy in clinical practice.* New York: Jason Aronson, 1978.
7. McDaniel SH, Hepworth J, Doherty WJ. *Medical family therapy.* New York: Basic Books, 1992.
8. Becvar DS, Becvar RT. *Family therapy.* Boston: Allyn & Bacon, 1988.
9. Benson, H. *The relaxation response.* New York: Morrow, 1975.
10. Keller, E. Bzdek, V. Effects of therapeutic touch on tension headache pain. *Nursing Research* 35:101–106, 1986.
11. Heidt, P. Effects of therapeutic touch on anxiety levels of hospitalized patients. *Nursing Research* 30:32–37, 1981.
12. Krieger, D. Therapeutic touch: An ancient but unorthodox nursing intervention. *Journal of NYS Nursing Association* 6:6–10, 1975.
13. Gugne, D. and Toye, RC. The effects of therapeutic touch and relaxation therapy in reducing anxiety. *Archives of Psychiatric Nursing* 3:3, 184–189, 1994.
14. Yalom, ID. *The theory and practice of group psychotherapy* (3rd ed). New York: Basic

Books, 1985.

15. Benner D, Wrubel J. *The primacy of caring*. California: Addison-Wesley, 1989.

16. Kleinman A. *The illness narratives: Suffering, healing and the human condition*. New York: Basic Books, 1988.

17. Rolland, J. Toward a psychosocial typology of chronic and life threatening illness. *Family Systems Medicine* 2:245–262, 1984.

18. Janosik AH, Phipps LB. *Life cycle group work in nursing*. CA: Wadsworth Health Sciences Division, 1982.

19. Frost MH, et al. An analysis of factors influencing psychosocial adjustments to cardiomyopathy. *Cardiovascular Nursing* 30:1, 1994.

Index

Note: Page numbers followed by *f* designate figures; those followed by *t* designate tables.